Bone Marrow IHC

Dedication

I dedicate this book to my husband Goran
and to my children Lino, Jakov, Marija Milena, and Marta Danica
—*Emina Emilia Torlakovic, MD, PhD*

Affiliations

Emina Emilia Torlakovic, MD, PhD
Associate Professor
Department of Pathology and Laboratory Medicine
Royal University Hospital University of Saskatchewan
Saskatoon, SK Canada

Professor Kikkeri Naresh, MBBS, CCP, MD, FRCPath
Consultant Haematopathologist
Department of Histopathology
Hammersmith Hospital
London
UK

Richard D Brunning, MD
Professor Emeritus
Department of Laboratory Medicine and Pathology
University of Minnesota
Minneapolis, MN USA

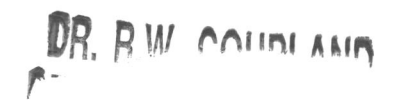

Bone Marrow IHC

Emina Emilia Torlakovic, MD, PhD

Kikkeri N Naresh, MBBS, CCP, MD, FRCPath

Richard D Brunning, MD

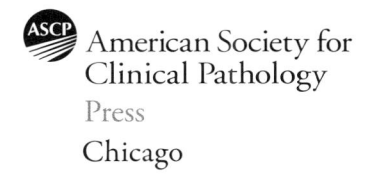

American Society for
Clinical Pathology
Press
Chicago

Publishing Team
Erik Tanck (design and production)
Joshua Weikersheimer (publishing direction)

Notice
Trade names for equipment and supplies described herein are included as suggestions only. In no way does their inclusion constitute an endorsement or preference by the American Society for Clinical Pathology. The ASCP did not test the equipment, supplies, or procedures and therefore urges all readers to read and follow all manufacturers' instructions and package insert warnings concerning the proper and safe use of products.

Copyright © 2009 by the American Society for Clinical Pathology.
All rights reserved. No part of this publication may be reproduced, stored in a retrieval system, or transmitted in any form or by any means, electronic, mechanical, photocopying, recording, or otherwise, without the prior written permission of the publisher.

13 12 11 10 09   5 4 3 2 1

Printed in Hong Kong

Abbreviations

Ab – antibody
Ag – antigen
ALL – acute lymphoblastic leukemia
ALPS – autoimmune lymphoproliferative syndrome
AMF – acute myelofibrosis
AMKL – acute megakaryoblastic leukemia
AML – acute myeloid leukemia
APMF – acute panmyelosis with myelofibrosis
B-ALL – B-cell acute lymphoblastic leukemia
BM – bone marrow
cHL – classical Hodgkin lymphoma
CLL – chronic lymphocytic leukemia
CLL/SLL – chronic lymphocytic leukemia/small lymphocytic lymphoma
CML – chronic myeloid leukemia
CMML – chronic myelomonocytic leukemia
DLBCL – diffuse large B-cell lymphoma
DS – Down syndrome
EBV – Epstein-Bar virus
EGIL – European Group for the Immunologic Classification of Leukemia
ET – essential thrombocythemia
FISH – fluorescent in situ hybridization
FL – follicular lymphoma
HCL – hairy cell leukemia
HIER – heat-induced epitope retrieval
IHC – immunohistochemistry
ISH – in situ hybridization
LF – lactoferrin
LPL – lymphoplasmacytic lymphoma
LZ – lysozyme
MCD – mast cell disease
MCL – mantle cell lymphoma
MCT – mast cell tryptase
MDS – myelodysplastic syndrome
MGUS – monoclonal gammopathy of undetermined significance
MPD – myeloproliferative disease
MPO – myeloperoxidase
MZL – marginal zone lymphoma
OMIM – Online Mendelian Inheritance in Man
PROW – Protein Reviews on the Web (http://mpr.nci.nih.gov/PROW/)
PTCL – peripheral T-cell lymphoma
RA – refractory anemia
RAEB – refractory anemia with excess blasts
RARS – refractory anemia with ringed sideroblasts
RCMD – refractory anemia with multilineage dysplasia
T-ALL – T-cell acute lymphoblastic leukemia

TABLE OF CONTENTS

Preface xiii

Acknowledgements xiv

Chapter 1
Introduction 1

References 2

Chapter 2
The Role of Tissue Processing In Bone Marrow Immunohistochemistry ... 3

2.1 **BM Biopsy Fixation** 3
2.2 **Decalcification** 5
2.3 **Embedding** 5
2.4 **Tissue Sectioning** 5
2.5 **Antigen Retrieval** 5
2.6 **Turnaround Time** 6
2.7 **Protocols** 11
    Protocol for Bone Marrow Processing and Staining Used at Hammersmith Hospital 11
    Protocol for Bone Marrow Processing and Staining Suitable for Rapid Turnaround Time 11
    References 11

Table of Contents

Chapter 3
Cluster of Differentiation Markers. ... 13

3.1	CD1a	13
3.2	CD2	16
3.3	CD3	17
3.4	CD4	24
3.5	CD5	27
3.6	CD7	31
3.7	CD8	32
3.8	CD9	36
3.9	CD10	38
3.10	CD14	44
3.11	CD15	51
3.12	CD16	54
3.13	CD20	57
3.14	CD21	64
3.15	CD22	68
3.16	CD23	69
3.17	CD25	75
3.18	CD30	78
3.19	CD31 (PECAM)	81
3.20	CD33	84
3.21	CD34	88
3.22	CD35	95
3.23	CD45 (CD45RA)	97
3.24	CD45 (CD45RO)	102
3.25	CD56	104
3.26	CD57	107
3.27	CD61 and CD42b	109
3.28	CD68	114
3.29	CD79a	119
3.30	CD99	123

Table of Contents

3.31	CD117	128
3.32	CD123	133
3.33	CD138	134
3.34	CD235a (Glycophorin A)	140
	References	142

Chapter 4
Other Common Markers . . . 153

4.1	Myeloperoxidase	153
4.2	Hemoglobin A (HgbA)	157
4.3	Mast Cell Tryptase	161
4.4	Terminal Deoxynucleotidyltransferase (TdT)	167
4.5	Factor 8-Related Antigen (von Willebrand Factor)	174
4.6	Pax-5	178
4.7	PU.1	185
4.8	Fli-1	191
4.9	Cyclin D1	194
4.10	Lysozyme	199
4.11	Bcl-6	201
4.12	Immunoglobulins	203
4.13	Ki-67	209
4.14	Cytotoxic Molecules	211
4.15	Stromal Markers	213
4.16	MUM1	221
4.17	TRAP	224
4.18	Bcl-2	226
	References	229

Table of Contents

Chapter 5
Special Diagnostic Considerations 237

5.1	**Acute Leukemia**.	237
5.2	**Metastatic Tumors**.	247
5.3	**Recommended Panels**	253
	References.	254

Index. 256

PREFACE

Bone Marrow IHC is intended to provide a collection of illustrations of various immunohistochemical tests that are routinely used in diagnostic practice. The choice of tests and the frequency of use vary greatly depending not only on the type of practice and personal experience, but also on availability of the tests. The menus of primary antibodies that can be applied to bone marrrow (BM) biopsy are logarithmically growing, and the number of published articles describing newly available tests is following the trend. Despite the advance of flow cytometry and molecular methods, immunohistochemistry remains an integral part of the diagnostic evaluation of most BM biopsies and is not likely to become less important in the future. The intrinsic value of the in situ tests will be difficult to replace by any other type of evaluation. This work does not include descriptions and possible uses of all currently available markers, but results of the most common markers are depicted in detail. Some not so commonly used markers are also portrayed to illustrate results that can be expected and help in their interpretation, which may be difficult if the range of expected outcomes is unfamiliar. The number of rare diseases and unusual findings may be overrepresented because of the greater need for immunohistochemistry studies in such cases. Also, some representative cases were used to illustrate several different markers solely for practical reasons. The comments associated with the findings and their interpretation are, however, based on the literature and wider experience and were not deduced from such individual samples except where it is explicitly stated to be the case.

Bone Marrow IHC does not promote or recommend use of any particular test, testing method, protocol, primary antibody, or other material and methods, but rather focuses on the results with optimized protocols. It cannot be overemphasised that the path to optimization and standardization of any test starts with agreed on expected/optimal results. The great majority of images in this book are, in our opinion, examples of what results may be expected with optimal methods, with the assumption that any method and/or reagent that can produce such results is acceptable. Some suboptimal results are also illustrated to depict certain common problems. Most BM biopsies that are illustrated here were fixed in 10% buffered formalin, aceto-zinc-formalin fixative, or B5, and most were decalcified by rapid decalcifier or Gooding and Stewart's decalcification fluid (10% formic acid and 5% formaldehyde). All but a few tests used the EnVision+ detection system simply because this is what is currently used, but with the clear acknowledgment that many other detection systems could produce the same if not better results. When any other method is used for detection, it is stated in the figure legend. The great majority of antibody clones or polyclonal antibodies that are illustrated here are listed and were evaluated by NordiQC (www.nordiqc.org). The names "PROW," "Entrez Gene," and "OMIM" are used throughout the text to designate the following Web sites as a source of information: http://mpr.nci.nih.gov/PROW, http://www.ncbi.nlm.nih.gov/sites/entrez, and http://www.ncbi.nlm.nih.gov/omim, respectively.

A number of internet sites serve those who study bone marrow protein expression by immunohistochemistry. Search at http://www.proteinatlas.org offers IHC images of relatively high quality showing various proteins that can be evaluated in TMA samples. Hematopoietic tissue markers are searchable at http://www.tissuemarkers.org.uk/htm/search.php. It includes many good images, but not all markers are illustrated, and most do not show bone marrow expression patterns.

ACKNOWLEDGEMENTS

We are indebted to many colleagues and collaborators who made this book possible. Professor Dr. Jan Nesland, Head of the Department of Pathology, The National Hospital–The Norwegian Radium Hospital, University of Oslo, Norway, was generous in his support and professional mentorship that created a platform for learning and experience in diagnostic immunohistochemistry as well as reasearch applications. About one third of the images included in the Atlas are from the cases E. Torlakovic evaluated while working at the Norwegian Radium Hospital. We are aslo indebted to laboratory technologists Grette Mykkelbost, Eva Gustavson, and Don Trihn, whose dedication to patient care, technical expertise, hard work, and perfectionism have facilitated the application of various new techniques and antibodies to bone marrow biopsies at the Norwegian Radium Hospital. In particular, gratitude is due to Grette Mykklebost, a collaborator and a friend, who was eager to quickly adopt not-so-routine methods like double and triple immunohistochemistry applications and any combination of immunohistochemistry and in situ hybridization and whose commitment to excellence in all things is unprecedented. E. Torlakovic currently works with Shannon Klassen and her team whose working motto could be "nothing is impossible in immunohistochemistry" and who is able to accomodate 3 months of developmental testing into a couple of weeks.

The authors thank the biomedical scientists in the department of histopathology, Hammersmith Hospital, London, UK, particularly Donna Horncastle and Kay Elderfield for maintaining high standards of bone marrow trephine biopsy processing, sectioning, immunohistochemistry, and in situ hybridization.

On a more personal level, we thank our families for their loving patience and support.

—*Emina Emilia Torlakovic*
—*Kikkeri N Naresh*
—*Richard D Brunning*

Chapter 1

INTRODUCTION

The bone marrow (BM) core biopsy technique, as performed commonly today along the posterior superior iliac spine, was first described by McFarland and Dameshek in 1958 [McFarland 1958]. Besides critical and indispensable morphologic examination, results of such biopsies can be evaluated with histochemical, immunohistochemical, and molecular methods [Kubic 1989; Fend 2008; Fend 2007; Fend 2005; Kremer 2005]. The role of immunohistochemistry (IHC) in the evaluation of the BM biopsy is growing despite parallel advancements in flow cytometry and molecular genetics. One reason is that IHC appears to be a simple procedure and can be reliably performed on routinely fixed, decalcified, and paraffin-embedded trephine biopsy specimens [Fend 2008; Kremer 2005]. It is also probably the cheapest medical test, considering the abundance of information it provides in the diagnostic process; in some cases, it serves well for the purpose of evidence-based medical practice.

The need for immunohistochemical stains is determined by the clinical circumstances and the preliminary morphologic findings [Bain 2001]. The need for immunohistochemical analysis or the selected panels may be very different if flow cytometry results are available at the time of the biopsy. Immunohistochemical tests in diagnostic practice are not fully standardized. This is particularly true for BM IHC. Therefore, individual laboratory experience regarding the quality of the results can vary. This applies not only to differences among laboratories, but also to variable success with different tests in the same laboratory, in addition to daily variations on a single test because of various preanalytical, analytical, and postanalytical factors, none of which can be ignored [Pileri 1993; Jack 1993; Curran 1980]. These important technical considerations of the BM IHC are discussed in more detail in chapter 2.

Not so long ago the review of the immunohistochemical evaluation of neoplasms in BM biopsies using monoclonal antibodies (mAbs) reactive in paraffin-embedded tissues included fewer than 10 such primary antibodies [Kubic 1989]. Only 3 antibodies were used in a study by West et al [West 1986]. Today, more than 100 mAb can be used in the evaluation of the BM biopsy, and about 30 may be considered to be in routine use [Kremer 2005]. For example, in the evaluation of acute leukemia with flow cytometry, a minimum of 10 antibodies are recommended for the first line panel. When flow cytometry is not available or cannot make a definitive diagnosis, the same rules should be followed in IHC evaluation because most if not all mAb (albeit different primary antibodies or different clones) can be used in paraffin-embedded tissues with satisfactory results [Bain 2002; Béné 2005; Pileri 1999]. The panels should be chosen based not only on morphologic evidence, but also on clinical evidence because some lesions may be missed based solely on morphologic examination. At a minimum, we recommend CD3 and CD20 for BM biopsies performed for staging of non-Hodgkin or Hodgkin lymphoma [Pittaluga 1999]. We also recommend, at a minimum, CD34 and 1 good megakaryocyte marker for evaluation of biopsies for myelodysplasia, which is probably a common practice [Horny 2007].

BM biopsies may be very small and may also have crush artifact. Biopsy specimens are also sometimes fragmented or processing can result in many artifacts. All of these aforementioned factors could make morphologic evaluation difficult [Bishop 1992]. Occasionally IHC may be very helpful and can facilitate interpretation of such suboptimal biopsy specimens. However, immunohistochemical analyses do not fully compensate for suboptimal sampling because some lesions simply are not present in biopsy specimens that are unilateral or of inadequate length [Brunning 1975; Jatoi 1999; Wang 2002].

Interpretation of IHC results is not always simple and should consider many variables including techniques used (including both preanalytical and analytical steps) and current state of knowledge regarding the expected distribution and levels of expression of certain antigens and their biological significance. The interpretation of the results is also significantly biased by individual background training in BM pathology and personal experience. Highly sensitive biotin-free IHC visualization methods and more powerful antigen retrieval methods have been applied to BM evaluation only during the last decade [Shi 1999]. Former "optimal results" cannot be applied anymore; we need to adapt to new standards, which, unfortunately, are not fully decided or agreed on at present, and be prepared for new developments and changes in the near future.

In diagnostic IHC, the tests are ordered with an aim to get answers to specific diagnostic questions. Every test in the panel has a specific purpose and plays a role in diagnostic evaluation. It is highly recommended that all IHC results be included in pathology reports. However, evaluation of stained slides usually also reveals additional information that is not directly relevant to our diagnostic question. This additional information in non-lesional tissue does not need to be included in the reports, but it may occasionally uncover important biological concepts. Some of this additional information is included in the Text. The purpose of this inclusion is to accurately illustrate expected results of the IHC tests, the familiarity of which may also help accurate diagnostic interpretation. **T1.1** summarizes the expected localization of all diagnostically informative IHC staining for all markers discussed in this Text.

T1.1 Localization of Selected Diagnostically Informative IHC Markers

	Marker	Comments
Nuclear	TdT, cyclin D1, Bcl-6, MUM1, Pax-5, PU.1, BOB1, Oct2, Parvovirus B19, Ki-67, NPM1, p53, Fli-1	Cytoplasmic localization can also be observed with different frequency for most of the typically nuclear markers since they are all synthesized in the cytoplasm before they are transported in the nuclei. Cytoplasmic NPM1 expression is aberrant. This is considered a positive reaction.
Cytoplasmic	Bcl-2, vimentin, cytokeratin, hemoglobin A, S-100, CD68, CD163, immunoglobulin (cIg), von Willebrand factor (vWF, FIVIII-ra), myeloperoxidase, lysozyme, mast cell tryptase, mast cell chymase, TIA-1, granzyme B, perforin, desmin, smooth muscle actin, TRAP, chromogranin, NSE, B72.3, neurofilaments	Submembranous concentration of the Ag may produce pseudomembranous pattern (frequently observed with cytokeratin). Nuclear staining is also frequently observed for S-100 and hemoglobin A.
Membranous	Most CD antigens, immunoglobulins (sIg), HLA-DR, glycophorins, CA-125, EMA	For most CD markers, Golgi-type or diffuse cytoplasmic localization is acceptable because of the physiological processing of the Ag in these localizations. Cytoplasmic CD10 and even possible nuclear localization are seen in neutrophils. CD15 and CD30 may be identified as only Golgi-type and/or diffuse cytoplasmic in classical Hodgkin lymphoma cells. By IHC, CD79a, CD61, and CD42b are also almost always cytoplasmic or cytoplasmic only. EMA is similarly cytoplasmic only in many cells. CD34 is often present in cytoplasmic vesicles of blasts with or even without appreciable membranous staining by IHC. VCAM-1 (CD106) most of the time shows predominant diffuse cytoplasmic and Golgi-type positivity by IHC in stromal cells of the bone marrow.

References

Bain BJ, Barnett D, Linch D, Matutes E, Reilly JT; General Haematology Task Force of the British Committee for Standards in Haematology (BCSH), British Society of Haematology. Revised guideline on immunophenotyping in acute leukaemias and chronic lymphoproliferative disorders. *Clin Lab Haematol* 2002;24(1):1-13.

Bain BJ. Bone marrow trephine biopsy. *J Clin Pathol* 2001;54(10):737-42.

Béné MC. Immunophenotyping of acute leukaemias [review]. *Immunol Lett* 2005;98(1):9-21.

Bishop PW, McNally K, Harris M. Audit of bone marrow trephines. *J Clin Pathol* 1992;45(12):1105-8.

Brunning RD, Bloomfield CD, McKenna RW, Peterson LA. Bilateral trephine bone marrow biopsies in lymphoma and other neoplastic diseases. *Ann Intern Med* 1975;82(3):365-6.

Curran RC, Gregory J. Effects of fixation and processing on immunohistochemical demonstration of immunoglobulin in paraffin sections of tonsil and bone marrow. *J Clin Pathol* 1980;33(11):1047-57.

Fend F, Bock O, Kremer M, Specht K, Quintanilla-Martinez L. Ancillary techniques in BM pathology: molecular diagnostics on bone marrow trephine biopsies [published online ahead of print October 18, 2005] [review]. *Virchows Arch* 2005;447(6):909-19.

Fend F, Kremer M. Diagnosis and classification of malignant lymphoma and related entities in the bone marrow trephine biopsy [review]. *Pathobiology* 2007;74(2):133-43.

Fend F, Tzankov A, Bink K, et al. Modern techniques for the diagnostic evaluation of the trephine bone marrow biopsy: methodological aspects and applications [published online ahead of print January 4, 2008]. *Prog Histochem Cytochem* 2008;42(4):203-52.

Horny HP, Sotlar K, Valent P. Diagnostic value of histology and immunohistochemistry in myelodysplastic syndromes [published online ahead of print July 2, 2007]. *Leuk Res* 2007;31:1609-16.

Jack AS, Roberts BE, Scott CS. Processing of trephine biopsy specimens. *J Clin Pathol* 1993;46(3):285-6.

Jatoi A, Dallal GE, Nguyen PL. False-negative rates of tumor metastases in the histologic examination of BM. *Mod Pathol* 1999;12(1):29-32.

Kremer M, Quintanilla-Martínez L, Nährig J, von Schilling C, Fend F. Immunohistochemistry in bone marrow pathology: a useful adjunct for morphologic diagnosis [published online ahead of print October 18, 2005] [review]. *Virchows Arch* 2005 Dec;447(6):920-37.

Kubic VL, Brunning RD. Immunohistochemical evaluation of neoplasms in bone marrow biopsies using monoclonal antibodies reactive in paraffin-embedded tissue. *Mod Pathol* 1989;2(6):618-29.

McFarland W, Dameshek W. Biopsy of BM with the Vim-Silverman needle. *JAMA* 1958;166(12):1464-6.

Pileri SA, Ascani S, Milani M, et al. Acute leukaemia immunophenotyping in bone-marrow routine sections. *Br J Haematol* 1999;105(2):394-401.

Pileri SA, Roncador G, Ceccarelli C, et al. Antigen retrieval techniques in immunohistochemistry: comparison of different methods. *J Pathol* 1997;183(1):116-23.

Pittaluga S, Tierens A, Dodoo YL, Delabie J, De Wolf-Peeters C. How reliable is histologic examination of BM trephine biopsy specimens for the staging of non-Hodgkin lymphoma? A study of hairy cell leukemia and mantle cell lymphoma involvement of the bone marrow trephine specimen by histologic, immunohistochemical, and polymerase chain reaction techniques. *Am J Clin Pathol* 1999;111(2):179-84.

Shi S-R, Guo J, Cote RJ, et al. Sensitivity and detection efficiency of a novel two-step detection system (PowerVision) for immunohistochemistry. *Appl Immunohistochem Mol Morphol* 1999;7(3):201.

Wang J, Weiss LM, Chang KL, et al. Diagnostic utility of bilateral bone marrow examination: significance of morphologic and ancillary technique study in malignancy. *Cancer* 2002;94(5):1522-31.

West KP, Warford A, Fray L, Allen M, Campbell AC, Lauder I. The demonstration of B-cell, T-cell and myeloid antigens in paraffin sections. *J Pathol* 1986;150(2):89-101.

Chapter 2
THE ROLE OF TISSUE PROCESSING IN BONE MARROW IMMUNOHISTOCHEMISTRY

Immunohistochemistry (IHC) was developed as a technique to evaluate histologic or a cytologic expression of various antigens (Ags) or proteins in situ. Answers provided by IHC are complex and provide various levels of information about Ag expression including:

1. qualitative identification of the presence or absence of the Ag;
2. quantitative determination of the levels of expression;
3. determination of subcellular localization of the protein; and
4. assessment of the distribution in different cell types in the tissue.

The results usually provide far more information than some other tests intended for protein identification/expression (Western blotting, enzyme-linked immunosorbent assay [ELISA], spectrophotometry). For the hematopathologist, IHC translates into immunohistology because it uncovers immunobiology or molecular histology of the tissues. However, suboptimal protocols result in difficulties in assessing all of the aforementioned aspects of IHC. While these 4 aspects of IHC results can be evaluated even with single antibody (Ab) staining, multiplex IHC developing for clinical applications will increase our insight into protein expression distribution in the tissues and enhance diagnostic precision.

IHC does not compete with flow cytometry. Flow cytometry has various applications, and immunophenotyping of BM aspirate is particularly important. Flow cytometry is the gold standard in the analysis of membrane antigen expression. Flow cytometry is also very powerful in detection of cytoplasmic and nuclear antigens. It enables quantitative detection of coexpression of several antigens at the same time, which is difficult to do using routine IHC. Therefore, both methods are often necessary in a study of BM diseases. It was recently suggested that automated IHC of the peripheral blood and BM smears may be used when there is no suitable sample for flow cytometry [Happerfield 2000]. This may be sensible in occasional cases, but regular use would require additional positive and negative controls that differ from those for paraffin-embedded tissues. The choice of methods for immunophenotyping in BM samples has to be determined in each individual case. Generally, acute leukemia and small B-cell lymphoproliferative diseases are a priori indications for flow cytometric analysis, which may be complemented with additional IHC analyses.

Factors that influence IHC can be broadly classified as preanalytical (tissue processing), analytical (IHC protocols), and postanalytical (interpretation). Tissue processing is a crucial factor for IHC, which greatly influences the success of the Ag demonstration [Leong 2004; Taylor 2006; Yakizi 2007]. This is emphasized in BM IHC because in this procedure, tissue processing is less standardized than in other types of specimen processing. Various fixatives and decalcification methods are used in different laboratories, usually based on personal preference of the leading hematopathologist or methods established in the past. Whatever method of tissue processing is used, one needs to consider its effects on preservation of cytologic details of the constituent cells and of epitope antigenicity, which are both of paramount importance. Nucleic acid preservation should also be considered. Tissue morphology is a very important factor in the interpretation of IHC results. It can be altered by many factors including the quality of the biopsy specimen; hemorrhage and crush artefacts cannot be corrected even in the most exquisitely processed sample. Furthermore, the promptness of fixation, the type of the fixative, appropriate buffers, and other steps in tissue processing may also alter tissue morphology. Even in a single institution, factors linked to tissue processing, including the length of fixation or decalcification, often vary from case to case. This is influenced by the time during the day when the biopsy is performed; for example, often biopsies performed late on Friday are left in the fixative for a longer period. The promptness of fixation and the type of fixative used is a major factor influencing antigen preservation. Delayed fixation or drying of the biopsy sample can also produce irreversible damage to both morphology of the cells and antigenicity of epitopes. Similarly, epitopes can be irreversibly damaged by increasing the temperature to above 60°C at any point during tissue processing (except during controlled Ag retrieval step). These factors are compounded in laboratories or institutions that receive tissue samples processed in other hospitals or laboratories that perform IHC testing on samples processed elsewhere by using various different tissue processing protocols [Leong 2004]. BM biopsy requires separate, strictly defined, and controlled protocols for tissue processing followed by appropriately optimized IHC protocols that are validated for institution-specific tissue processing.

2.1 BM Biopsy Fixation

Several factors affect the fixation process, including volume of the fixative, penetration of the fixative in the tissue, and time of fixation. Buffering is also important because fixation is best at neutral pH (pH = 6-8). Phosphate buffer is used for formalin. Black polarizable formalin-heme pigment formation indicates acidity of the tissue and suboptimal buffering. Nuclear shrinkage and cellular clumping suggest delayed fixation. Some fixatives that can be used for BM core biopsies are listed in **T2.1**. Many laboratories use formalin fixation followed by EDTA or acid decalcification.

Compared with formalin fixation, mercurial fixatives such as B5 and Zenker result in improved morphologic findings, which are still inferior to those obtained with plastic embedding and semithin sections [Mullink 1985; Gala 1997; Nagasaka 2000; Werner 1992; Toth 1999]. However, mercurial fixatives may have deleterious effects on some Ags. For instance, CD30 may be more difficult to demonstrate in B5-fixed tissues than in formalin-fixed tissues. In contrast, B5 fixation may also improve preservation of some antigens, for instance, the well-known positive effects on immunoglobulin and CD15. While B5 is certainly a good fixative for BM biopsy and has been used for a long time, the use of mercurial fixatives may yield poor nucleic acid preservation, result in additional procedures, and raise concerns about the disposal of the mercury-containing solutions. Formalin fixation results in overall better Ag and nucleic acid preservation than picric acid– or mercury-based fixatives, which is a definite advantage in light of the expanding clinical repertoire of molecular tests applied to BM biopsy specimens.

The length of fixation is critical for optimal fixation effects of formalin on the epitopes and nucleic acid preservation. Although small biopsy specimens are penetrated by formalin in 2 hours, the fixation process involves penetration as well as a chemical reaction; the cross-linking by formalin requires longer than 2 hours even in small biopsy specimens [Fox 1985; Goldstein 2003]. The alcohol used in the dehydration process will continue the denaturing process, but the primary fixative characteristics that determine morphology, staining, and epitope and nucleic acid preservation will not be complete. Also, some of the alcohol fixation characteristics, which are often suboptimal for IHC, will be introduced in an inversely proportional ratio of formalin fixation time to alcohol fixation time. In addition, the decalcification process, to which a BM biopsy is exposed before the tissue processing is continued in alcohols, is particularly harmful to the epitopes if the fixation process is not complete.

Bonds et al [2005] compared B5 with 5 other fixatives and showed that acetic acid–zinc-formalin (AZF) was overall comparable in staining and morphologic detail. Furthermore, the study also showed that the AZF fixative resulted in superior Ag preservation and that the RNA and DNA were also found to be well-preserved for in situ hybridization and molecular analysis. During formalin fixation, formaldehyde introduces hydroxymethylene cross-links among proteins, and between proteins and nucleic acid. On the other hand, the mechanism by which zinc, which appears to be a crucial component in the success of the AZF fixative, exerts its effects is currently unclear. Even in the AZF cocktail, formalin is essential for optimal morphology. The AZF-fixed paraffin-embedded BMTB specimens are also optimal for the use of the Giemsa, silver and Perls stains [Naresh 2006].

T2.1 Different Fixatives Used for Processing Bone Marrow Biopsy Specimens

Fixative	Fixation Time	Comment
Zenker fixative	4-24 hours	Good morphology Contains mercuric chloride
B5 fixative	4 hours; not more than 6 hours	Good morphology Overall good epitope preservation Contains mercuric chloride
Bouin fixative	4-12 hours; optimal is 6 hours	Rarely used Contains picric acid Not recommended for IHC
Lowy formalin mercuric chloride acid solution	20 hours	1-step fixation/decalcification procedure Contains mercuric chloride Many Ags well preserved
Schäfer's fixative	6-10 hours (can be up to 72 hours)	Allows histochemical detection of tartrate-resistant acid phosphatase and naphthol AS-D chloroacetate esterase and a specific platelet esterase A broad panel of Ags is well preserved Usually followed by EDTA decalcification Discriminates mineralized and nonmineralized bone even after decalcification
10% neutral buffered formal-saline	6-24 hours; optimal is 18 hours*	Commonly used Good for most purposes Nucleic acids may be degraded during the decalcification
AZF	20-24 hours	Excellent for morphology and epitope preservation If followed by formic acid decalcification also good nucleic acid preservation

Ag = antigen; AZF = aceto-zinc-formalin; IHC = immunohistochemistry.
*2 hours fixation in formalin is often used to shorten turnaround time. The bone marrow biopsy specimen is suboptimally fixed in such protocol.

2.2 Decalcification

The presence of bone in BM biopsy requires either decalcification or the use of special blades such as tungsten-carbide knives that can cut undecalcified bony tissues. Decalcification is an additional important variable in BM IHC that can alter epitopes. Some epitopes are more resistant to the decalcification step than others. Several different methods of decalcification of BM biopsy are in use T2.2. Timing of the decalcification step is critical for epitope preservation. The more aggressive the decalcification medium, the faster the biopsy specimen is processed and the faster the epitopes are destroyed. Because the turnaround time (TAT) is of major concern in many institutions, rapid decalcifying solutions are used. It is of great importance that the tissue is well fixed before it is decalcified and the decalcification step is timed precisely. Exact timing of the more gentle (and slower) decalcifying solutions is less critical.

Lowy formalin mercuric chlorid acid solution is a 1-step fixation/decalcification procedure, but it is not widely used because of the toxic mercuric chloride component [Gaulier 1994].

The calcium chelator EDTA, which is widely used for BM biopsy processing, is slow and takes at least 24 hours and up to 48 to 72 hours, but the application of an ultrasonic bath can help hasten this process to 8 to 12 hours [Milan 1981; Reineke 2006]. Acid decalcification using hydrochloric acid, nitric acid, acetic acid, or formic acid is generally faster, but is thought to result in some destruction of Ags, nucleic acids, and tissue architecture [Arber 1997]. However, the deleterious effects can be circumvented by shortening the period of acid decalcification [Gebhard 2001; Brown 2002]. Some protocols, which use AZF fixative, recommend a short formic acid decalcification. It should, however, be noted that many of the adverse effects of fixation and decalcification can be corrected to a certain extent by the use of Ag retrieval techniques [Loyson 1997]. The process of decalcification reduces the amount of stainable iron in BM biopsy sections [DePalma 1996; Gatter 1987].

2.3 Embedding

BM biopsies are embedded either in paraffin or resin. Resin embedding and sectioning with tungsten carbide knives can result in improved morphology [Gatter 1987]. Recent modifications of the plastic embedding procedure have shown that IHC can be performed on resin-embedded semithin sections [Krenacs 2005]. It appears that the main criticisms of this procedure are the requirements for specialized technology, specially trained technologists, as well as additional costs associated with it. Admittedly, most pathologists and technologists are not familiar with this technique. However, resin-embedded semithin sections remain the gold standard for BM biopsy cytomorphology, and any alternate method should aim to provide comparable cytologic detail. Obtaining sections from paraffin-embedded decalcified BM biopsy specimens of a quality similar to resin-embedded semithin sections has been a real challenge.

2.4 Tissue Sectioning

Thin sectioning, preferably by an experienced histotechnologist, is a key variable in ensuring excellent quality slides both for morphology and immunostaining. Sections should not be cut thicker than 5 µm because the interpretation becomes difficult if not impossible in the presence of 2 cell layers. In principle, the sections should be cut as thin as possible and 1 to 2 µm sections can be achieved by experienced histotechnologists.

2.5 Antigen Retrieval

There are no special requirements regarding Ag retrieval from the BM biopsy specimen. The only specific consideration is that BM aspirate clot specimens may provide less robust Ag retrieval than BM core biopsy specimens because the epitopes are better preserved in nondecalcified tissues. On the other hand, tissue fixation in the

T2.2 Different Decalcification Procedures Used for Processing Bone Marrow Biopsy Specimens

Decalcification Procedure	Decalcification Time	Comments
RDO (commercially available dilute solution of hydrochloric acid in coal tar base)	1 hour exactly	Timing is important May affect epitope and RNA preservation
Surgipath Decalcifier II	1-1.5 hours	Timing is important May affect epitope and RNA preservation
5%-10% Nitric acid	2 hours	May affect morphologic, epitope, and RNA preservation
Hydrochloric acid–formic acid solution	2.5 hours	May affect morphologic, epitope, and RNA preservation
Gooding and Stewart decalcification fluid (10% formic acid and 5% formaldehyde)	6 hours	Optimal, but may encounter TAT issues
5% Formic acid	12-18 hours (overnight)	May affect epitope preservation and encounter TAT issues
5% EDTA	up to 48-72 hours	Optimal, but may encounter TAT issues

TAT = turnaround time.

clot specimen may be suboptimal if large blood clots were placed in fixative. Fixative penetration through such large clotted blood fragments is slow and many times suboptimal because some laboratories fix the clots for the same length of time as the matching core biopsy specimen, which is often many times smaller than the clot. The suboptimal fixation will display poor morphologic features and poor Ag localization after Ag retrieval. The significance of suboptimally fixation of clot specimens is twofold:

1. they may detach from the glass slide during the Ag retrieval step; and
2. they may show inferior epitope preservation which cannot be rescued by Ag retrieval.

Generally speaking, most Ag retrieval protocols are the same as in any other tissue and their choice usually depends more on the epitope to be detected than the type of the tissue. The "DeCal Retrieval Solution" (BioGenex, San Ramon, CA) is a solution of saturated sodium hydroxide in methanol and has been developed specifically for decalcified tissues. The Ag retrieval is done at room temperature for 30 minutes in a DeCal Retrieval Solution designed to unmask Ags in formalin-fixed, acid-decalcified tissues embedded in paraffin, in particular BM biopsies; however, the entire procedure with all required washes takes about 1 hour [Shi 1993] and it has not been validated for most markers that are in use in hematopathology.

2.6 Turnaround Time

Some processing protocols are very quick, but show suboptimal tissue and Ag preservation. Others procedures are slower, but result in better tissue preservation. However, this rule does not always apply. Some shorter protocols may result in better overall performance than longer ones. Despite the clinical requirements that are linked to the diagnostic indication for a BM biopsy, the TAT requirement varies hugely among different centers. BM biopsy is mostly accompanied by a BM aspirate, which is evaluated morphologically the same day, often also with flow cytometry, and occasionally with histochemical methods within a few hours. Therefore, in some centers, the need for rapid processing of the BM biopsy is not emphasized. Currently, fixation and decalcification procedures on BM biopsy specimens widely differ, resulting in a TAT varying from 24 to 26 hours to more than 5 days. An approximate comparison of different methods is summarized in T2.3. Using the Hammersmith protocol (see p. 11), results of H&E, Giemsa, reticulin and Perls staining are available within 48 hours, and the initial panel of IHC test results is ready within 72 hours of sample receipt. This method uses procedures that are generally similar to other standard tissue processing protocols. Alternatively, shorter protocols are available, but may compromise morphology and to some extent IHC results. We agree with those who point out that "the patient is likely to benefit from the right result, rather than the rapid one" [Yaziji 2007].

In institutions with a high proportion of BM biopsy samples involved by neoplastic diseases, IHC is required in a large number of cases. In such laboratories, IHC panels can be planned based on the clinical diagnosis, and the required number of unstained sections for each panel can be cut at the time of initial sectioning. Some laboratories may opt to design small IHC panels for each type of clinical question. For example, in staging of non-Hodgkin lymphoma, CD3 and CD20 may be used routinely in each case. Immunostains and in situ hybridization can be performed on the automated systems for most tests. These measures can somewhat improve the TAT in longer tissue processing protocols. F2.1 to F2.11 illustrate IHC results typically found in the BM biopsy specimen fixed in either AZF or 10% neutral-buffered formal saline solution (18-24 hours) and decalcified using Gooding and Stewart decalcification fluid (10% formic acid and 5% formaldehyde). Most of the images in this book illustrate formalin-fixed BM biopsy specimens, with a few B5-fixed tissue specimens.

For most IHC tests, optimal results are possible with almost any fixative, but the achievable endpoints may be somewhat different for different epitopes. The choice of the primary Abs, good selection of Ag retrieval protocols, and use of highly sensitive detection systems can greatly improve results of IHC staining irrespective of the type of commonly used BM tissue fixation. However, this fact prevented a reduction in the number of tissue processing protocols needed for standardization and application of extralaboratory quality control systems. Extralaboratory quality control is needed for the BM IHC biopsy specimen as much as it is needed for any other tissue biopsy specimen. More uniform tissue processing would be of great help when BM biopsy specimens are evaluated at other centers or laboratories. True standardization of diagnostic IHC in anatomic pathology is not yet achieved [Goldstein 2007]. Developing like standards for BM biopsies will be even more difficult.

T2.3 Comparison of TAT for Different Bone Marrow Biopsy Protocols

#	Fixation	Decalcification	Embedding	TAT (hours)	Morphology	IHC	ISH
1	Formalin (rapid)	Acid (rapid)	Paraffin	~24	+ / ++	++	Suboptimal
2	Formalin	Acid (short)	Paraffin	~48	++	+++	Suboptimal
3	Formalin	EDTA	Paraffin	~72-96	++	+++	+++
4	AZF	Gooding and Stewart	Paraffin	~48	+++	+++	+++
5	Formalin	EDTA	Epoxy resin	~48	+++	++	

AZF = aceto-zinc-formalin; IHC = immunohistochemistry; ISH = in situ hybridization; TAT = turnaround time.

IHC Results (AZF or 10% Neutral Buffered Formal Saline Fixed Tissue)

F2.1 Parvovirus B19 in erythroid hypoplasia

This bone marrow (BM) biopsy specimen is from a patient with previous renal transplantation admitted with marked anemia and reticulocytopenia. The BM specimen shows markedly abnormal erythroid precursors **A**, which are highlighted by glycophorin-C immunohistochemistry **B**. Giant proerythroblasts are shown. Immunostaining with parvovirus B19 viral capsid proteins VP1 and VP2 identifies several infected erythroid precursors (**C** and **D**).

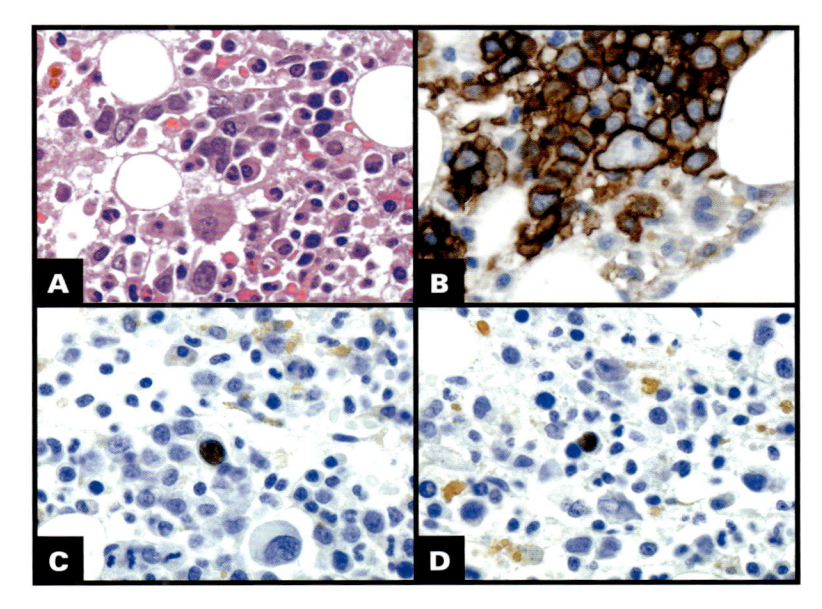

F2.2 Glycophorin C in early erythroid precursors

This specimen is from a patient with a myelodysplastic syndrome with megaloblastoid dyserythropoiesis **A**. A proportion of the erythroid cells appears to express CD117 **B**. Some of the cells show nuclear lobation and bi/multinucleation. These features are highlighted by glycophorin C immunohistochemistry, which also confirms that the abnormal cells are of erythroid lineage (**C** and **D**).

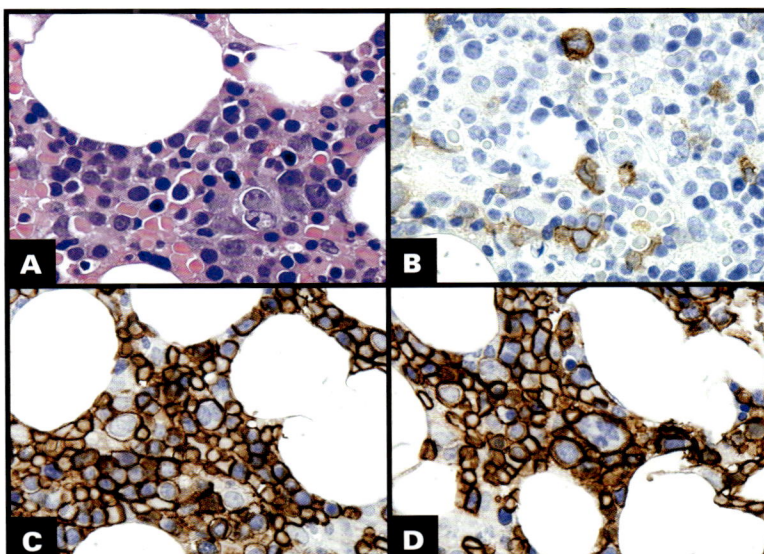

F2.3 HLA-DR is not expressed in acute promyelocytic leukemia (APL)

This BM biopsy specimen shows APL. The leukemic cells have deeply indented nuclei and the cytoplasm was heavily granulated **A**. The cells express myeloperoxidase **B**. Characteristically, these blasts are negative for both HLA-DR **C** and CD34 **D** [Brunning 2001].

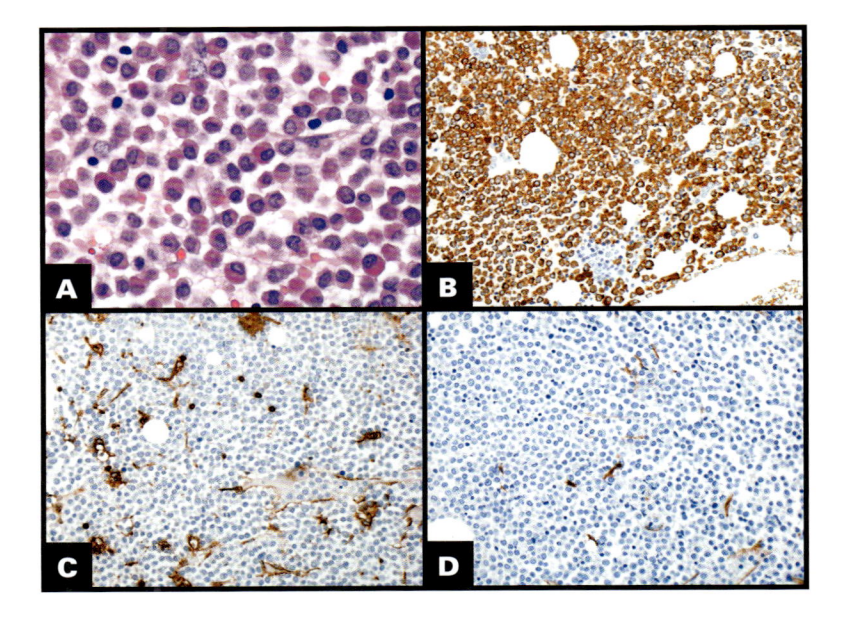

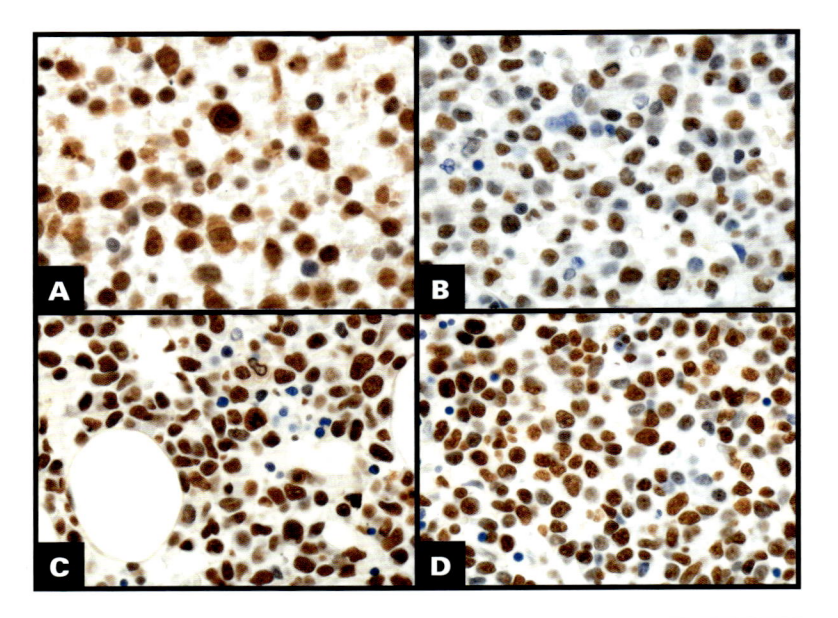

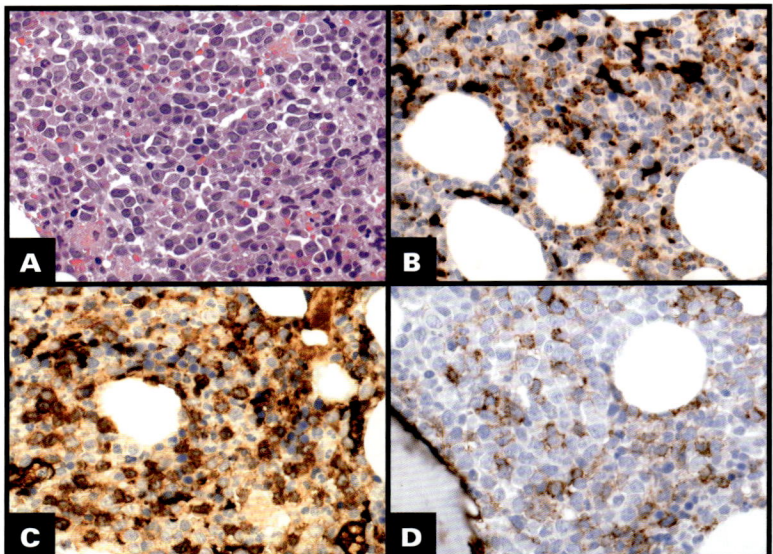

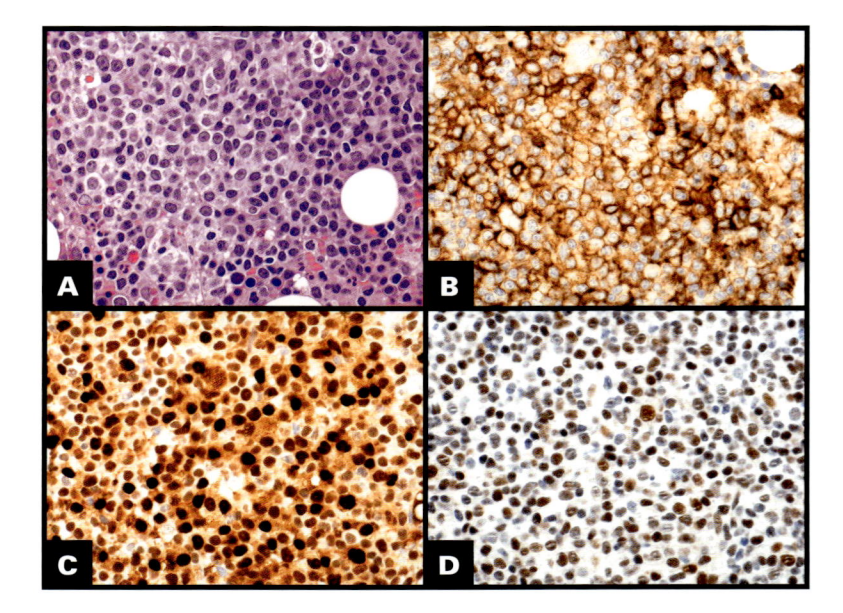

F2.4 Nucleophosmin (NPM) in acute myelogenous leukemia (AML); monoclonal antibody (mAb) for NPM (clone 376 was a generous gift from Professor Brunangelo Falini)

The bone marrow biopsy specimen illustrated in **A** and **B** is from a patient with AML showing nuclear and cytoplasmic expression of NPM **A** and only nuclear expression of nucleolin **B**. Cytoplasmic expression of NPM is abnormal; however, it may identify a good prognostic subset of AML. AML with nuclear expression of NPM only is shown in **C** and nuclear expression only of nucleolin in **D**. Lack of cytoplasmic NPM expression implies lack of NPM mutations. The antibody recognizes both the wild-type NPM and the NPM leukemic mutants. mAb against nucleolin (C23, Santa Cruz Biotechnology, Santa Cruz, CA) is used as a control. Except in mitotic cells, nucleolin expression should be restricted to the nucleus in all cell types [Falini 2006]. However, use of IHC detection of NPM for prediction of likelihood of complete remission and prolonged survival was recently challenged [Kronoplev 2008].

F2.5 Comparison of CD68 and CD163

This bone marrow biopsy specimen is from a patient with chronic myelomonocytic leukemia (CMML) **A**. The CD68R (PGM-1) antibody highlights mainly monocytic/histiocytic cells as follows: phagocytic histiocytes show diffuse dense cytoplasmic staining, which is often vacuolated; dendritic histiocytes show long dendritic processes; monocytes show dark, coarse cytoplasmic granules; and promonocytes often have finer cytoplasmic granules. Promonocytes have slightly larger nuclei, less prominent nuclear indentation, and often a more prominent nucleolus **B** and **C**. CD163 is also expressed by the monocytic/histiocytic cells. In this case, the proportion of cells stained by CD68R and CD163 are nearly comparable. CD68R is detected in a greater proportion of cells than CD163. The monocytic/myelomonocytic cells of CMML may also show aberrant expression of CD56 in a proportion of the cells **D** [Ngo 2008].

F2.6 CD38, MUM1, and p53 in chronic lymphocytic leukemia (CLL)

This bone marrow biopsy specimen is from a patient with CLL with nodular and interstitial infiltrates of lymphoid cells. Proliferation centers are present **A**. The neoplastic lymphocytes expressed CD38 **B**, MUM1 **C** and p53 **D**. These markers have been associated with poor prognosis in CLL [Cordone 1998; Ito 2002; Patten 2008].

IHC Results (AZF or 10% Neutral Buffered Formal Saline Fixed Tissue)

F2.7 t(14;19)(q32;q13)+ small B-cell leukemia characterized as a B-cell chronic lymphocytic leukemia (CLL)–like disorder with CD5+ cells and a low CLL score

This bone marrow biopsy specimen is from a patient with peripheral blood lymphocytosis. On flow cytometry, the cells were CD22+, CD79b+, and FMC7+. Both sIg and CD20 were strongly positive, while CD5 and CD23 were negative. The CLL score was 0. The IgVH gene was unmutated. There is an interstitial infiltrate **A** of small B-lymphoid cells which express CD20 **C** and show weak/focal expression of CD5 **D**. They were negative for CD10, CD23, and cyclin D1. The malignant cells are BCL-3 positive with a nuclear pattern **B**. The karyotype showed evidence of trisomy12 and t(14;19)(q32;q13). Fluorescence in situ hybridization analysis confirmed the involvement of the BCL3 and IgH loci in the translocation. This identifies a distinct nosological entity termed t(14;19)(q32;q13)+ small B-cell leukemia characterized as a B-cell CLL-like disorder with CD5+ cells and a low CLL score [Reid 2008].

F2.8 DBA.44 and TRAP in hairy cell leukemia (HCL)

This posttreatment bone marrow biopsy specimen is from a patient with HCL showing residual disease. The H&E slide **A** shows the typical cytomorphology of HCL cells with indented or monocytoid nuclei and no obvious nucleoli, moderate amounts of pale staining or clear cytoplasm, and a prominent cell membrane. On CD20 **B** and DBA44 **C** immunostains, the membrane of the HCL cells typically shows a ruffled appearance. This feature is better appreciated when the infiltrate is not "heavy." The cells also express tartrate resistant acid phosphatase (TRAP) **D**.

F2.9 Immunoglobulin light chain demonstration by in situ hybridization

This hypocellular bone marrow biopsy specimen is involved by myeloma. The cytomorphology of the tumor cells was lymphoid-like **A**. They expressed cyclin D1 **B**. In addition, they were positive for CD138 and CD20. Light-chain immunohistochemistry results were difficult to interpret and hence in situ hybridization (ISH) was performed, which showed that the neoplastic cells did not express κ Ig light chain mRNA **C** and showed strong positivity for λ mRNA **D**.

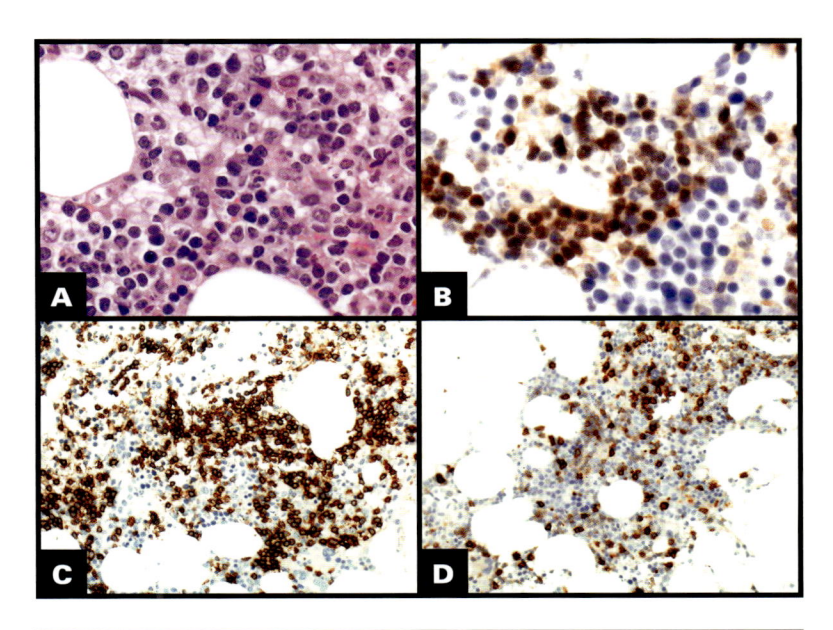

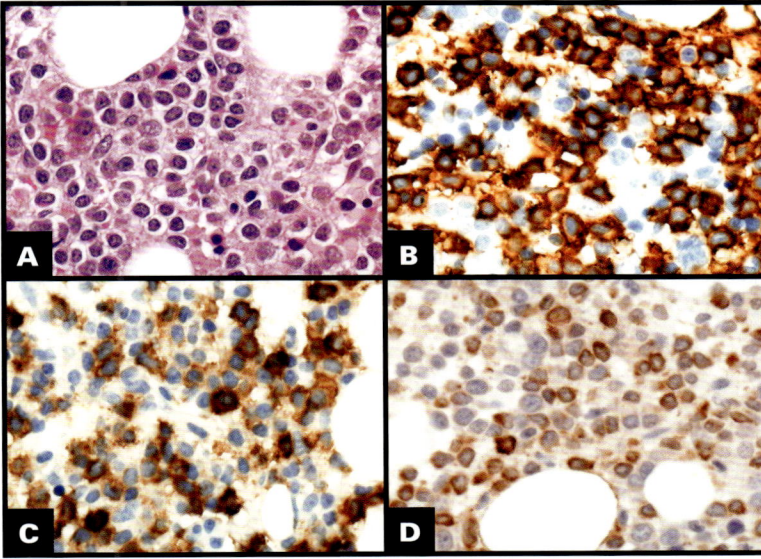

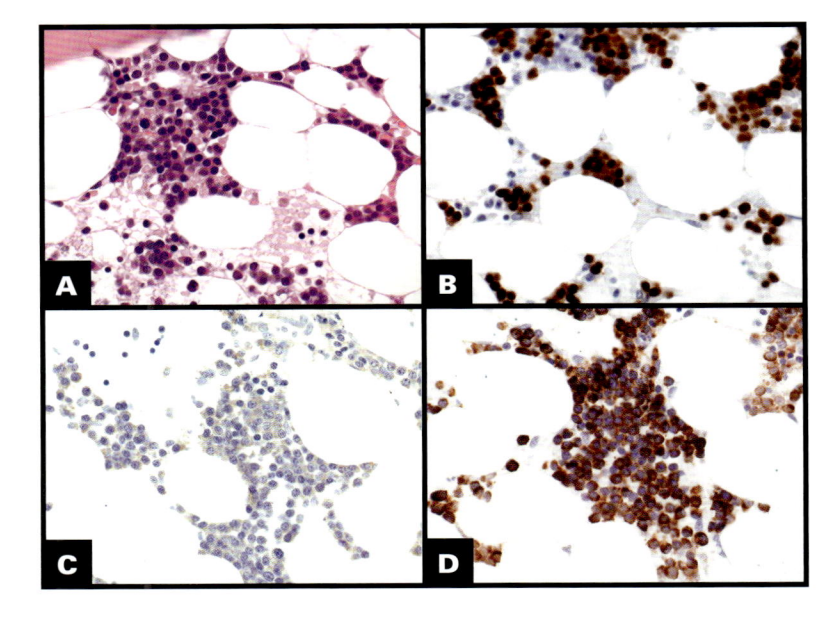

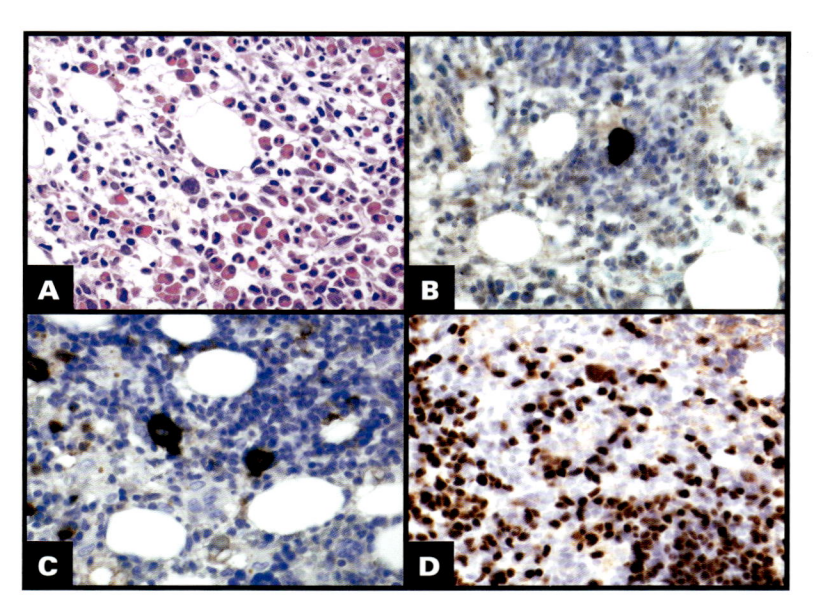

F2.10 Epstein-Barr virus (EBV) in situ hybridization (ISH) in classical Hodgkin lymphoma (cHL)

This bone marrow biopsy specimen shows focal involvement by cHL. The initial H&E section **A** showed only occasional mononuclear Hodgkin cells amidst abundant eosinophils. On the deeper sections used for immunohistochemistry and ISH, the neoplastic cells were more numerous and were accompanied by small lymphoid cells. The large atypical cells (Reed-Sternberg cells) were positive for EBV mRNA in ISH test conducted with the EBER1 probe **B**. The cells were also positive for CD30 **C** and PAX5 **D**.

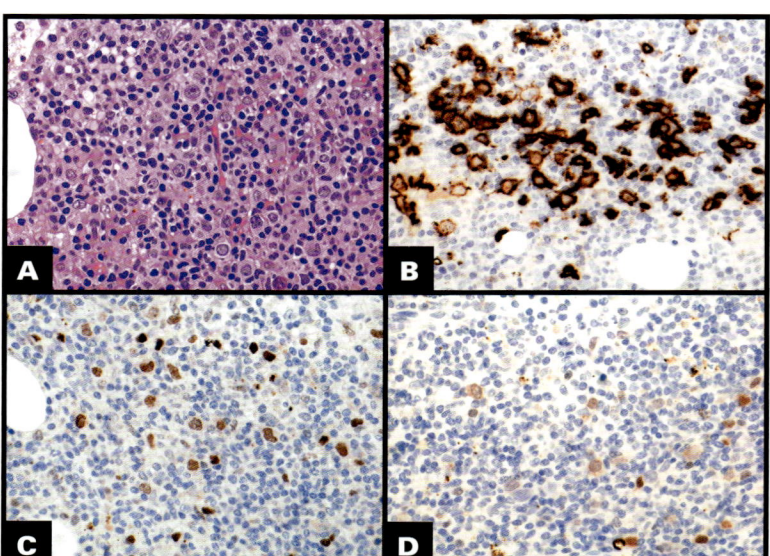

F2.11 OCT2 and BOB1

This bone marrow biopsy specimen shows focal involvement by atypical lymphoid infiltrate composed of lymphoid cells of varying size **A**. The smaller lymphoid cells were mostly CD3+ T cells. The larger lymphoid cells expressed CD45, CD20 **B**, CD79a, CD30, PAX5, BCL6, MUM1, Ki-67, OCT2 **C** and BOB1 **D**. BOB1 expression is weaker than OCT2 expression (possibly because of suboptimal antigen preservation). Expression of both OCT2 and BOB1 is usually not a feature of neoplastic cells of classical Hodgkin lymphoma, where the immunoglobulin transcriptional machinery is abrogated [Stein 2001].

In conclusion, there are several good protocols for BM biopsy tissue processing. However, this is an evolving field. In 1985, Mullink et al [Mullink 1985] compared suitability of different fixation and decalcification methods for BM IHC. They found that fixation in a mercuric chloride–formaldehyde mixture followed by decalcification in acetic acid–formaldehyde-saline proved to be the best procedure at the time for Ag preservation and retention of morphologic detail. As new fixation, decalcification, and Ag retrieval procedures are described and new primary Abs and ever more sensitive detection methods are introduced at a fairly rapid pace, the process of validating the impact of tissue processing on IHC for different Ags/Abs is a continuous one. New studies similar to the study by Mullink et al are required. Because of the uncertainty about which BM biopsy tissue protocol may be best for all possible IHC tests, histochemical, and molecular applications, each currently used protocol may continue to be used. All of the protocols applied to BM biopsy need fine tuning for each individual institution's circumstances, including scheduling of BM biopsy procedure, availability of technical personnel, and TAT issues. Minor modifications to accommodate individual needs generally do not significantly hamper the results, but all methods of BM biopsy processing should be validated before they are introduced into routine practice. The validation process may be complex because of the multiple steps involved in tissue processing. Efforts toward developing fewer (optimally 1, but not more than 3-4) standard BM biopsy processing protocols are necessary. This will help in the sharing of IHC and other protocols across different centers and enable extralaboratory quality control testing in BM IHC procedures. Standardized tissue processing also may be a necessary requirement for conducting multi-institutional research studies and clinical trials.

2.7 Protocols

Protocol for Bone Marrow Processing and Staining Used at Hammersmith Hospital
[Naresh 2006]

Fixative. The AZF fixative (12.5 g zinc chloride, 150 mL concentrated formaldehyde, 7.5 mL glacial acetic acid, and up to 1000 mL distilled water) is prepared in bulk and aliquotted into 20 mL universal containers with corrosive hazard labels. These aliquots are sent to the hematology departments and other inpatient and clinic locations where BM biopsies are performed. The hematologist is instructed to place the freshly obtained trephine biopsy specimen directly into AZF fixative and transport it immediately to the histopathology department.

Fixation. Once received in the laboratory, the BM biopsy specimens are left overnight in the AZF fixative. The following morning (after 20-24 hours), the solution is decanted (using a strainer) and the biopsy specimen is washed in distilled water for 30 minutes.

Decalcification. The water is replaced by Gooding and Stewart decalcification fluid (10% formic acid and 5% formaldehyde). The biopsy specimens are left to decalcify for about 6 hours before being processed and embedded in paraffin using procedures similar to those used for other specimens.

Comment. This protocol provides excellent preservation of morphology, epitopes for IHC, and RNA for in situ hybridization.

Protocol for Bone Marrow Processing and Staining Suitable for Rapid Turnaround Time

Fixative. 10% buffered formalin.

Fixation. Minimum of 2 hours. If possible, the BM biopsy specimen is left in 10% buffered formalin until decalcification needs to be started (usually midafternoon). This way, many BM biopsies are fixed in formalin for 4 hours or longer before decalcification.

Decalcification. The bone marrow biopsy specimen is decalcified in RDO, Rapid Decalcifier (Apex Engineering, Aurora, IL) for exactly 1 hour. A shorter period will produce suboptimal decalcification of the bone marrow biopsy specimen. Longer incubation will induce epitope degradation and is not recommended. The decalcification step must be timed precisely.

Comment. While 2-hour fixation in formalin usually produces interpretable results, both morphology and epitope preservation are known to be affected. The decalcification step is less harmful to the tissue if the tissue is well fixed.

References

Arber JM, Weiss LM, Chang KL, Battifora H, Arber DA. The effect of decalcification on in situ hybridization. *Mod Pathol* 1997;10(10):1009-14.

Bonds LA, Barnes P, Foucar K, Sever CE. Acetic acid-zinc-formalin: a safe alternative to B-5 fixative. *Am J Clin Pathol* 2005;124(2):205-11.

Brown RS, Edwards J, Bartlett JW, Jones C, Dogan A. Routine acid decalcification of bone marrow samples can preserve DNA for FISH and CGH studies in metastatic prostate cancer. *J HistochemCytochem* 2002;50(1):113-5.

Brunning RD, Matutes E, Flandrin G, et al. Acute myeloid leukaemia with recurrent genetic abnormalities. In: Jaffe ES, Harris NL, Stein H, Vardiman JW, eds. *World Health Organization Classification of Tumours Pathology & Genetics Tumours of Haematopoietic and Lymphoid Tissues*. Lyon, France: IARC Press; 2001:81-8.

Cordone I, Masi S, Mauro FR, et al. p53 expression in B-cell chronic lymphocytic leukemia: a marker of disease progression and poor prognosis. *Blood* 1998;91(11):4342-9.

DePalma L. The effect of decalcification and choice of fixative on histiocytic iron in bone marrow core biopsies. *Biotech Histochem* 1996;71(2):57-60.

Falini B, Martelli MP, Bolli N, et al. Immunohistochemistry predicts nucleophosmin (NPM) mutations in acute myeloid leukemia. *Blood* 2006;108(6):1999-2005.

Fox CH, Johnson FB, Whiting J, Roller PP. Formaldehyde fixation. *J Histochem Cytochem* 1985 Aug;33(8):845-53.

Gala JL, Chenut F, Hong KB, et al. A panel of antibodies for the immunostaining of Bouin's fixed bone marrow trephine biopsies. *J Clin Pathol* 1997;50(6):521-4.

Gatter KC, Heryet A, Brown DC, Mason DY. Is it necessary to embed bone marrow biopsies in plastic for haematological diagnosis? *Histopathology* 1987;11(1):1-7.

Gaulier A, Fourcade C, Szekeres G, Pulik M. Bone marrow one step fixation-decalcification in Lowy FMA solution: an immunohistological and in situ hybridization study. *Pathol Res Pract* 1994;190(12):1149-61.

Gebhard S, Benhattar J, Bricod C, Meuge-Moraw C, Delacretaz F. Polymerase chain reaction in the diagnosis of T-cell lymphoma in paraffin-embedded bone marrow biopsies: a comparative study. *Histopathology* 2001;38(1):37-44.

Goldstein NS, Hewitt SM, Taylor CR, Yaziji H, Hicks DG; Members of Ad-Hoc Committee On Immunohistochemistry Standardization. Recommendations for improved standardization of immunohistochemistry. *Appl Immunohistochem Mol Morphol* 2007 Jun;15(2):124-33.

Goldstein NS, Ferkowicz M, Odish E, Mani A, Hastah F. Minimum formalin fixation time for consistent estrogen receptor immunohistochemical staining of invasive breast carcinoma. *Am J Clin Pathol* 2003 Jul;120(1):86-92.

Happerfield LC, Saward R, Grimwade L, et al. Automated immunostaining of cell smears: an alternative to flow cytometry. *J Clin Pathol* 2008;61(6):740-43.

Ito M, Iida S, Inagaki H, Tsuboi K, et al. MUM1/IRF4 expression is an unfavorable prognostic factor in B-cell chronic lymphocytic leukemia (CLL)/small lymphocytic lymphoma (SLL). *Jpn J Cancer Res* 2002;93(6):685-94.

Knonoplev S, Nguyen M, Huang X, et al. Cytoplasmic expression of nucleophosmin does not predict favorable prognosis in AML patients. Abstract 1192. *Mod Pathol* 2008;216(supplement 1):260A-261A.

Krenacs T, Bagdi E, Stelkovics E, Bereczki L, Krenacs L. How we process trephine biopsy specimens: epoxy resin embedded bone marrow biopsies. *J Clin Pathol* 2005;58(9):897-903.

Kunze E, Middel P, Fayazzi A, et al. Immunohistochemical staining of plastic (methyl-methacrylate)-embedded bone marrow biopsies applying the biotin-free tyramide signal amplification system. *Appl Immunohistochem Mol Morphol* 2008;16(1):76-82.

Leong AS. Pitfalls in diagnostic immunohistology. *Adv Anat Pathol* 2004;11(2):86-93.

Loyson SA, Rademakers LH, Joling P, Vroom TM, van den Tweel JG. Immunohistochemical analysis of decalcified paraffin-embedded human bone marrow biopsies with emphasis on MHC class I and CD34 expression. *Histopathology* 1997;31(5):412-9.

Milan L, Trachtenberg MC. Ultrasonic decalcification of bone. *Am J Surg Pathol* 1981;5(6):573-9.

Mullink H, Henzen-Logmans SC, Tadema TM, Mol JJ, Meijer CJ. Influence of fixation and decalcification on the immunohistochemical staining of cell-specific markers in paraffin-embedded human bone biopsies. *J Histochem Cytochem* 1985;33(11):1103-9.

Nagasaka T, Lai R, Chen YY, et al. The use of archival bone marrow specimens in detecting B-cell non-Hodgkin's lymphomas using polymerase chain reaction methods. *Leuk Lymphoma* 2000;36(3-4):347-52.

Naresh KN, Lampert I, Hasserjian R, et al. Optimal processing of bone marrow trephine biopsy: the Hammersmith protocol. *J Clin Pathol* 2006;59(9):903-11.

Ngo N, Lampert IA, Naresh KN. Bone marrow trephine morphology and immunohistochemical findings in chronic myelomonocytic leukaemia [published online ahead of print March 26, 2008]. *Br J Haematol*

Patten PE, Buggins AG, Richards J, et al. CD38 expression in chronic lymphocytic leukemia is regulated by the tumor microenvironment [published online ahead of print March 7, 2008]. *Blood*

Reid A, Naresh K, Wagner S, MacDonald D. Interphase FISH using a BCL3 probe to diagnose the t(14;19)(q32;q13)-positive small B-cell leukemia. *Leuk Lymphoma* 2008;49(2):356-8.

Reineke T, Jenni B, Abdou MT, et al. Ultrasonic decalcification offers new perspectives for rapid FISH, DNA, and RT-PCR analysis in bone marrow trephines. *Am J Surg Pathol* 2006;30(7):892-6.

Shi SR, Tandon AK, Haussmann RR, Kalra KL, Taylor CR. Immunohistochemical study of intermediate filament proteins on routinely processed, celloidin-embedded human temporal bone sections by using a new technique for antigen retrieval. *Acta Otolaryngol* 1993;113(1):48-54.

Stein H, Marafioti T, Foss HD, et al. Down-regulation of BOB.1/OBF.1 and Oct2 in classical Hodgkin disease but not in lymphocyte predominant Hodgkin disease correlates with immunoglobulin transcription. *Blood* 2001;97(2):496-501.

Stuart-Smith SE, Hughes DA, Bain BJ. Are routine iron stains on bone marrow trephine biopsy specimens necessary? *J Clin Pathol* 2005;58(3):269-72.

Taylor CR, Levenson RM. Quantification of immunohistochemistry--issues concerning methods, utility and semiquantitative assessment II. *Histopathology* 2006 Oct;49(4):411-24. Review.

Toth B, Wehrmann M, Kaiserling E, Horny HP. Immunophenotyping of acute lymphoblastic leukaemia in routinely processed bone marrow biopsy specimens. *J Clin Pathol* 1999;52(9):688-92.

Werner M, Kaloutsi V, Walter K, Buhr T, Bernhards J, Georgii A. Immunohistochemical examination of routinely processed bone marrow biopsies. *Pathol Res Pract* 1992;188(6):707-13.

Yaziji H, Taylor CR. Begin at the beginning, with the tissue! The key message underlying the ASCO/CAP Task-force Guideline Recommendations for HER2 testing. *Appl Immunohistochem Mol Morphol* 2007 Sep;15(3):239-41.

Chapter 3
CLUSTER OF DIFFERENTIATION MARKERS

The CD nomenclature was established in 1982 at the first International Workshop and Conference on Human Leukocyte Differentiation Antigens (HLDA) in Paris, France. Human Cell Differentiation Molecules is an organization that runs HLDA (human leucocyte differentiation antigens) workshops and names and characterizes CD molecules [hcdm.org 2008]. The main purpose of this system was to facilitate classification of the monoclonal antibodies (mAbs) generated against T-cell surface molecules on leukocytes. The characteristic approach of the HLDA workshops was multilaboratory blind analysis of antibodies, which has provided independent validation of antibody specificity and usability, and has enabled scientists and clinicians alike to confidently use these reagents in research, diagnosis, and therapy [Schlossman 1994]. The "CD" is an abreviaton for "cluster of differentiation" because cluster analysis was used to identify clusters of antibodies (Abs) expressed at various stages of differentiation. At the 8th HLDA conference, HLDA was replaced by HCDM, which stands for "human cell differentiation molecules" because CD nomenclature is no longer reserved only for leukocytes, but has expanded to other cells types. Molecules CD1 to CD350 have been characterized at the HLDA/HCDM workshops [Zola 2005].

An antigen is designated its own CD if it shows reactivity with at least 2 mAbs. Also, some CD molecules carry a provisional indicator "w" if this CD shows reactivity with only a single mAb or it is not well characterized. A study of the subset of the CD molecules in human bone marrow biopsy evaluation is illustrated here.

3.1 CD1a

CD1a is 1 of the 5 CD1 proteins encoded by CD1A, CD1B, CD1C, CD1D, and CD1E genes (PROW) [McMichael 1979]. In contrast to other species, humans express just a single example of each of the CD1 molecules, that is, no isoforms are made [Calabi 1989]. CD1a is not really expressed before the thymocyte stage of T-cell development [Blom 2006]. Therefore, no normal early T-cell precursors should express CD1a in the bone marrow (BM). Any specific expression should be considered pathological even though in some cases it is reactive/activated T cells that express this antigen, not necessarily the neoplasic T cells. Therefore it is said that up to 10% of adult BM cells may express CD1a as measured with flow cytometry [Keren 2001]. Immunohistochemistry (IHC) shows no CD1a+ cells even when activated T cells are present . CD1a is not used very frequently in the evaluation of BM biopsy specimens. However, there are 2 diseases for which CD1a may be useful: precursor T-cell lymphoblastic leukemia also refered to as T-cell acute lymphoblastic leukemia (T-ALL) and Langerhans cell histocytosis (LCH). Precursor T-ALL is usually immunophenotyped with flow cytometry, but in LCH, CD1a is very useful for primary diagnosis or staging, and it is the most specific marker [McClain 2004]. CD1a is very useful to confirm the presence of Langerhans cells even if a small number of neoplastic cells is present in the biopsy specimen. The other freqently used marker in the diagnosis of LCH is S-100, but it is less specific and may be difficult to interpret when only a small number of positive cells is found.

F3.1.1 CD1a in a 20-year-old man with thrombocytopenia and no definite pathologic bone marrow findings

CD1a is not detectable in the normal BM. It is not detectable before thymic stage. It is found on cortical thymocytes (CD4+ CD8+) and it is absent on mature peripheral blood T cells, but intracytoplasmic CD1a can be found on activated T cells. Very rare positive cells in this BM biopsy specimen are presumed to be activated T cells.

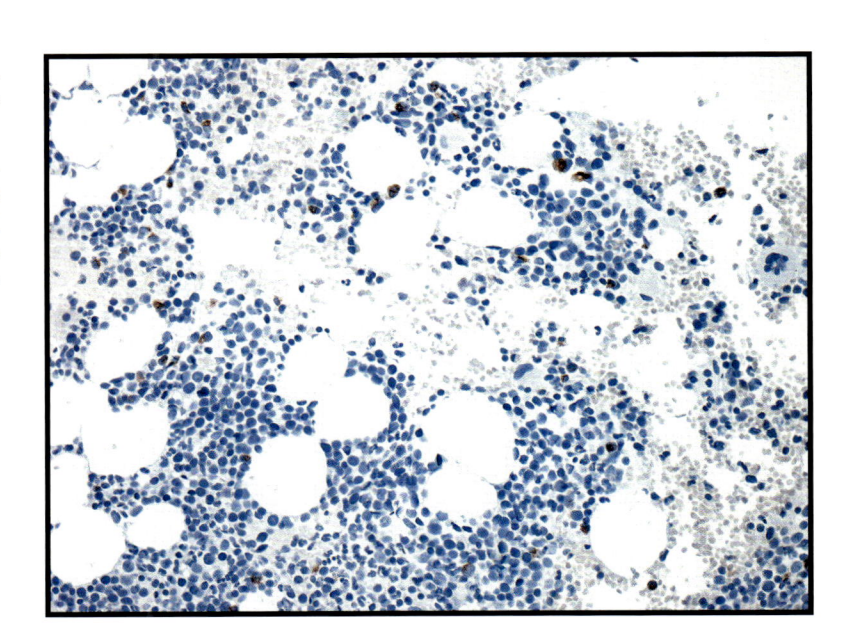

3: Cluster of Differentiation Markers

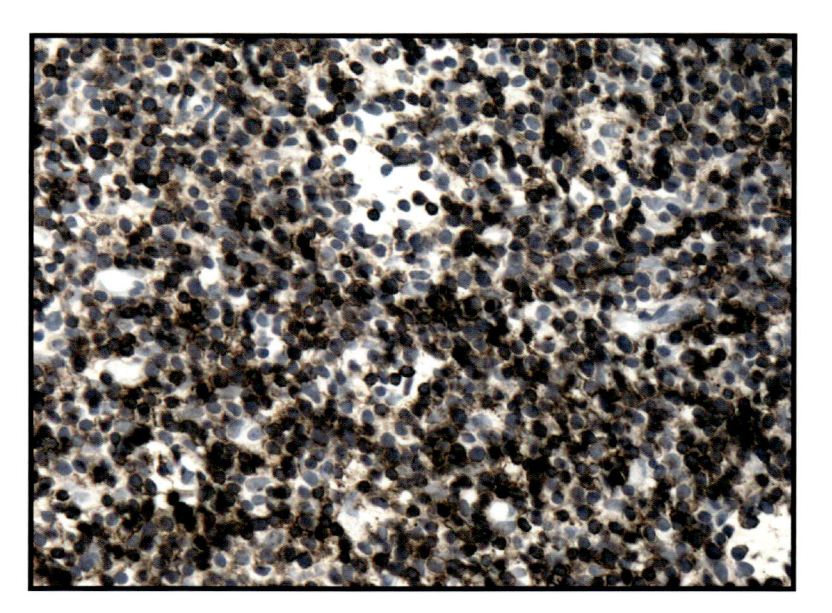

F3.1.2 CD1a in type B1 thymoma

This biopsy is from a 42-year-old man with B1 thymoma and myasthenia gravis. This subtype of thymoma is also known as "organoid" because of its resemblance to normal cortex of the thymus; therefore, the finding of benign precursor T cells with variable CD1a is expected. It is evident in many cells that the positivity is clearly membranous with focal or minor cytoplasmic expression of the CD1.

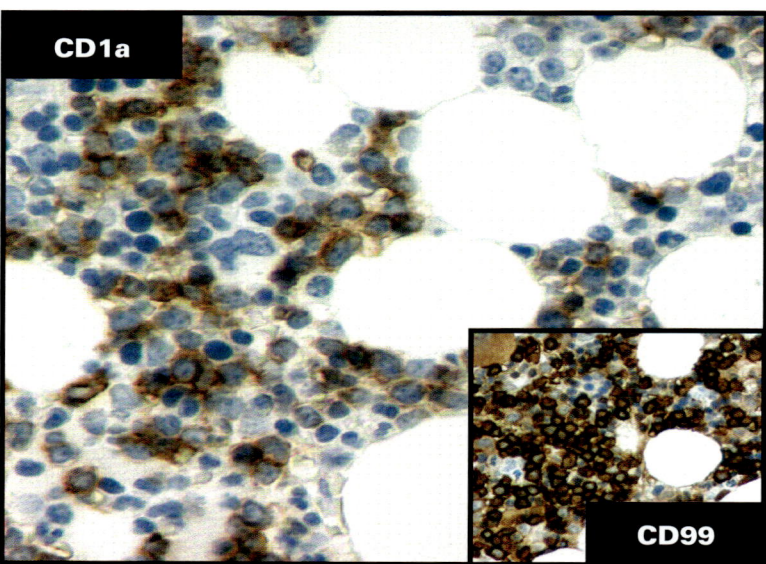

F3.1.3 CD1a in precursor T-cell acute lymphoblastic leukemia (T-ALL) involving the bone marrow

This BM biopsy specimen is from an 11-year-old boy with an anterior mediastinal mass, thrombocytopenia, and anemia. In contrast to benign precursor T cells, it is not unusual to find a predominantly cytoplasmic pattern of CD1a expression in precursor T-ALL. However, the expression may be weak or even undetectable on immunohistochemistry. CD99 staining (inset) and TdT (not shown) often better highlight the number of malignant cells.

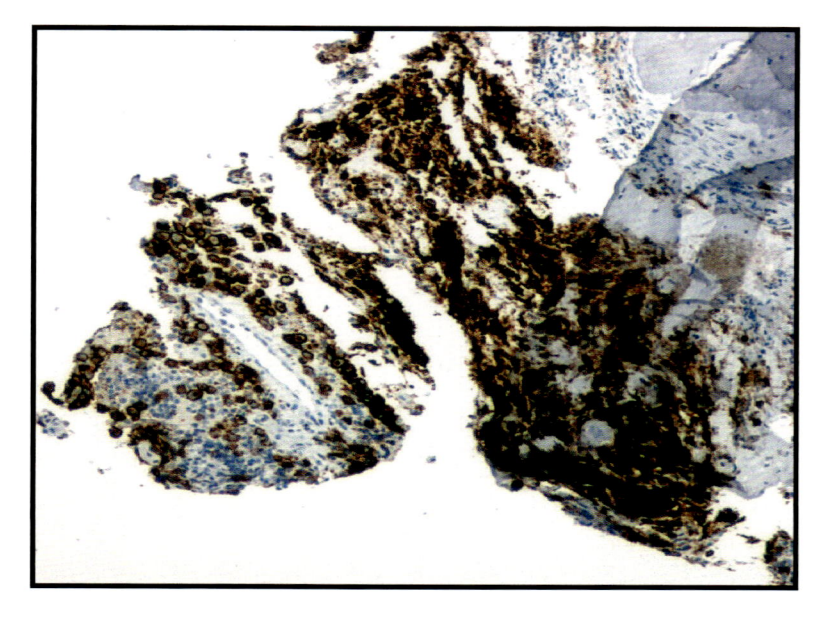

F3.1.4 CD1a in Langerhans cell histocytosis (LCH)

If LCH presents as a primary bone lesion, as in this biopsy specimen from the vertebrae from a 14-year-old boy, the biopsy is usually performed with a bone needle core in which all technical considerations are the same as in a regular bone marrow core biopsy from the iliac spine. CD1a is a more specific marker than S-100 for labeling both benign and neoplastic Langerhans dendritic cells.

F3.1.5 CD1a in Langerhans cell histocytosis (LCH) in the same case as in F3.1.4

Higher magnification shows Golgi-type, cytoplasmic, and membranous positivity for CD1a. CD1a is the most specific test for identification of LCH in various sites. This is particularly true for the bone marrow biopsy because no normal structures express CD1a and precursor T-ALL is generally not in the differential diagnosis.

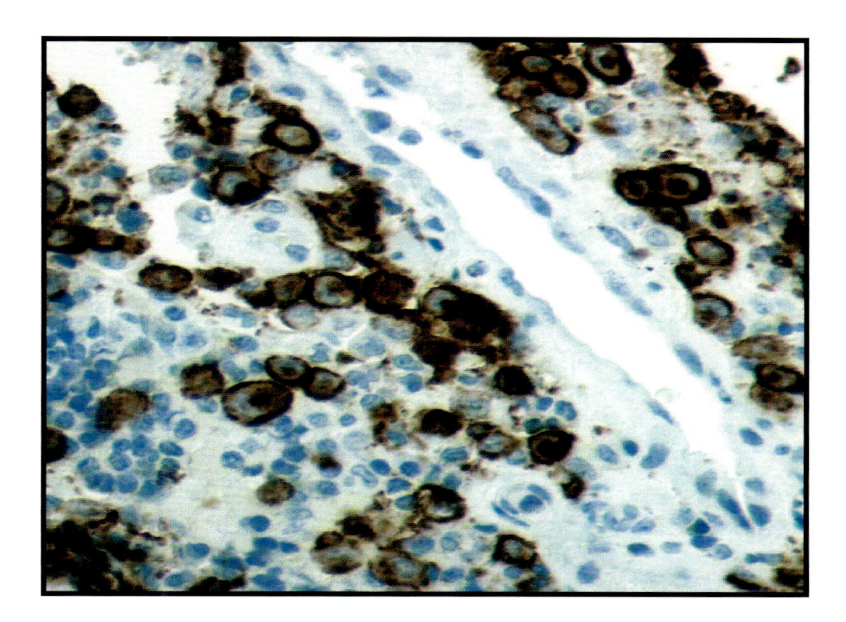

F3.1.6 CD1a in Langerhans cell histocytosis (LCH) in the same case as in F3.1.4. and F3.1.5

Smaller number than illustrated here of randomly dispersed positive cells is sufficient finding for definitive diagnosis of LCH in the bone or bone marrow biopsy. This is because of the very selective distribution of CD1a in the human tissues. S-100 may also be used to further corroborate the diagnosis of LCH.

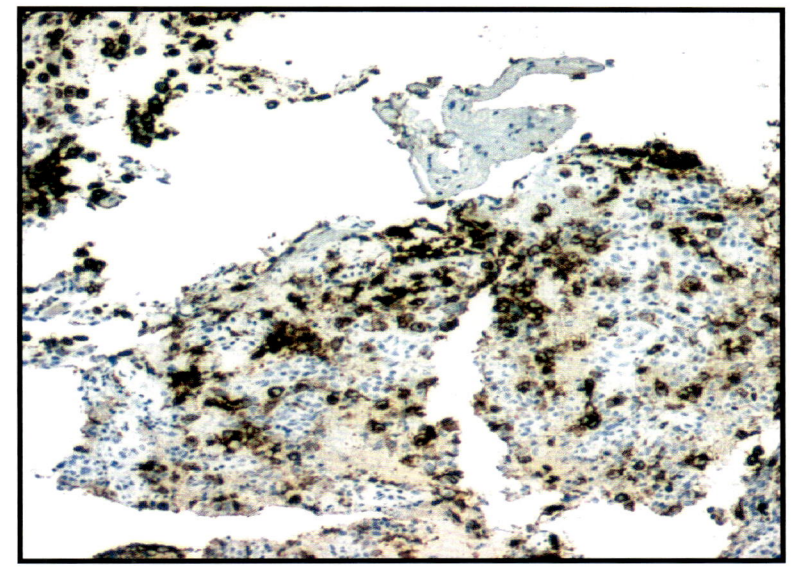

3.2 CD2

CD2 is also known as CD2R, E-rosette receptor, T11, and lymphocyte-function antigen-2 (LFA-2) (PROW). CD2 is a surface antigen (Ag) that is expressed on all T cells as well as on natural killer (NK) cells and a subpopulation of thymic B cells (OMIM) [Punnonen 1993]. Its main function is a costimulatory role by binding to CD58 on antigen-presenting cells [Bierer 1989b]. While frequently used in flow cytometry, detection of CD2 by IHC is rarely needed in the evaluation of a BM biopsy specimen. It is used to characterize a potentially abnormal T-cell population, detect CD2+ neoplastic mast cells, and evaluate the presence of acute leukemia if flow cytometric analysis is not available [Ohshima 1999; Escribano 1995; Gore 1991; Braylan 2001]. Acute myeloid leukemia (AML) with CD2 was found associated with pseudo-Chèdiak-Higashi anomaly and it was also identified as an adverse prognostic marker in adult de novo AML when CD2/inv(16)+ cases were excluded [Lee 2006; Chang 2006; Perea 2005].

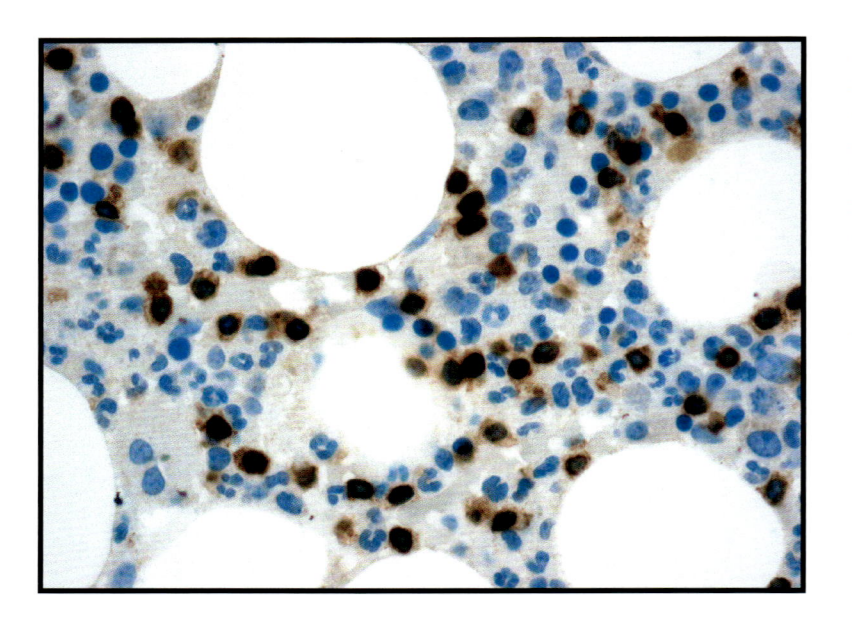

F3.2.1 CD2 in histologically unremarkable bone marrow specimen

This BM biopsy specimen is from a 45-year-old woman with extranodal diffuse large B-cell lymphoma. The BM biopsy specimen for restaging is negative. T cells were not increased, as demonstrated with CD3, but the number of CD2+ cells shown here is slightly higher than the number of the CD3+ cells. The expression of the Ag appears cytoplasmic rather than membranous. One cannot exclude poor localization of the signals.

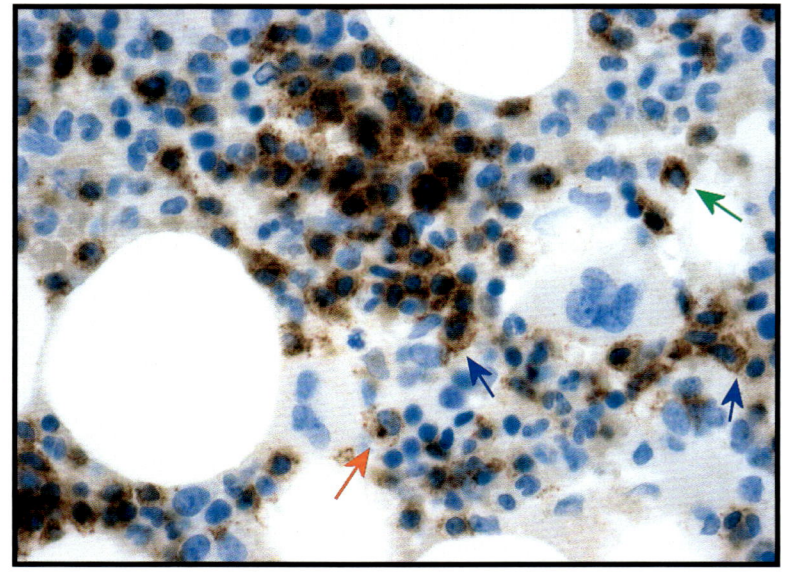

F3.2.2 CD2 in peripheral T-cell lymphoma (PTCL)

Malignant cells show variable expression of CD2 in regard to intensity of staining and the localization of the signals. There is a Golgi-type or perinuclear dotlike pattern (red arrow), membranous pattern (blue arrows), and cytoplasmic pattern (green arrow). In addition, many of the cells show weak diffuse signals.

F3.2.3 CD2 in peripheral T-cell lymphoma (PTCL)
Variable expression of CD2 is also present in this case of PTCL. There is a neoplastic cell in mitosis (arrow). The overall "dirty" appearance is because of the granular cytoplasmic pattern and marked variation in the intensity of the staining. However, there is an excellent signal-to-noise ratio and the staining is specific. Flow cytometry showed almost no cells positive for CD2, which may be because of its predominant cytoplasmic localization.

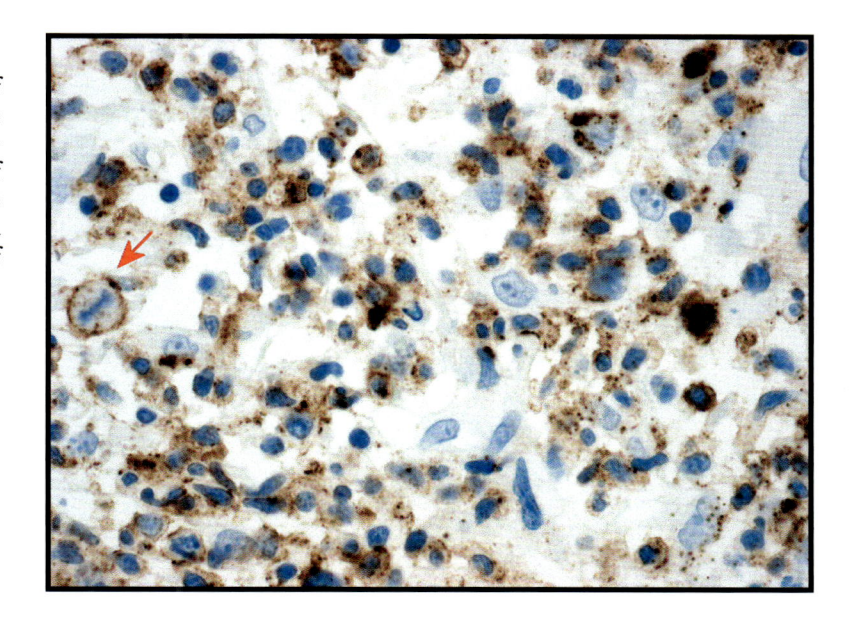

3.3 CD3

The T-cell receptor (TCR) is a complex of ligand-binding subunits of the receptor, the α and β TCR chains, CD3, and ζ chains. Furthermore, human CD3, also known as T3, consists of at least 4 proteins: γ, δ, ε, and ζ (OMIM). Polyclonal sera against the CD3 molecule that can be used for detection of CD3 in paraffin-embedded tissues were reported in 1987 [Mason 1987]. At present, both monoclonal and polyclonal anti-CD3 antibodies can be used for this purpose. MT-1 and UCHL-1 antibodies should not be used for the identification of T cells [Chadburn 1994]. In fact, CD43 (MT-1) is considered a sensitive myeloid marker if T lineage can be excluded [Hudock 1994]. Importantly, CD3 ε is not restricted to T cells, because activated human natural killer (NK) cells express intracytoplasmic CD3 ε polypeptides. CD3 ε is also present in the cytoplasm of fetal thymic T/NK bipotential progenitor cells, suggesting that it constitutes a component of the NK differentiation program [Biassoni 1988]. This is important because anti-CD3 antibodies also detect CD3 ε chain; cytoplasmic reactivity for CD3 does not necessarily represent evidence of T-cell lineage. Cytoplasmic CD3 reactivity is regularly found in extranodal NK/T-cell lymphoma nasal type [Gaal 2000]. Precursor T cells also typically express cytoplasmic CD3 (cCD3) before membranous CD3 can be identified [Campana 1989; Haynes 1995; Blom 1999]. Therefore, cCD3 is incorporated in acute leukemia panels for flow cytometry. In immunohistochemistry, no separate test is needed, but awareness that the localization of the signals may be critical for the interperetation of the results and final diagnosis.

F3.3.1 CD3 in normal bone marrow (BM)
The T cells are not increased in number. The CD3+ cells are small and there is no nuclear atypia. Of importance, no cutoff point has been established to differentiate between potentially neoplastic and reactive T cells. Membranous expression is specific for T cells because in this localization, the CD3 is a part of the T-cell receptor complex.

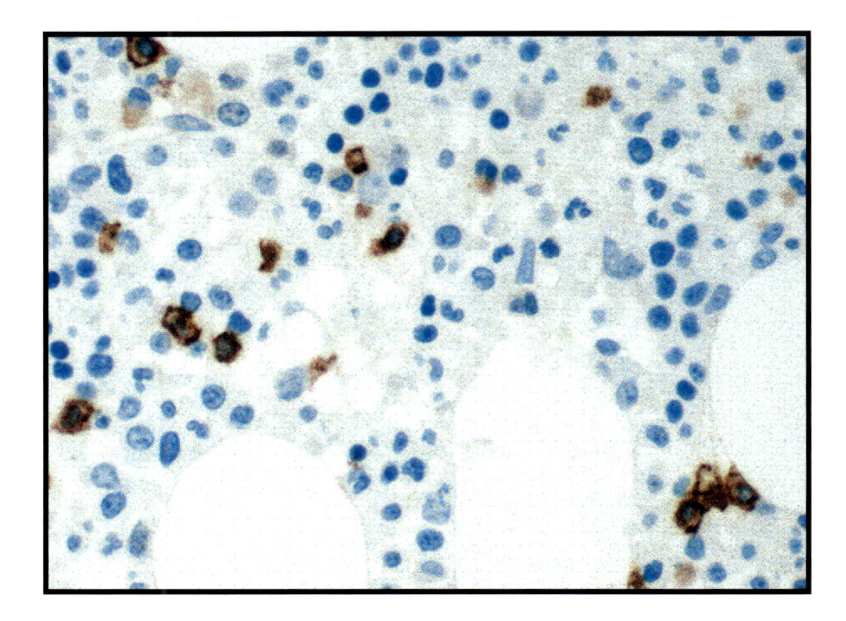

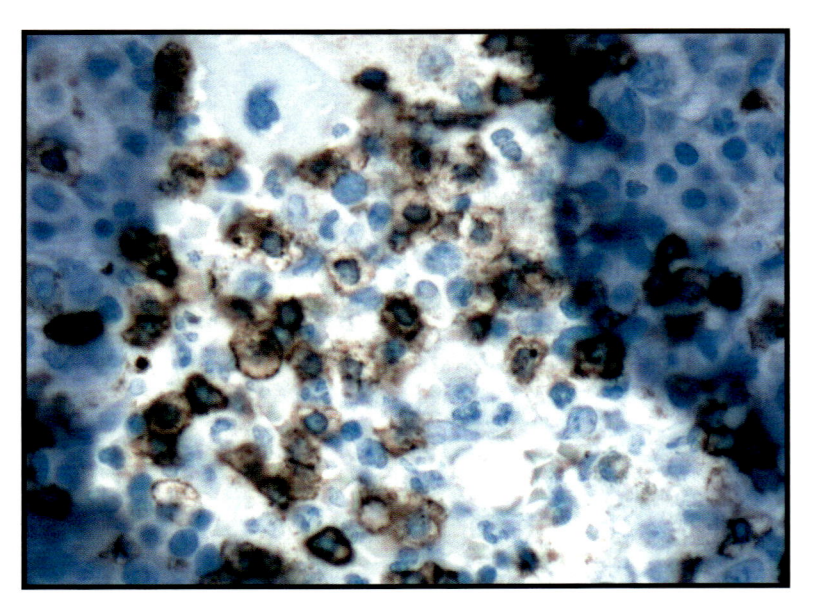

F3.3.2 CD3: Activated T cells

The patient has multiple myeloma. The CD3+ T cells have relatively low nuclear-cytoplasmic ratio and no definite nuclear atypia. With such morphologic findings and clinical history, despite the large T cells, it is unlikely that cells would be neoplastic. The T-cell receptor-γ gene rearrangement study showed a polyclonal T-cell population. Bone trabeculae are detached and interfere with the reading, which is common in bone marrow immunohistochemistry.

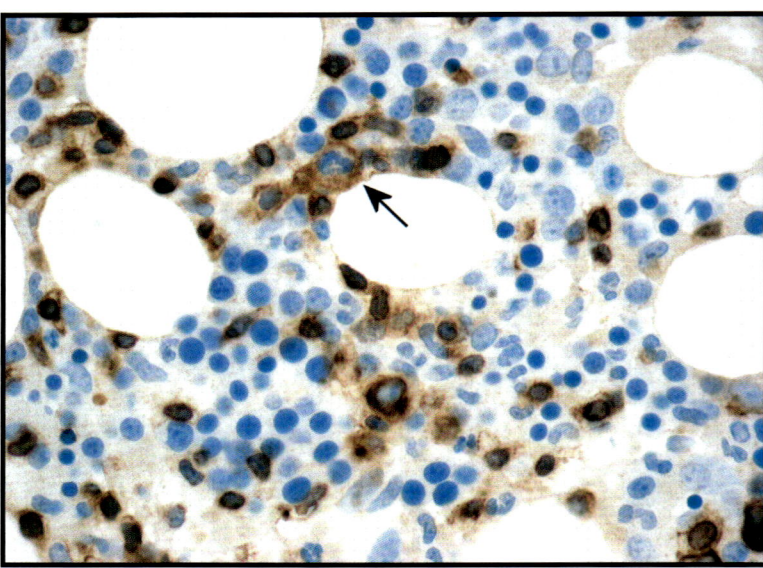

F3.3.3 CD3: Activated T cells

In this patient with follicular lymphoma in the bone marrow, the T cells were large, with nuclear atypia and the number of T cells is moderately increased. Some of the CD3+ cells were in mitosis (arrow). However, no clinical or molecular evidence of a T-cell lymphoproliferative disease was present. No loss of pan-T antigens or acquisition of CD56 or CD57 is detected and most of these cells expressed CD8.

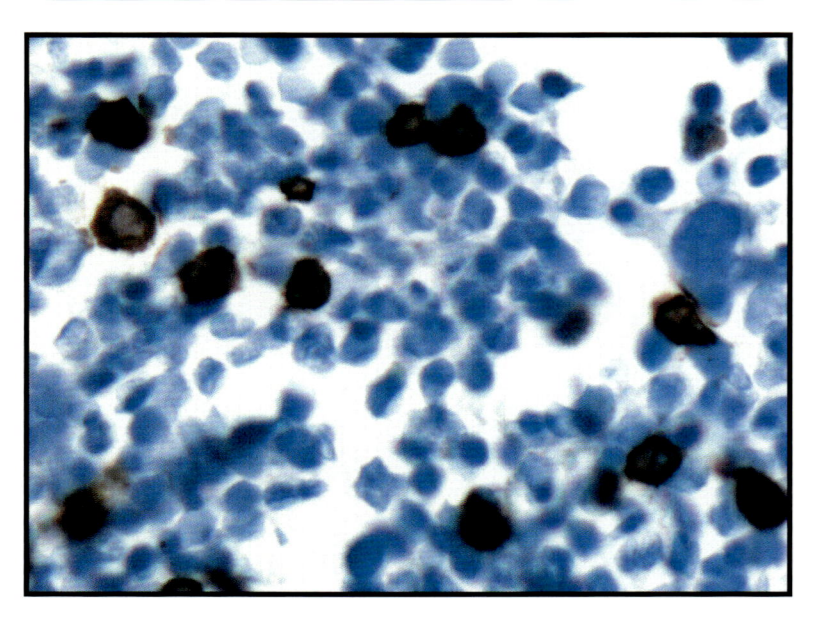

F3.3.4 Cytoplasmic CD3 in reactive T cells

The biopsy specimen is from a 28-month-old boy with acute myelogenous leukemia 14 days after induction chemotherapy. No leukemic cells were present. The T cells were marked by strong cytoplasmic expression of CD3 suggesting T-cell regeneration and increased content of reactive T cells. The myeloid leukemic clone was CD34+ and did not express CD3 or TdT. There is no morphologic evidence of leukemic blasts, CD34+ cells were not increased, and TdT is only slightly increased in this biopsy.

F3.3.5 CD3 in reactive T cells in bone marrow involved by follicular lymphoma (FL)

The T cells are increased and have atypical morphology. The immunophenotype is not abnormal and they were polyclonal in a TCR-γ gene rearrangement PCR assay. It was concluded that the T-cell population was reactive.

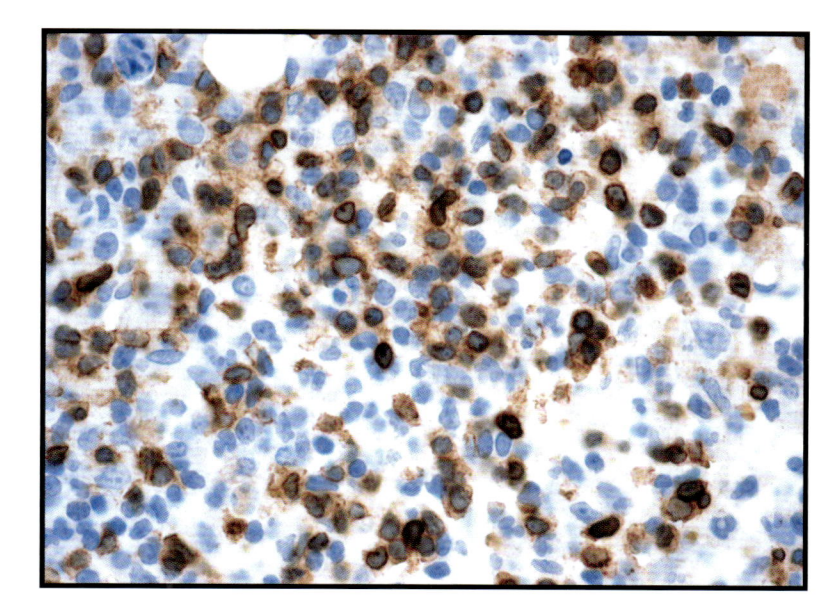

F3.3.6 CD3 in reactive T cells in adult

This bone marrow biopsy specimen is from a 57-year-old man who had widely metastatic adenocarcinoma. The BM is not involved. The T cells are somewhat increased and have reactive changes including overall increase in size, slightly decreased nuclear-cytoplasmic ratio, downregulated surface CD3, and increased cytoplasmic CD3.

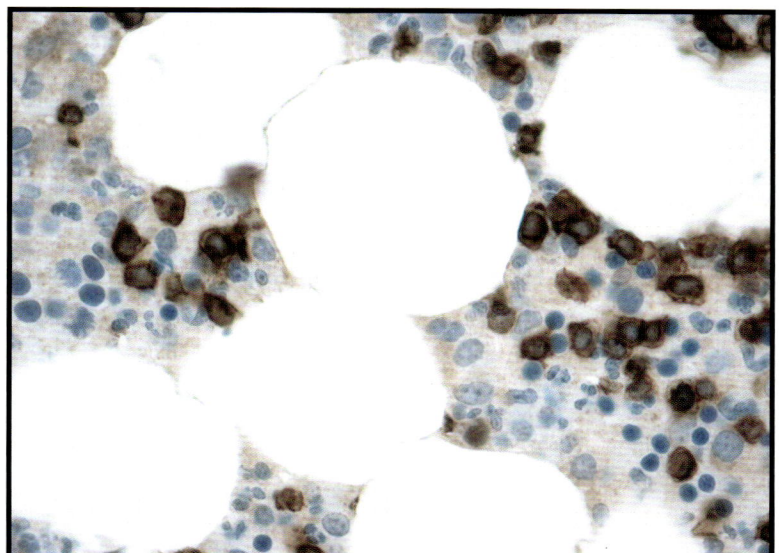

F3.3.7 Cytoplasmic CD3 expression in acute biphenotypic leukemia

This biopsy specimen is from a 57-year-old woman with acute biphenotypic leukemia diagnosed with flow cytometry. Expression of cytoplasmic CD3 can be demonstrated in some cases by using immunohistochemistry. In many cells, the expression assumes localized cytoplasmic pattern and also a dotlike pattern, which is most likely limited to the Golgi area. This was found only in a clot section and could not be demonstrated in the decalcified core biopsy specimen.

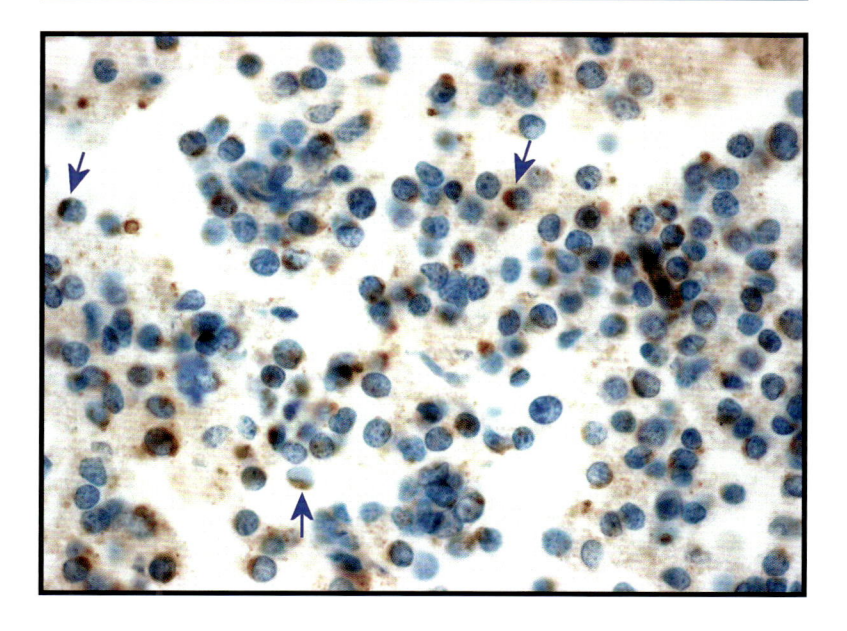

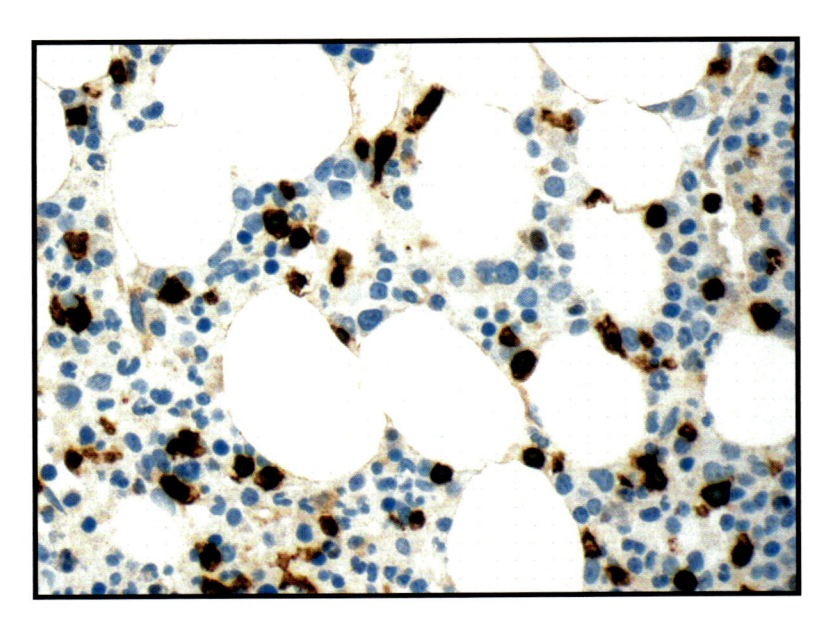

F3.3.8 CD3 in slightly atypical T cells of unknown biological significance

This biopsy specimen is from a 56-year-old man with weight loss, with no evidence of malignant lymphoma or other malignancy. CD3 is cytoplasmic and membranous and there is slight cytological atypia. The molecular analysis revealed an oligoclonal T-cell population by T-cell receptor–γ gene rearrangement polymerase chain reaction assay. The significance of these cells is unclear, but they are most likely reactive T cells.

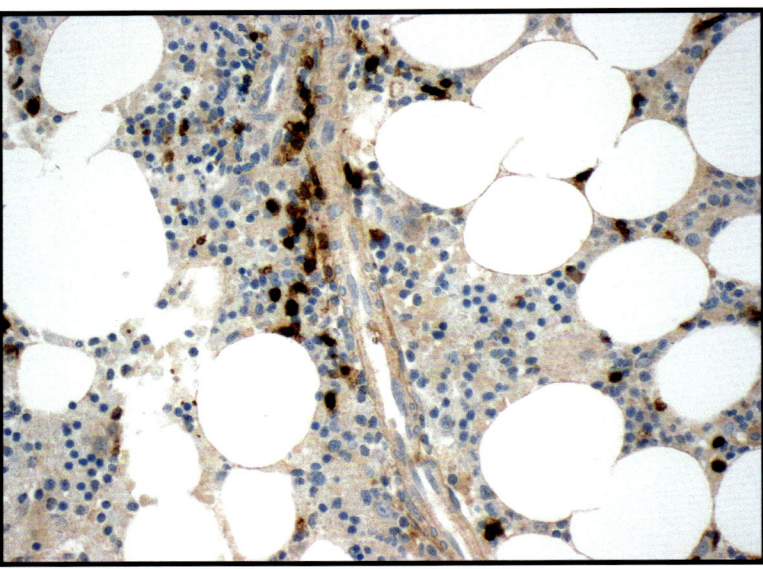

F3.3.9 Perivascular CD3+ cells

Occasionally, CD3 will demonstrate T cells mainly in a perivascular location. These are usually CD4+ cells; CD8+ cells are more randomly distributed in the bone marrow. Most cells in benign small interstitial lymphoid aggregates are also CD4+ cells, but some CD8 cells are usually present.

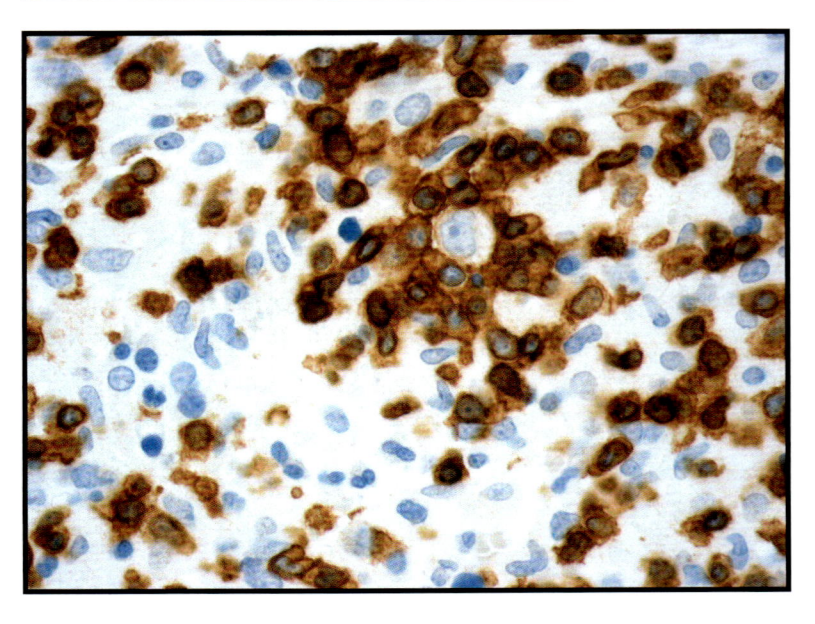

F3.3.10 CD3 in bone marrow involved by classical Hodgkin lymphoma (cHL)

This biopsy specimen from a 32-year-old woman with stage IV cHL shows focal evidence of cHL. There is minimal fibrosis, which is rare. These areas are screened for by using CD3 only. When the rosettes of T cells may be found around the larger cells, CD30, Pax-5, and CD15 were used for the confirmation of the diagnosis. Note the reactive appearance of the benign T cells.

3.3　CD3

F3.3.11　CD3 in peripheral T-cell lymphoma (PTCL)

This patient has a PTCL involving the bone marrow. As is obvious in comparison with **F3.3.10**, **F3.3.5**, and **F3.3.6**, it is difficult to distinguish this infiltrate from the florid reactive T-cell population. Additional immunophenotypic and molecular studies are almost always required in an evaluation of the T-cell lesions.

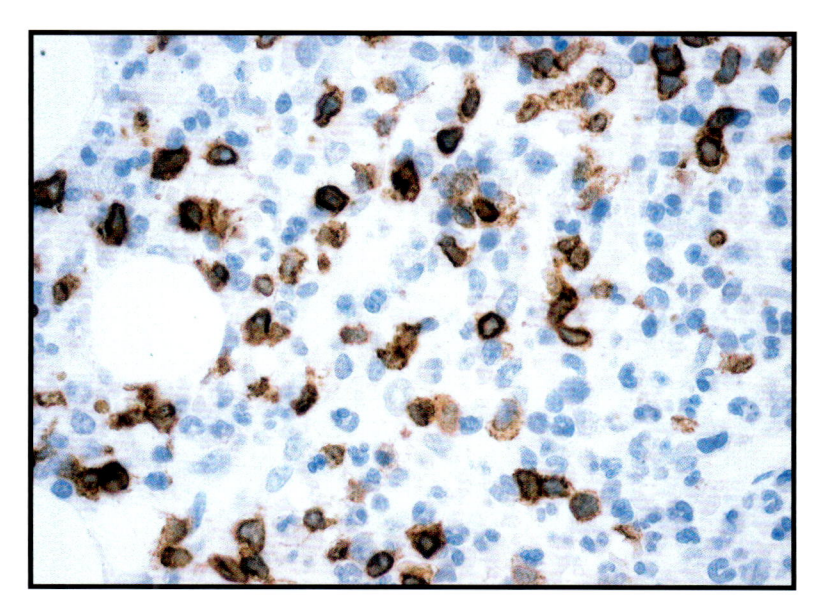

F3.3.12　CD3 in peripheral T-cell lymphoma (PTCL)

This biopsy specimen is from a 48-year-old man with primary nodal PTCL (not otherwise specified). The bone marrow infiltrates are rather obvious and involve about 70% of the specimen; the CD3 expression is weak in the neoplastic population. In addition to a weak membranous positivity, indistinct cytoplasmic granular and focally fine filamentous patterns are present.

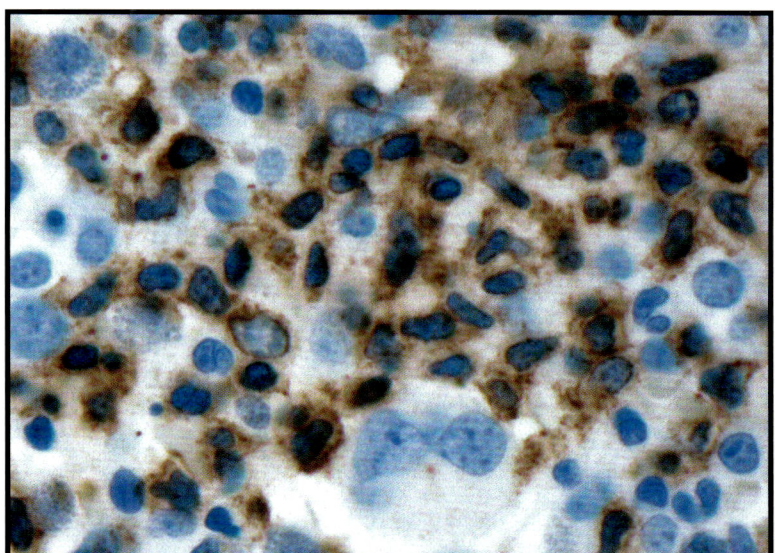

F3.3.13　CD3 in acute promyelocytic leukemia

In most myeloid leukemias T cells do not comprise a significant component. However, in some cases of myeloid leukemia and also in myelodysplastic syndromes, lymphocytosis may occur. When present, it may assume the pattern of large lymphoid aggregates as seen in this case. Very few B cells are present in this aggregate.

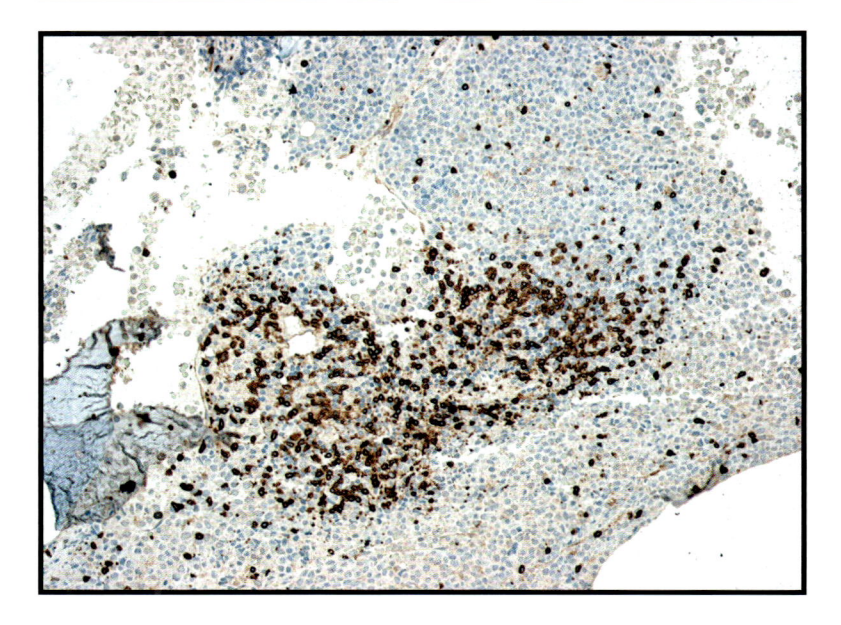

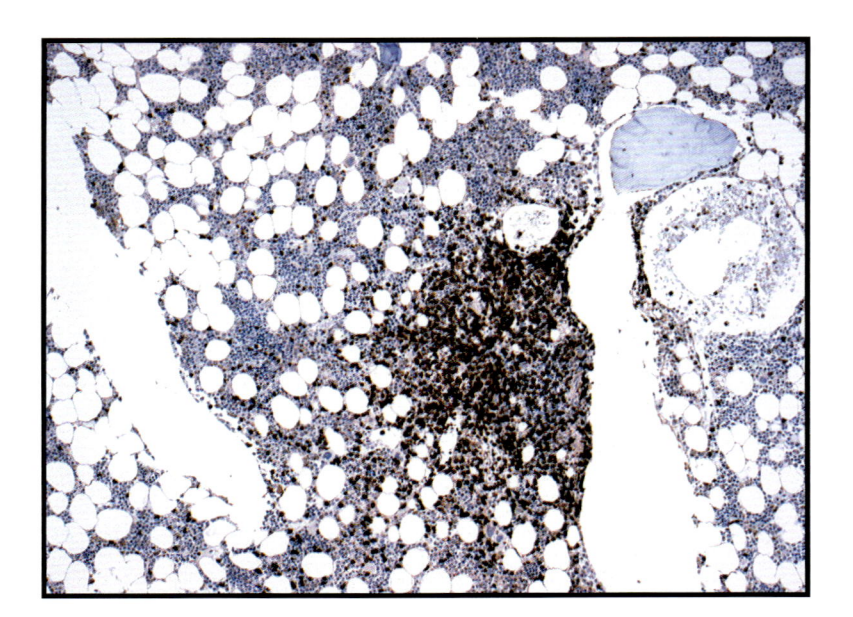

F3.3.14 CD3 in an atypical lymphoid aggregate in a human immunodeficiency virus (HIV)+ male patient

This biopsy specimen is from a 48-year-old patient who presented with weight loss and fever and was found to be HIV+. Bone marrow culture did not yield any microorganisms. However, large lymphoid aggregates with predominant T-cell CD8+ population were found.

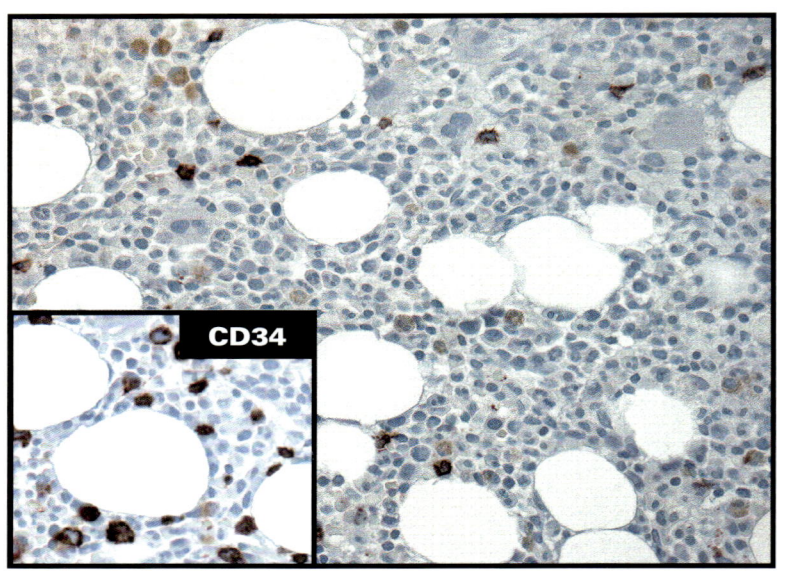

F3.3.15 CD3 in a 5-month-old male infant with increased hematogones and slightly hypocellular bone marrow (BM)

BM T cell dynamics do not necessarily follow the B-cell changes. In this BM specimen, the B cells showed left shift and increased numbers, but this was not the case for T cells. The infant had a soft tissue lesion of the leg that was eventually found to be a benign vascular tumor. The finding of increased hematogones was associated with a slight increase in CD34+ cells (inset).

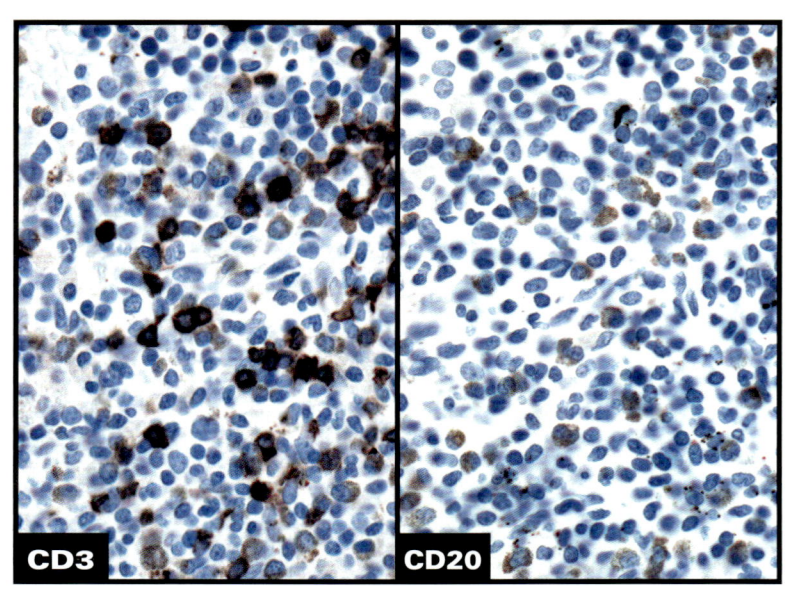

F3.3.16 CD3 and CD20 in interstitial lymphoid aggregates

The patient is a 54-year-old woman with nodal diffuse large B-cell lymphoma. The marrow did not contain large B cells and the number of CD20+ cells was very low. Note numerous CD3−/CD20− small lymphocytes in the aggregates, which is an abnormal finding. Further investigation revealed multiple lymphoid aggregates of CD79a+, IgM+, λ+ small lymphocytes. Because only minimal evidence of IgM was found in serum, this was interpreted as most consistent with marginal zone lymphoma.

3.3 CD3

F3.3.17 CD3 in chronic myeloid leukemia (CML)

CML is not characterized by lymphocytosis. Neither T cells nor B cells are increased. The morphologic features of the T cells are usually unremarkable, with small lymphocytes showing no evidence of activation. The T cells have random and even distribution. In CML, B cells often show more variation in morphologic features and distribution.

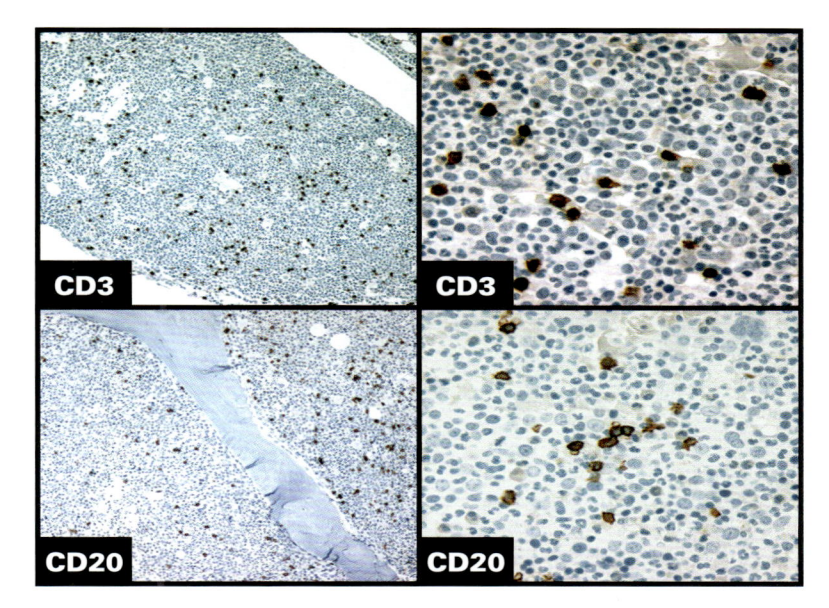

F3.3.18 CD3 in precursor T-lymphoblastic leukemia

This biopsy specimen is from an 11-year-old boy with precursor T-lymphoblastic leukemia. The cytoplasmic CD3 expression is evident as an accentuation of the perinuclear cytoplasm. While the level of expression is rather high, note that membranous positivity is difficult to appreciate in most cells. This is a typical finding in precursor T-lymphoblastic leukemia.

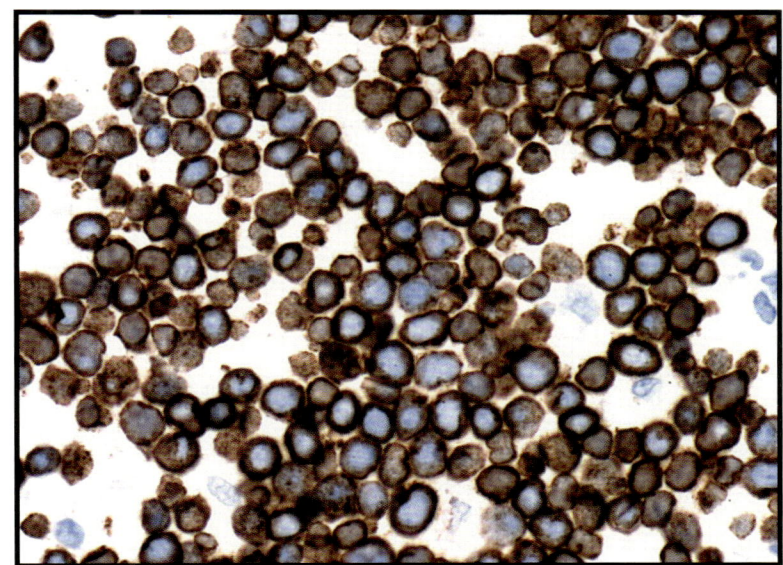

F3.3.19 CD3 in benign T cells infiltrating lymphoplasmacytic lymphoma (LPL)

The malignant B cells are negative. The T cells show very strong staining, which is difficult to localize. The sections are very thick and the strong membranous staining is overwhelming. Therefore membranous staining can be distinguished from weak cytoplasmic staining (arrows) in few lymphocytes only. F3.3.19 and F3.3.20 illustrate the fact that the interpretation of the localization of CD3 expression may be difficult in tissue sections.

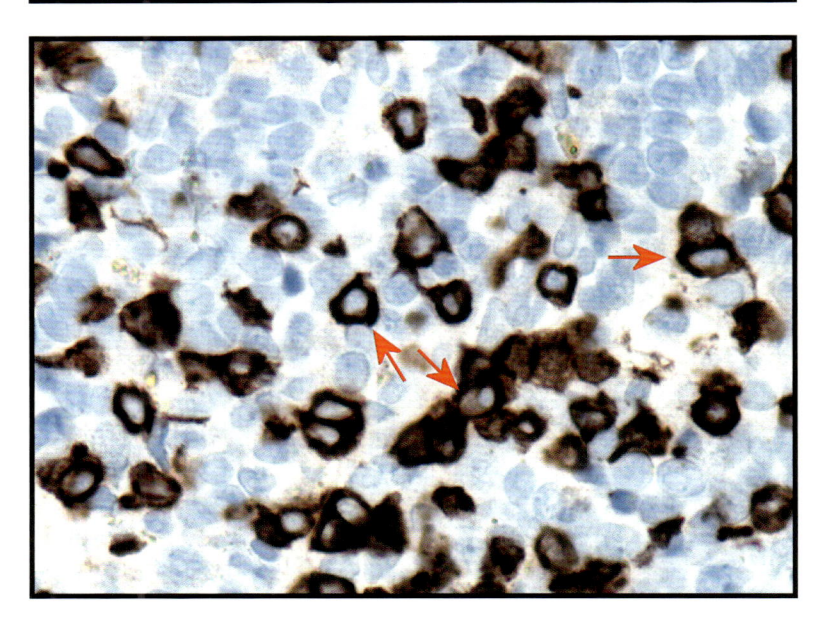

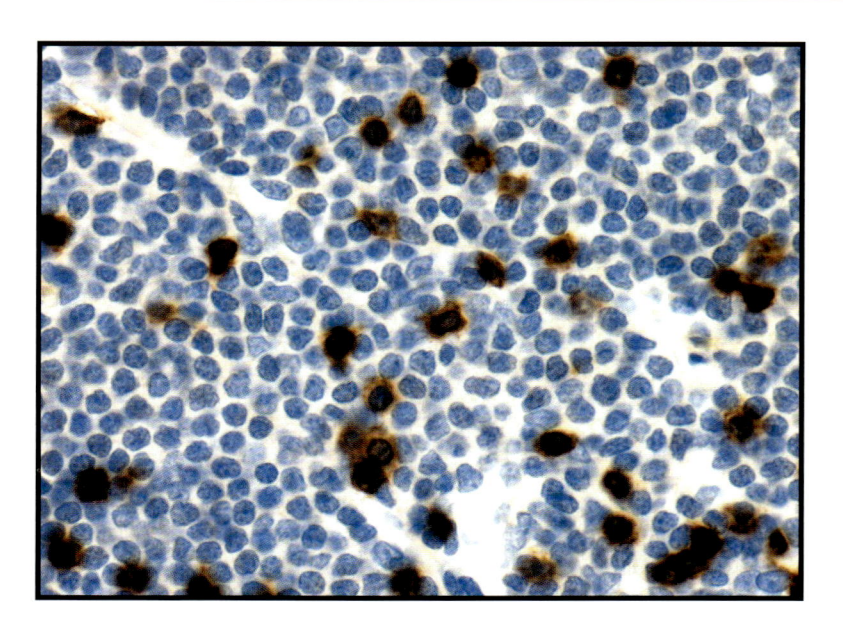

F3.3.20 CD3 in benign T-cells infiltrating mantle cell lymphoma

The T cells appear to show predominant cytoplasmic localization of the signals, which is unexpected in mature T cells. At times the localization of the antigen is hampered by the characteristics of the primary antibody (Ab). Similar results were relatively common when using some polyclonal Abs and may not be seen when using some monoclonal Abs. It is important to observe the distribution of the signals when a new Ab is used to avoid misinterpretation.

3.4 CD4

CD4, also known as L3T4 and W3/25, is a coreceptor in MHC class II–restricted antigen-induced T-cell activation (PROW, 1). CD4 is also an HIV-receptor [Sattentau 1988]. It is expressed by thymocyte subsets, mature helper T cells, monocytes, and macrophages. Expression of CD4 by a subpopulation of megakaryocytes has also been reported [Basch 1990]. CD4+/CD56+ hematodermic neoplasm is a tumor of plasmacytoid dendritic cells and is regularly CD4+ [Kato 2001; Peetrella 2002]. In general, dendritic cells can express CD4 and also CD8 antigen [Vremec 2000].

In the BM, the CD4/CD8 ratio of T cells is usually reverse from that in peripheral blood [Shin 1992]. CD4 detection by IHC in the BM biopsy can be used to characterize various T-cell lymphoproliferative diseases and histiocytic disorders [Schmidt-Wolf 1992; Attygalle 2002; Rakozy 2001; Yoshida 2008]. In T-cell large granular lymphocyte leukemia, the benign T cells localize at the periphery of the reactive B-cell aggregates [Osuji 2007]. In general, benign CD4 cells in the normal BM are scant and appear to be found mainly in perivascular localization, in contrast to CD8+ T cells, which tend to be randomly distributed in the BM interstitium. CD4 is also expressed in endothelial cells of the BM and some sites of extramedullary hematopoiesis [Couvelard 1996; Cines 1998].

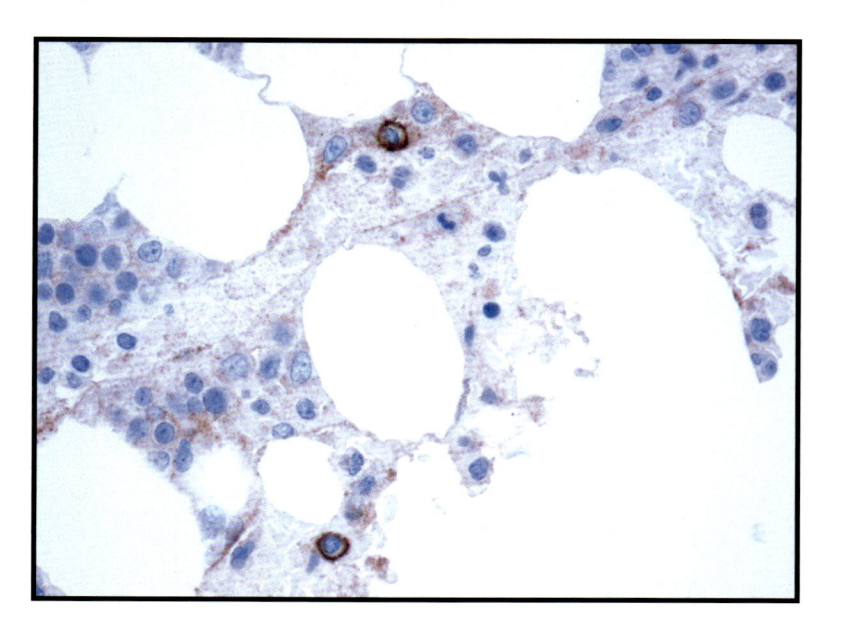

F3.4.1 CD4 in T lymphocytes in normal B5-fixed bone marrow (BM; ADVANCE)

This BM biopsy specimen is from a normal donor. Rare T cells with strong membranous CD4 expression can be detected. These are mature T-helper cells. There is also a very weak staining of the sinusoidal endothelial cells. CD4 is also expressed on the sinusoidal lining cells of the liver. It is not clear if this is due to the fact that both BM and liver are organs that support hematopoiesis [Couvelard 1996; Cines 1998].

F3.4.2 **CD4 in normal bone marrow (BM; ADVANCE)**

This BM biopsy specimen is from a healthy donor. Infrequent ill-defined clusters of CD4+ lymphocytes are detected in loose perivascular distribution. Occasional larger mononuclear cells with weaker expression of CD4 may represent a monocyte rather than CD4+ T-lymphocyte (center). Similar to **F3.4.1**, rather weak endothelial cell staining is also noted (red arrow).

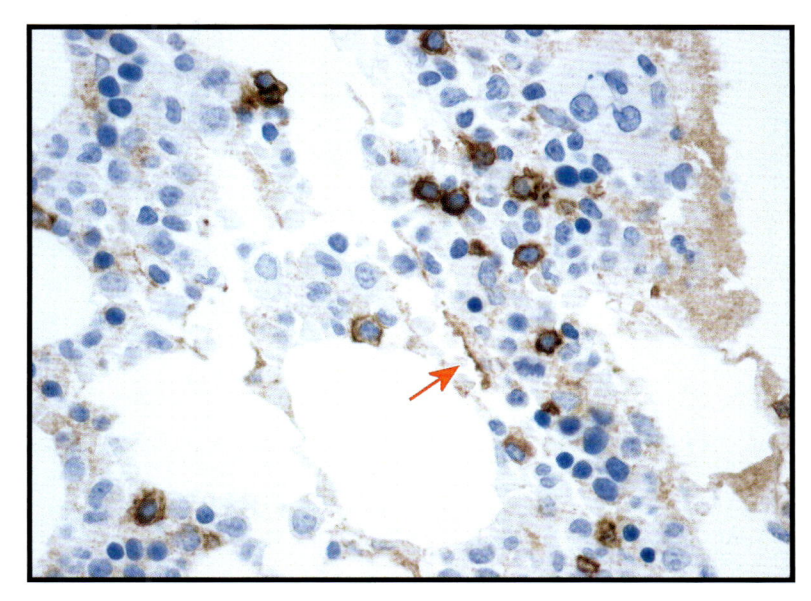

F3.4.3 **CD4 in sinusoidal endothelial cells (ADVANCE)**

In this area, sinusoidal endothelial cells showed strong staining with CD4 (red arrow). A single CD4+ T-cell is also present (blue arrow). One cell with Golgi-type staining and diffuse weak cytoplasmic staining is also present (green arrow).

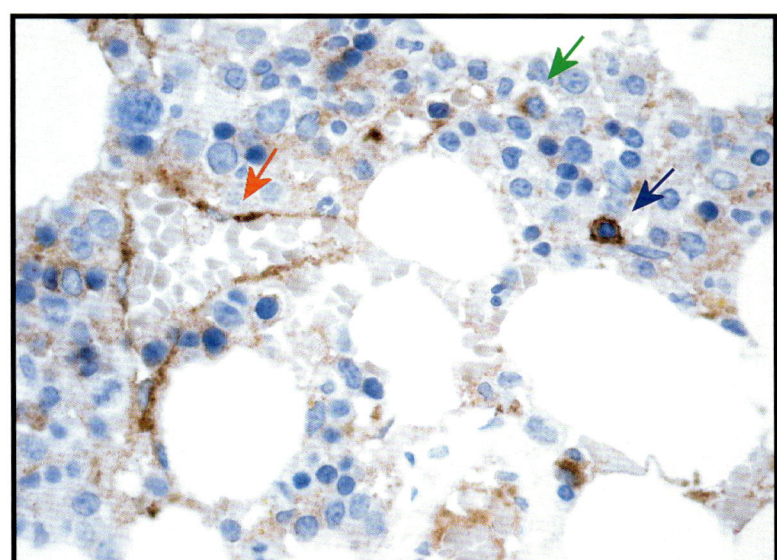

F3.4.4 **CD4 in a benign lymphoid aggregate**

This biopsy specimen is from a 45-year-old man with refractory anemia with excess blasts. There were a few small to medium-sized lymphoid aggregates composed almost exclusively of T cells. The T cells are also increased throughout the interstitium. The aggregates contain CD4+ cells, while the more randomly distributed T cells are CD8+ cells. Suboptimal hematoxylin staining, being too pale in this case, could cause difficulty in the interpretation of the results.

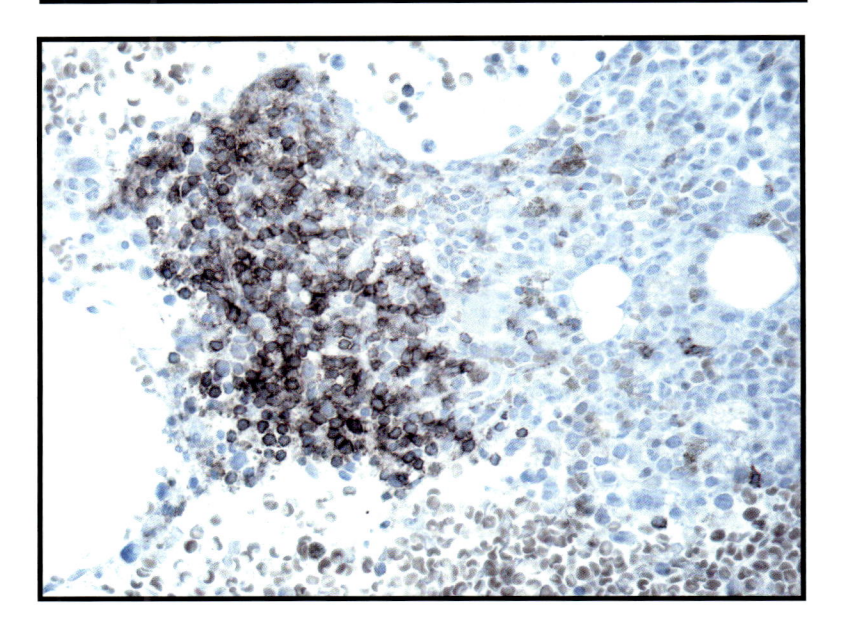

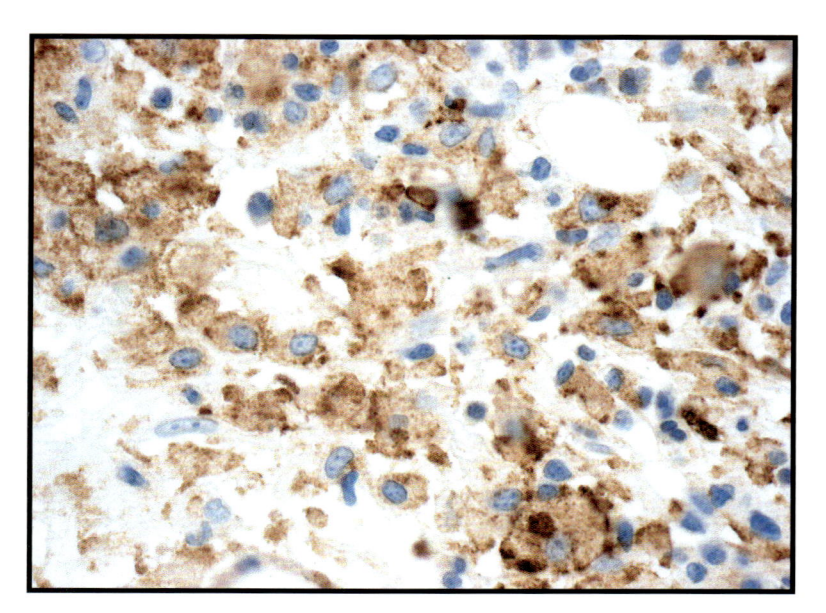

F3.4.5 CD4 in epithelioid histiocytes

CD4 can be identified on the surface, weakly in the cytoplasm, and also in the Golgi area in both benign and malignant histiocytes. This biopsy specimen is from a 27-year-old man with hemophagocytic syndrome associated with peripheral T-cell lymphoma. The histiocytes did not appear "hemophagocytic" in all areas.

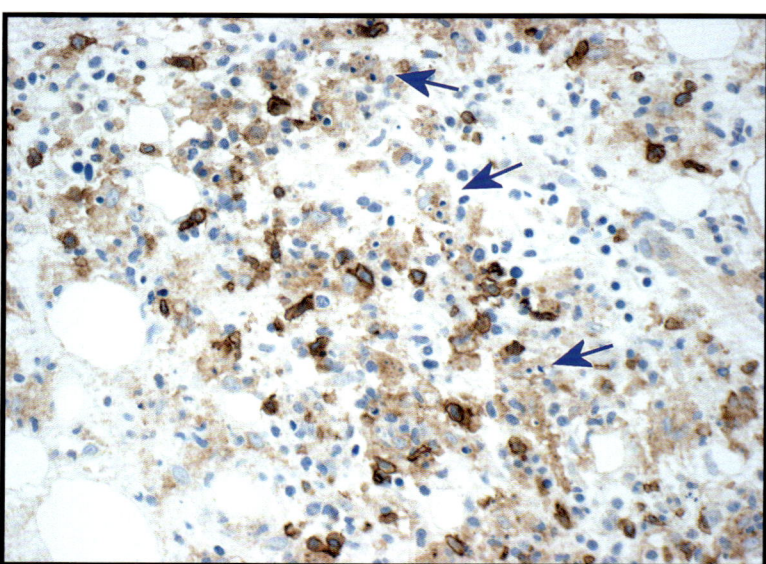

F3.4.6 CD4 in hemophagocytic histiocytes

Same patient as in **F3.4.5**. Arrows point to hemophagocytic macrophages. The staining of CD4 in the histiocytes and macrophages is weaker than in CD4+ T cells. Occasional strongly staining cells are T cells and are probably malignant (the peripheral T-cell lymphoma was CD4+).

3.5 CD5

CD5 is also known as Leu-1, Ly-1, T1, and Tp67 (PROW). CD5 is a a human T-cell surface glycoprotein and a pan-T-cell marker. Its expression is lower in thymocytes than on mature T cells and it is also lower in CD8+ T cells than in CD4+ T cells [Beyers 1992]. CD5 is the phenotypic marker of a B-cell subpopulation (B1a cells) involved in the production of autoreactive antibodies, which in normal conditions are the most abundant B-cell population in coelomic cavities. Antibodies produced by B1a cells are the first-line defense against encapsulated bacteria. Thymic B-cell progenitors are B1b cells and also express CD5 [Duan 2006; Ceredig 2002]. CD5 expression was also detected in various epithelial tissues [Tateyama 1999].

CD5 modulates lymphocyte signaling through the antigen-specific receptor complex (TCR and BCR). In thymocytes and B1a cells, CD5 appears to provide inhibitory signals, while in peripheral mature T lymphocytes it acts as a costimulatory signal receptor. After BM transplantation, a large proportion of circulating T cells lacks CD5 expression, but these cells are nevertheless functional [Bierer 1989a].

On average, BM frozen sections have 9% T cells, which in addition to CD3, express other pan-T-cell markers including CD5 [Shin 1992]. Up to 5% of BM TdT+ mononuclear cells belong to the T-lymphoid lineage by virtue of expression of CD5 [Gore 1991; Smith 1989]. CD5 is typically expressed by chronic lymphocytic leukemia (CLL) and mantle cell lymphoma, but it may occasionally be detected in other small B-cell lymphoproliferative diseases [Pezzella 2000; Sundeen 1992; Chen 2000; Cabezudo 1999; Moreau 1997]. In marginal zone lymphoma (MZL), the presence of CD5 may be a marker of persistent or recurrent disease, for dissemination to the marrow and other extranodal sites, and for leukemic involvement of the peripheral blood [Ferry 1996]. About 10% of lymphoplasmacytic lymphomas are reported to express CD5 [Hunter 2005]. While only a small subset of aggressive diffuse large B-cell lymphomas expresses CD5, expression of this marker is described in one third of cases of the intravascular diffuse large B-cell lymphoma subtypes (DLBCL), which may present in the BM [Estalilla 1999; Matsue 2008]. CD5+ B-ALL is an exceedingly rare and aggressive disease with only 3 cases reported in the literature [Peterson 2007]. Rarely, CD5+ B-cell lymphomas may also coexpress CD10 [Barekman 2001].

F3.5.1 CD5 in histologically normal bone marrow (BM)

This biopsy specimen is from a 39-year-old man with suspected paraneoplastic syndrome; the malignancy was not discovered even after extensive clinical and radiological evaluation. The BM biopsy specimen had only mild focal lymphocytosis. Rare T cells had large, abundant cytoplasm with strong membranous expression of CD5. At the time of this writing, 4 years later, the patient is well.

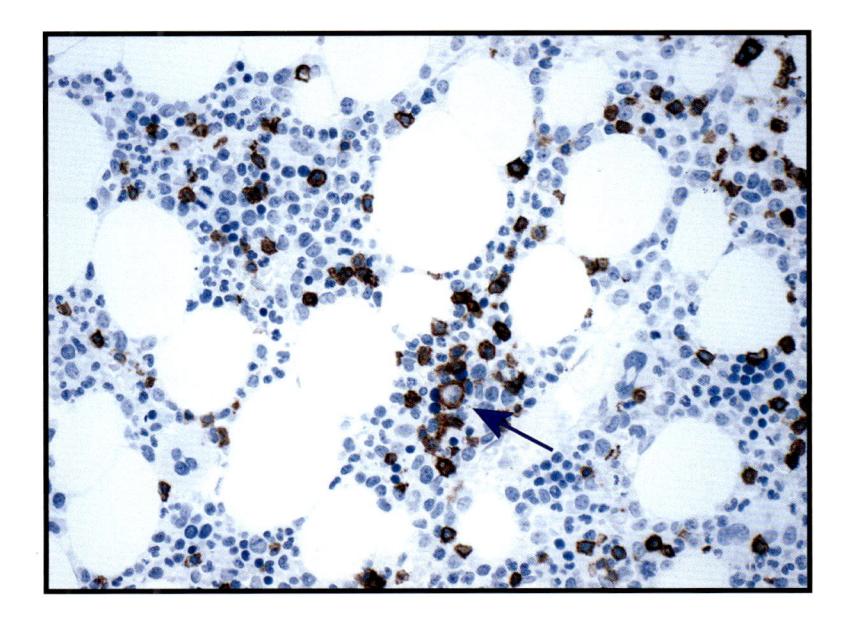

3: Cluster of Differentiation Markers

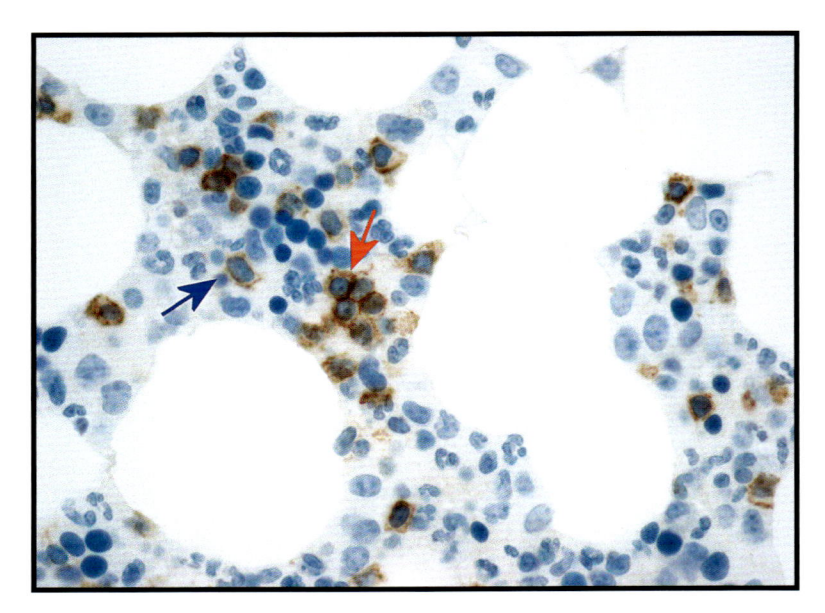

F3.5.2 CD5 in activated T cells

This bone marrow biopsy specimen is from a 43-year-old man with classical Hodgkin lymphoma. The BM is not involved. The T cells had an activated appearance and some pan-T-cell markers were downregulated including CD5. The expression was mainly weak and membranous (blue arrow). The nuclei had an "open chromatin" and some had small nucleoli (red arrow).

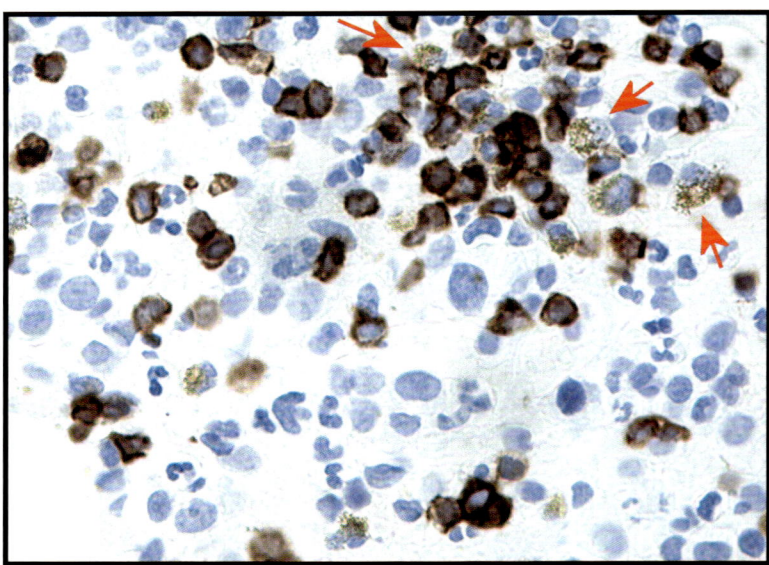

F3.5.3 CD5: Membranous and cytoplasmic expression

This biopsy specimen is from a patient with multiple myeloma, with reactive T cells showing predominant membranous expression of CD5. Some cytoplasmic staining is also present. The T cells are frequently associated with eosinophils (here recognized as faintly refractile granular cells; red arrows).

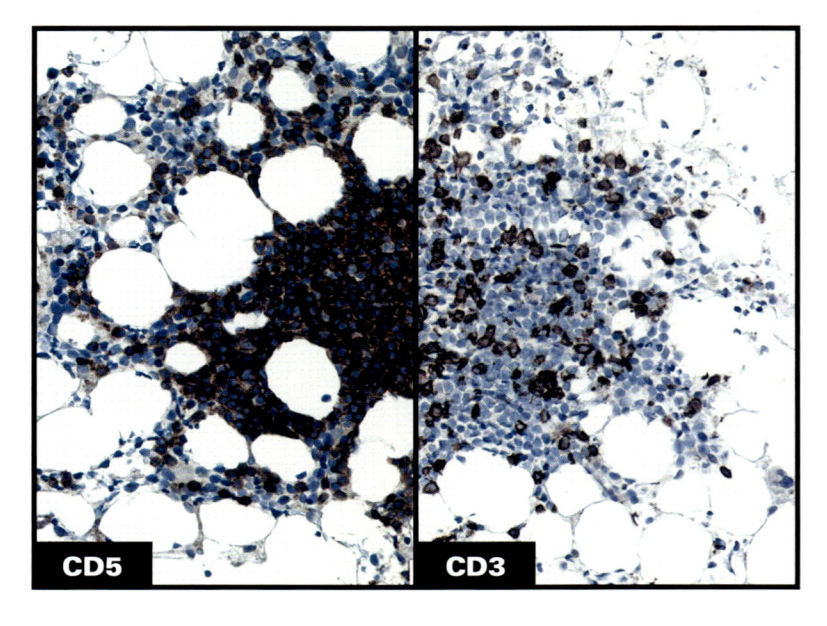

F3.5.4 Interpretation of CD5 expression in B-cell lymphoma

This biopsy specimen illustrates focal involvement with CLL. CD5 expression in B-cell lymphoma can be interpreted only in comparison with CD3 expression to exclude T cells. In some cases, the interpretation is rather obvious because the distribution of T cells is distinct and the number of T cells is low.

F3.5.5 CD5 expression in B-cell lymphoma

In this case of mantle cell lymphoma (MCL), which is clearly CD5+, the lymphocytes have the morphology of large cleaved cells, which is sometimes designated as "large cell variant of MCL" or "anaplastic variant of MCL." Some variation in CD5 expression is present with weak expression in left lower half and strong expression in right upper half. Some of the smaller cells with strong expression were probably small reactive T cells. Excessive heat-induced epitope retrieval produced poor localization of the Ag.

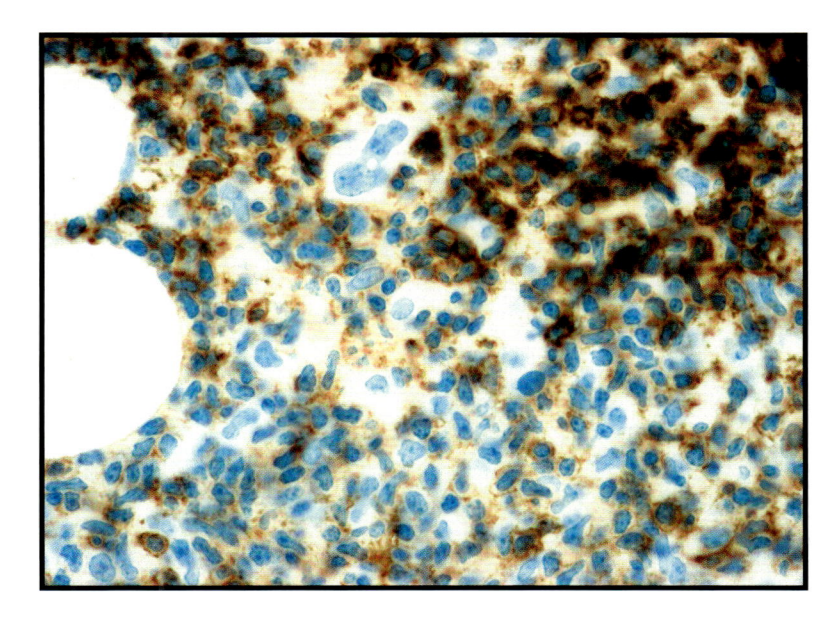

F3.5.6 CD5 in peripheral T-cell lymphoma (PTCL)

The bone marrow biopsy specimen is from a patient with a nodal PTCL. Focal T cells with atypical morphology are found, but it would be difficult to interpret this biopsy specimen as positive for PTCL because of the small number of T cells. Their marked variation in size, nuclear morphology, and the presence of atypical mitoses all favor malignant lymphoma. This diagnosis of BM involvement by PTCL was confirmed by detection of monoclonal T-cell receptor–γ gene rearrangement with polymerase chain reaction in the BM aspirate specimen.

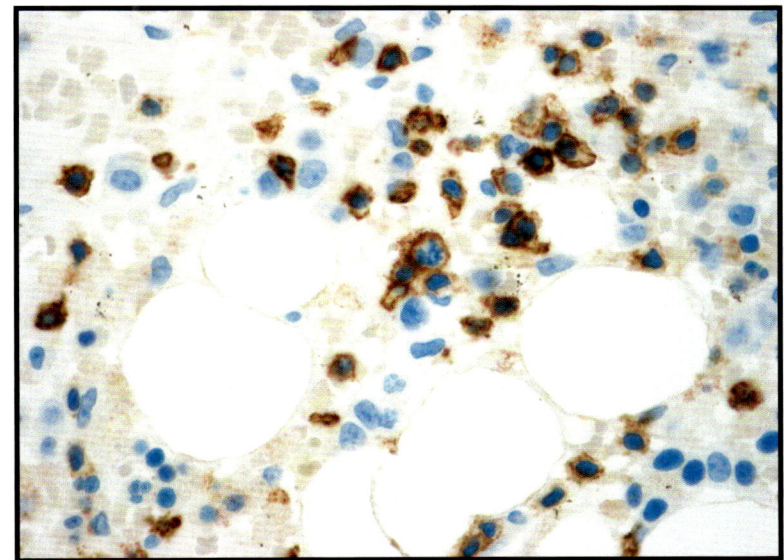

F3.5.7 CD5 in peripheral T-cell lymphoma (PTCL)

This bone marrow biopsy specimen is clearly involved by CD3+ PTCL. It is very helpful when CD5 is not expressed in PTCL (as shown here) and there is a major discrepancy between the CD3 and CD5 expression. This is uncommon. Weak expression is also present in activated T cells, which can assume rather atypical morphology. Such "loss" or "downregulation" of CD5 should be interpreted with great caution. In this field, only rare cells are CD5+ and they may be either benign or malignant T cells.

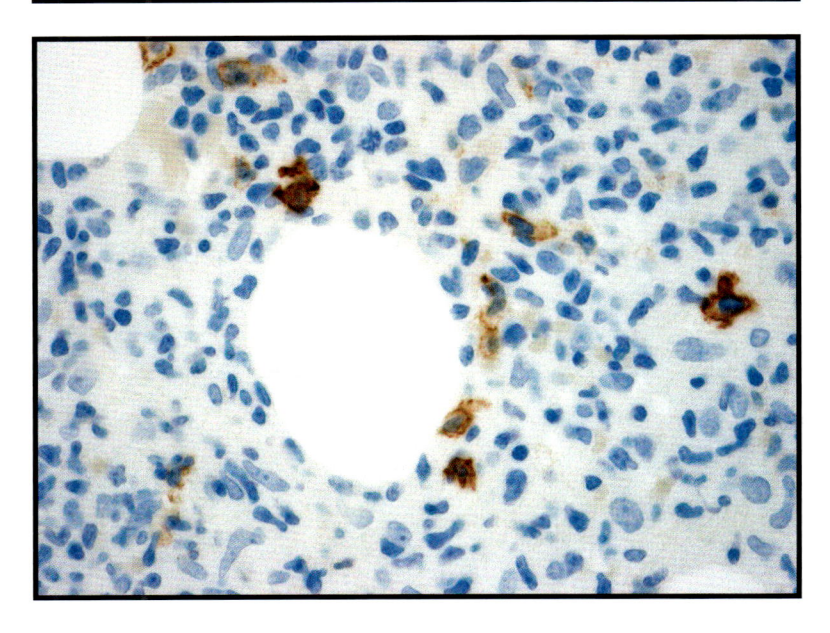

3: Cluster of Differentiation Markers

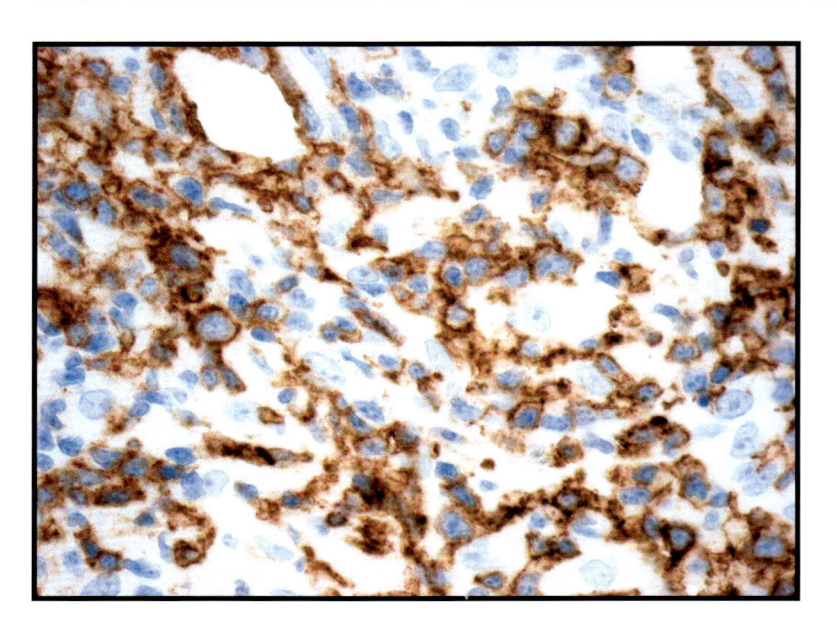

F3.5.8 CD5 in peripheral T-cell lymphoma (PTCL), moderate expression

This biopsy specimen is from a 27-year-old man with hemophagocytic syndrome. An atypical and monoclonal (by PCR test) T-cell infiltrate was noted on the biopsy specimen, and the diagnosis of PTCL with hemophagocytic syndrome was established. Large and atypical cells are not unusual in reactive lesions, but they are usually uniform. It is very difficult to use morphology in the diagnosis of PTCL in the BM biopsy because reactive cells can be morphologically atypical (see **F3.3.5** and **F3.3.6** for comparison).

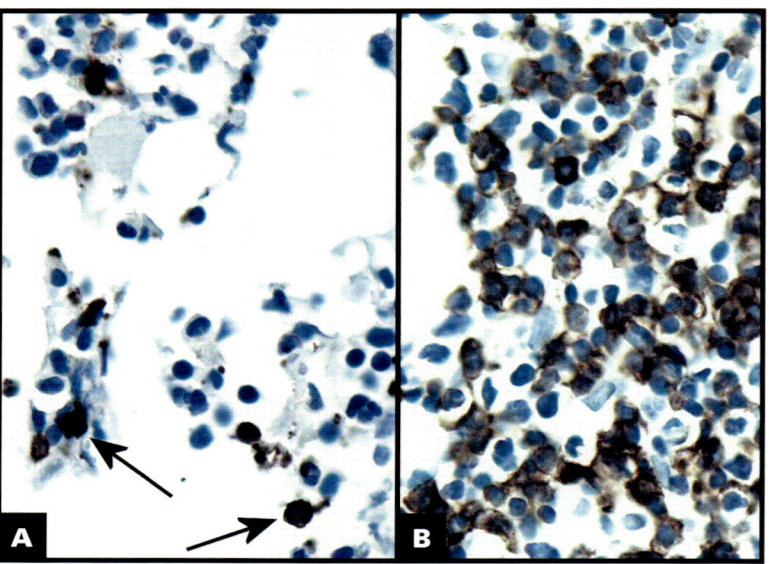

F3.5.9 CD5 in follicular lymphoma (FL)

This bone marrow biopsy specimen is from a patient with FL and diffuse large B-cell lymphoma. Only FL was found in the BM biopsy. While it is clear that these T cells are activated T cells, note that in the lymphoid aggregates of follicular lymphoma, the T cells have more atypical morphology **B** than in the rest of the same BM biopsy **A**. Only subtle differences are noted in the appearance of activated T cells and neoplastic T cells in the peripheral T-cell lymphoma in **F3.5.8**.

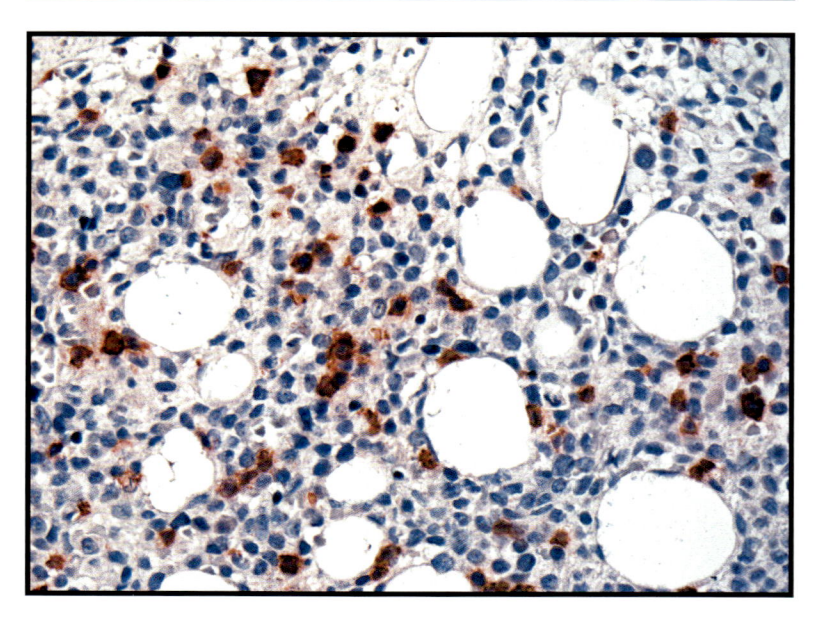

F3.5.10 CD5 demonstrating benign T cells in bone marrow (BM) biopsy with hairy cell leukemia (fast red chromogen)

Some laboratories prefer red chromogen. With improved sensitivity of the red chromogens, the color that will be used depends mainly on price and personal preference. The results finally reflect overall optimization of the procedure. In this particular case, the excessive antigen background is probably due to an excess of the primary antibody.

3.6 CD7

CD7 is also known as Tp41 and is a cell surface glycoprotein expressed by thymocytes and mature T cells (OMIM). It plays an essential role in T-cell interactions and also in T-cell/B-cell interaction during early lymphoid development [Nishimura 2006; Chang 2007; Osada 1988; Yoshikawa 1991; Schanberg 1991]. Because it is expressed very early in T-cell development, CD7 is a sensitive marker of precursor T-ALL. It plays a role in demonstrating T cells in T-cell lymphomas. The lack of CD7 expression is typical for mycosis fungoides, which is not relevant to BM evaluation. In addition, the detection of CD7 with multiparameter flow cytometry in immature cells in myelodysplastic syndromes has been claimed to represent an adverse prognostic factor [Font 2006; Font 2008; van de Loosdrecht 2007; Ogata 2005; Ogata 2002]. Flow cytometry is used to evaluate the CD34+ myeloid blasts for aberrant expression of CD7 or CD56. It was shown that patients with immunophenotypically abberant myeloid blasts are at risk for transfusion dependency and/or progressive disease independent of other known risk factors [van de Loosdrecht 2007]. Identification of such rare events with IHC is neither practical nor possible at this time.

F3.6.1 CD7 in reactive T cells

This biopsy specimen is from a 42-year-old woman with a history of rheumatoid arthritis and pancytopenia. The bone marrow is normocellular to focally hypocellular and T cells are slightly increased. No other pathological findings were detected. The T cells had an "activated appearance" with variable amount of cytoplasm. Pan-T-cell antigens can be significantly downregulated in an activated T-cell population, as shown here for CD7.

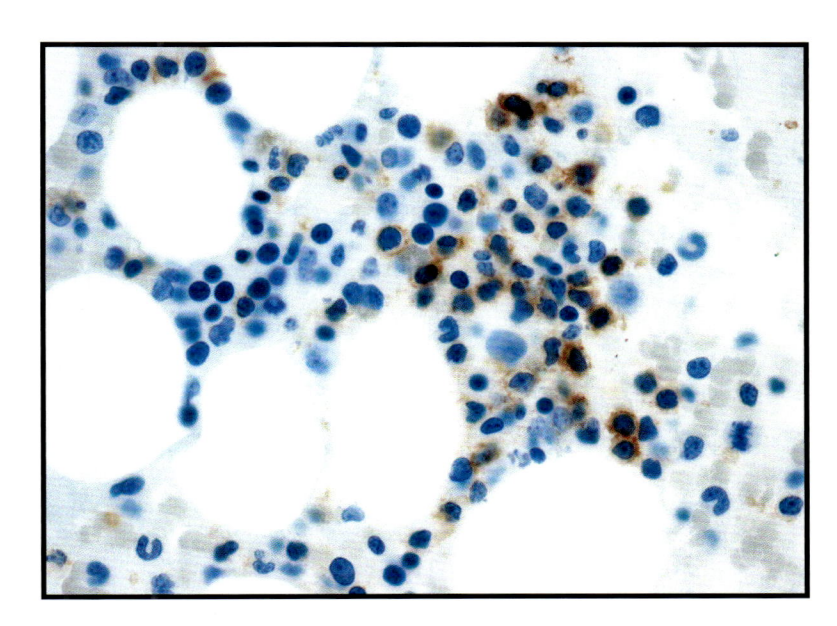

F3.6.2 CD7 in refractory anemia with excess blasts

CD7 is detected in rare cells. Some are obviously small lymphoid cells and are presumed to be T cells. Others, with more abundant cytoplasm are difficult to interpret. They are most likely activated T cells, but aberrant expression of CD7 in myeloid cells cannot be entirely excluded in a patient with a myelodysplastic syndrome. Morphologic features in this case strongly favor reactive lymphocytes rather than myeloblasts.

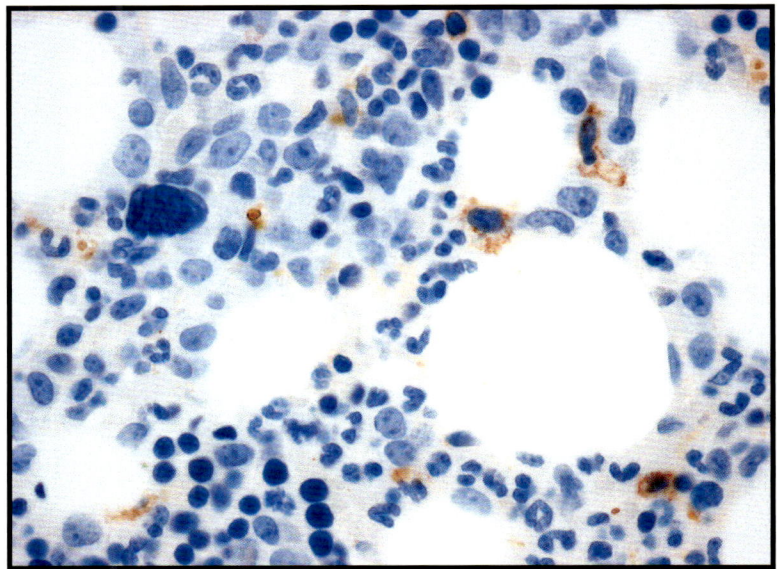

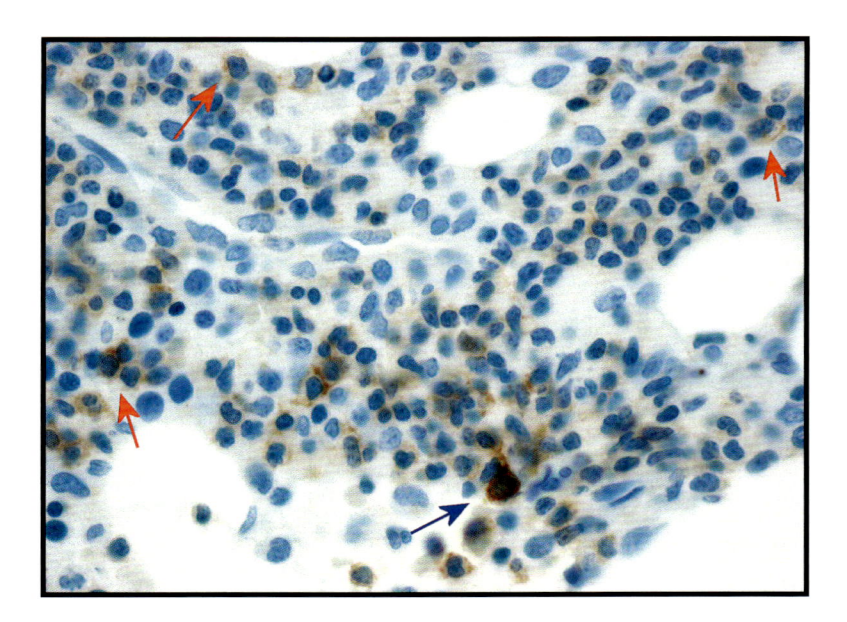

F3.6.3 CD7 in peripheral T-cell lymphoma

Only a single cell shows strong expression of the CD7 antigen (blue arrow). Numerous malignant T cells are negative and a minor subpopulation shows weak membranous expression (red arrows). About 70% of the cells in this field are strongly positive for CD3. While activated T cells may also downregulate CD7, such marked downregulation is more characteristic of a neoplastic T-cell infiltrate.

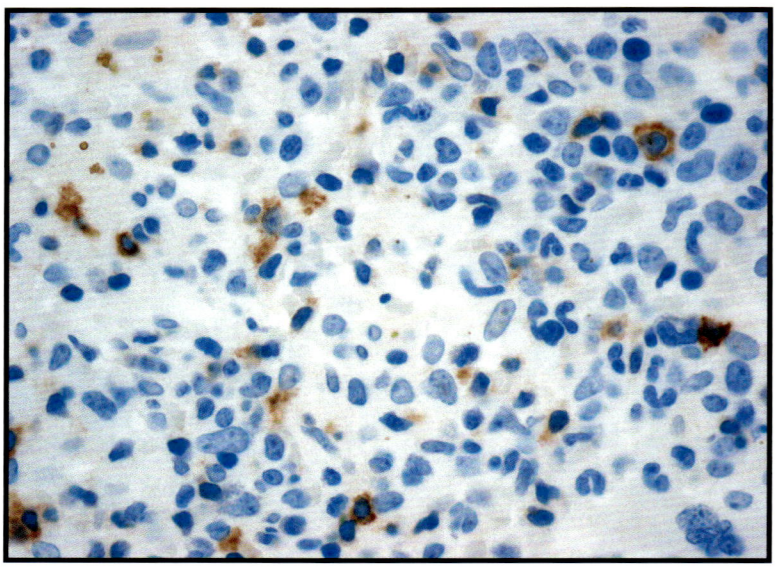

F3.6.4 CD7 in peripheral T-cell lymphoma

Different case from that shown in **F3.6.3**. As demonstrated in this case, a complete loss of CD7 may be observed in some peripheral T-cell lymphomas. The negative finding can only be used if there is an appropriate internal control. Rare lymphoid cells show strong expression of the CD7 and confirm that this is not a false-negative result. These rare strongly positive cells could also be lymphoma cells, but are more likely to represent a small benign T-cell population.

3.7 CD8

CD8 is a cell surface glycoprotein found on most cytotoxic T cells. It functions as a coreceptor in recognition of the antigens presented by antigen-presenting cells in the context of class I MHC molecules. It is found as either a homodimer (CD8-α-α) or heterodimer (CD8-α-β) (OMIM). Recently, CD8 has been identified on macrophages, mast cells, and dendritic cells [Hirji 1999; Hirji 2000]. CD8 is expressed by the dendritic cells of lymphoid origin, while myeloid dendritic cells that are derived from a CD14+ monocytic precursor do not express CD8 [Wu 1996; Wu 1998]. The CD4 to CD8 ratio is reversed in the BM from that of peripheral blood [Shin 1992]. Generally, CD8+ T cells are present diffusely in the interstitium of the BM as well as together with CD4+ T cells in perivascular localization and lymphoid aggregates. Even though CD8+ T cells are normally found in the BM, there is evidence that in different BM tumors some of the T cells are so-called tumor infiltrating lymphocyte (TIL) clones [Grube 2007; Mellstedt 2006]. Postthymic T-cell malignancies are uncommon in the Western hemisphere. Consequently, CD8+ lymphomas and leukemias are also uncommon. However, typically CD8+ lesions that can involve the BM are precursor T-ALL (CD4+/CD8+ or CD4-/CD8+), T-cell large granular lymphocyte leukemia, and various other CD8+ peripheral T-cell lymphomas [Osuji 2007; Evans 2000; Fend 2007; Dogan 2004].

3.7 CD8

F3.7.1 CD8 in histologically normal bone marrow

This biopsy specimen is from a 14-year-old girl with a history of recently treated classical Hodgkin lymphoma (cHL). The BM was not involved. The BM is somewhat hypocellular for the patient's age, but the number of CD8+ small lymphoid cells, presumed benign cytotoxic/suppressor T cells, appears normal. CD8+ lymphocytes are a normal finding in the BM and are usually more numerous than CD4+ cells. They are regularly seen evenly distributed in the interstitium of the BM.

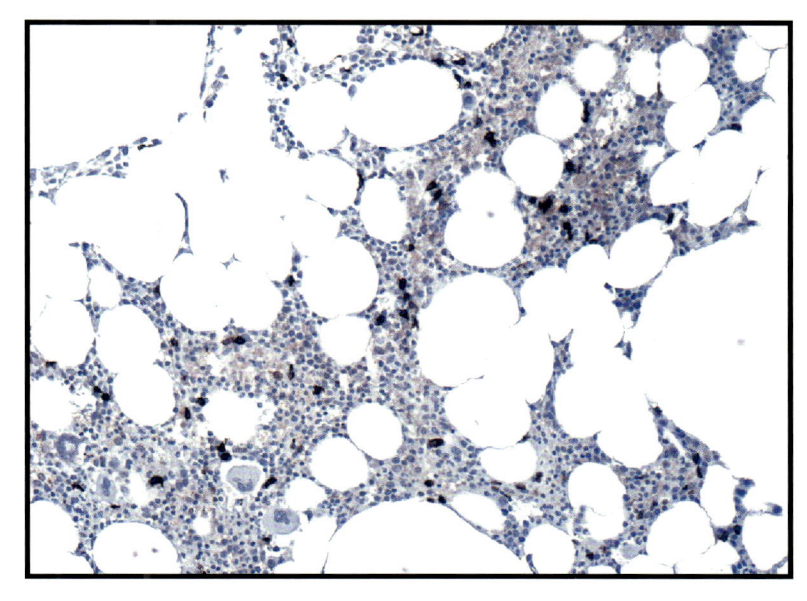

F3.7.2 CD8 in the interstitial T cells and endothelial cells (ADVANCE)

While the T cells express membranous CD8, the endothelial cells in a B5-fixed BM biopsy specimen appear to show specific expression of very strong membranous and possibly also weak cytoplasmic reactivity.

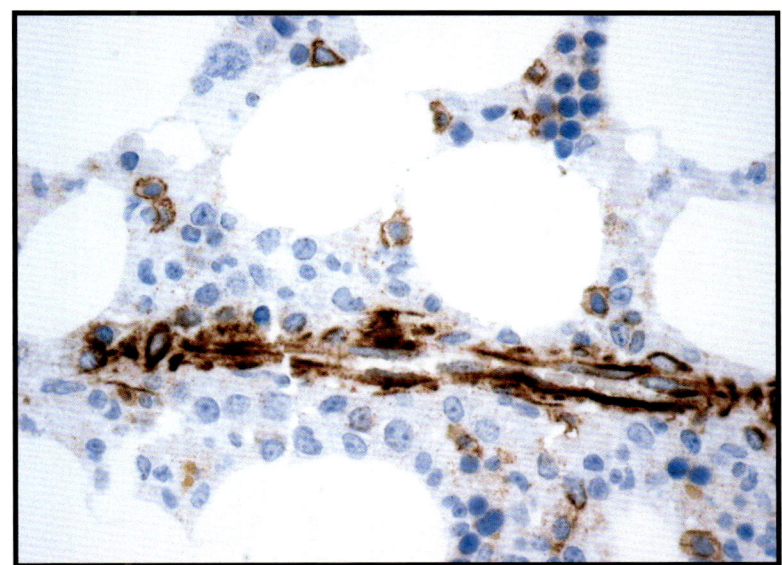

F3.7.3 CD8 in endothelial cells (ADVANCE)

The CD8 in endothelial cells appears segmentally expressed. This figure illustrates that the strongest expression in the endothelial cells is associated with perivascular CD8+ cells. The nature of the more peripheral CD8+ cells is not clear. They could be smooth muscle cells, pericytes, or even CD14+ perivascular monocytes. Otherwise, the CD8 in endothelial cells is weakly expressed in a dotlike membranous pattern.

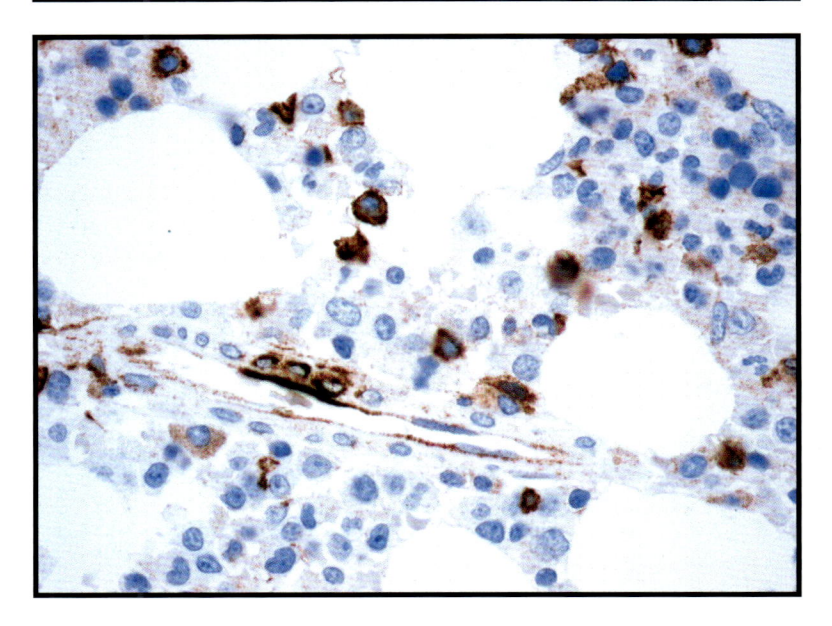

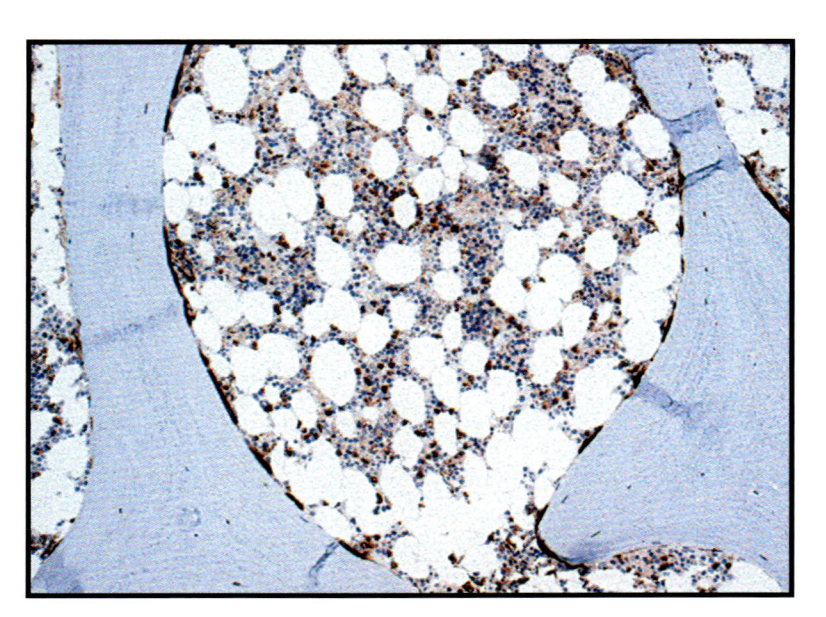

F3.7.4 CD8 in endosteal lining cells (ADVANCE)

This bone marrow biopsy specimen is obtained for staging of cHL in a 23-year-old woman with nodular sclerosis type of HL. In B5-fixed tissues, several stromal cells show reactivity with CD8. The periodic reactivity in endosteal lining cells resembles segmental reactivity in endothelial cells (see **F3.7.3**). The periodic CD8 expression is not universally present. The biological significance of this phenomenon has not been evaluated yet. Crossreaction with CD8-like epitopes has not been excluded.

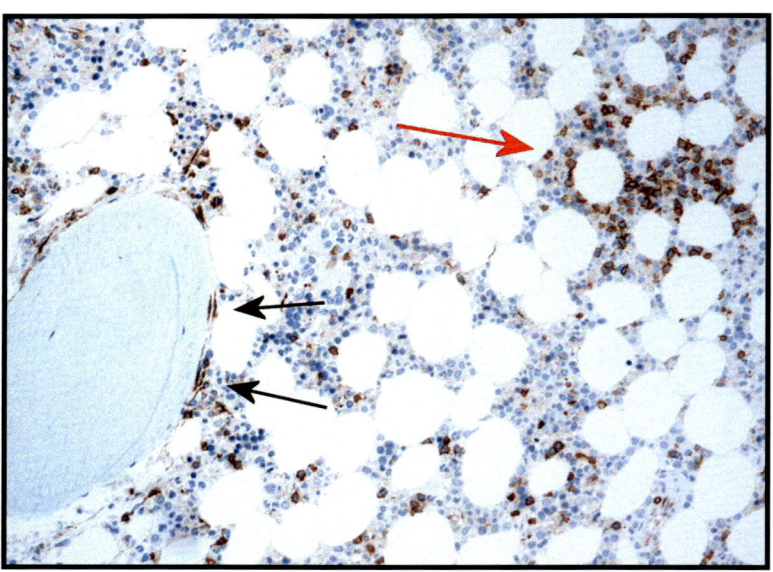

F3.7.5 CD8 in endosteal lining cells (ADVANCE)

The endosteal lining cells show segmental "dual/parallel" expression (black arrows). Note the focal interstitial clustering rather than true lymphoid aggregate with expanding borders, the latter being more often seen with CD4+ T cells (red arrow).

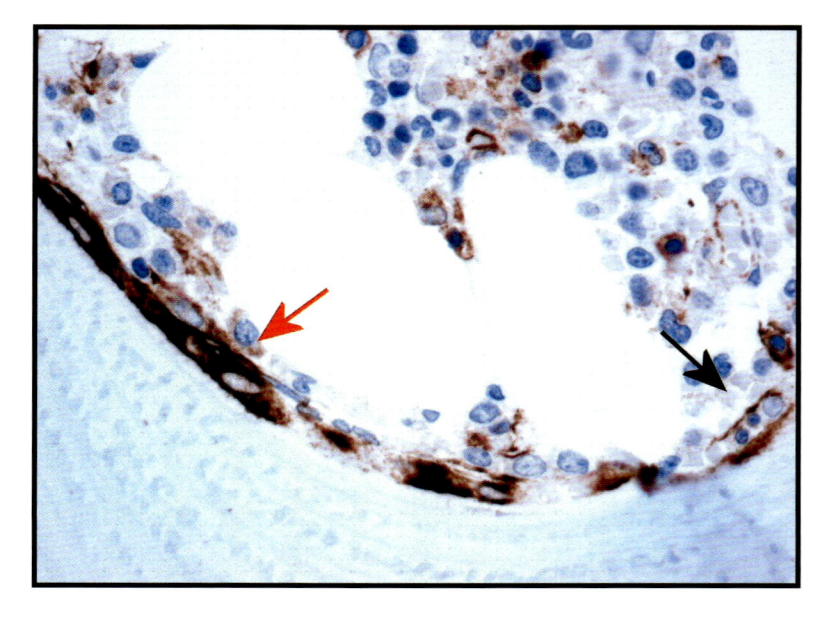

F3.7.6 CD8 expression in endosteal lining cells (ADVANCE)

In some areas the CD8 positivity is found in dual population of endosteal lining cells (red arrow, see also **F3.7.5**). Possibly both osteoblasts and endothelial cells are stained in such areas (black arrow).

3.7 CD8

F3.7.7 CD8 in refractory anemia with excess blasts; CD8 lymphocytosis of uncertain biological significance

The blast percentage was 9%. In addition, the patient also had increased CD8 lymphocytes and monoclonal polymerase chain reaction product by T-cell receptor–γ gene rearrangement study. Because there was no other evidence of a T-cell lymphoproliferative disease, the patient was not treated for T-cell lymphoma. A few months later, the T-cell clonality was no longer detectable. Some background staining is evident, but does not interfere with the interpretation.

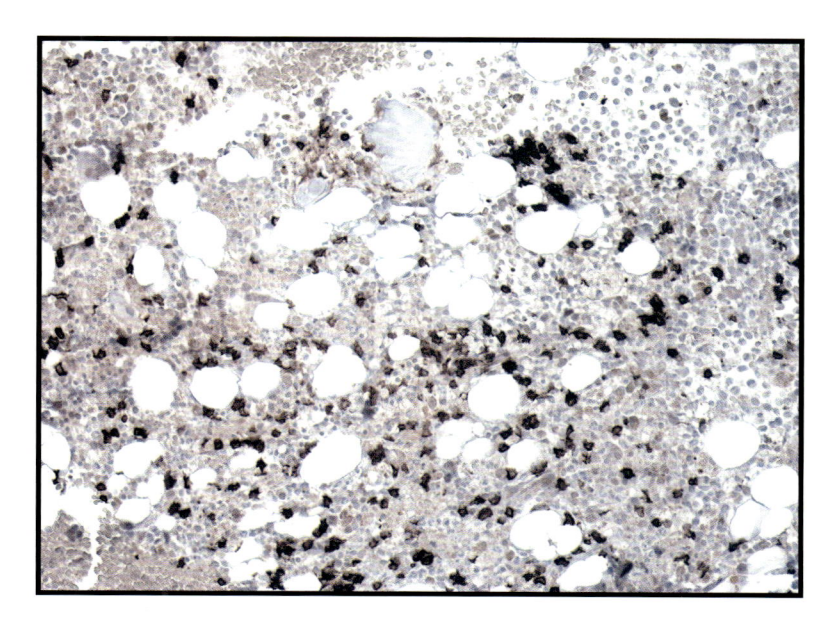

F3.7.8 CD8 in peripheral T-cell lymphoma in a 68-year-old woman

Both membranous and Golgi-type expression of CD8 are evident in this peripheral T-cell lymphoma. The cellular morphology is clearly atypical, but great caution has to be exercised in using this feature to diagnose such cells as malignant because reactive CD8 cells also can show very atypical morphology. This was not a problem in this case because the patient had primary nodal disease.

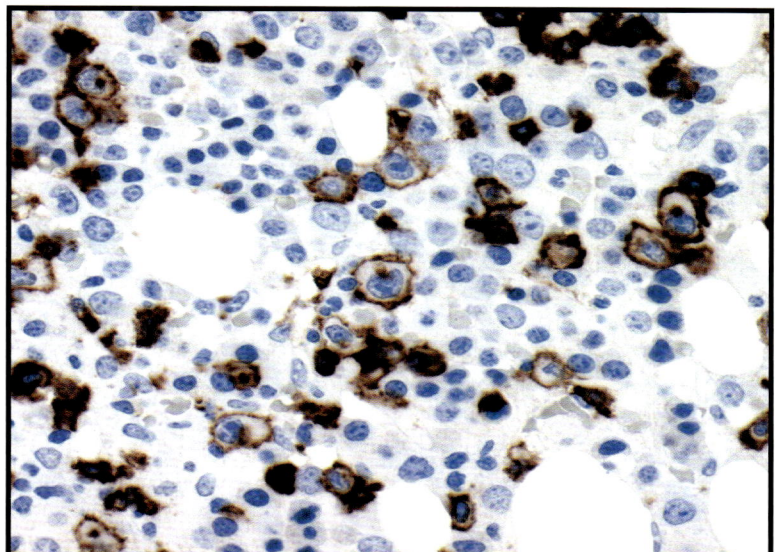

F3.7.9 CD8 in T-cell large granular lymphocytic leukemia (T-LGL)

Malignant cells have relatively low nuclear-cytoplasmic ratio and no definite nuclear atypia. In the bone marrow, because of similarities with either myeloid cells or erythroid cells, such cells are easily missed or grossly underestimated on morphologic examination of H&E sections, which is similar to BM involvement by marginal zone lymphoma. Interstitial pattern with or without intravascular pattern of involvement is typical.

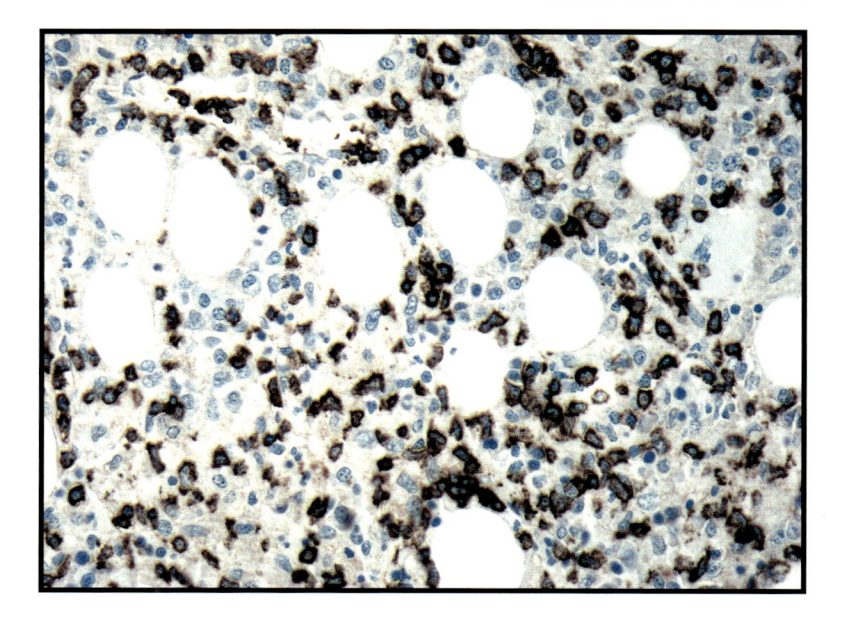

3.8 CD9

CD9 is also known as DRAP-27, MRP-1, and p24. It is a receptor for diphteria toxin. It is expressed by megakaryocytes and platelets, early B cells and the blasts of precursor B-ALL, activated B cells, plasma cells, activated T cells, eosinophils, basophils, mast cells, endothelial cells, brain and peripheral nerves, vascular smooth muscle, and cardiac muscle, and epithelial cells (PROW) [Wright 1994; 1996; 2006; Escribano 1998; Valent 1989. It has been reported to be expressed by human adipose tissue–derived stromal cells [Gronthos 2001]. Because of its ubiquitous distribution, CD9 detection on the BM biopsy specimen with IHC has not been widely used in diagnostic hematopathology. CD9 may be decreased in plasma cell dyscrasia [Barrena 2005].

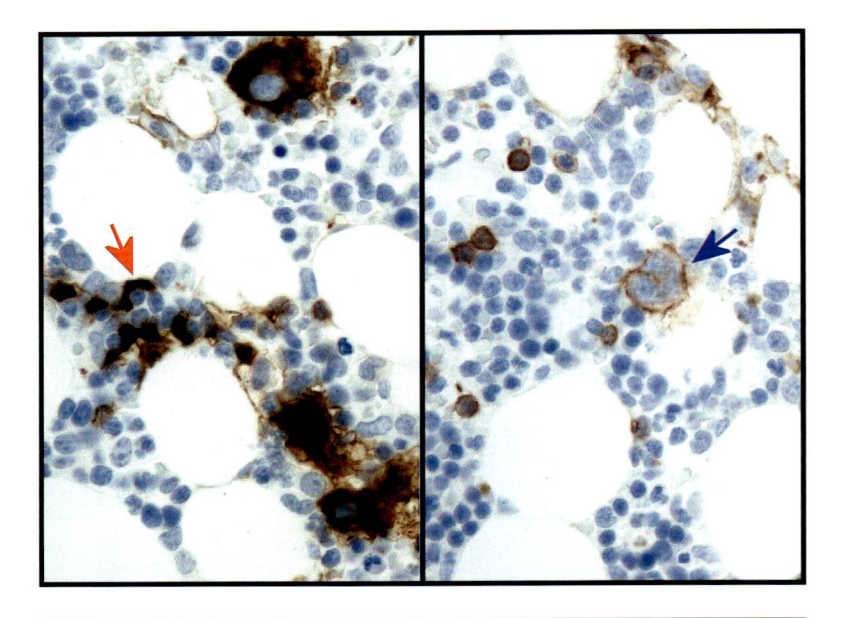

F3.8.1 CD9 in megakaryocytes and platelets

CD9 is generally strongly expressed in megakaryocytes and platelets (red arrow). Occasional megakaryocytes with higher nuclear-cytoplasmic ratio may show membranous expression of CD9 (blue arrow).

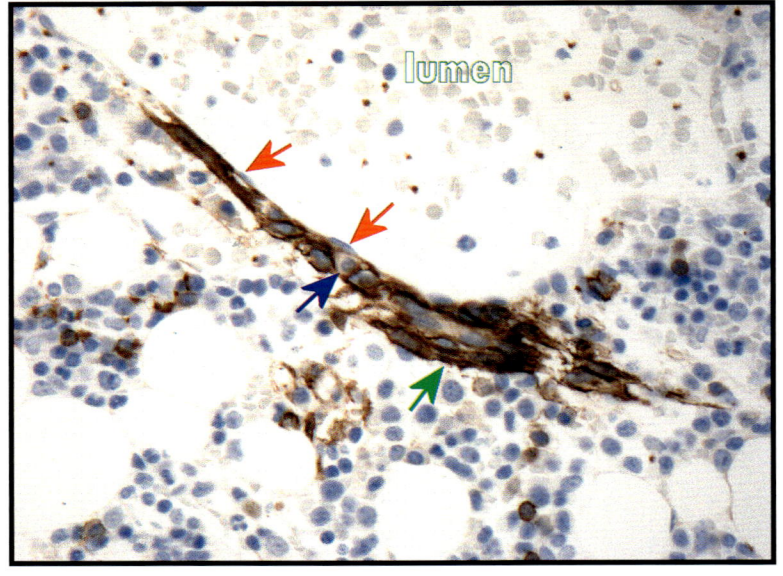

F3.8.2 CD9 expression in vessels

Vascular smooth muscle and pericytes express CD9 (green arrow). Endothelial cells were also described as positive, but they appear negative in the illustrated vessel (red arrow). A few perivascular plasma cells are also present and weakly express CD9 (blue arrow).

3.8   CD9

F3.8.3 CD9 in small lymphoid cells and plasma cells

CD9 is expressed in precursor B cells (blue arrows point to possible precursor B cells) and is downregulated when CD10 is no longer expressed. It is re-expressed in normal plasma cells (red arrow).

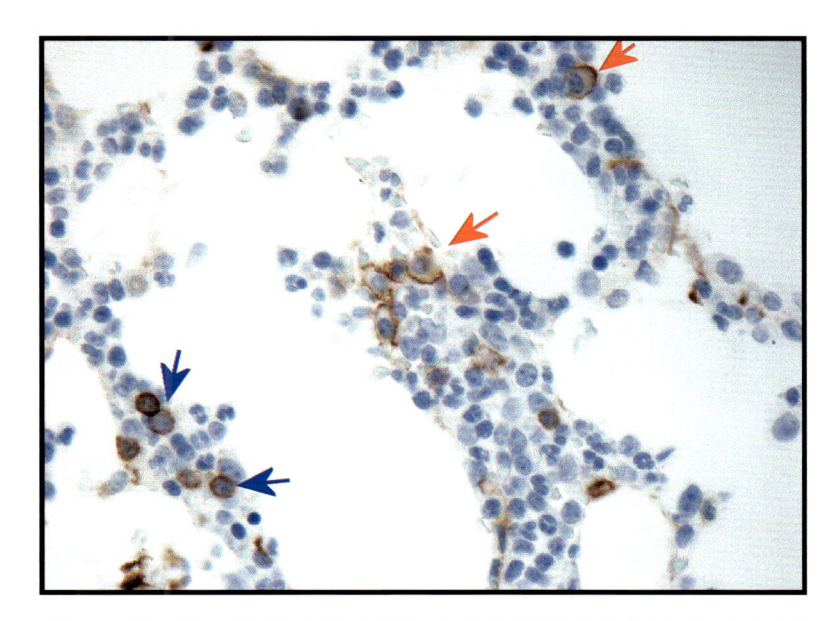

F3.8.4 CD9 in mast cells

Rare mast cells are present in this bone marrow biopsy. Mast cells show strong membranous expression (red arrows).

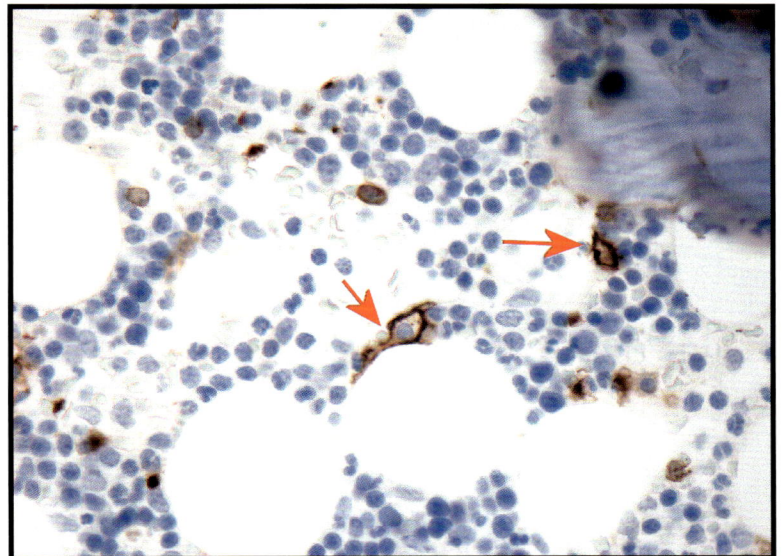

F3.8.5 CD9 in endothelial cells and pericytes

CD9 is expressed in endothelial cells and pericytes (left). It also appears to be expressed focally by endosteal lining cells (red arrow).

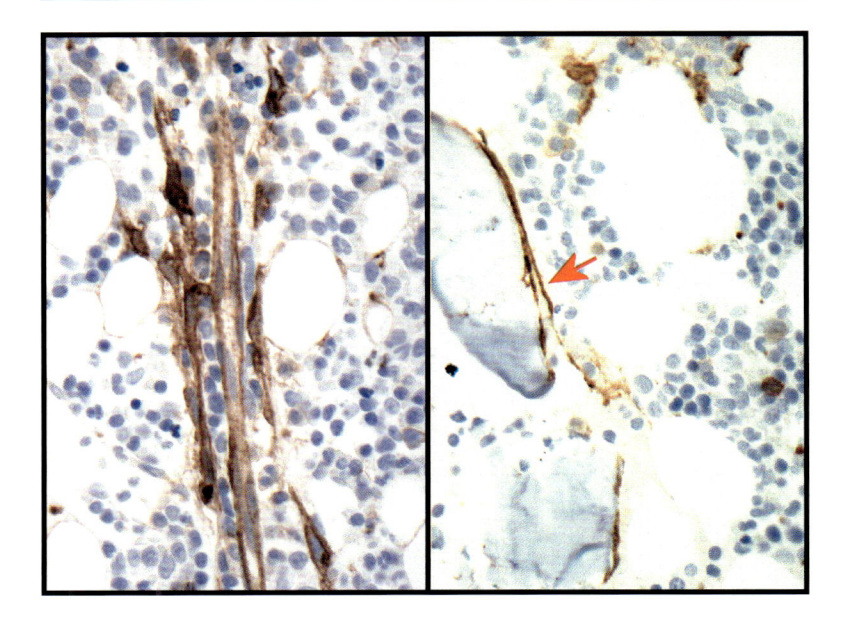

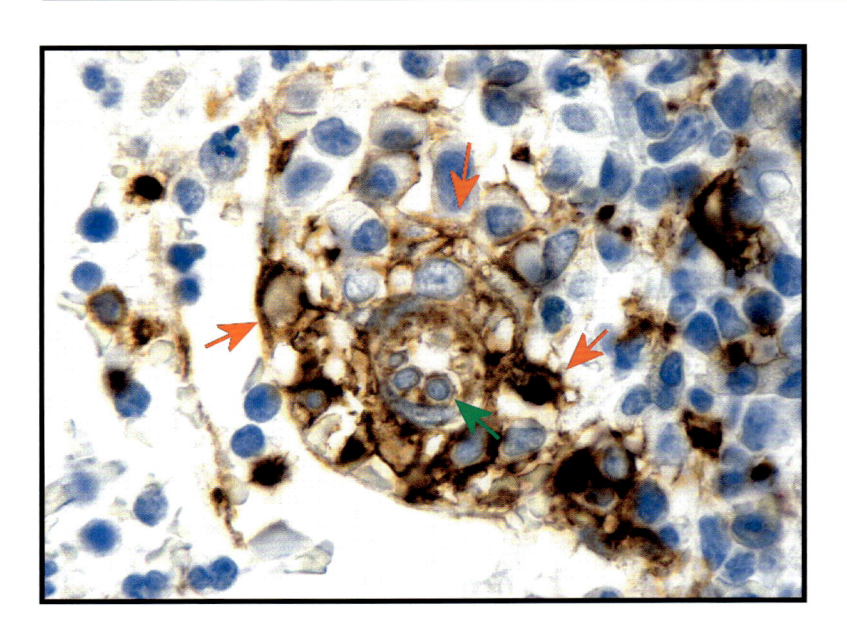

F3.8.6 CD9 in BM stromal cells

Endothelial cells show very weak expression in this small artery (green arrow). Vascular smooth muscle is positive as expected. In addition, there are a few BM stromal cells that appear to express CD9 (red arrows).

3.9 CD10

CD10 is a membrane metallo-endopeptidase (MME) and is also known as common acute lymphocytic leukemia antigen (CALLA), neprilysin (NEP), enkephalinase, atriopeptidase, endopeptidase-2, neutral endopeptidase, and kidney-brush-border neutral proteinase [Torlakovic 2007].

Despite its designation as CALLA, CD10 is also normally expressed in several types of cells in the BM. It is expressed by a normal lymphoid precursor [Muehleck 1983; Longacre 1989; Rimsza 2000]. In reactive conditions CD10+ lymphoid precursors, in particular of B lineage, may be markedly increased [Davis 1994; McKenna 2001]. Postmitotic neutrophils also express CD10 to a variable degree [Elghetany 2002]. An estimated 25% of maturing BM neutrophils are CD10− [McCormack 1988]. It is expressed uniformly in adipocytes, but only if very sensitive methods of detection are used. It is also expressed by a subset of CD10+ dendritic stromal cells, which form a niche for maturation of B cells [Torlakovic 2005]. CD10 is usually evaluated with flow cytometry in acute leukemia, but CD10 can also be demonstrated in this disease with IHC [Bavikatty 2000]. Even though CD10 is typically expressed in FL, its expression appears to be downregulated once the FL cells exit the environment of the follicular dendritic cells [Eshoa 2001]. Unequivocal demonstration of CD10 in paratrabecular infiltrates is uncommon. However, CD10 is usually positive even in the BM if FL forms neoplastic follicles with follicular dendritic cells [Torlakovic 2002a; Torlakovic 2002b]. It is also detected in some cases of angioimmunoblastic T-cell lymphoma [Attygalle 2002]. However, CD10 and Bcl-6 expression are frequently lacking in the neoplastic cells of angioimmunoblastic T-cell lymphoma lesions—similar to their decreased expression in follicular lymphoma [Tan 2007]. Flow cytometric detection of CD10 was reported to be somewhat more sensitive than IHC in DLBCL [Xu 2002]. CD10 has been found to be decreased in neutrophils in chronic myeloid leukemia [Cruse 2007]. CD10 is typically expressed in ALL, Burkitt lymphoma, follicular lymphoma, a subset of diffuse large B-cell lymphomas, and angioimmunoblastic T-cell lymphoma. It is an important marker in evaluation of leukemias and lymphomas in the BM [Schwonzen 1992; Shin 1992; Kröber 2000; Pezzella 2000; Kaufmann 1999].

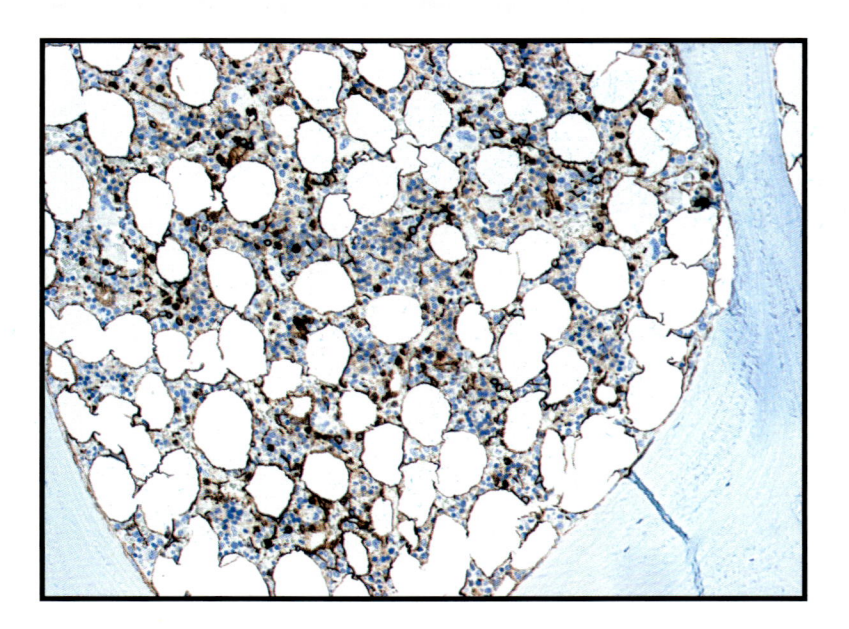

F3.9.1 CD10 at low magnification (ADVANCE)

In the bone marrow 4 elements regularly express CD10: immature lymphoid cells, adipocytes, dendritic extensions of CD10+ stromal cells, and neutrophils. Sometimes, rare plasma cells can express CD10. At 50× magnification, the appearance is rather complex. Less sensitive detection systems do not stain all adipocytes, but other cell populations are usually well demonstrated in an optimized CD10 protocols.

F3.9.2 CD10 (EnVision+)

EnVision+ is several times less sensitive than ADVANCE and adipocytes are either negative or at best variably positive. Other cells that express CD10 appear to be positive.

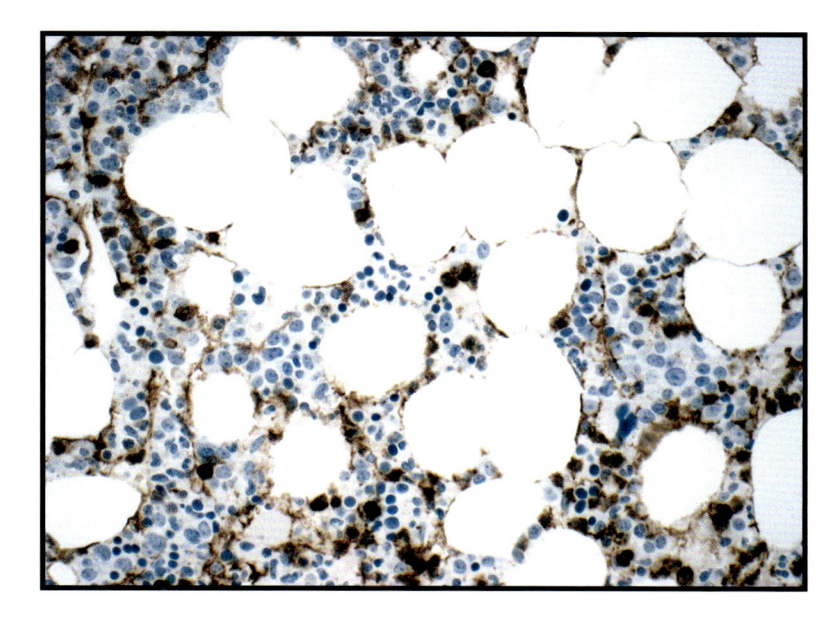

F3.9.3 CD10 in maturing lymphocytes (ADVANCE)

CD10 is clearly demonstrated in immature lymphoid cells. They are always found attached to the CD10+ dendritic extension of the stromal cells or on the surface of the adipocytes. This feature may be helpful in interpreting CD10 in the bone marrow biopsy specimen from patients with ALL when looking for residual leukemic cells, which form rounded aggregates and generally do not show this peculiar association with CD10+ dendritic extensions or adipocytes. However, this feature has not been systematically evaluated in a large number of patients.

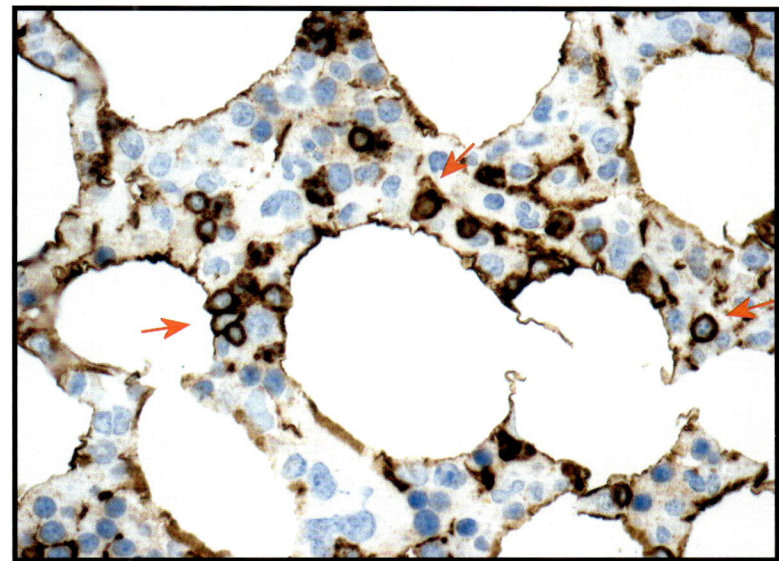

F3.9.4 CD10 in neutrophils (ADVANCE)

Several neutrophils are identified in the center (red arrows). Neutrophils express CD10, but this feature was described as significantly variable. Typically and in contrast to maturing lymphoid cells, the entire cell appears to stain, and nuclei are difficult to see. Only postmitotic neutrophils express CD10. Therefore, CD10 expression is typical of only mature neutrophil forms. Some benign plasma cells can also be found to express surface CD10 (black arrows).

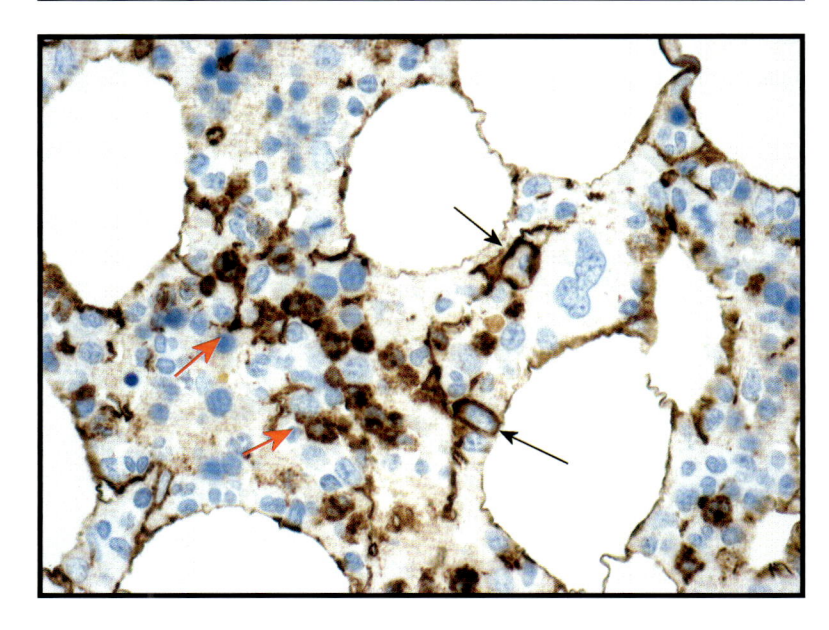

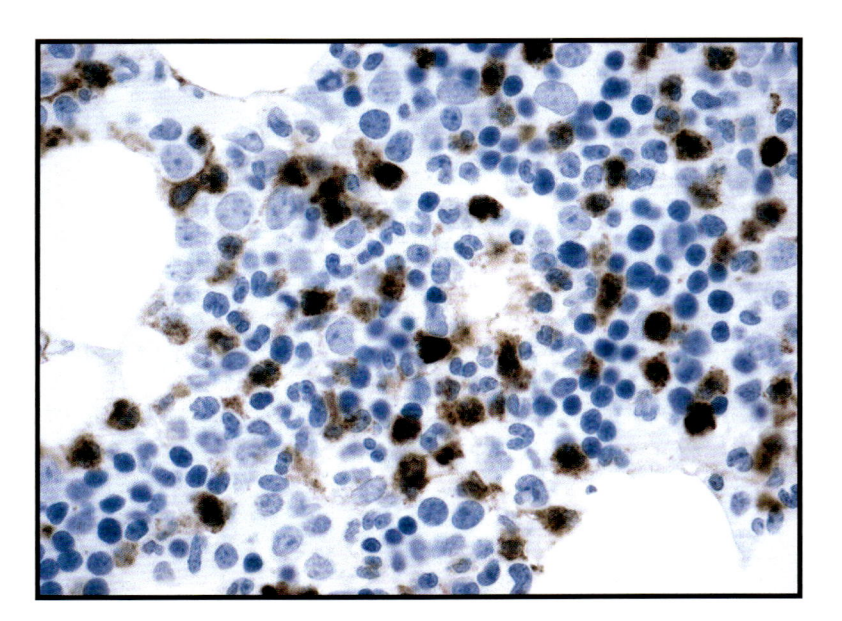

F3.9.5 CD10 in neutrophils (EnVision+TM)

Mostly neutrophils are demonstrated. Adipocytes and dendritic stromal cells did not stain for the most part. However, as can be clearly appreciated, the neutrophils appeared to express high levels of CD10. Typically, nuclear detail cannot be easily discerned because the expression appears to be granular cytoplasmic and possibly nuclear.

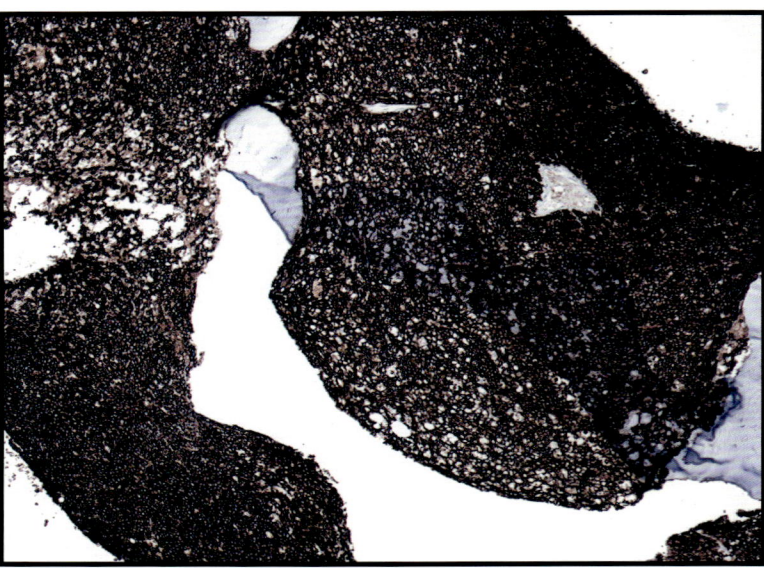

F3.9.6 CD10 expression in a precursor B-cell lymphoblastic leukemia

CD10 is expressed in both precursor T-cell and B-cell lymphoblastic leukemias. As shown here, the level of expression is usually very high. CD10 is re-expressed on the germinal center cells in B-cell development, but is it highly variable both in benign and malignant germinal centers. The intensity of staining like one depicted here is generally not seen in the benign germinal centers, but more often in low-grade follicular lymphoma.

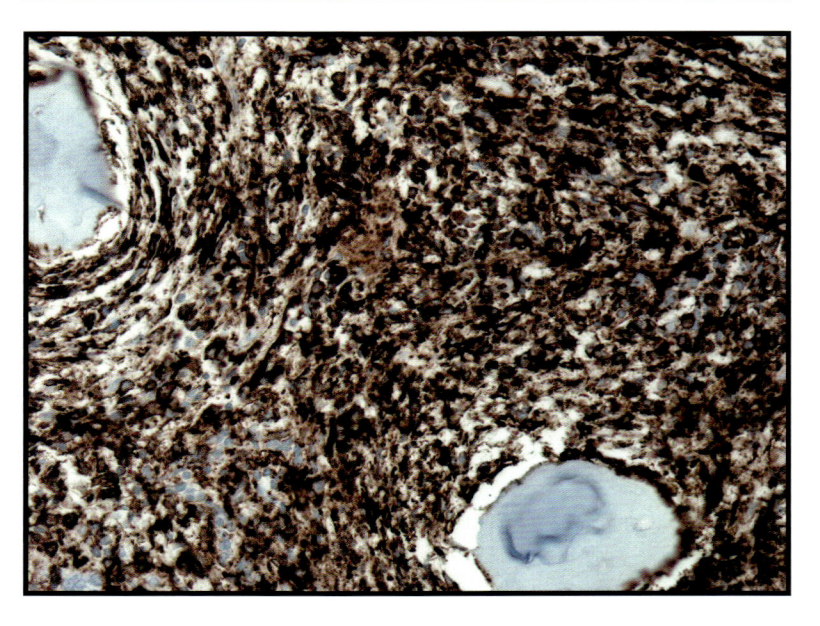

F3.9.7 CD10 in precursor B-cell acute lymphoblastic leukemia 14 days after chemotherapy

In this 14-month old infant, the leukemic cells lost CD34, TdT, and Pax-5 expression after chemotherapy. Even though almost all cells were blasts, only CD10 and CD20 were detectable.

F3.9.8 CD10 in acute lymphoblastic leukemia 14 days after induction chemotherapy

Occasional groups of CD10+ small lymphoid cells are found in groups and intravascularly (as shown here). These cells also had TdT and CD34 expression, confirming that they are residual leukemic cells. Also, the association with CD10+ dendritic cells or adipocytes was notably lacking (compare with F3.9.3).

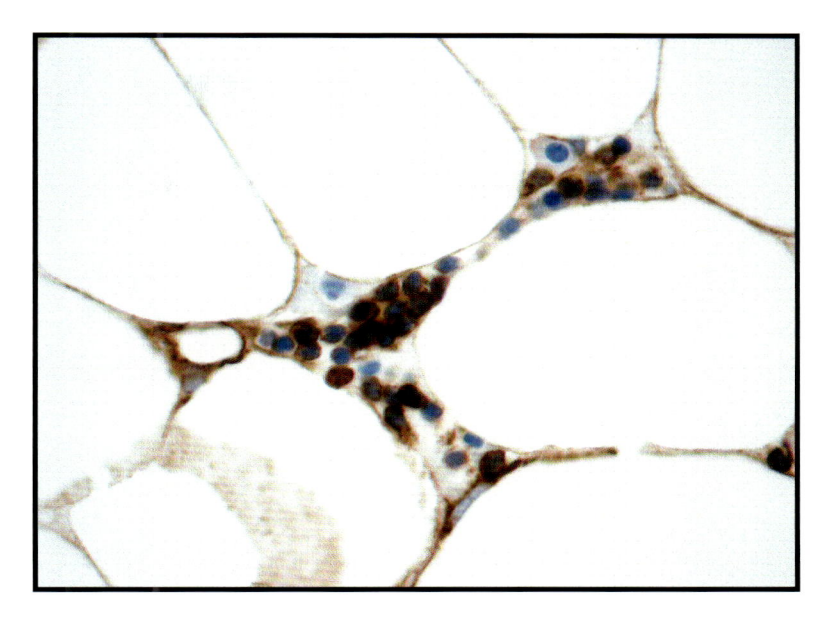

F3.9.9 CD10 in hematogones induced around lymphoid aggregate of lymphoplasmacytic lymphoma

Small CD10+ lymphoid cells correlate with TdT+ cells that appeared to concentrate around neoplastic lymphoid aggregates only. It is presumed that these cells represent hematogones, which express variable levels of TdT and CD10 representing non-neoplastic B-cell maturation. This feature has not been systematically studied and can be considered "controversial" even though expression of CD34 and TdT is observed.

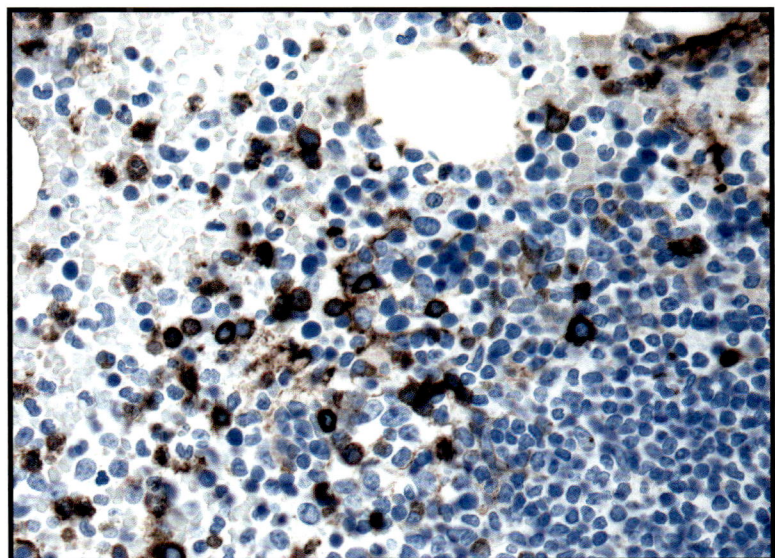

F3.9.10 CD10 in plasma cells

In this case of multiple myeloma, the plasma cells show surface and Golgi-type expression of CD10. This is a rare finding in myeloma.

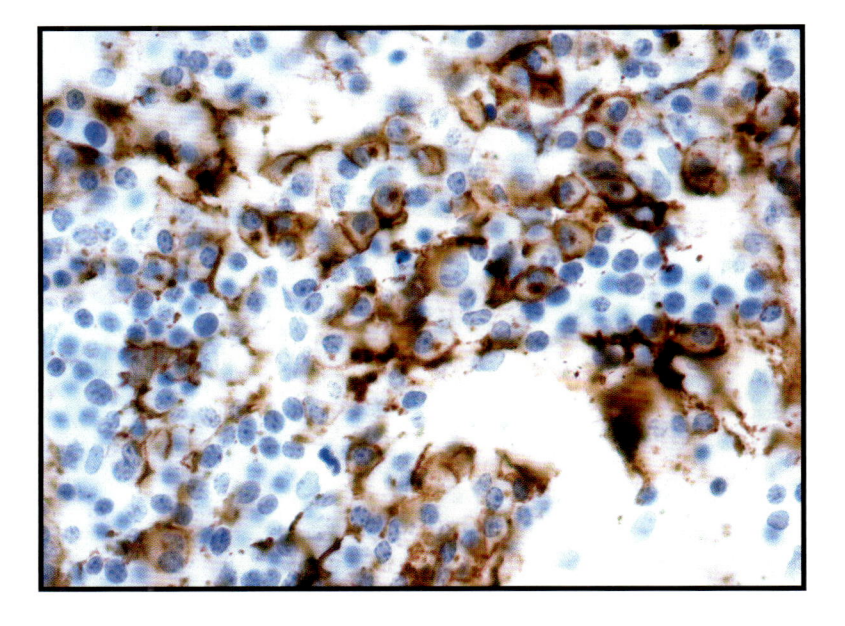

3: Cluster of Differentiation Markers

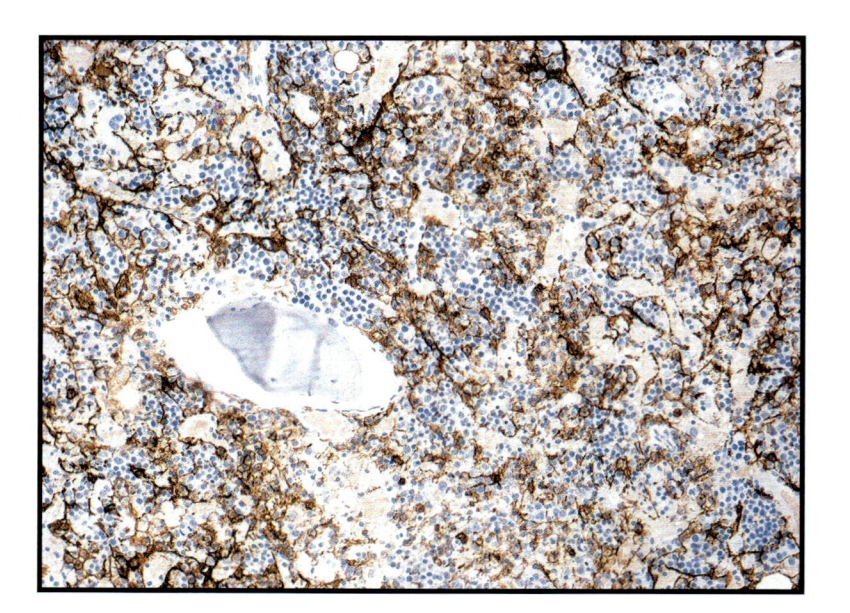

F3.9.11 CD10 stromal induction, core biopsy

In some neoplastic processes, the BM reacts with proliferation of CD10+ dendritic stromal cells. This was a diffuse and very prominent finding in a 61-year-old woman with multiple myeloma. The biological role of this phenomenon has not yet been evaluated.

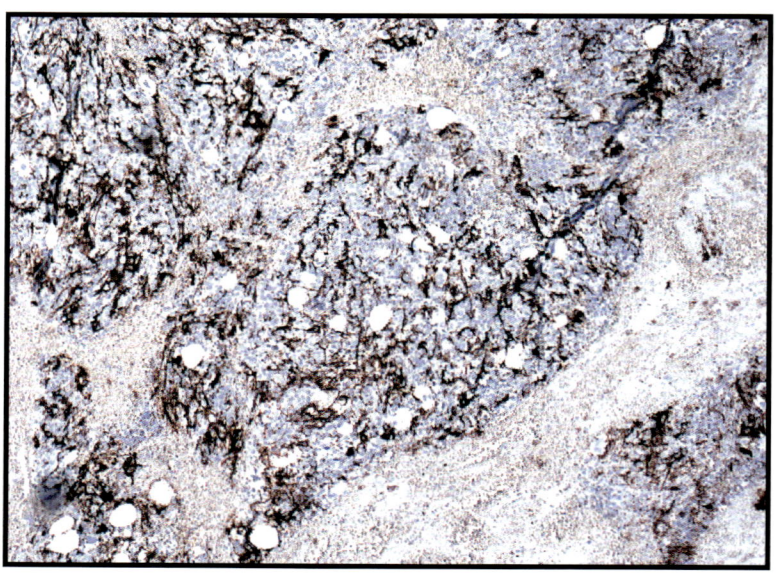

F3.9.12 CD10 stromal induction, clot section

The patient was a 37-year-old man who presented with stage IV classical Hodgkin lymphoma. Despite the focal involvement, a diffuse marked increase in CD10+ stromal cells was noted. The significance, if any, of this finding is not clear.

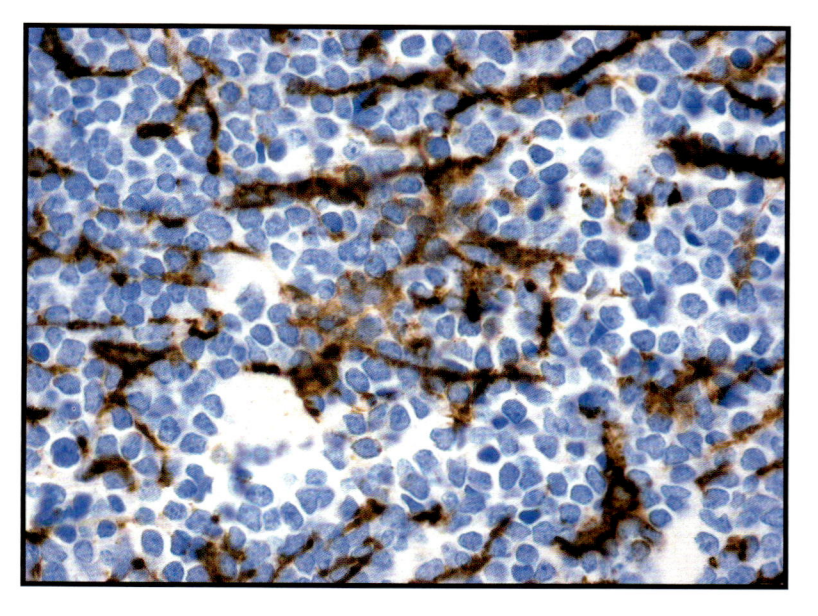

F3.9.13 CD10 in stromal cells of an undifferentiated acute myeloid leukemia

The leukemic cells do not express CD10 and the stromal dendritic cells appear only slightly increased in content, but the intensity of CD10 expression is possibly higher than that in a non-neoplastic bone marrow. The nuclei of the CD10+ stromal cells are clearly visible in several cells, which contributes to a general appreciation of their overall morphology.

3.9 CD10

F3.9.14 CD10 in dendritic stromal cells

CD10+ stromal cells do not correlate with the stromal pattern of reticulin staining. It is very likely that these cells are not involved in bone marrow reticulin production and deposition.

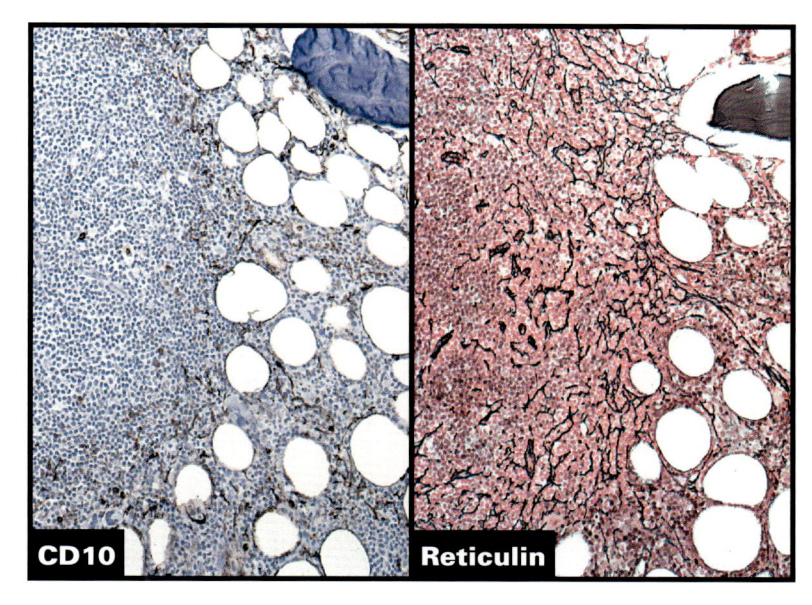

F3.9.15 CD10 in follicular lymphoma (FL)

This demonstrates a very case of FL in which CD10 can be demonstrated in paratrabecular lymphoid aggregates and some neoplastic cells present interstitially. The bony trabecula detached from its original position, which is now represented as an empty space along the scant lymphoid aggregate.

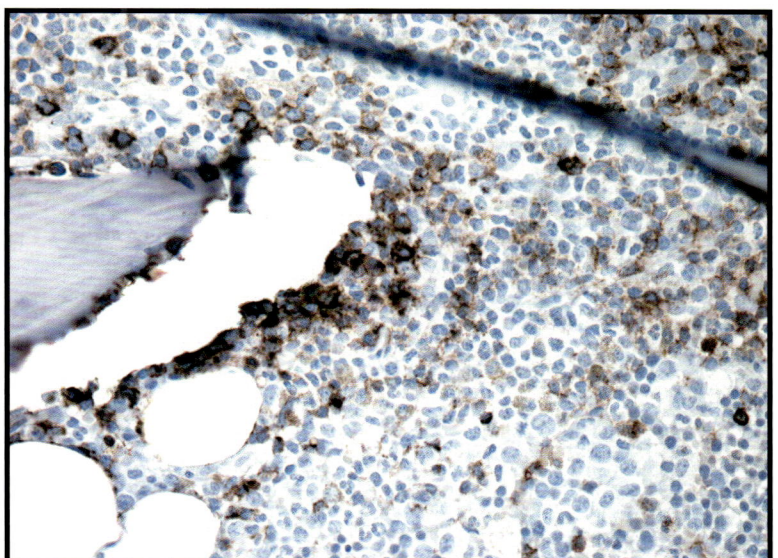

F3.9.16 CD10 in follicular lymphoma with pure follicular pattern and wide "mantles"

This patient had evidence of transformation to diffuse large B-cell lymphoma in the peripheral lymph node biopsy. However, in the bone marrow only interstitial follicles were identified. Wide pseudo-mantle zones were present with surrounding CD3+ lymphocytes. The CD10+ cells in the small germinal centers were also strongly Bcl-6+ and Bcl-2+ indicating follicular colonization of the benign follicles by follicular lymphoma cells.

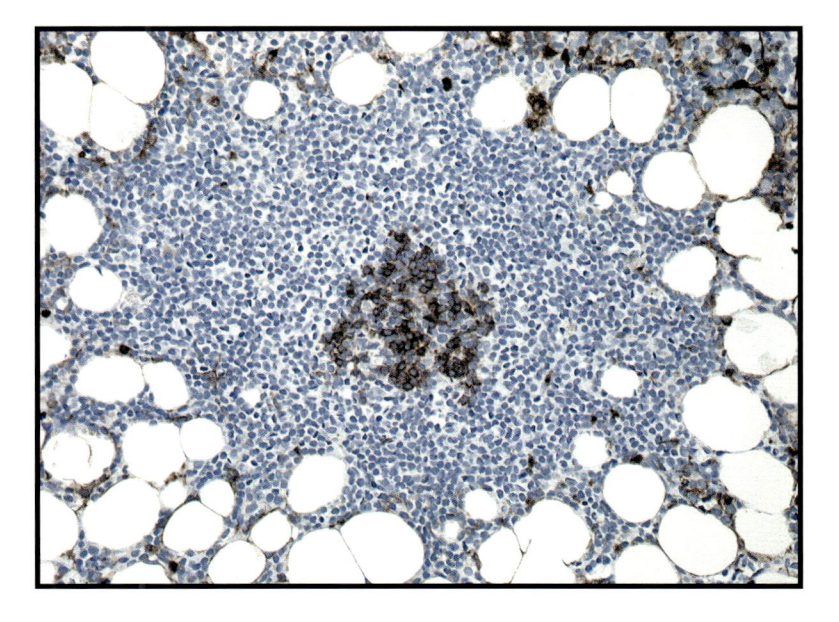

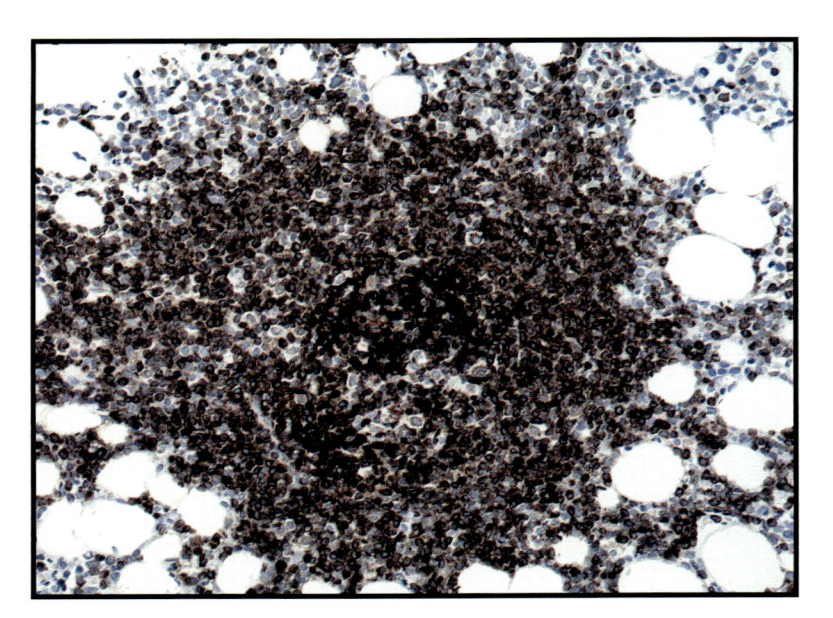

F3.9.17 Bcl-2 in a B-cell lymphoid follicle (see F3.9.16)

The Bcl-6+ and CD10+ cells of this and all other interstitial lymphoid follicles in this bone marrow biopsy specimen were also strongly Bcl-2+. The expression of Bcl-2 was stronger than in the germinal center than in mantle cells or the T cells, which is frequently the case in follicular colonization by follicular lymphoma.

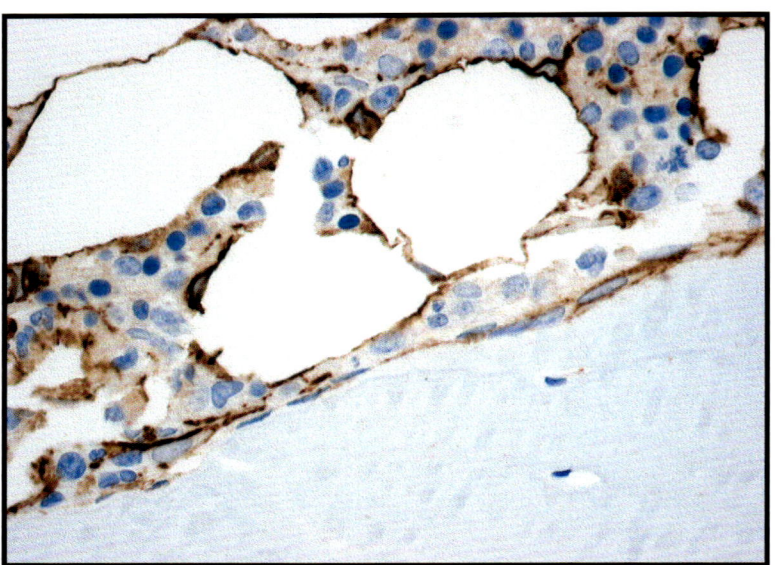

F3.9.18 CD10 in endosteal lining cells (ADVANCE)

CD10 seems also expressed, albeit unevenly, by the endosteal lining cells, possibly inactive osteoblasts. Osteocytes are always negative. A bone marrow biopsy in this adult male patient did not show any definite pathological findings.

3.10 CD14

CD14 is a receptor for endotoxin and is expressed by monocytes (CD14+/CD11c+), macrophages (CD14+/CD11c−), and weakly on the surface of mature granulocytes, but not neutrophil precursors (PROW). Myeloid dendritic cells (CD1a+ and CD1c+) are mainly CD14−, but this is inconsistent. Also, plasmacytoid dendritic cells (CD123+) generally do not express either CD11c or CD14 [Takeuchi 2007]. CD14 was demonstrated in paraffin-embedded tissue only recently, thus enabling investigators for the first time to identify different CD14+ cell types in situ with excellent morphologic features.

In the BM, monocytes and macrophages are expected to express CD14 [Baldus 1998; Lee 1988]. However, CD14 is also a marker of some dendritic cells including Langerhans cells and follicular dendritic cells [Petrasch 1990]. While CD14 is used as a highly sensitive marker in the detection of monocytic differentiation with flow cytometry, the IHC results for CD14 in the BM core biopsy may not be as useful [Horny 2007b]. It was reported that myelomonocytic diseases like chronic myelomoocytic leukemia may show loss of CD14 expression and that cytochemical detection of monocytic differentiation by using α-naphthylacetate esterase is more sensitive than that of flow cytometric detection of CD14 expression [Dunphy 2004; Eshoa 1999]. While CD14 is a highly sensitive marker of mature and normal monocytic cells, it is not expressed in most acute myelomonocytic leukemias and acute monoblastic leukemia as detected on flow cytometry [Platzer 2004]. CD14 detection by IHC needs to be further evaluated in various diseases to determine its value for diagnostic purposes.

3.10 CD14

F3.10.1 CD14 overview in histologically normal bone marrow

Rare randomly distributed cells are seen, probably corresponding to monocytic lineage. In addition, macrophages, which appear as relatively large cells because of an abundant cytoplasm (red arrow pointing to 2 cells) and perivascular monocytic cells are demonstrated (blue arrow).

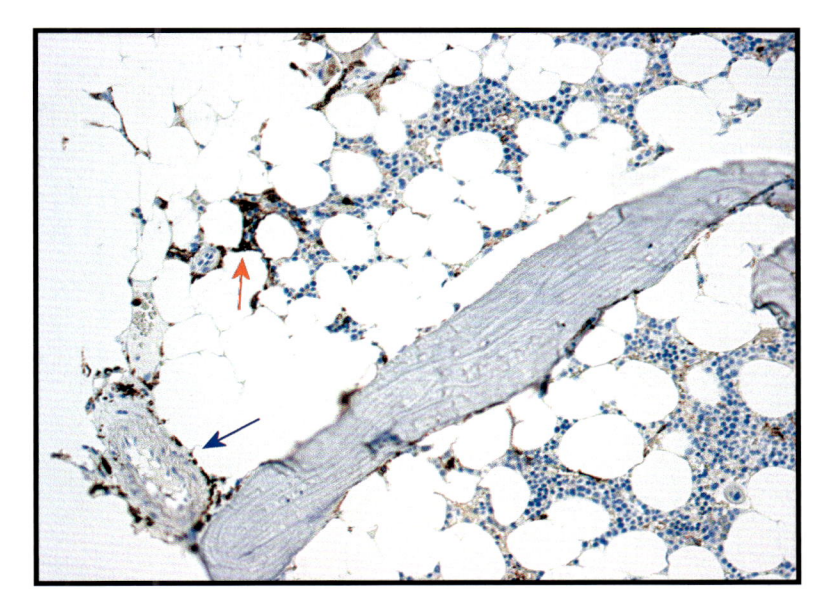

F3.10.2 CD14 in a histologically normal bone marrow (BM)

CD14 is labeling occasional monocytes and rare weakly stained stromal dendritic cells. Macrophages are generally difficult to find in a normal BM. Just like some other cell types, in some BM biopsies, the CD14+ monocytes appear to have nonrandom distribution and affinity to associate with adipocytes ("nipple sign").

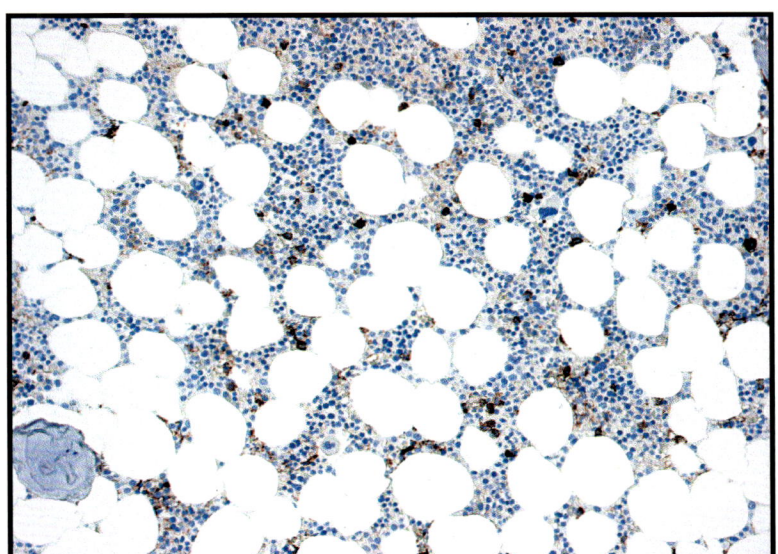

F3.10.3 CD14 in interstitium

These cells with ruffled surfaces are not always present. They are detected here in a reactive bone marrow in a patient with classical Hodgkin lymphoma stage I. Surface ruffles are identical to those seen in B-cell maturation when CD20+ cells are migrating into BM sinusoids (see F3.13.4 and F3.13.5). It is presumed that the cells in this field represent active migration of the monocytic cells, but there is no proof for this contention.

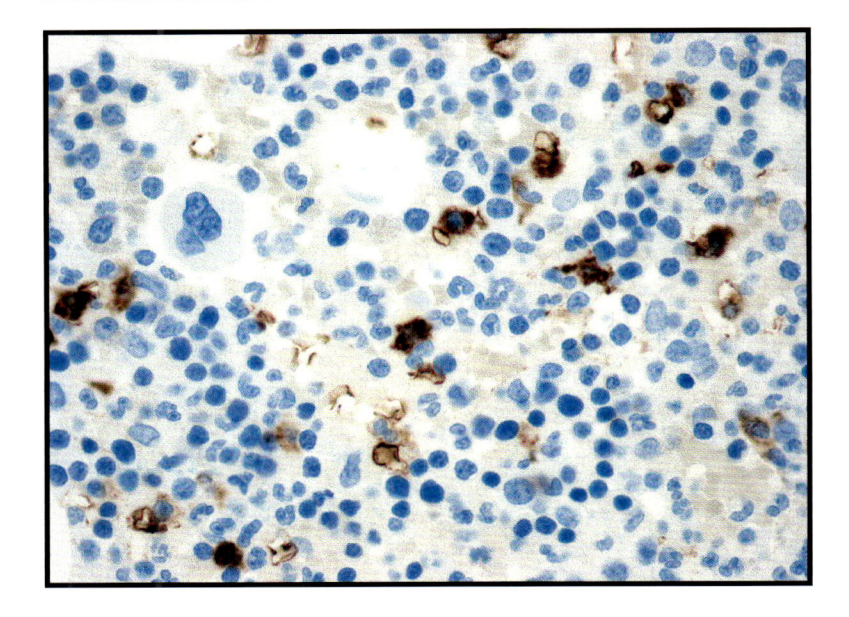

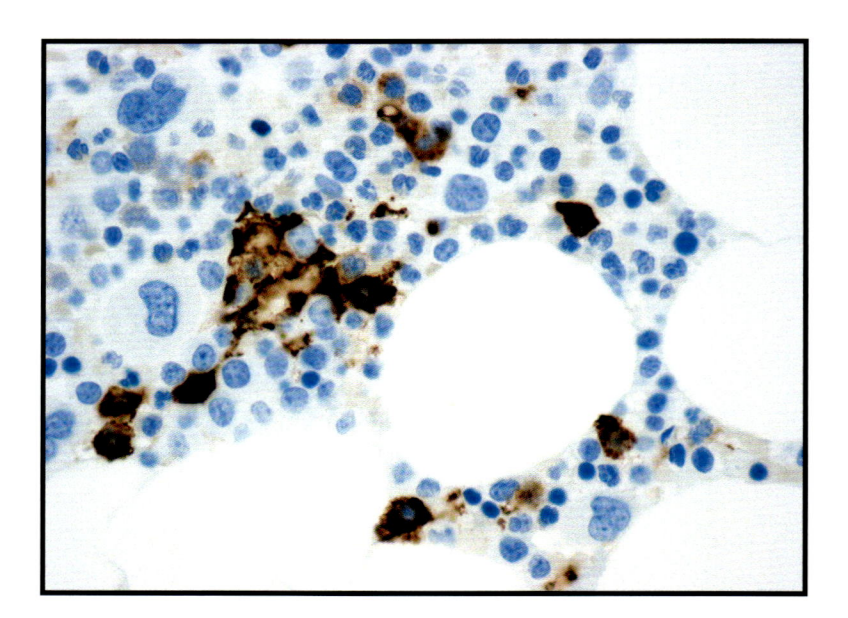

F3.10.4 CD14 in macrophages or bone marrow dendritic cells in normal bone marrow

Rare large cells with very low nuclear-cytoplasmic ratio are detected by CD14. It is assumed that these represent marrow macrophages or a subtype of marrow dendritic cells because their cell outlines are impressed by surrounding cells. Smaller cells are most likely monocytes. Cells with similar morphology but in much higher numbers are also detected by using anti-VCAM antibodies.

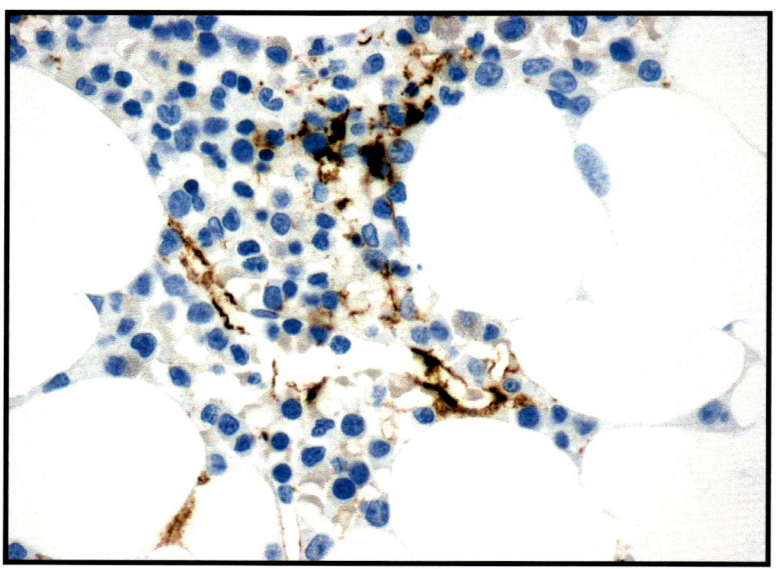

F3.10.5 CD14 in endothelial cells

The great majority of endothelial cells do not express CD14. However, in normal bone marrow, rare vascular spaces are lined by CD14+ cells. Even in these areas, the positivity is only focal. The biological background and significance of this finding is not clear. Crossreactivity with CD14-like molecules in endothelial cells cannot be excluded.

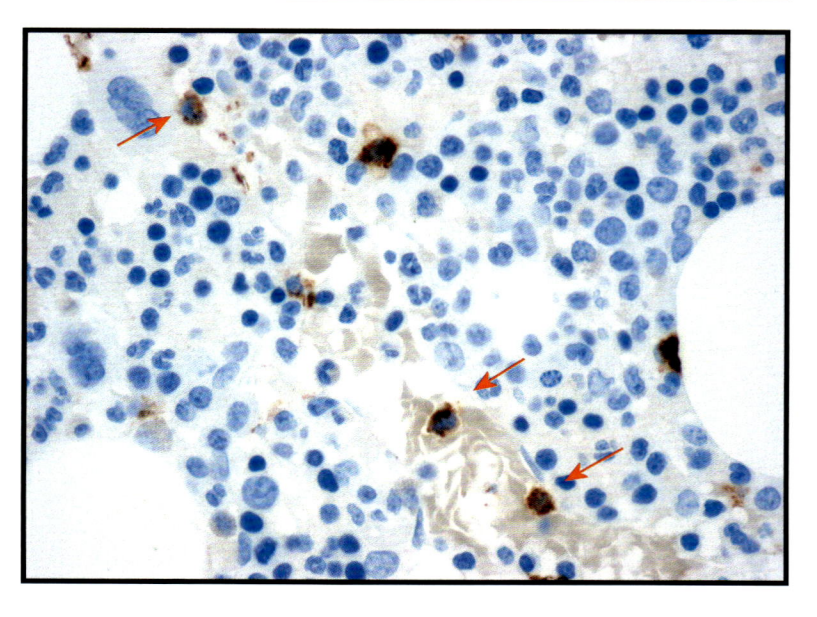

F3.10.6 CD14 in circulating monocytes

Vascular spaces of any bone marrow biopsy specimen can be expected to display a few positive mononuclear cells corresponding to circulating monocytes. In this image, 3 such cells are detected (red arrows). Also, the 2 positive cells in the BM interstitial space are most likely rare BM monocytes. In normal BM, CD14+ monocytes comprise up to 7% of all cells and most of the time they are lower than that.

3.10 CD14

F3.10.7 CD14: dendritic pattern

This image illustrates infrequent foci in the normal BM that display a "dendritic pattern." The cell body of the CD14+ dendritic processes is not evident. The delicate cell extensions engulf several cell types including in this example, both myeloid and erythroid cells. Megakaryocytes appear in contact only by random association. Rare marrow monocytes are also demonstrated (blue arrows).

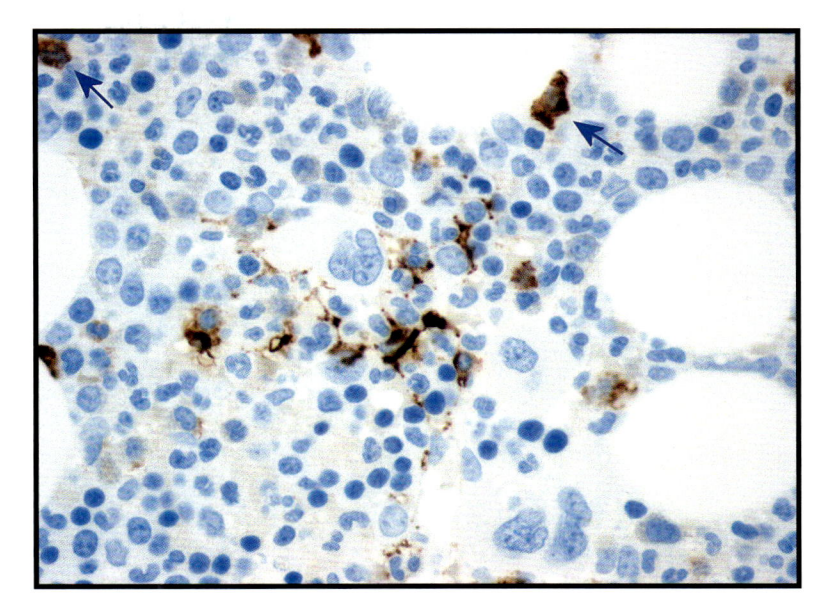

F3.10.8 CD14 in hypocellular bone marrow (BM)

The patient was a 34-year-old woman with presumed aplastic anemia. The overall marrow cellularity was less than 5%. The BM CD14+ cells were similar to those in a normocellular BM, appearing overrepresented in this hypocellular BM. Because no studies with CD14 in aplastic anemia have been reported, it is not certain that this image is a typical finding in this entity.

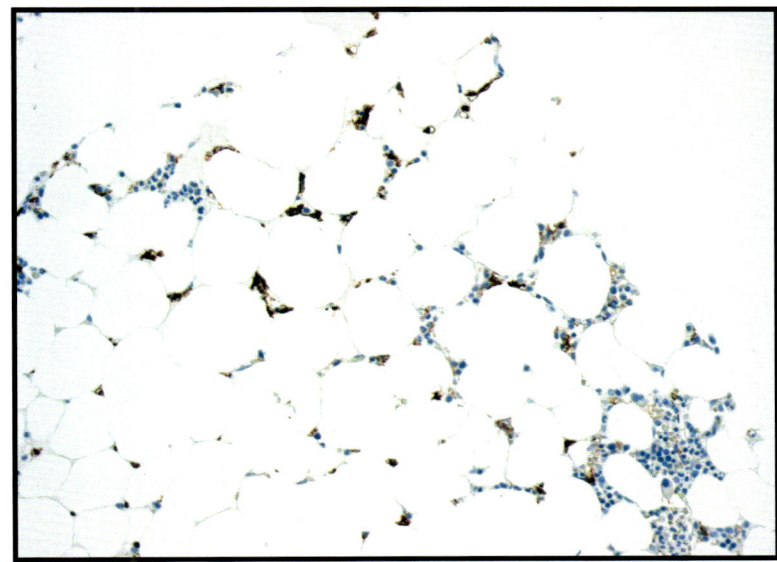

F3.10.9 CD14 in perivascular mononuclear cells

Perivascular monocytic cells are demonstrated. These cells are a normal finding. Further studies are needed to elucidate the biologic significance of this population. They are present in most organs including the bone marrow. See also **F4.7.2** and **F4.11.3**.

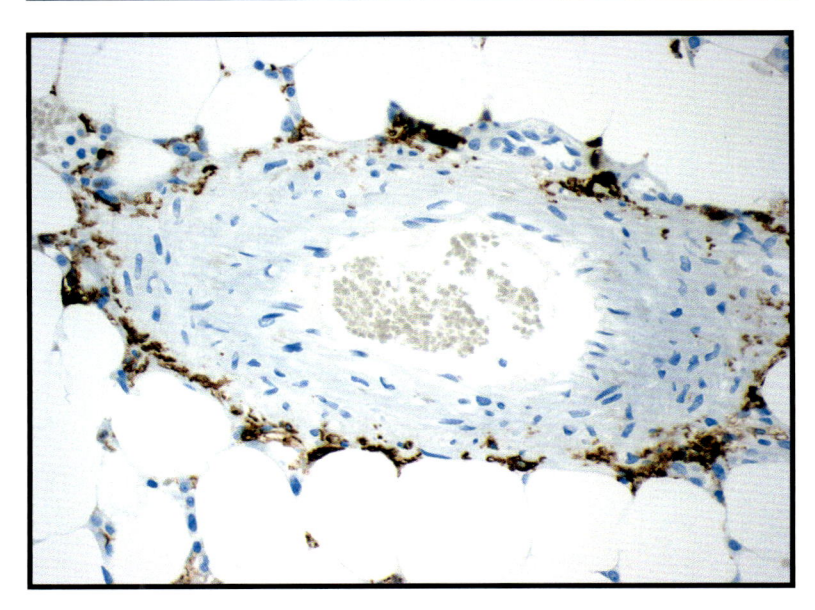

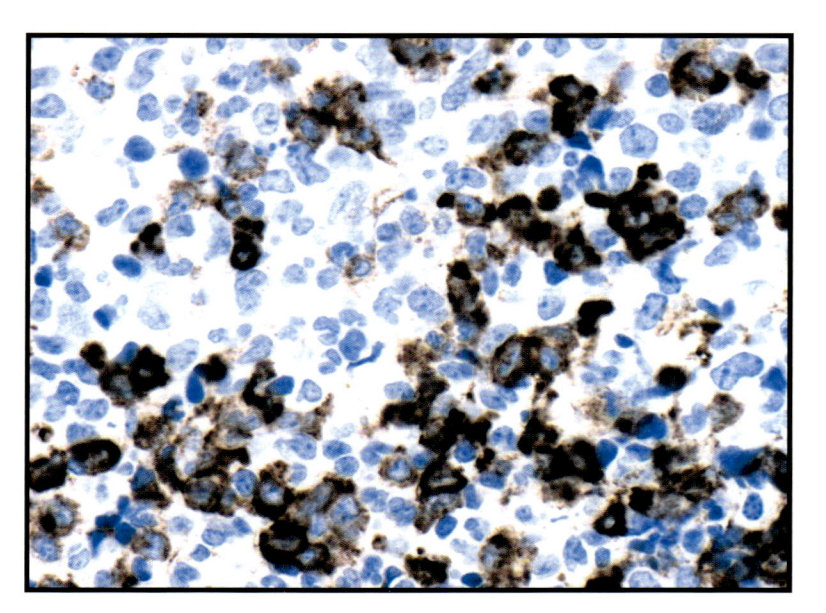

F3.10.10 CD14 in chronic myelomonocytic leukemia (CMML)

Hypercellular bone marrow specimen from this 67-year-old man shows an increased population of CD14+ cells. There was no previous history of hematologic disease. The BM showed 8% blasts. The strongly positive cells are mature monocytes because monoblasts in this and other diseases with increased monoblasts, are likely to be CD14–. Cytochemistry for α naphthylacetate esterase appears to be more sensitive for monoblastic cells in various conditions.

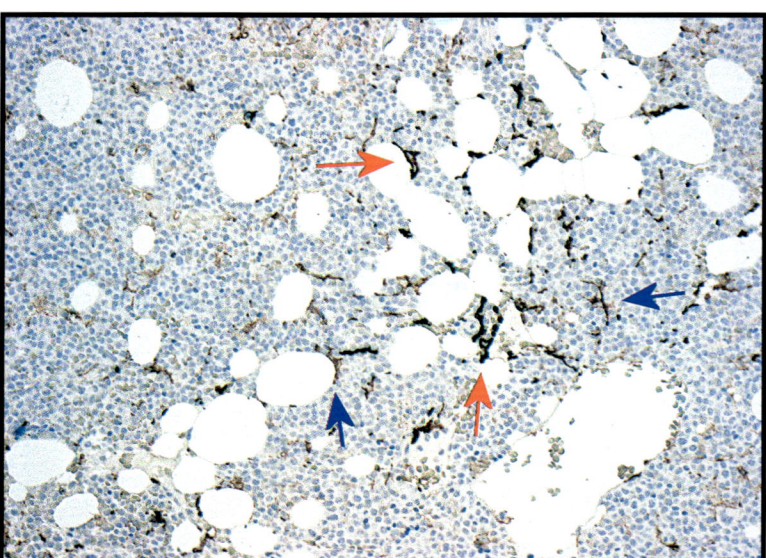

F3.10.11 CD14 in acute promyelocytic leukemia

The leukemic promyelocytes are negative. Unusually strong focal expression of CD14 is found in the dendritic extensions of stromal cells, some of which appear clearly related to adipocytes. The biological background and significance, if any, is unclear. Very little is known about bone marrow stromal cells in different diseases.

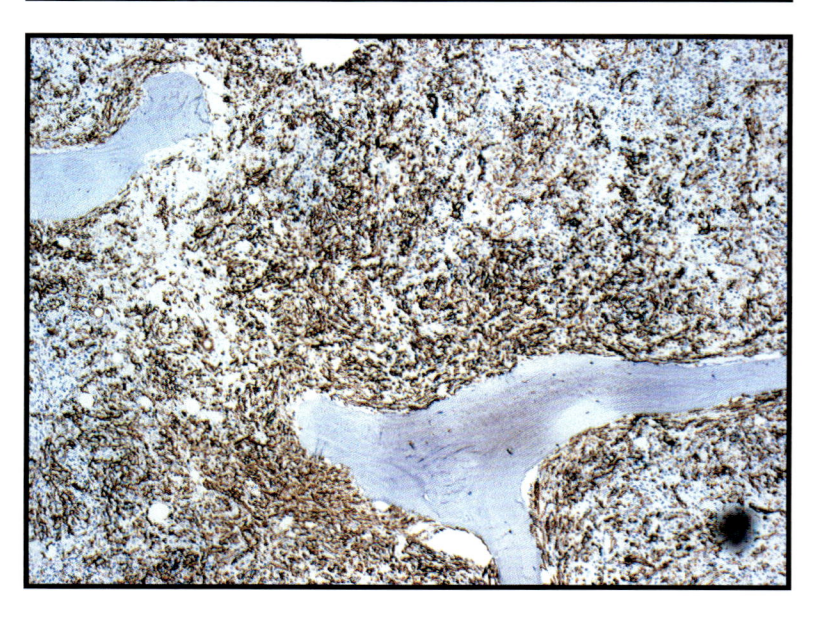

F3.10.12 CD14 in macrophages and dendritic cells in peripheral T-cell lymphoma (PTCL) with hemophagocytic syndrome

In this bone marrow biopsy specimen that is involved by PTCL, the number of CD14+ cells is markedly increased. In addition to BM macrophages, it appears that the CD14+ dendritic cell population is also a significant component. In some areas the density of the CD14+ cells is much lower (right upper corner).

3.10 CD14

F3.10.13 CD14 in peripheral T-cell lymphoma with hemophagocytic syndrome

An area with lower density of CD14+ cells is illustrated. The expression of CD14 varies in both cells with dendritic morphology and macrophages with or without obvious hemophagocytic activity.

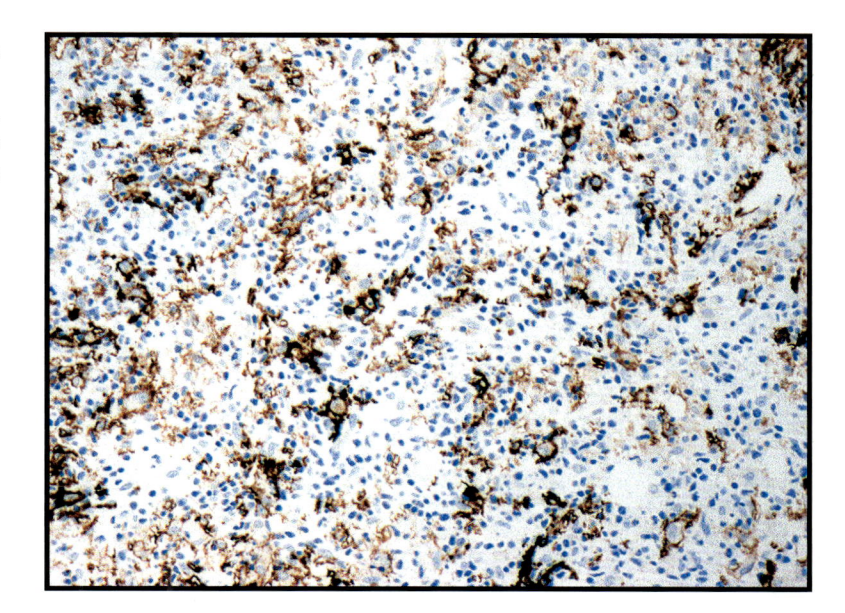

F3.10.14 CD14 in peripheral T-cell lymphoma with hemophagocytic syndrome

Large macrophages are markedly increased. Hemophagocytic content is found only in a few cells in this area. Compare this area with the area seen in **F3.10.15**, in which macrophages are closely intermixed with predominant spindled/dendritic cells.

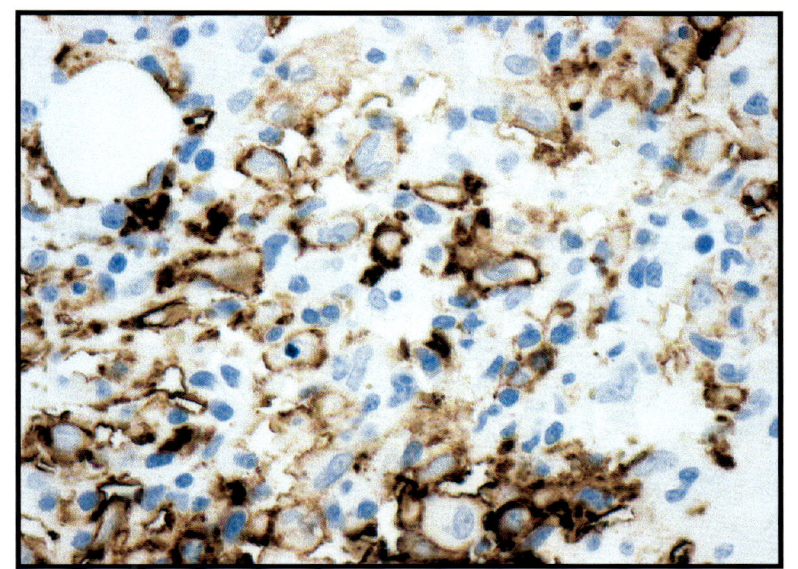

F3.10.15 CD14 in peripheral T-cell lymphoma with hemophagocytic syndrome

Areas like this are very difficult to interpret. There appears to be a closely intermixed population of macrophages, spindled cells, and cells with dendritic extensions. It is not clear whether these represent various functional stages of the same prototypic CD14+ stromal cell or they represent different stromal cells, all of which express CD14.

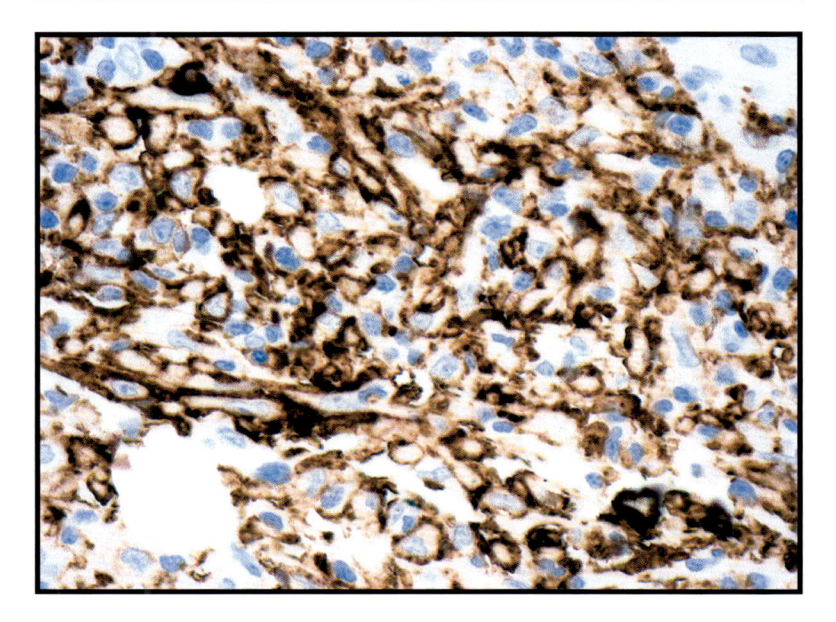

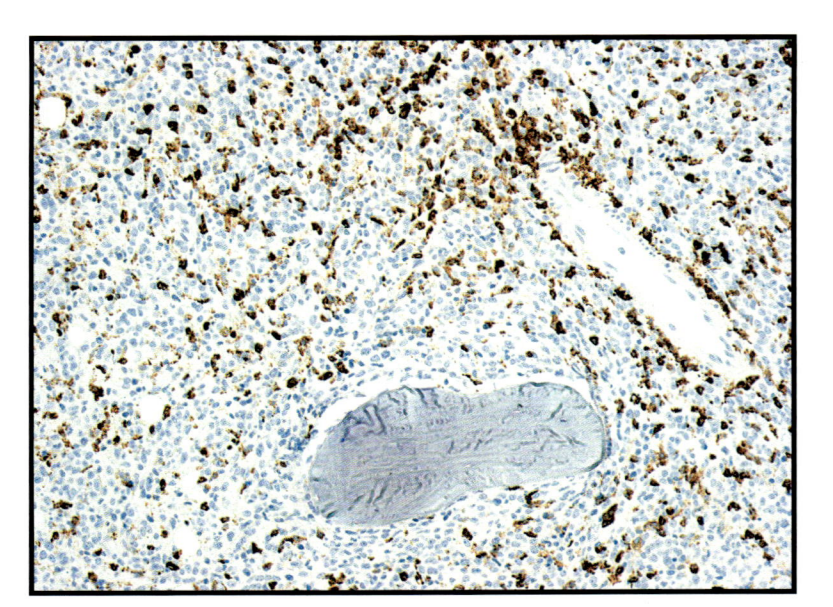

F3.10.16 CD14 in acute promyelocytic leukemia (APL)

This biopsy specimen is from a 72-year-old woman with APL. The usual perivascular CD14+ monocytic cells are present, but bone marrow macrophages with short dendritic extensions appear markedly increased and are evenly distributed throughout the BM. The leukemic cells of APL do not express CD14. See also **F3.10.17**.

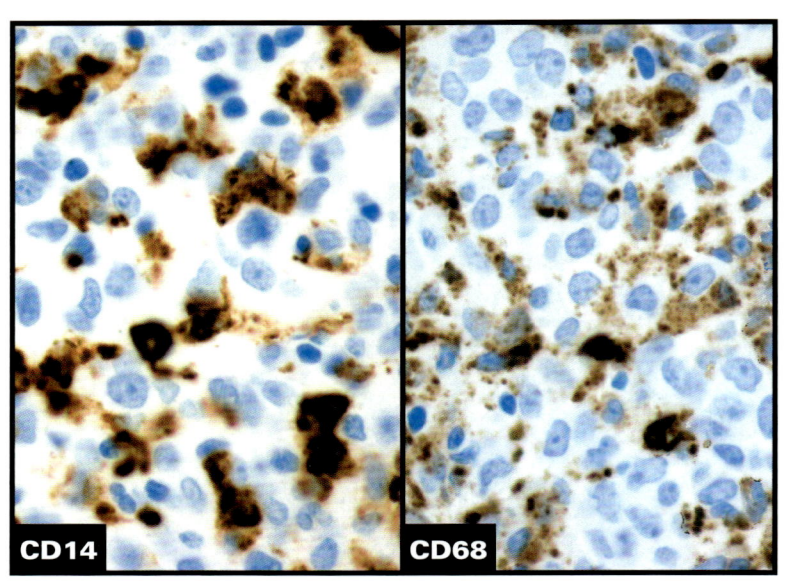

F3.10.17 CD14 and CD68 (PG-M1) in acute promyelocytic leukemia

The same case as in **F3.10.16**. These strongly stained cells are probably macrophages or a subtype of a stromal dendritic cell, which is either markedly increased or in which there is CD14 upregulation as a response to/interaction with tumor cells. Dendritic extensions appear shorter with CD14 than CD68 staining, indicating a different distribution of these antigens in the marrow macrophages. Alternatively (less likely), these represent 2 different populations of stromal cells.

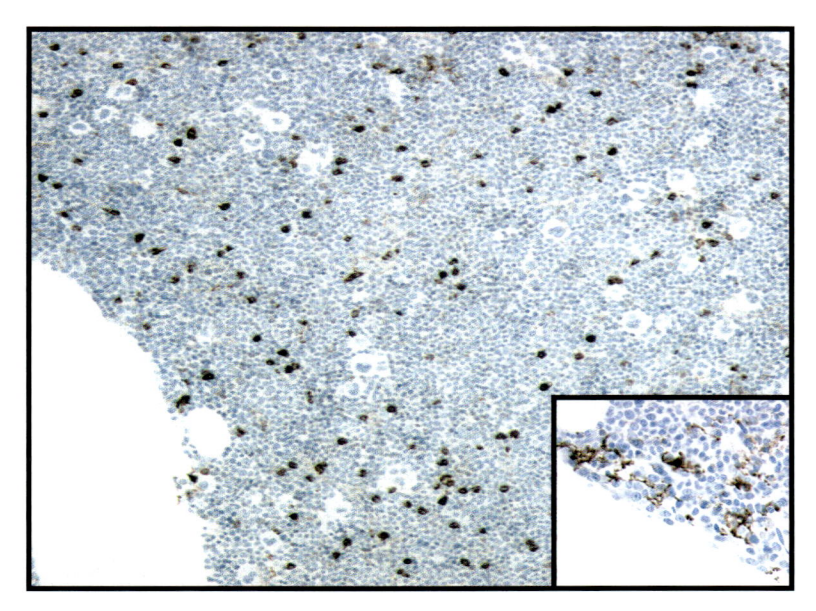

F3.10.18 CD14 in chronic myeloid leukemia (CML)

Monocytes are generally not increased in CML. The overall absolute content is probably comparable to the normal BM (see **F3.10.2**). Weakly stained CD14+ dendritic cells are present (see inset, right lower corner), but most of the time appear close to the bony trabeculae, rather than being randomly distributed as is the case in the normal BM or some acute leukemias.

3.11 CD15

CD15 is also known as nonsialated Lewis x, FUT4, ELFT, FCT3A, and FUC-TIV. It has a role in embryonic development, where it was termed "stage-specific embryonic antigen 1 (SSEA-1)" because it is one of the embryonic stem cell markers with an important role in adhesion and migration of the cells in the preimplantation embryo [Fox 1983]. CD15 is a myeloid marker that is expressed in mature human neutrophils, monocytes, and promyelocytes [Nakayama 2001]. Its expression can be induced in T cells [Azuma 2007]. It is most commonly used to detect classical Hodgkin lymphoma or sometimes as a second-choice marker to distinguish between mesothelioma and adenocarcinoma [Hsu 1984; Yaziji 2006]. The CD15 antigen is expressed on approximately 90% of human circulating granulocytes, and 30% to 60% of circulating monocytes; it is not present on normal lymphocytes. CD15 antigen is also expressed on Reed-Sternberg cells of Hodgkin disease, on lymphocytes of T-cell lymphomas including mycosis fungoides, and on some leukemias. CD15 plays a role in mediating phagocytosis, bactericidal activity, and chemotaxis. CD15 is downregulated in chronic myeloid leukemia [Yaziji 2006]. In AML, expression of CD15 is associated with, but not limited to AMLs with a monocytic component [Dunphy 2001]. Therefore, in the BM, the CD15 expression is evaluated in acute leukemia and classical Hodgkin lymphoma. Any other use is uncommon.

F3.11.1 CD15 in histologically normal bone marrow

Neutrophils and precursors are positive. Erythroid cells and megakaryocytes as well as lymphoid cells and all stromal cells are negative. With optimal staining, the normal BM is strongly stained because of the predominance of neutrophil series.

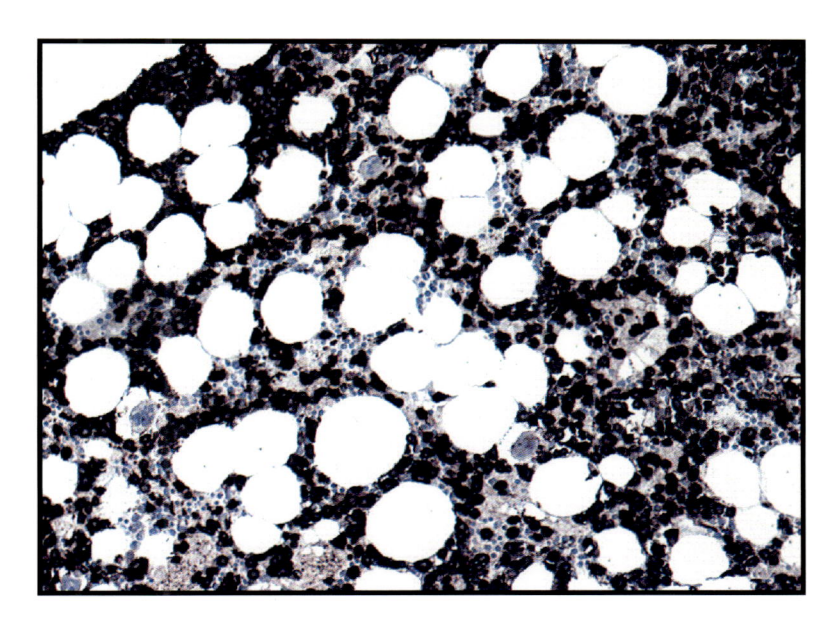

F3.11.2 CD15 in bone marrow with mild erythroid hyperplasia

CD15, as well as myeloperoxidase, can be used for determining the myeloid-erythroid ratio. This biopsy specimen showed mild erythroid hyperplasia, in an estimated myeloid-erythroid ratio of approximately 1:1.

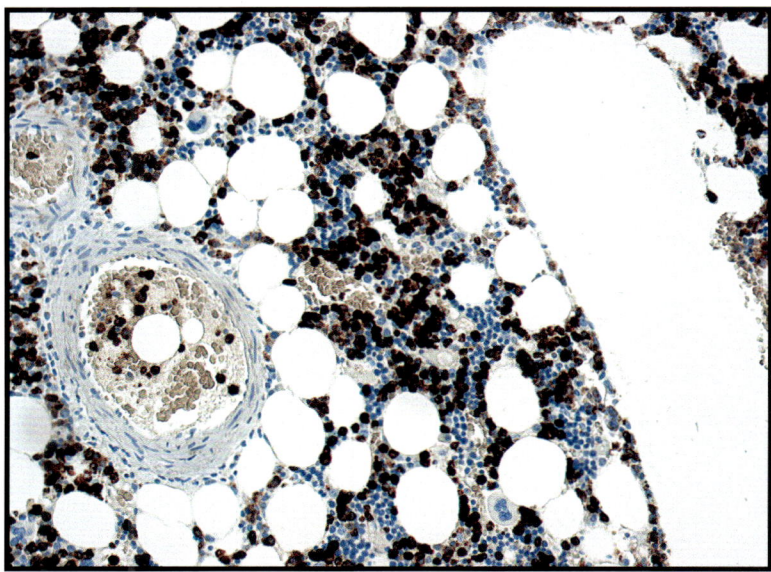

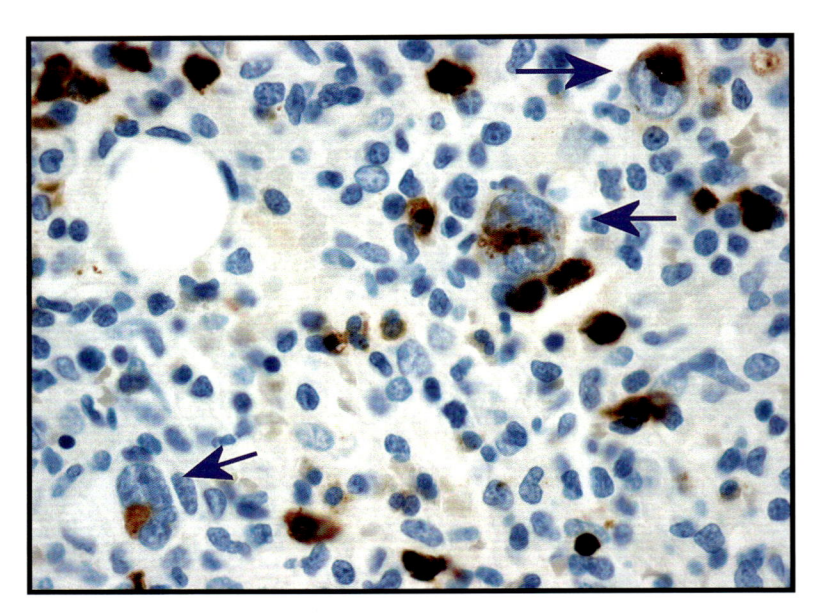

F3.11.3 CD15 in classical Hodgkin lymphoma (cHL)

Arrows point to Hodgkin cells, which were all positive for CD15. Illustrated is a rare case that did not show bone marrow fibrosis associated with involvement by cHL. In such cases, it is critical to demonstrate malignant cells by their immunophenotype because marrow megakaryocytes offer strong competition regarding morphologic appearance. CD15 epitope appears better preserved in B5-fixed tissue, but procedures may be optimized to perform as well in formalin-fixed tissue.

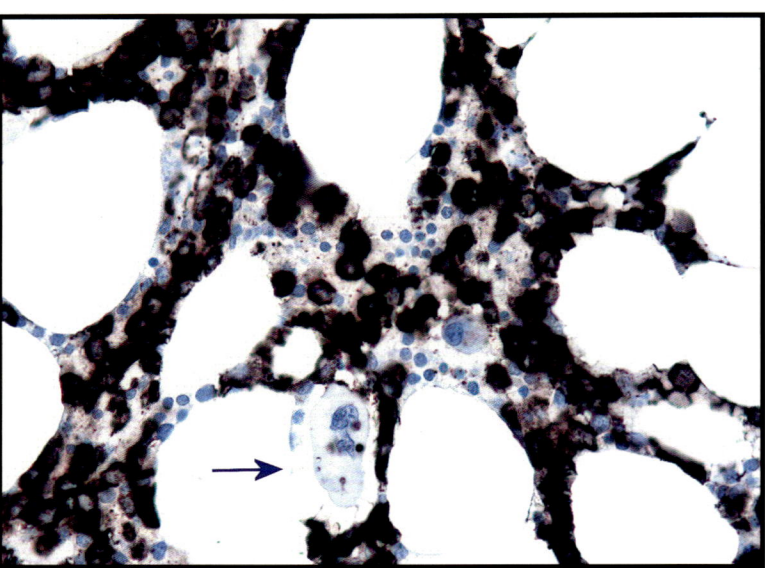

F3.11.4 CD15 with antigen diffusion

In any bone marrow with large content of neutrophils, some antigen diffusion is possible and it occasionally may be seen in the megakaryocytes (arrow). When evaluating such cells in the context of classical Hodgkin lymphoma, they should not be confused with Hodgkin cells.

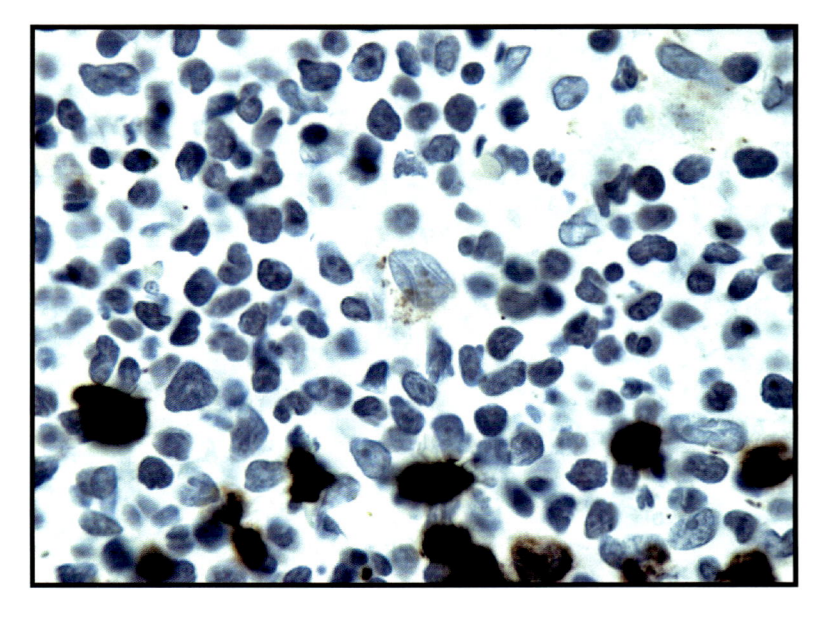

F3.11.5 CD15 in histiocytic and dendritic cells

Some dendritic cells in the lymphoid aggregates, benign or malignant, in the bone marrow or in other tissues, may express variable levels of CD15. However, this patient had classical Hodgkin lymphoma in the lymph node and this BM contained small lymphoid aggregates. Other large cells with borderline positivity for CD15 are CD30− and are most likely histiocytic or dendritic cell. Such cells should not be confused with Hodgkin cells.

F3.11.6 CD15 in acute myeloid leukemia (AML), minimally differentiated

Myeloperoxidase (MPO) was not detected in this case of AML. CD15+/MPO− immunophenotype would not be unusual in monoblastic leukemia, but in this case there was no cytochemical evidence of monocytic differentiation. Flow cytometry confirmed the diagnosis (CD117+, CD33+). No Auer rods were found. This case illustrates the fact that CD15 (left) and MPO (right) are not interchangeable. Also, higher specificity for myeloid differentiation of the MPO is not substituted by CD15, as seen in the European Group for the Immunologic Classification of Leukemia (EGIL) scores used to weigh evidence of lineage differentiation in acute leukemias (MPO=2, CD15=0.5).

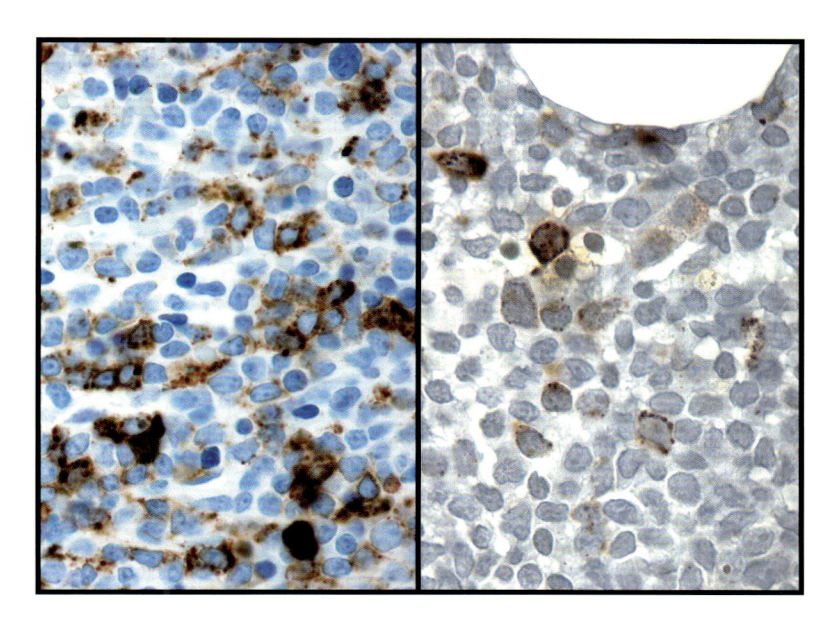

F3.11.7 CD15 in biphenotypic acute leukemia (acute lymphoblastic leukemia/acute myeloid leukemia)

This 72-year-old man with acute biphenotypic leukemia also had bone marrow fibrosis and only a few cells were aspirated. The aspirate clot specimen was evaluated and showed dotlike positivity in the blasts for CD15 (left) and no reactivity with anti-myeloperoxidase antibodies (right) in the paucicellular clot section. The leukemic cells were positive for myeloid markers CD33, CD11b, CD14, and lymphoid markers TdT, cCD3, CD2, and CD7 on flow cytometry.

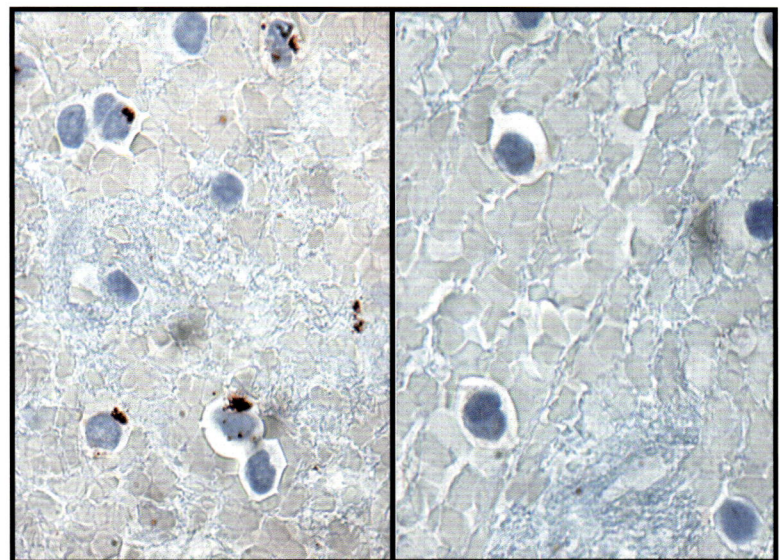

F3.11.8 CD15 in acute myeloid/erythroid leukemia

Acute erythroid leukemia rarely shows expression of myeloid antigens, although no large studies have been done. In this case, rare cells with Golgi-type positivity could be found (red arrows). Many other cells show peculiar brown dots over the nuclei and in the scant cytoplasm (blue arrows), which is insufficient evidence to interpret this as true CD15 positivity.

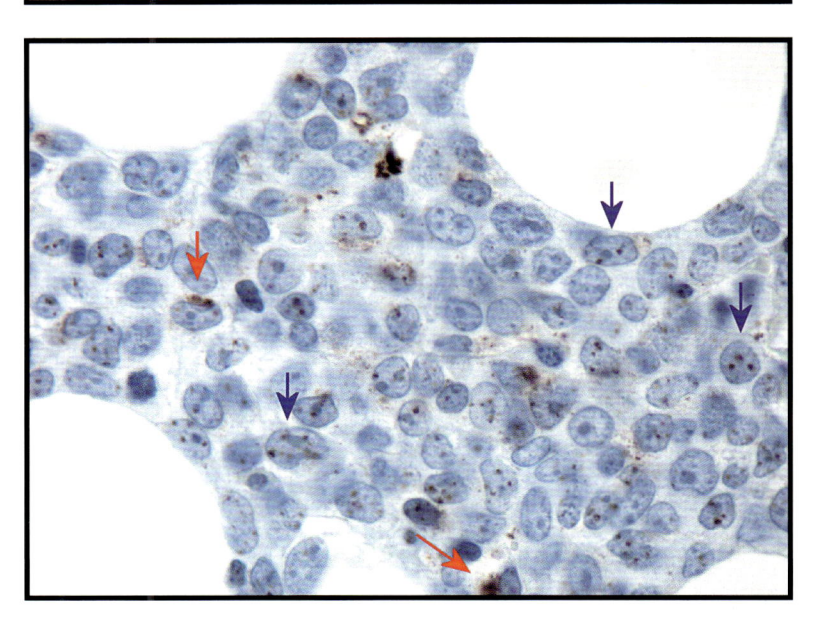

3.12 CD16

CD16 is a Fc gama receptor IIIa (CD16a), which is expressed by NK cells and macrophages and also IIIB (CD16b), which is expressed by granulocytes (PROW). The CD16 antibodies that react in paraffin-embedded tissue detect all of the above and therefore, NK cells, macrophages, and granulocytes will be positive. Specification of the Ab reactivity needs to be evaluated before the results are interpreted. In contrast to CD10, which is expressed only in postmitotic mature neutrophils, CD16 expression is acquired during the metamyelocyte stage and levels gradually increase with continuing morphologic maturation [Terstappen 1990]. Eosinophils generally do not express CD16. However, expression of CD16 on the surface of eosinophils can be found on activated eosinophils in the peripheral blood [Davoine 2004]. BM macrophages are also reported as both strongly positive for CD16 and CD4 and negative for CD16 and CD4 [Lee 1991; Köller 1996]. This contradiction is probably because of the method of marrow macrophage selection for the studies. Those that are strongly positive for CD4 were isolated from erythroid islands [Lee 1991] and those that were reported as CD4 negative were selected on flow cytometry after BM culture with granulocyte-macrophage colony-stimulating factor (GM-CSF) and macrophage colony-stimulating factor (M-CSF) [Köller 1996]. Various appearances of the BM macrophages in chronic myelomonocytic leukemia have been illustrated by Orazi et al [2006].

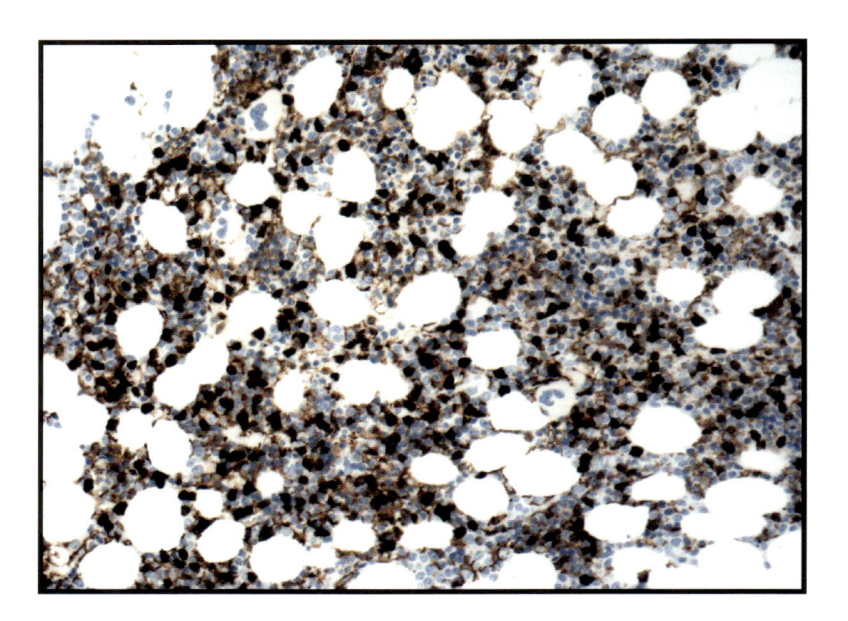

F3.12.1 CD16 in histologically normal bone marrow

The staining intensity is high in many cells and the pattern of distribution is rather complex. Megakaryocytes are clearly negative and neutrophils clearly positive. Monocytes, macrophages, and natural killer (NK) cells can not be identified with certainty even though they are presumed to be positive and present in this BM specimen.

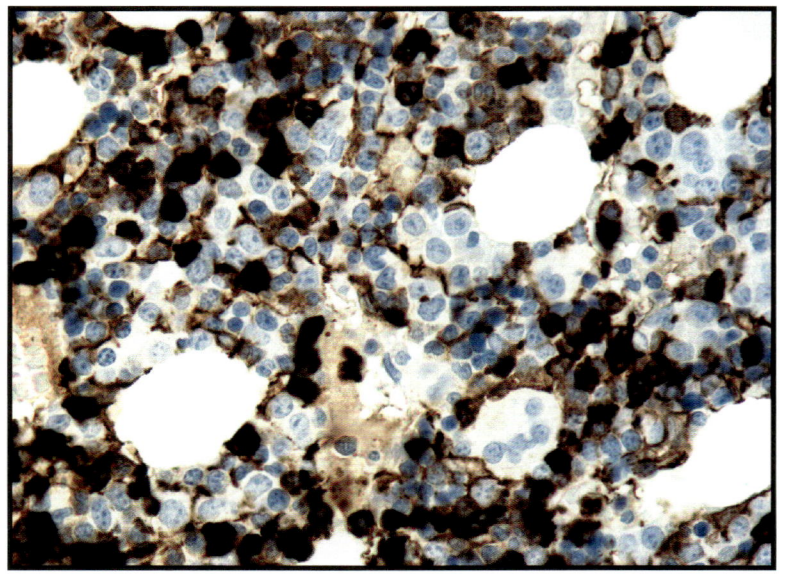

F3.12.2 CD16 in histologically normal bone marrow

Note the following 2 patterns: cytoplasmic and membranous staining. The most mature neutrophils show strong cytoplasmic expression, but are also known to have surface positivity as detected with flow cytometry. Weak diffuse cytoplasmic and strong membranous staining appears to be more characteristic of macrophages/stromal dendritic cells, which are seen percolating in between the different cell types.

3.12 CD16

F3.12.3 CD16 in histologically normal bone marrow

An erythroid island (erythron) appears to contain very delicate intercellular positivity possibly related to its association with marrow macrophages (red arrow). These are probably the only marrow macrophages that also express high levels of CD4. In contrast to neutrophils, eosinophils do not show expression of CD16 (green arrow). However, CD16 is transiently expressed in some activated eosinophils and may have a role in eosinophil degranulation [2].

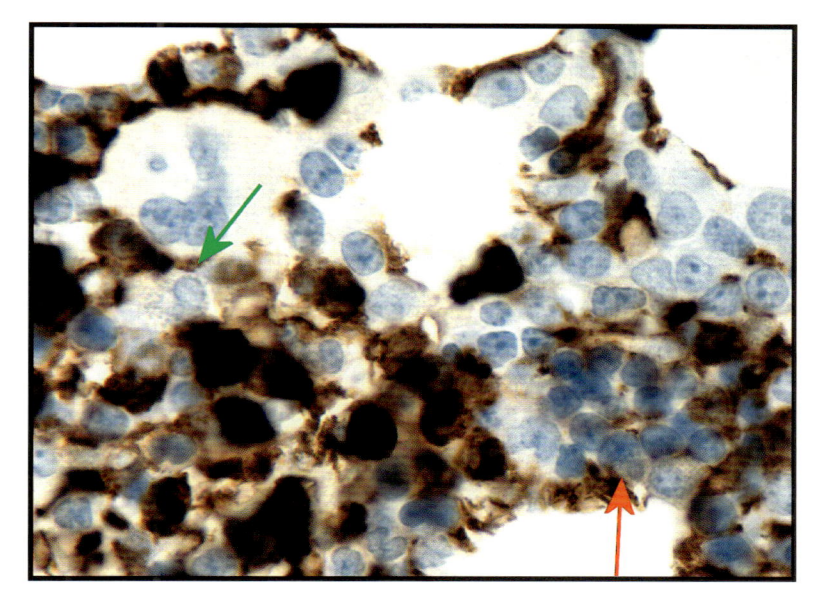

F3.12.4 CD16 in normal neutrophil maturation

CD16 is not expressed in early neutrophil precursors. Neutrophil precursors in the juxtatrabecular location in this reactive bone marrow are negative. Only a few dendritic extensions of the stromal cells can be seen in this area.

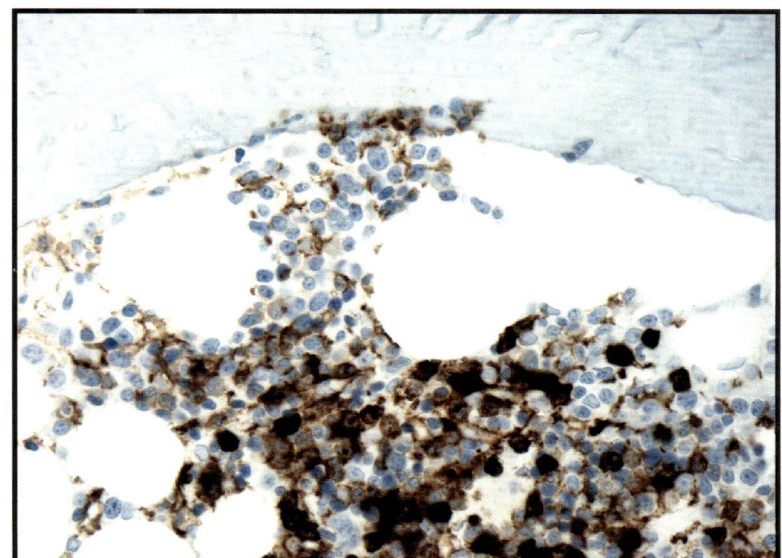

F3.12.5 CD16 in metamyelocytes, bands, and segmented neutrophils

CD16 is first noted in neutrophil metamyelocytes (red arrow). It increases as neutrophil maturation progresses and moderate positivity is noted in bands (blue arrow). Segmented neutrophils show very high levels of CD16 expression. Therefore, CD16 is considered a marker of neutrophil maturation.

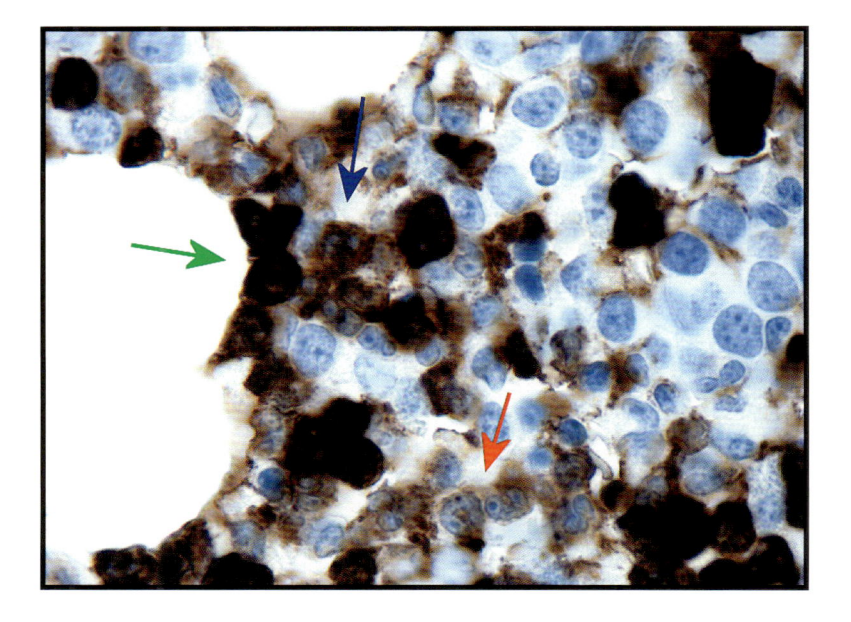

3: Cluster of Differentiation Markers

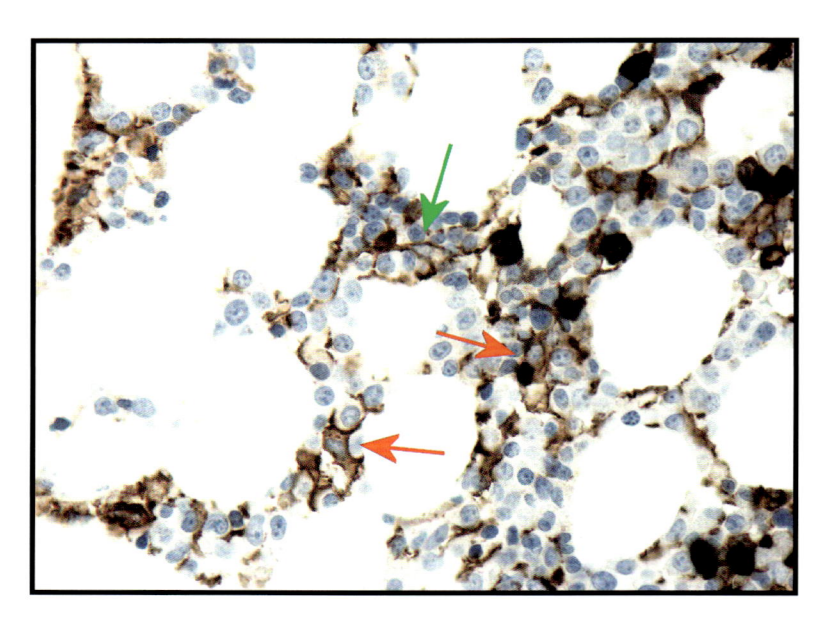

F3.12.6 CD16 in macrophages/dendritic cells

It is difficult to appreciate the macrophages and dendritic cells in areas rich in neutrophils. However, these can be observed as cells with irregular shape and complex cytoplasmic extensions (red arrows). The cytoplasmic CD16 is rather weak, while membranous expression stands out. However, most of the time only dendritic extensions can be detected (green arrow).

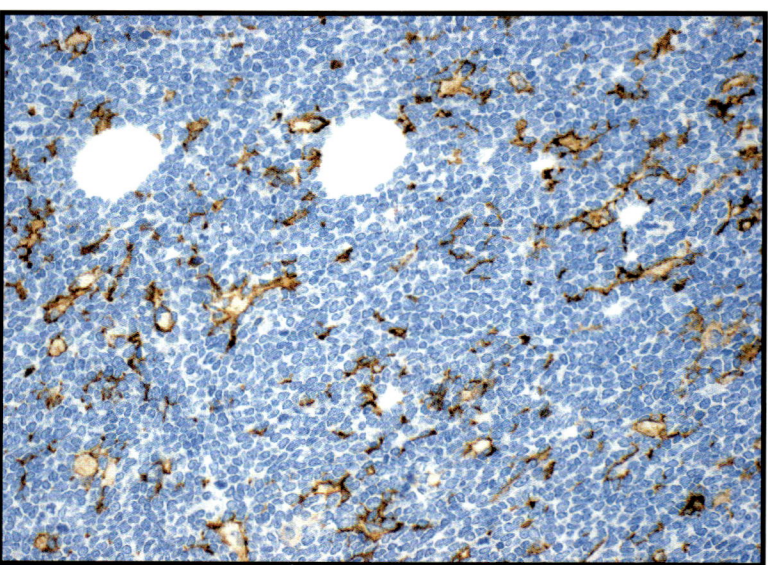

F3.12.7 CD16 in stromal cells in undifferentiated acute leukemia

These stromal cells with dendritic morphology are presumed to be bone marrow macrophages which are increased in this case of acute leukemia. However, they are not identified by using some other so-called monocyte/macrophage markers.

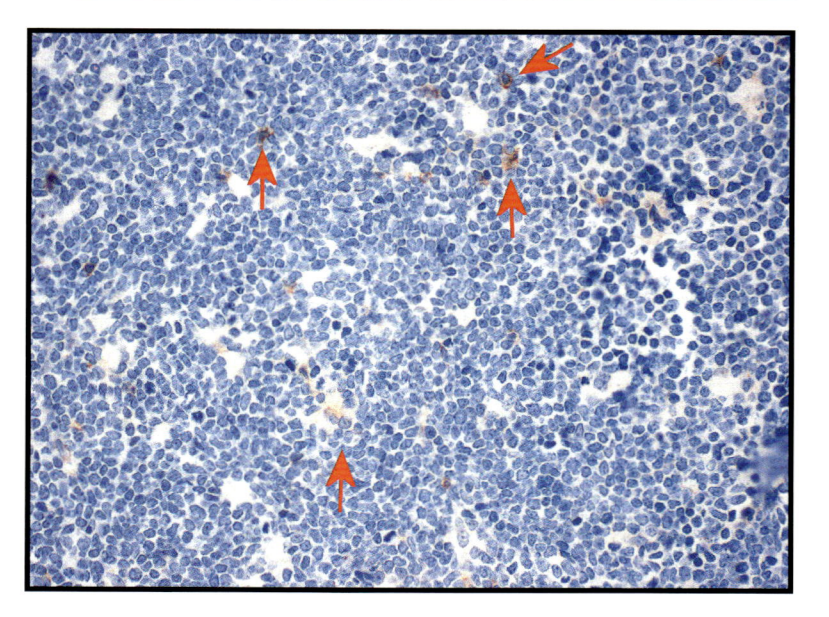

F3.12.8 CD4 in the same case as in F3.12.1

This biopsy specimen is from a 57-year-old woman with acute leukemia. While peripheral blood monocytes and tissue macrophages express CD4, not all bone marrow macrophages are consistently CD4+. CD16+ dendritic stromal cells are CD4− in this case. The BM macrophages that are associated with erythroid precursors are strongly positive for CD4, but this population appears absent in this BM specimen with no evidence of erythroid maturation.

F3.12.9 Comparison of CD16 and CD68 (PG-M1); same case as in **F3.12.1**

Both CD68 and CD16 are found in macrophages and are expected to be coexpressed. However, the antigen distribution is not the same. CD16 is predominantly a surface antigen, while CD68 is a lysosomal membrane glycoprotein in the cytoplasm. Lysosomes appear not to be present in the long dendritic extensions (for the most part), resulting in the more globular shape of the CD68+ cells. The leukemic cells are negative for both markers.

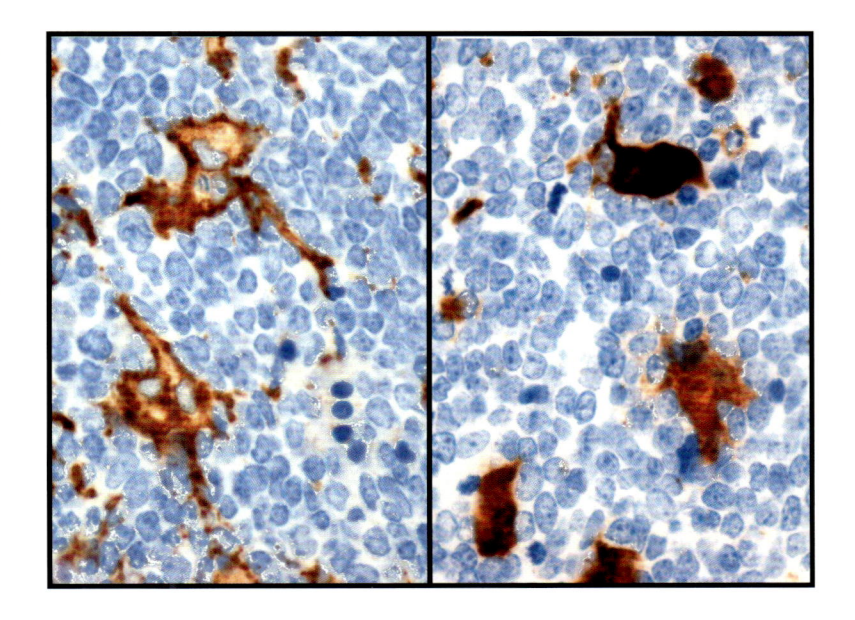

3.13 CD20

CD20 is also known as membrane-spanning 4-domains subfamily A member 1 (MS4A1), Leu-16, Bp35, B1, S7, and MGC3969 (OMIM). CD20 is a pan-B-cell marker because it is expressed early in the ontogeny of B-cell development and continues to be expressed until it becomes downregulated at the plasma cell stage [Matthias 2005; Loken 1987]. Generally, there are more mature T cells than mature B cells in normal BM [Shin 1992; Horny 1993]. An increased number of CD20+ cells in the BM may be seen because of either increased normal B-cell precursors (hematogones) or an increased mature B-cell population that infiltrates the BM due to various causes (ie, autoimmune disorders, polyclonal B-cell lymphocytosis, infection, or as a response to a nonlymphoid neoplasm in the BM) [Vandersteenhoven 1993; Bass 2001; Feugier 2004; Navone 1985]. Some benign plasma cells express CD20 and it is also expressed in CD20+ multiple myeloma [Robillard 2003].

Some general observations regarding CD20 expression are as follows:

1. In B cells, its expression most of the time parallels expression of CD45 and Pax-5.
2. It is a more specific marker of B-cell differentiation than CD79a.
3. In chronic lymphocytic leukemia, it is variably expressed, but generally weak.
4. In lymphoplasmacytic lymphoma, it is variable from case to case and could vary from cell to cell depending on the end of the spectrum and the extent of terminal B-cell differentiation.
5. It may not be detectable in some patients treated with anti-CD20 therapy either because of the presence of bound rituximab or, as described in some patients, the loss of CD20 expression in relapsed lymphoma [Haidar 2003; Seliem 2006; Foran 2001]. In theory, L26 (the most commonly used clone in IHC) detects cytoplasmic epitopes of the CD20, which are not bound or recognized by rituximab. Therefore, the negative results with L26 after rituximab therapy are caused by either the destruction of the CD20+ cells or clonal expansion of CD20− lymphoma cells. Rituximab is an IgG1 antibody. If the lymphoma expresses IgM or λ, detection of IgG or κ on the surface suggests bound rituximab. This implies that the cells remain CD20 positive and that rituximab is blocking detection.
6. By definition, it is not expressed in plasmablastic variant of DLBCL.
7. It is expressed in some cases of precursor B lymphoblastic leukemia (approximately 20% cases) and may occasionally be useful in detection of residual disease immediately after chemotherapy.
8. There is no real substitute for CD20 detection in the evaluation of malignant lymphoma. Pax-5 is gaining acceptance and is more widely used than before, but its significance rarely can be interpreted without reference to the CD20.
9. In many institutions, it is routinely used for evaluation of the BM biopsy for staging of non-Hodgkin lymphoma and Hodgkin lymphoma, acute leukemia panel, as well as in cases in which B-cell lymphoproliferative disease is considered (fever of unknown origin, history of autoimmune disease, etc).
10. In contrast to CD3, CD30, CD79a, and many other lymphoid markers, the "cytoplasmic CD20 expression" is not known to have any diagnostic meaning. However, the term "detection of cytoplasmic CD20" usually refers to "detection of cytoplasmic domain/epitope of CD20 by L26 mAb."
11. FMC7 mAb, which is used for flow cytometry detects a cholesterol-dependent epitope of CD20 and thus appears to be a sensitive indicator of the level of plasma membrane cholesterol and reveals a conformational state of CD20 that is regulated by cholesterol [Polyak 2003].
12. While rare B-cell lymphomas with CD20 expression have been described to express cytokeratin, epithelial tumors have not been described to express CD20 despite their relatively frequent expression of some other so-called leukocyte markers including CD5, CD79a, Pax-5, CD15, or CD10.

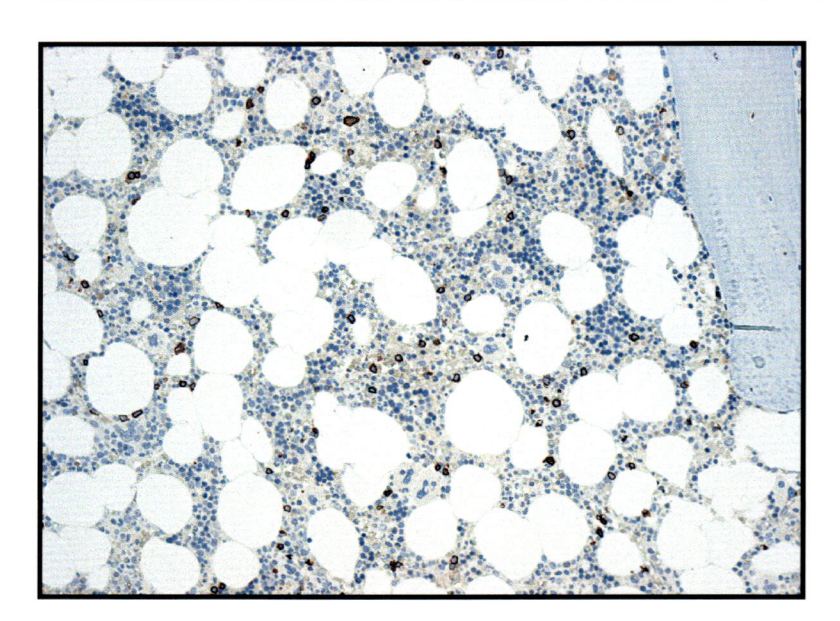

F3.13.1 CD20 in histologically normal bone marrow

While there are no morphologic abnormalities in this BM specimen from a 34-year-old man, the patient had nodal classical Hodgkin lymphoma; the number of B cells illustrated may not be entirely representative of asymptomatic healthy adults. However, this number and distribution of B cells should not be considered suspicious for a lymphoproliferative disease.

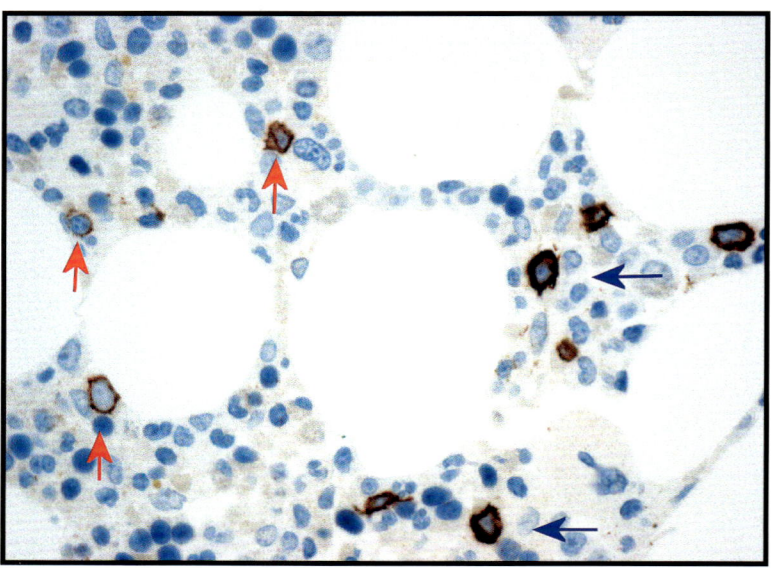

F3.13.2 CD20 in histologically normal bone marrow

The same patient as in **F3.13.1**. Some cells show strong membranous expression of CD20 (blue arrows), while others appear to show weaker and possibly cytoplasmic expression of CD20 (red arrows). It is presumed that the cells with weaker expression represent maturing B cells.

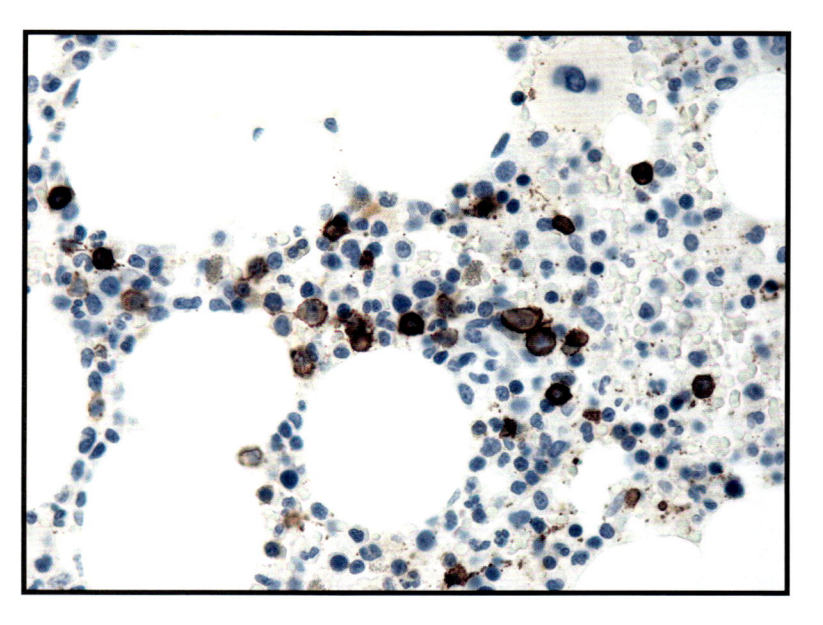

F3.13.3 CD20 in histologically normal bone marrow

This biopsy specimen is from a 37-year-old man with nodal nodular lymphocyte predominance Hodgkin lymphoma (NLPHL) stage I. The CD20+ B cells are increased, and in many areas, some larger cells with weaker expression of CD20 are noted. This should not be considered evidence of NLPHL in the BM because it clearly represents reactive change. Some of these cells may represent hematogones.

3.13 CD20

F3.13.4 CD20 in reactive bone marrow

The B cells are increased. However, they have a random distribution and do not aggregate. They are also frequently characterized by cytoplasmic ruffles (arrows), which in double staining with CD34, are present in cells that are just adjacent to sinusoids or are traversing into the vascular lumens. This could represent an indicator of an active migration into the circulation after maturation has been completed.

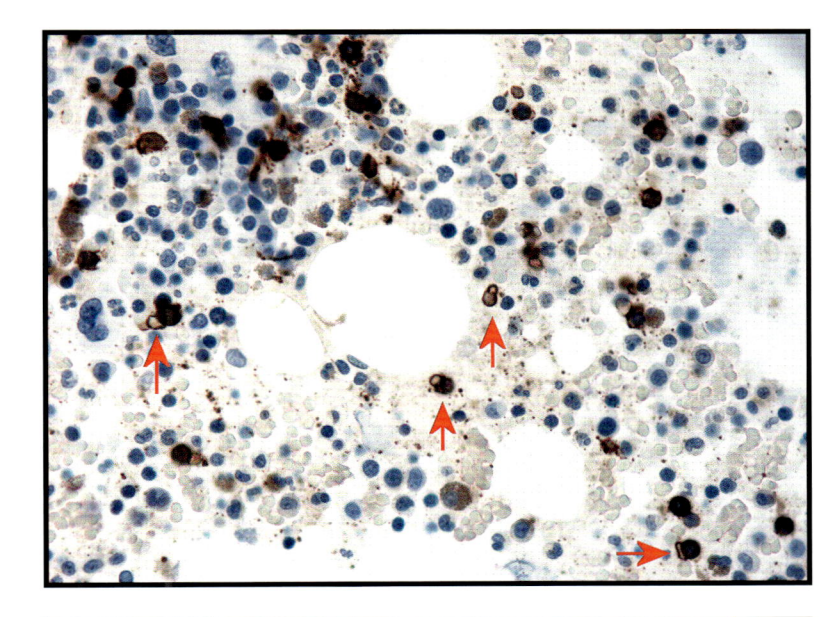

F3.13.5 CD20 in histologically normal bone marrow

Even in histologically unremarkable BM specimens, the cytoplasmic ruffles can often be found with CD20 antibody. Many cells with such cytoplasmic ruffles appear like cells with irregular cytoplasmic outline. The ruffles are not seen in each cross-section or plane of focus. Compare this with the CD14 staining shown in **F3.10.3**, where similar ruffles can be seen in monocytic cells. We have detected only these 2 epitopes that produce cytoplasmic ruffles.

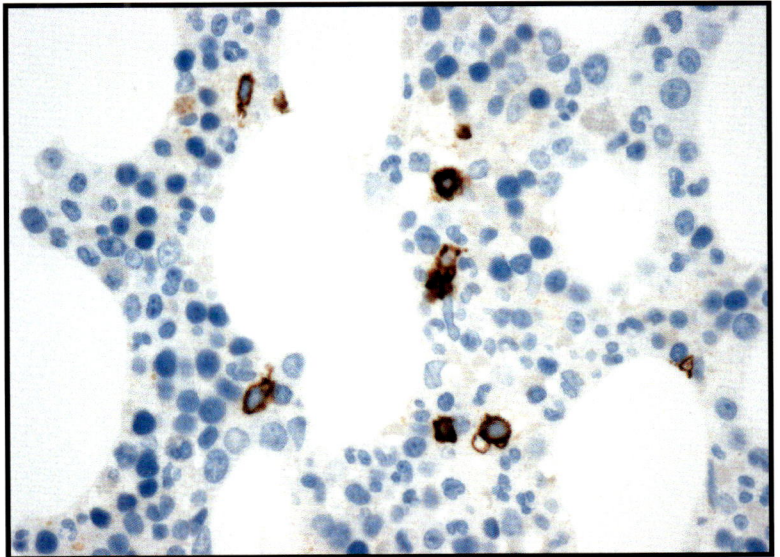

F3.13.6 CD20 in systemic lupus erythematosus

In autoimmune diseases, the content of B cells as well as plasma cells can be somewhat increased. Note that most cells have irregular cytoplasmic outlines because of the formation of ruffles. With CD20/CD34 double staining, most of these cells would be found in the vicinity of the sinusoids. This finding strongly favors a benign nature of the B cells.

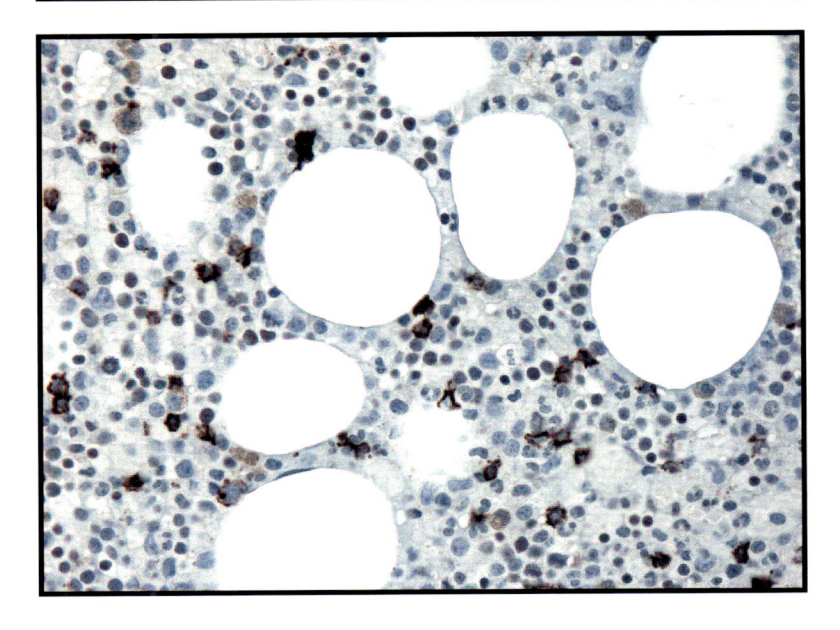

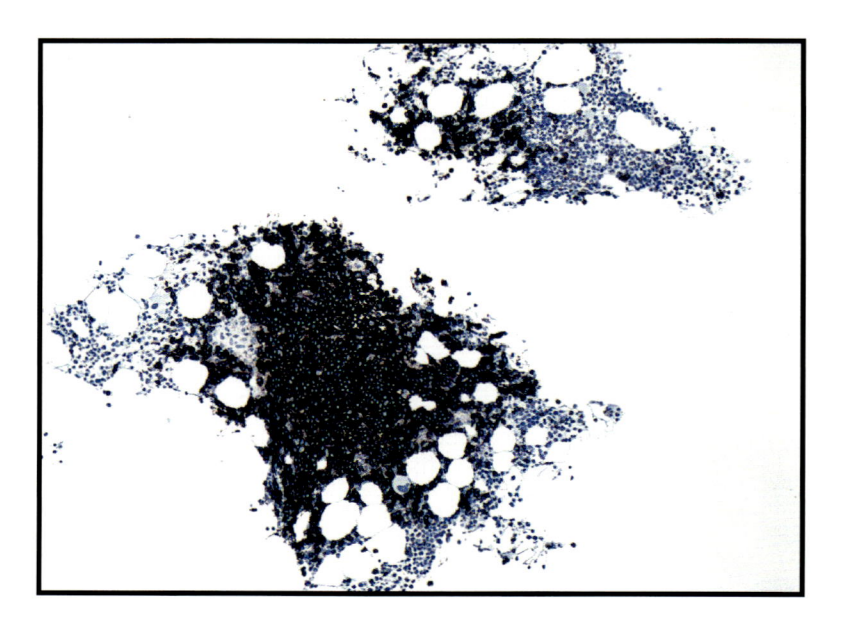

F3.13.7 CD20 in large lymphoid aggregates

These lymphoid aggregates were found only in the clot section; the 2.2-cm core biopsy section did not contain any. The patient was a 61-year-old man with mantle cell lymphoma. Such large CD20+ lymphoid aggregates are highly suggestive of malignancy and can be seen in different B-cell lymphoproliferative disorders.

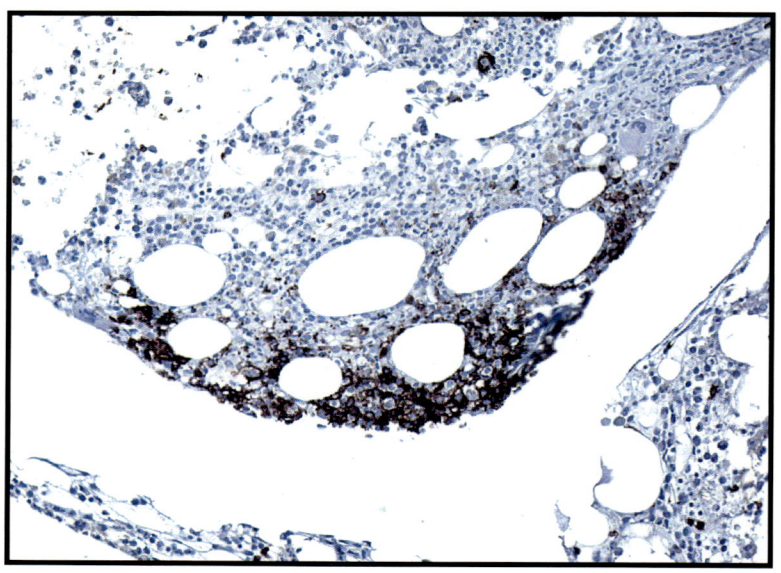

F3.13.8 CD20 in follicular lymphoma (FL)

In FL, it is typical to find paratrabecular aggregates. In contrast to juxtatrabecular aggregates, the width-to-length ratio of these aggregates is 2:5 or smaller. While the numerical value of the ratio is not critical, it is important that the B cells marginate along the bone and not just aggregate close to it. However, FL may also form interstitial lymphoid aggregates and other lymphomas may show a paratrabecular pattern. Chronic lymphocytic leukemia typically does not form paratrabecular lymphoid infiltrates.

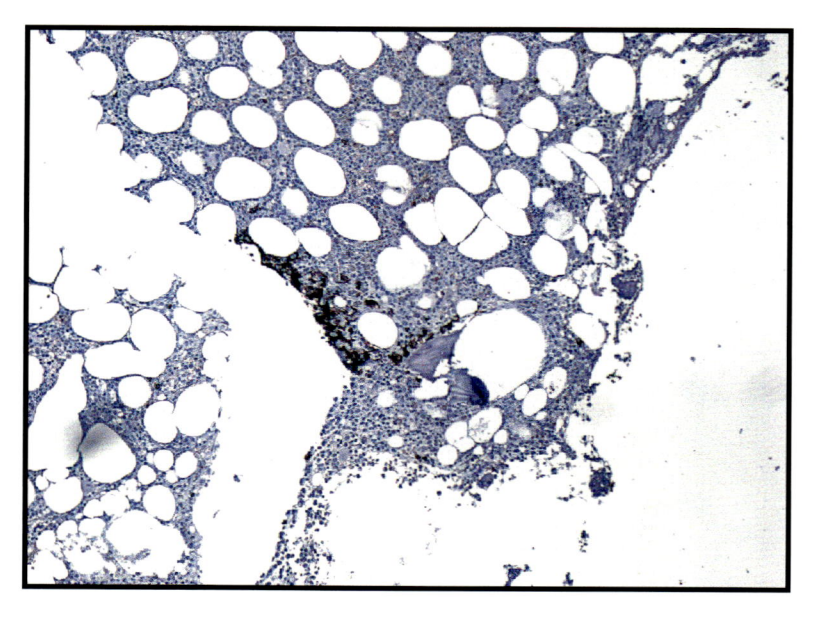

F3.13.9 CD20 in follicular lymphoma (FL)

In this 43-year-old woman with nodal FL grade 1, the 2.5-cm long bone marrow biopsy showed only a single small paratrabecular B-cell lymphoid aggregate. CD10 and Bcl-6 were negative in this area. However, this is sufficient to establish a diagnosis of "consistent with minimal evidence of FL" in the BM. Reactive or normal BM does not contain such distinct paratrabecular B cells. Such infiltrates generally cannot be appreciated with a morphologic examination alone.

F3.13.10 CD20 in a 55-year-old man with nodal follicular lymphoma

This biopsy specimen shows an ill-defined focal interstitial aggregate of small B cells. CD20+ aggregates of this type show focal fat infiltration rather than expanding borders. This finding may be problematic and needs to be interpreted with caution. These may be either reactive or malignant lymphoid infiltrations. The field shown may be a fat granuloma. This patient did not show any evidence of focally or diffusely increased B cells in the BM 4 months later.

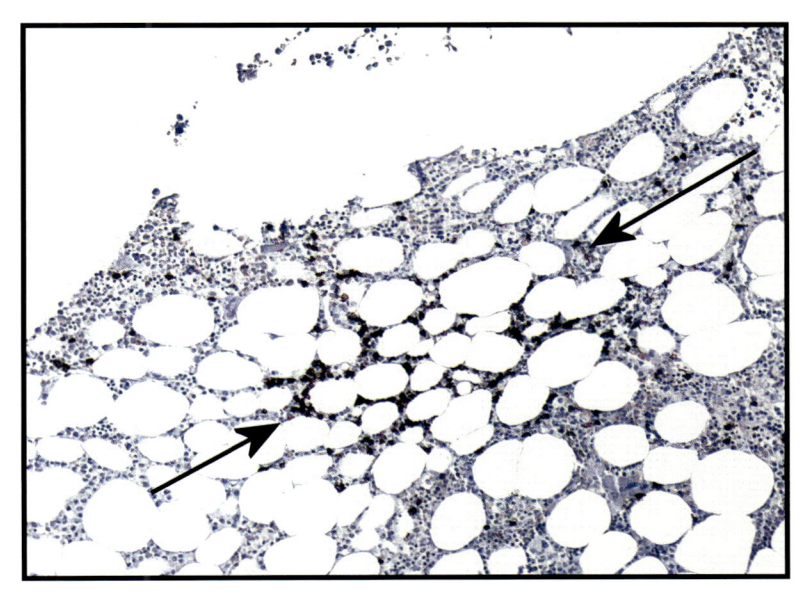

F3.13.11 CD20 in very small lymphoid aggregates

The patient was a 74-year-old with history of adenocarcinoma of the stomach. These small, ill-defined lymphoid aggregates were also CD23+, CD5+, and were interpreted as focal involvement by chronic lymphocytic leukemia. Bone marrow aspirate showed monoclonal B-cell population by PCR assay. Note that despite the small size and interstitial location, this would be an atypical finding for a benign lesion because the contours are not rounded and there is extension between the fat cells as well as great predominance of B cells.

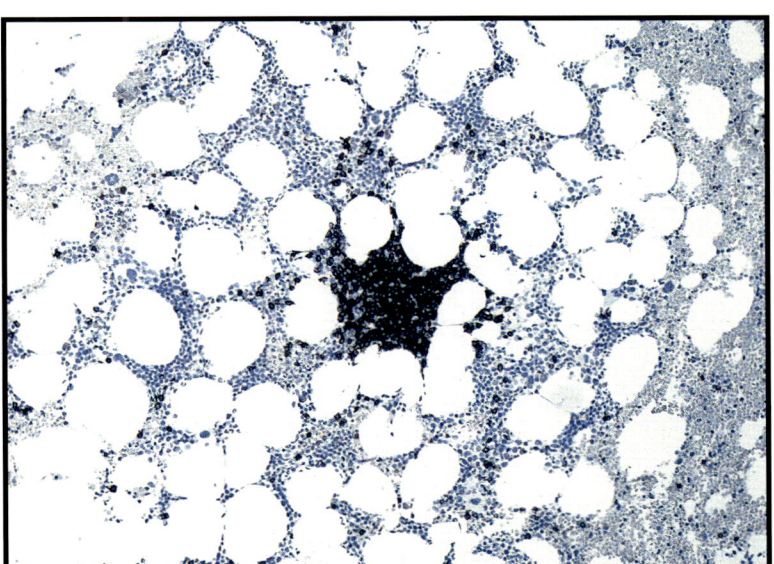

F3.13.12 CD20 in mantle cell lymphoma

Such very small interstitial clusters of B cells are frequently seen in mantle cell lymphoma, in particular when the involvement of the bone marrow is minimal. If cyclin D1 and CD5 can clearly be demonstrated as in this case, there is no difficulty in establishing a diagnosis. If the biopsy specimen was not screened with CD20 immunostaining, these inconspicuous clusters may have been missed.

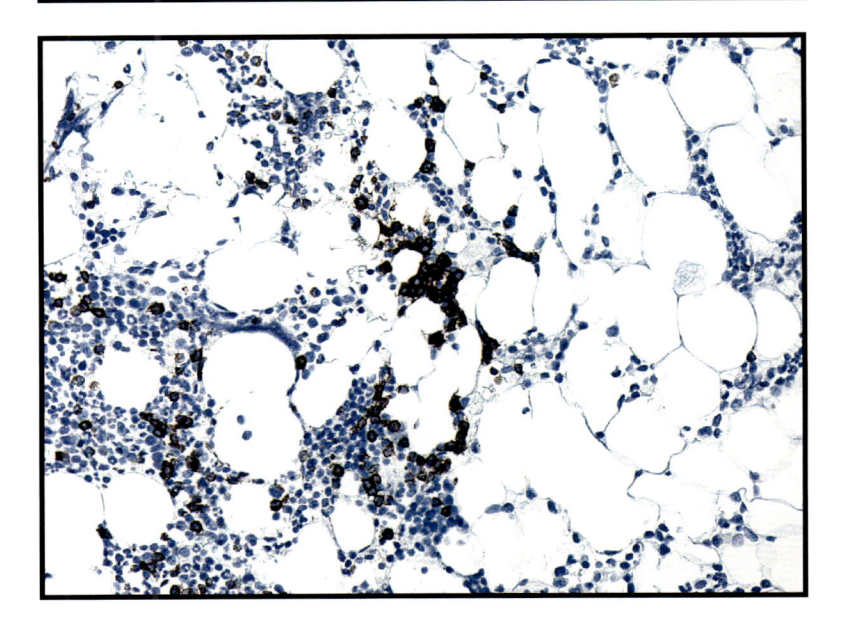

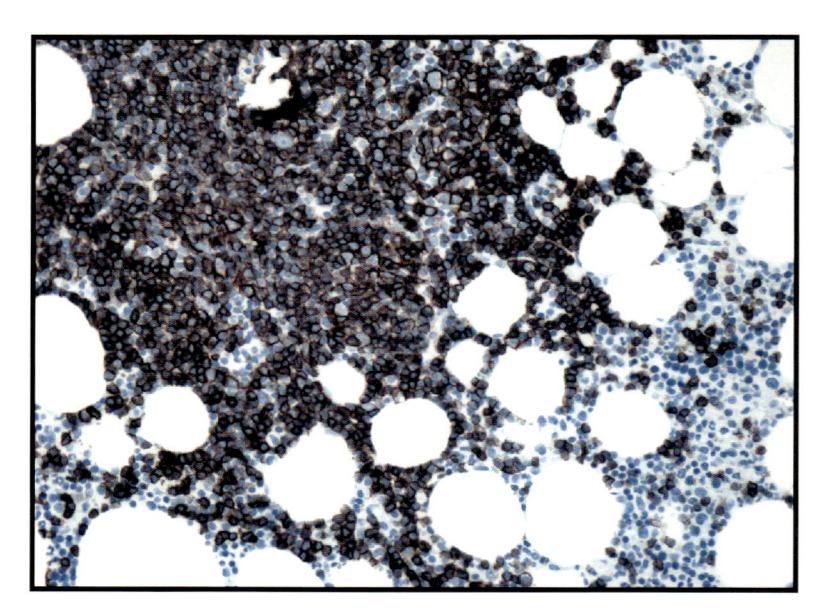

F3.13.13 CD20 in marginal zone lymphoma (MZL)

While strong overall, CD20 expression varies from cell to cell in this case of MZL. This variation in CD20 expression often reflects the variable extent of terminal B-cell differentiation from cell to cell. MZL involves the bone marrow in many different patterns, but the paratrabecular pattern is rare. An intrasinusoidal pattern is common, in particular in splenic MZL, but not specific and it is not invariably present. The size of the cells also may vary, but most cells should be small.

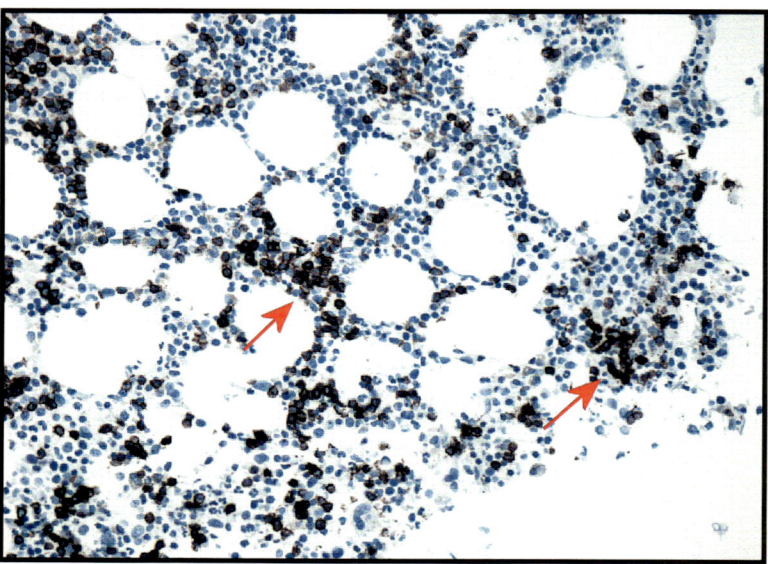

F3.13.14 CD20 in marginal zone lymphoma (MZL)

Same case as in F3.13.13. In some areas the cells are present in sinusoids (arrows). In many cases, no large lymphoid aggregates are present and this is the only evidence of bone marrow involvement. Because of a lower nuclear-cytoplasmic ratio than in many other small B-cell lymphoproliferative disorders and lack of frank nuclear atypia, these cells can be overlooked in routine stains. Therefore, CD20 immunohistochemistry is highly recommended in the evaluation of BM biopsy specimens in all patients with MZL.

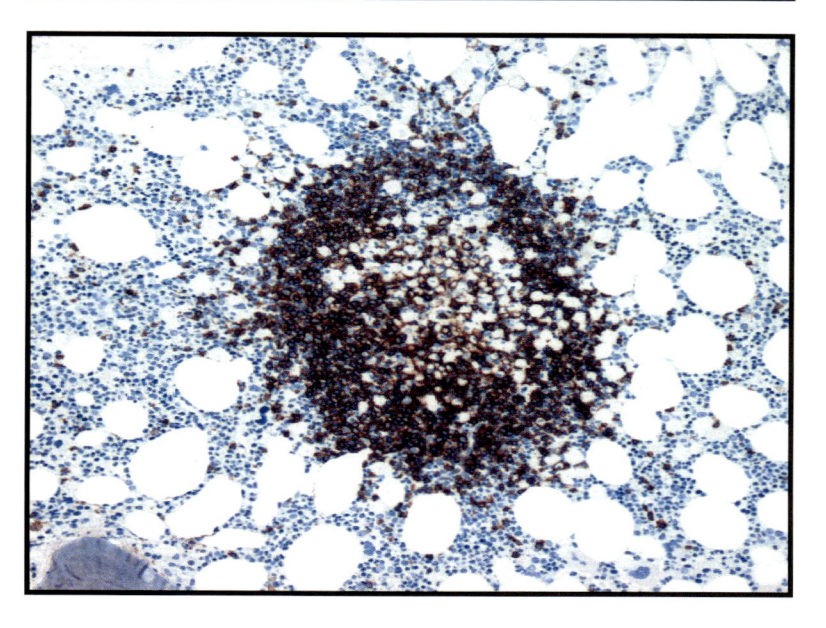

F3.13.15 CD20 in lymphoplasmacytic lymphoma (LPL)

LPL shows a spectrum of differentiation between mature B cells and terminally differentiated B cells, where CD20 is downregulated; the content of each varies greatly from case to case. In this example, the lymphoid nodules were populated with IgM+/κ+ plasma cells (CD20 negative center). MZL should be considered in the differential diagnosis, but clinically this was primary BM disease with very high serum IgM, which was incompatible with MZL.

F3.13.16 CD20 in diffuse large B-cell lymphoma treated with rituximab

It is claimed that opsonization of the CD20+ cells by rituximab should not cause false negative results with CD20 immunohistochemistry because L26 clone detects cytoplasmic component of the CD20 molecule. In this particular case, only weak cytoplasmic dotlike positivity is demonstrated (arrows). It is not clear whether the cells do not express surface CD20 or they appear to have no surface reactivity because of rituximab.

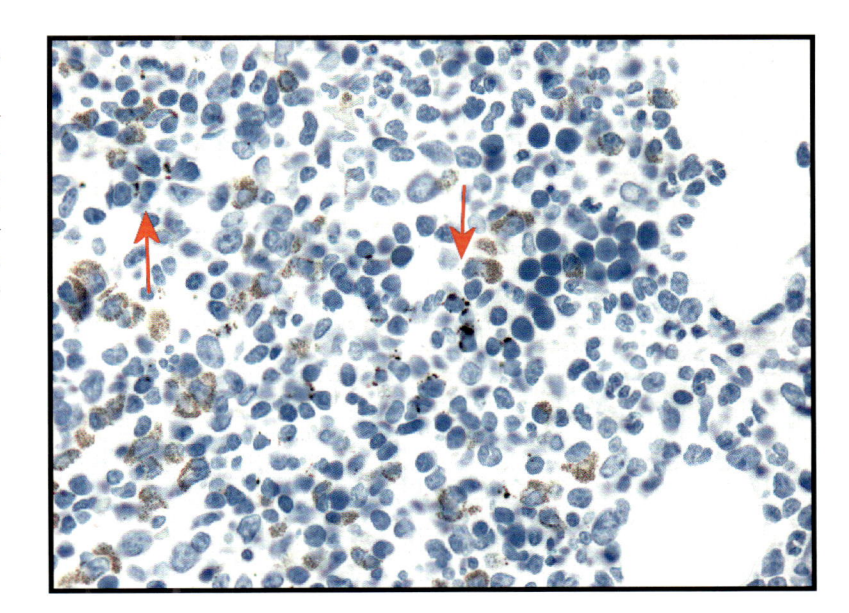

F3.13.17 CD20 in precursor B-cell lymphoblastic leukemia 14 days after induction chemotherapy

In this biopsy from a 28-month-old infant with precursor B-cell lymphoblastic leukemia at diagnosis, CD20 was not a significant marker. After induction chemotherapy, no CD34 or TdT were detected and only CD20 and CD10 remained expressed in blasts. Because aspirate smears were suboptimal, the demonstration of CD20 in almost all cells in the bone marrow was significant to confirm residual leukemia. It appears that this represents chemotherapy related change of immunophenotype.

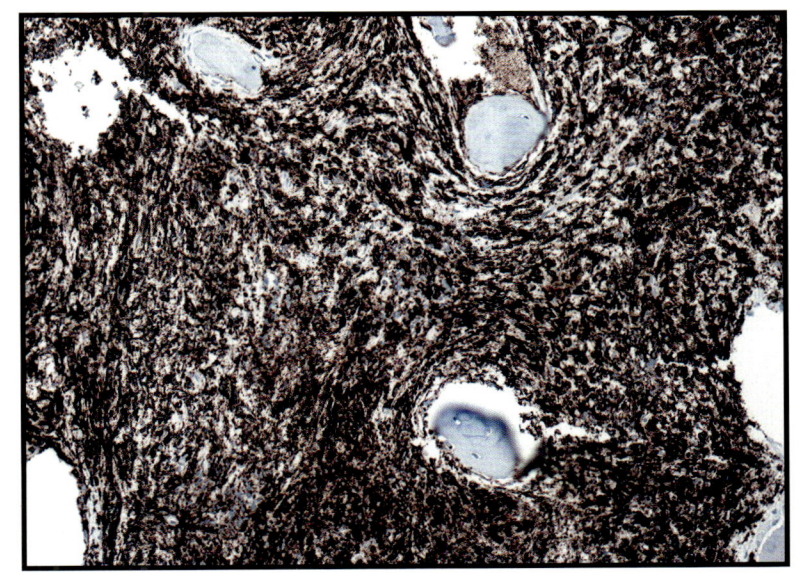

F3.13.18 CD20 in a fibrotic and crushed bone marrow biopsy specimen

This is a patient with myeloproliferative disease and a single large CD20+ lymphoid aggregate. The cells were negative for TdT, CD34, CD10, Bcl-6, CD5, CD23, and cyclin D1. The Ig light chains were negative and did not show monotypic B-cell population. Therefore, no definite evidence of an abnormal immunophenotype was demonstrated. IgH gene rearrangement study showed polyclonal population. This was diagnosed as reactive aggregate.

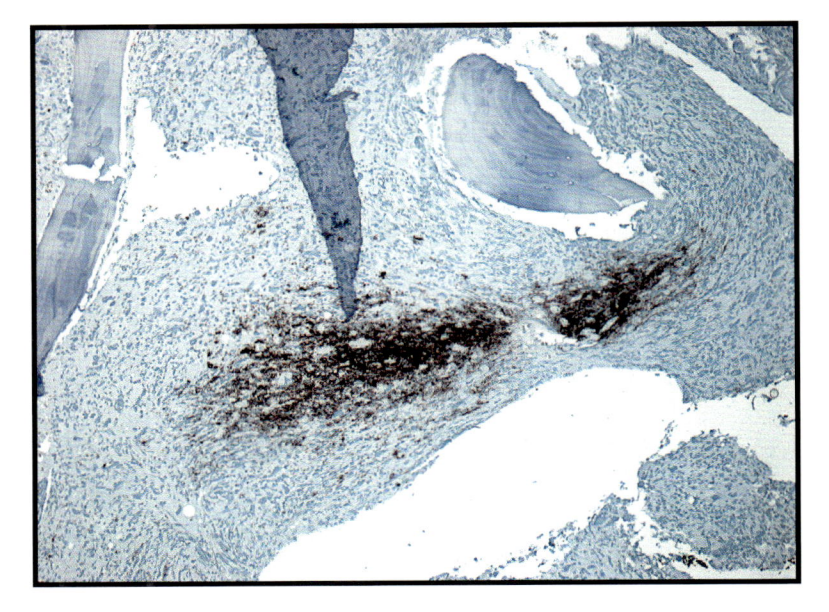

3.14 CD21

CD21 is a complement receptor (C3d, C3dg, and iC3b receptor) and Epstein-Barr virus (EBV) receptor (EBV-R) (OMIM). It is considered to be 1 of the regulators of complement activation and also as a pan-B-cell molecule [Yefenof 1976; Chapple 1990]. Similar to most "pan B-cell Ag", it is not really expressed by all B cells. It should be considered a B-cell maturation marker because B cells start expressing CD21 only after they lose CD10 expression. It is also lost after B-cell activation. Therefore, despite its designation as a pan B-cell marker, the expression in B cells is quite restricted. In the BM, it has been reported that as many as 50% of IgM+ B cells express CD21 [Chapple 1990; Loken 1988; Duperray 1990; Loken 1987]. This cannot be confirmed with IHC in the paraffin-embedded BM biopsy specimens because virtually no cells can be found with CD21 in the normal BM. CD21 is only detected in very rare cells in the form of cytoplasmic granular signals and it is not certain that the reactivity is specific.

While CD21 was found constantly negative in BM mast cells on flow cytometric analysis of the surface antigens, mRNA is expressed in a subset of BM and mucosal mast cells in mice [Escribano 1998; Andrásfalvy 2002]. Rare cells detected with CD21 Ab in the histologically normal BM in humans could therefore represent a subset of mast cells or immature mast cells. Alternatively, the anti-CD21 Ab crossreacts with a different epitope in the mast cells. It has been shown that CD21 is also the ligand for CD23 and the interaction between CD21/CD23 is involved in cell adhesion of human B lymphocytes [Aubry 1992]. In addition, the CD21 expression was also found in a subset of peripheral blood and thymic T cells [Fischer 1991; Delibrias 1994].

Strong expression of CD21, in its role as a dendritic cell marker, was reported in the BM involved by follicular dendritic cell sarcoma [Jiang 2006]. In CLL, strong CD21 expression has been linked with more aggressive disease [Gagro 1997]. Prolymphocytes in CLL express higher levels of CD21 than normal B cells or small CLL cells [Lopez-Matas 2000].

F3.14.1 CD21 in histologically normal bone marrow

Generally, no cells are detectable with CD21 antibody in paraffin-embedded tissues in the normal BM. Theoretically, B cells from the stage when surface Ig is first expressed and before they are activated express CD21. CD21 is acquired at a more mature stage of B-cell development, when CD10 is lost. However, as many as 50% of the IgM+ BM B cells have been shown to express CD21. This is not detectable on immunohistochemistry.

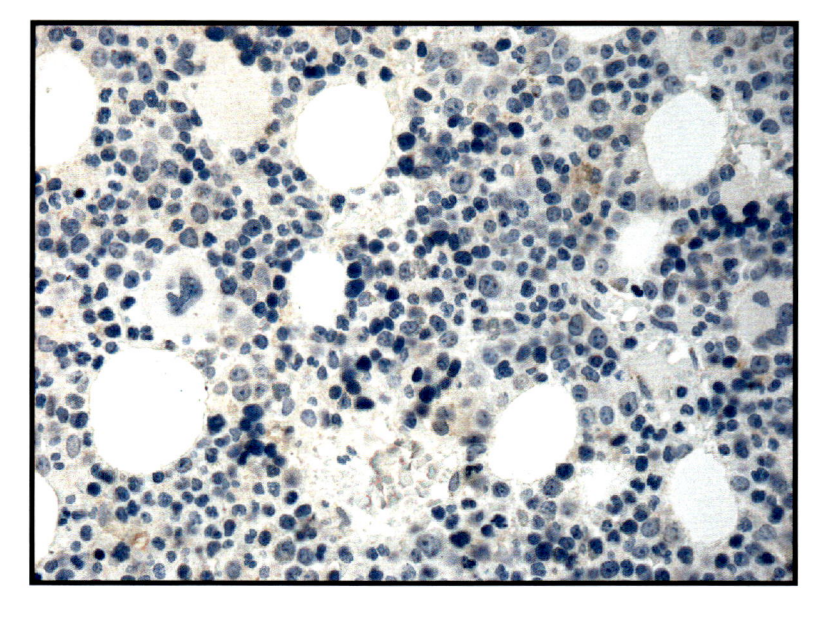

F3.14.2 CD21 in histologically normal bone marrow

Different patient from that in **F3.14.1**. Note that in this BM biopsy specimen, no cells can be detected to express CD21. This is most often the case in histologically normal BM biopsy specimens. Finding CD21 reactivity in the BM, just like finding CD23+ cells, usually designates a pathologic finding.

F3.14.3 CD21 weak expression in rare mononuclear bone marrow cell in a normal BM

The cell illustrated (center) in this image is an extremely rare finding. It may represent rare benign B cells in which CD21 can be detected with immunohistochemistry because of the high expression of this antigen.

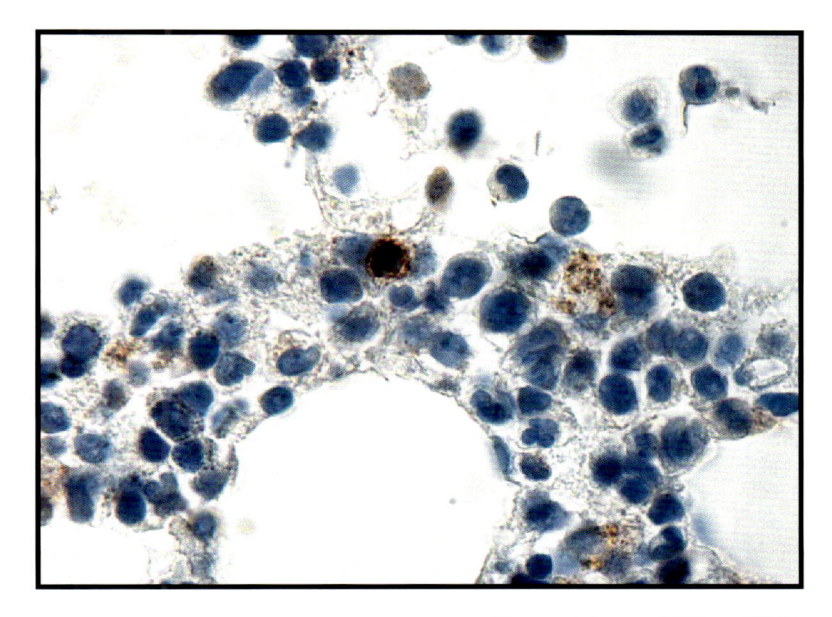

F3.14.4 Cytoplasmic CD21 in rare cells

Some bone marrow biopsy specimens, with or without pathologic findings, display rare cells with granular cytoplasmic CD21 positivity. This is possibly a subset or immature mast cells. Alternatively, this is just an artefact or crossreactivity of the primary antibody.

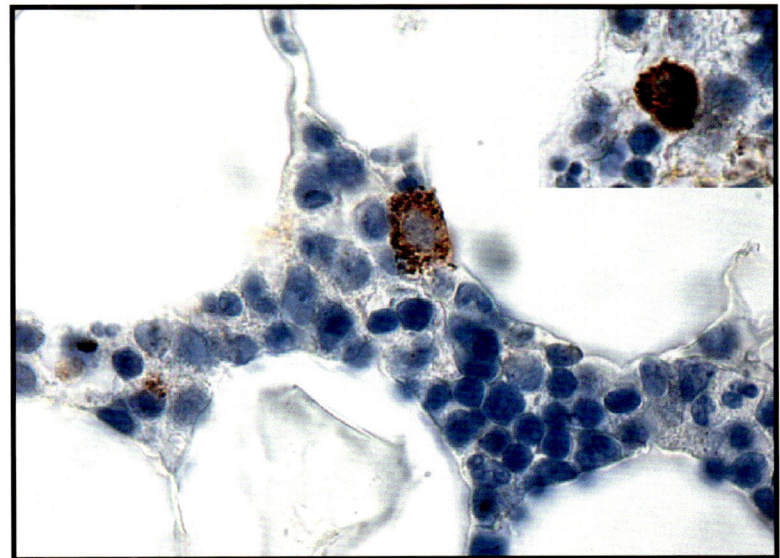

F3.14.5 CD21 in a reactive lymphoid aggregate

This bone marrow biopsy specimen was from a 72-year-old man with anemia and no evidence of lymphocytosis or lymphadenopathy. The specimen had a single lymphoid aggregate with a germinal center. In contrast to this case, most reactive and malignant lymphoid aggregates show no definite evidence of germinal center formation. No specific diagnosis was made. The germinal center cells were, as elsewhere, positive for Bcl-6 and CD10 and negative for Bcl-2. The CD21+ follicular dendritic cells are very prominent.

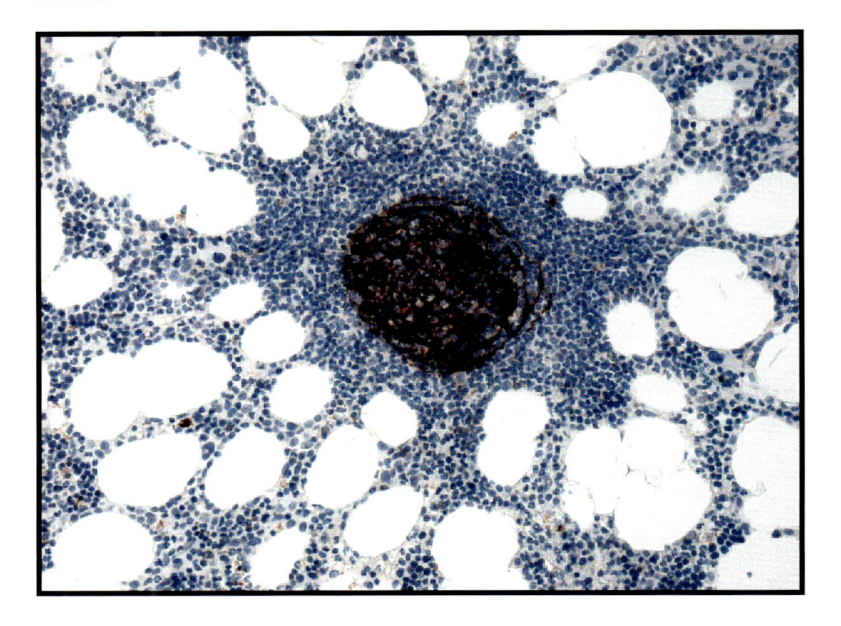

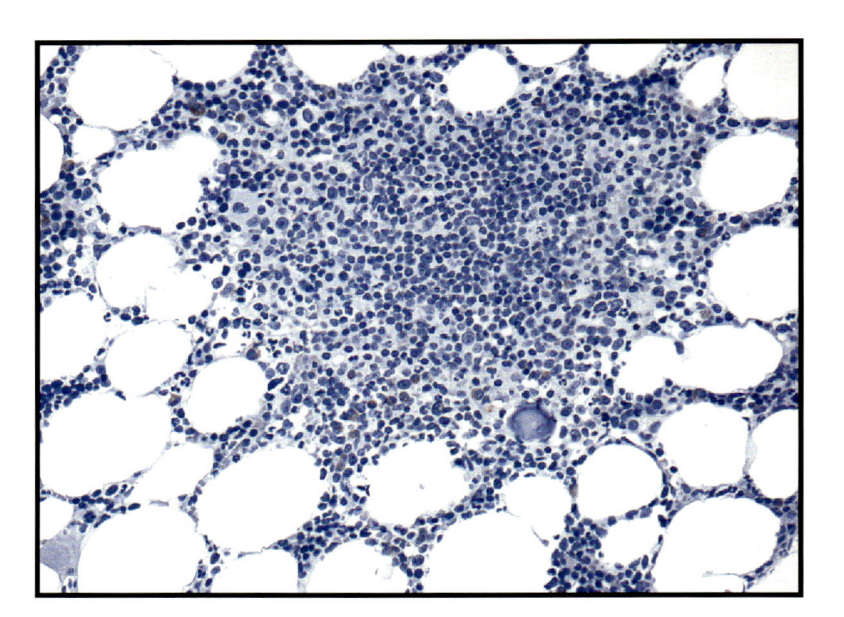

F3.14.6 CD21 in marginal zone lymphoma (MZL)

In contrast to reactive lymphoid aggregates with well-developed germinal centers, malignant lymphoid aggregates in the bone marrow many times show no evidence of follicular dendritic cells. This MZL did not express CD21, which was also confirmed on flow cytometry, but some MZLs may show expression of CD21 on immunohistochemistry including those involving the BM.

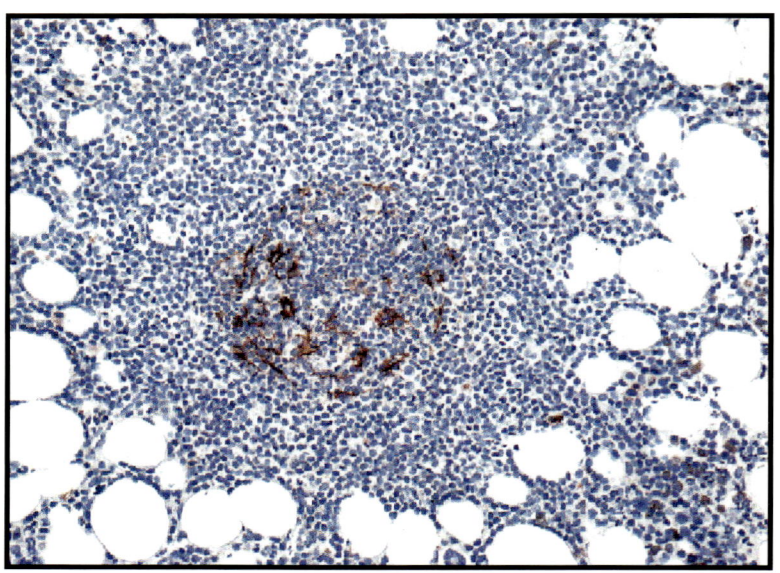

F3.14.7 CD21 in a follicular lymphoma (FL)

When FL creates interstitial lymphoid aggregates, follicular dendritic cells (FDCs) can be detected and they are often CD21+. Regarding the size of the malignant lymphoid aggregates, the number of CD21+ cells is often decreased compared with that in reactive germinal centers of this size. In reactive germinal centers, the number of CD21+ FDCs is usually proportional to the size of the germinal center, while this is clearly not observed in FL.

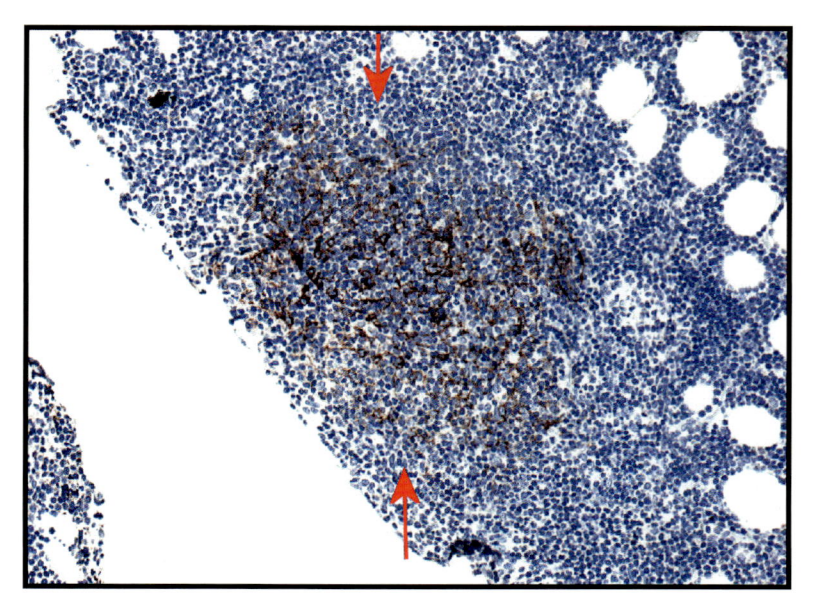

F3.14.8 CD21 in follicular lymphoma (FL)

Different patient than that in F3.14.7. This juxtatrabecular lymphoid aggregate shows numerous dispersed FDCs. This dispersed pattern and lack of clear borders between biological B-cell compartments (germinal center and possible follicular mantle) is typical of FL. Typically, in the same patient and the same organ, the CD21+ follicular dendritic cells show great variability in the intensity of staining and distribution.

3.14   CD21

F3.14.9 CD21 in follicular lymphoma

The same patient as in **F3.14.8**. Follicular dendritic cells (FDCs) in follicular lymphoma can be occasionally detected in the paratrabecular lymphoid aggregates in addition to interstitial and juxtatrabecular lymphoid aggregates. This image illustrates paratrabecular localization of the FDCs (red arrows) as well as juxtatrabecular lymphoid aggregate with FDCs (blue arrows).

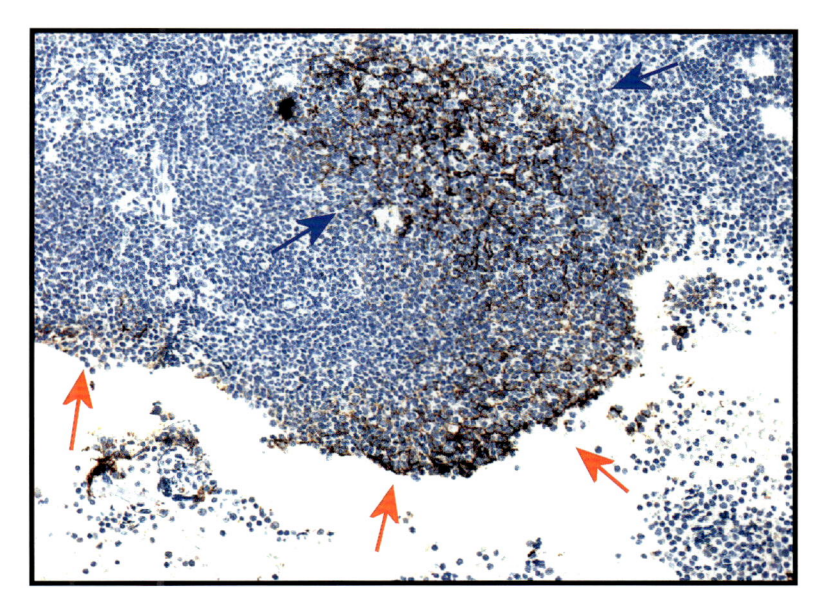

F3.14.10 CD21 in follicular lymphoma (FL)

The same patient as in **F3.14.8**. Follicular dendritic cells in FL can also be found in perivascular localization as illustrated (red arrows). This is not a common finding. This finding was associated with FL widely involving the BM. Air bubbles occasionally interfere with interpretation as seen here (blue arrowheads).

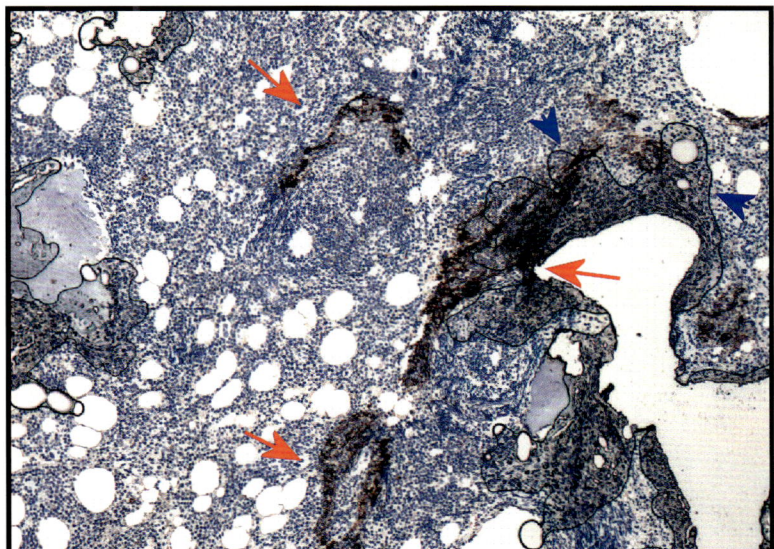

F3.14.11 CD21 in marginal zone lymphoma

This marginal zone lymphoma clearly expressed CD21 on flow cytometry. Only weak/borderline expression could be detected on CD21 immunohistochemistry. Better primary antibody for paraffin-embedded tissues may be developed in the future to better correspond to flow cytometric findings. This is illustrated to show that sometimes what appears to be weak and possibly nonspecific reactivity may indeed, in optimized protocols, reflect true expression of the antigen.

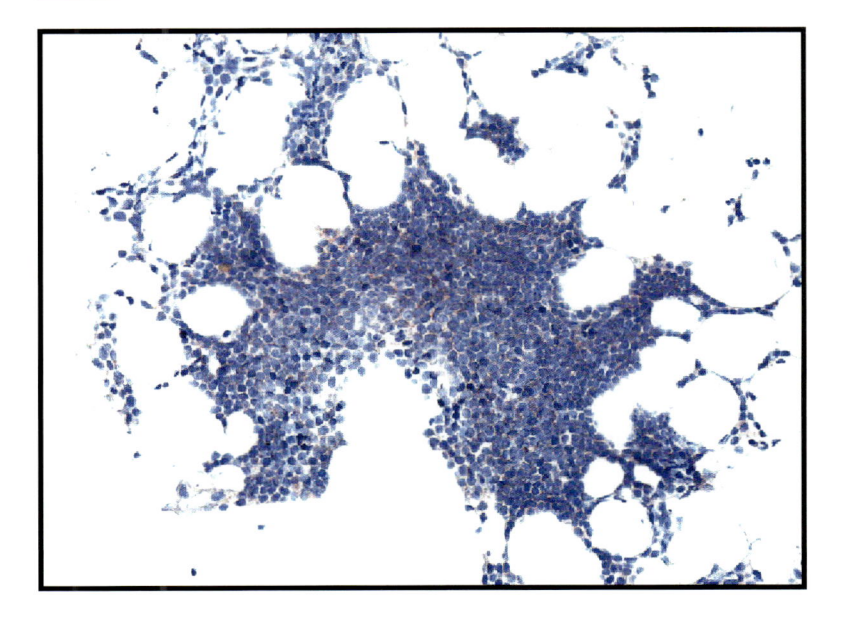

3.15 CD22

CD22 is also known as BL-CAM and Lyb8. Cytoplasmic expression is typically found on late pro- and early pre-B cells. Surface expression is found on mature B cells. CD22 belongs to adhesion and signaling molecules, but CD22-knockout mice have relatively normal B-cell development and response to thymus independent antigens (PROW). It mediates monocyte and erythrocyte adhesion and like CD2, it may facilitate antigen recognition by promoting antigen-nonspecific contacts with accessory cells [Stamenkovic 1990].

CD22 is considered a B-cell specific marker and the European Group for the Immunologic Classification of Leukemia (EGIL) scoring system designates a score of 2 if cytoplasmic CD22 is detected on flow cytometry [Bene 1995]. CD22 is also expressed by basophils. Therefore, it is not exclusively a B-cell marker and its expression in AML may not be really aberrant [Sato 2004]. Detection of both cytoplasmic and surface CD22 expression is widely used in flow cytometry, but IHC applications have been limited.

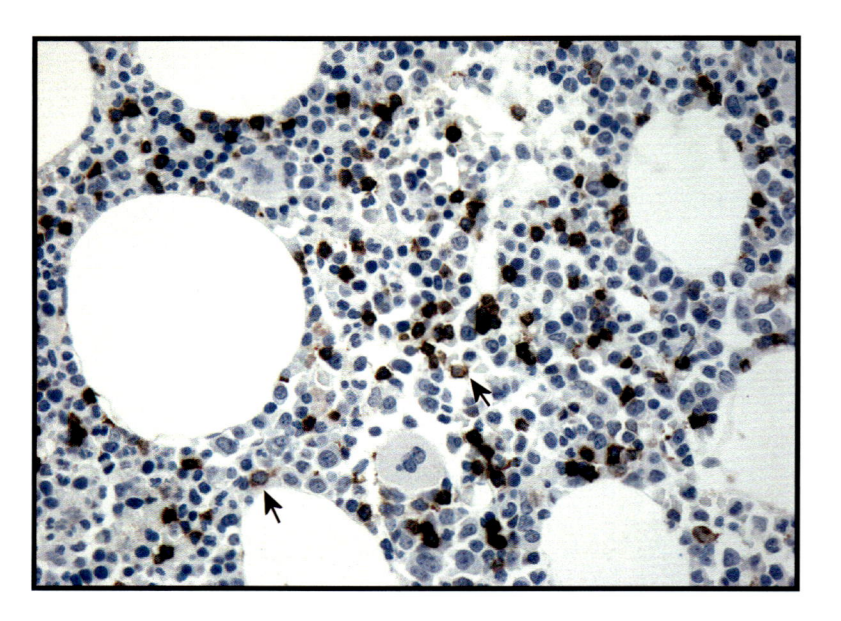

F3.15.1 CD22 in bone marrow with mild reactive changes

Only mild lymphocytosis was found in the BM biopsy specimen of a 57-year-old man with fever of unknown origin. Hematogones were somewhat increased, which is reflected in slightly increased CD22+ lymphocytes. These cells show almost perfect correlation with CD79a. In contrast to CD79a, mature plasma cells generally do not express CD22 detectable with immunohistochemistry. Arrows indicate weakly positive B-cell precursors.

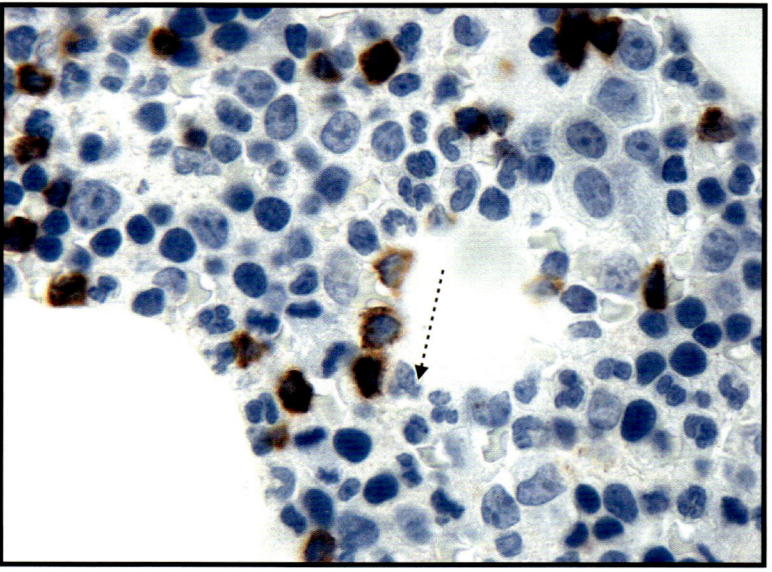

F3.15.2 CD22 in hematogones

This short row of CD22+ lymphoid cells shows gradual increase in the intensity of staining, suggesting possible evidence of B-cell maturation as they acquire increasing amounts of CD22. Such rows with increasing intensity of staining can also be demonstrated for CD20 antigen with immunohistochemistry. In contrast and as expected, decreasing intensity of staining for TdT can be shown in the same samples.

3.15 CD22

F3.15.3 CD22 (brown)+ CD10 (red)
An immature-appearing cell with blastlike features shows weak expression of CD22 (black arrow). This cell represents an early B-cell precursor. This stage is probably before CD10 is expressed. Red staining (CD10) highlights mainly stromal cells (red arrow) and 1 double-stained cell is also identified (blue arrow).

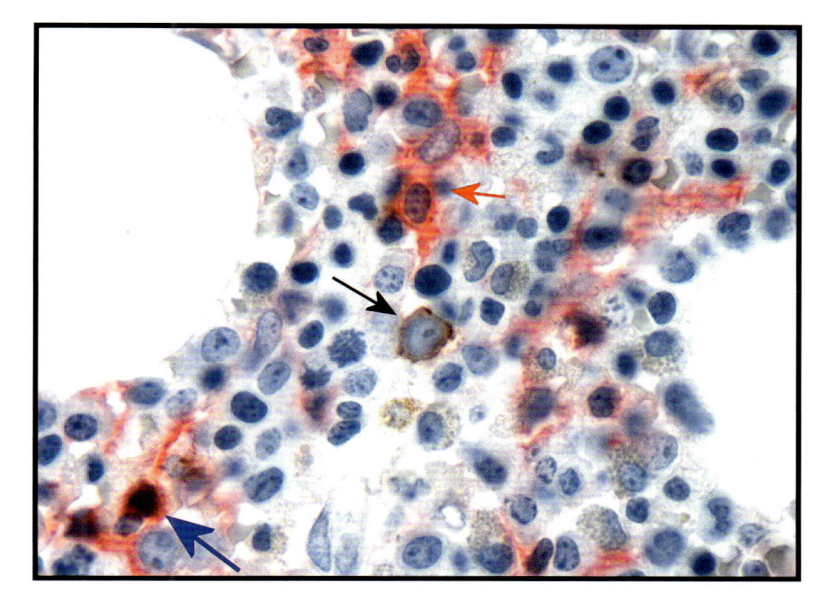

F3.15.4 CD22 (brown)+ CD34 (red)
3 of 4 strongly stained CD22+ cells are in direct contact with CD34+ endothelial cells. The cells illustrated here appear to have both cytoplasmic and membranous expression of CD22. The question remains as to how accurate is antigen localization in double-staining techniques. Rare cells show ill-defined dotlike positivity in the cytoplasm (black arrow). Coupled with immature-appearing nuclei, this may identify early B-cell precursors. Alternatively, this dotlike positivity may represent an artefact.

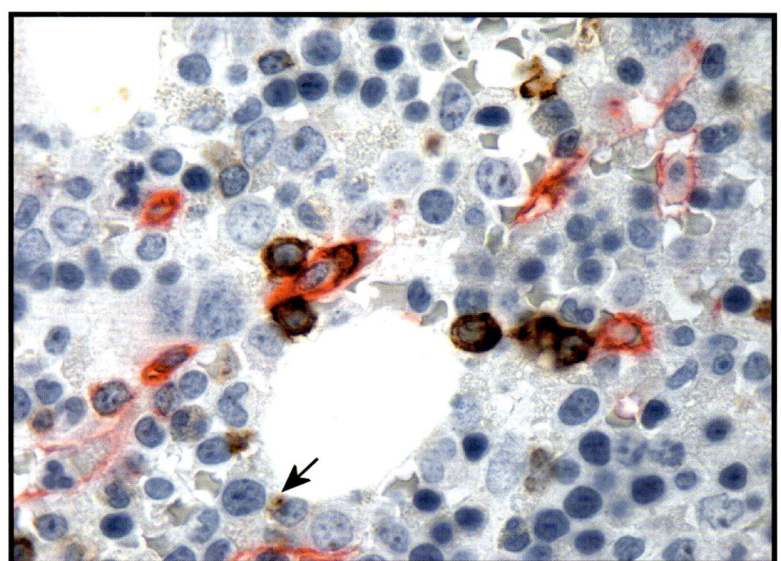

3.16 CD23

CD23 is also known as B6, BLAST-2, FceRII, Leu-20, and low-affinity IgE receptor (PROW). It has a role in regulation of IgE production [Aubry 1992]. CD23 is a key molecule for B-cell activation and growth. The truncated CD23 can be secreted to function as a potent mitogenic growth factor. It is expressed by B cells including some CD5+ cells and some CD10+ B cells, monocytes, follicular dendritic cells of the apical light zone as well as in some T cells, platelets, eosinophils, and neutrophils. While CD23 of macrophages, eosinophils, and platelets mediate IgE-dependent cytotoxicity and promote phagocytosis of IgE-antigen complexes, the function of CD23 on B lymphocytes remains unclear [Richards 1991]. Expression of CD23 and soluble CD23 has been associated with allergic diseases. Targeting CD23 with monoclonal antibody (lumiliximab) is a promising candidate therapy in allergic diseases [Rosenwasser 2005].

CD23 is mostly used as a marker of CLL, but other non-Hodgkin lymphomas may express CD23 including rare cases of mantle cell lymphoma [Garcia 2001; Schlette 2003; Chen 2006]. Therefore, in the evaluation of diffuse small B-cell lymphoproliferative disorders, a panel of markers is critical. In CLL, the CD23 expression frequently follows the pattern of CD20 being more strongly expressed in proliferation centers in prolymphocytoid cells and paraimmunoblasts than in other CLL cells [Lampert 1999]. The most benign condition in which CD23 is found is that of reactive lymphoid hyperplasia with formation of lymphoid follicles. The germinal centers contain CD23+ follicular dendritic cells; the B lymphocytes in the mantles of the lymphoid follicles can also show expression of CD23 if they are well developed, and if CD23 is detected with high sensitivity.

3: Cluster of Differentiation Markers

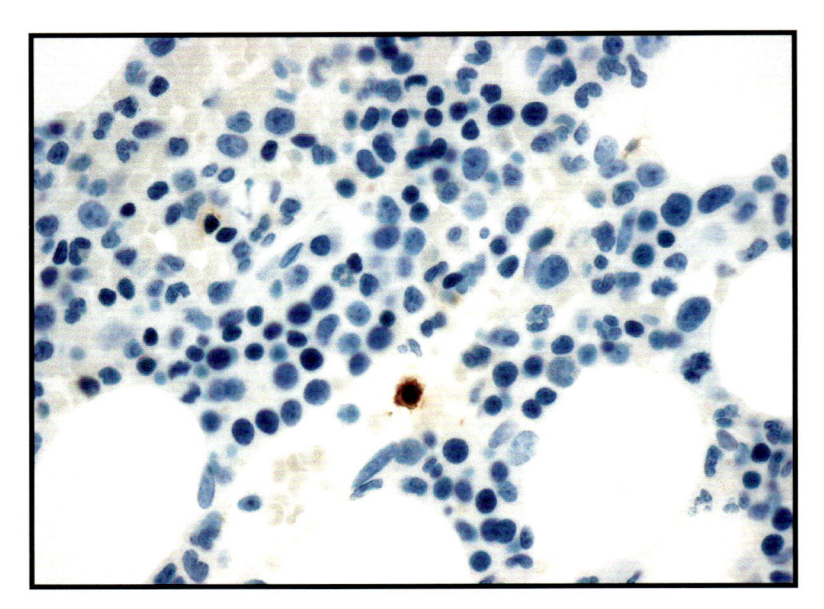

F3.16.1 CD23 in histologically normal bone marrow

In the normal BM specimen, generally very few B cells are positive for CD23 on immunohistochemistry. This is in contrast to flow cytometry, which reveals that about 60% of B cells in the BM express this antigen. By IHC, very rare CD23+ lymphocytes are found in the vascular spaces representing circulating CD23+ B cells as shown here.

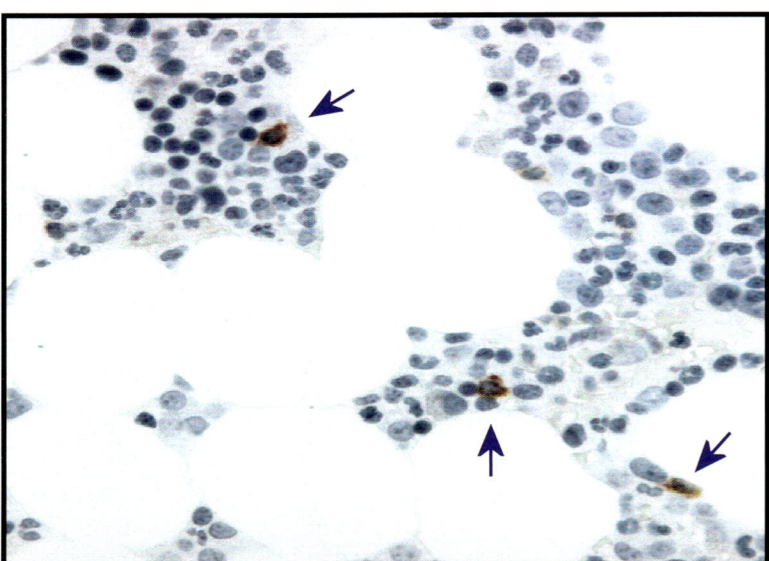

F3.16.2 CD23 in histologically normal bone marrow

This BM biopsy specimen with reactive changes shows rare CD23+ lymphocytes in the interstitium. The patient had a history of classical Hodgkin lymphoma. Both CD10+/CD23+ and CD5+/CD23+ populations are present in the normal BM. However, in contrast to chronic lymphocytic leukemia, the CD5+/CD23+ population is FMC7+.

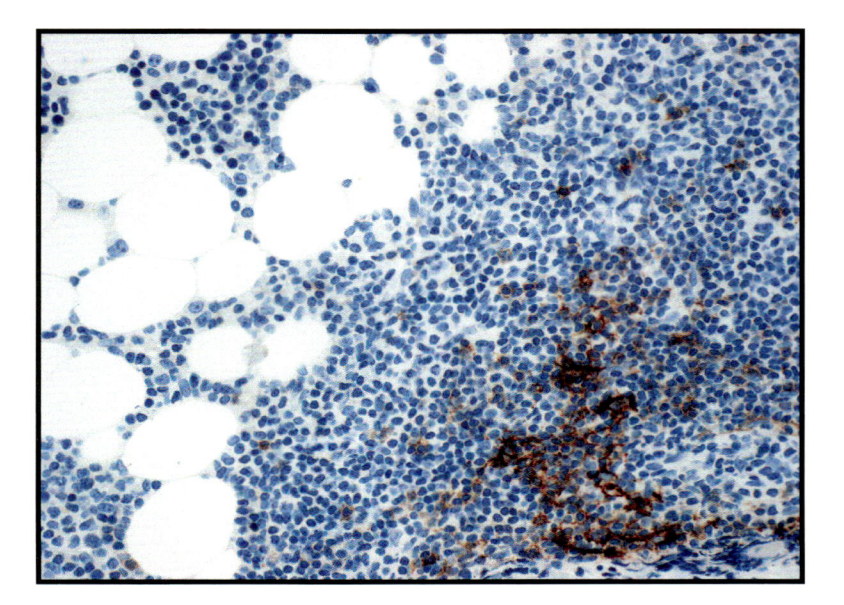

F3.16.3 CD23 highlighting follicular dendritic cells in the reactive lymphoid follicles

Reactive lymphoid aggregates with germinal centers always show some evidence of CD23+ follicular dendritic cells. In decalcified sections, it is more difficult to demonstrate CD23-weakly positive B cells in the follicle mantle. Rare cells in the mantle are stained in this example.

3.16   CD23

F3.16.4 CD23+ lymphocytes of unclear biological significance

This 34-year-old woman with normochromic normocytic anemia had a slightly hypocellular bone marrow specimen. The cause of anemia was not determined. Flow cytometric analysis did not show CD23+ lymphoproliferative disease and cytogenetic study findings were normal. Rare follicular dendritic cells and occasional CD23+ lymphocytes were present in a single lymphoid aggregate. The biological significance of this finding remains unclear.

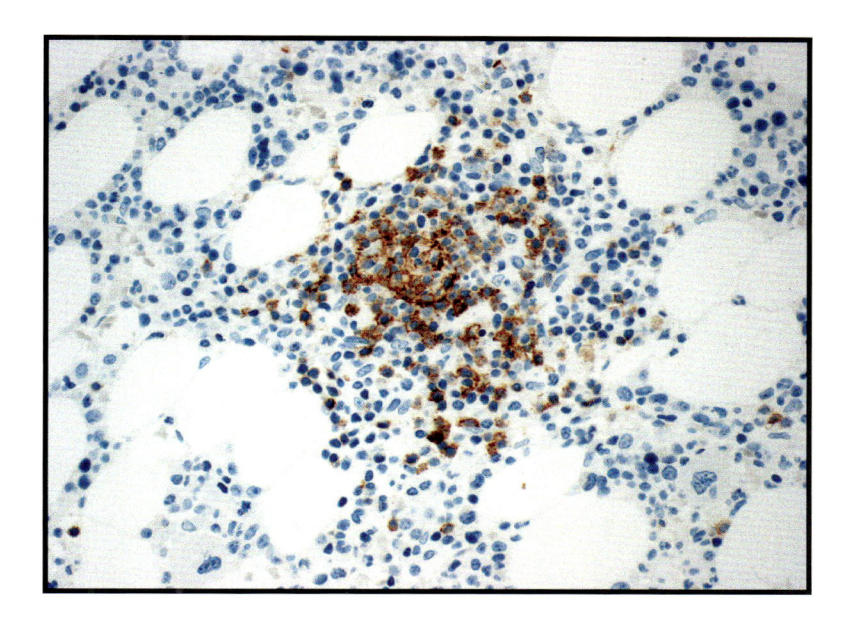

F3.16.5 CD23 in marginal zone lymphoma (MZL)

MZLs are considered to be CD23− small B-cell lymphomas. While in some cases, CD23 can be expressed, commonly many cells are negative on immunohistochemistry. Many CD20+ cells were identified in this area and many lymphocytes are identifiable on morphologic study, but only a small number showed weak expression of CD23 (compare with a single cell with strong expression labeled by red arrow).

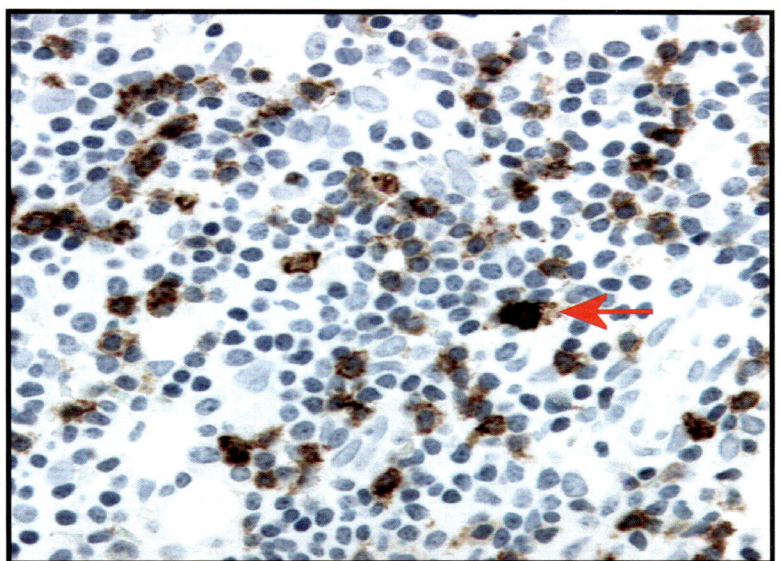

F3.16.6 CD23 in follicular lymphoma (FL)

CD23 is not expressed by most FLs. It has been described that when FL loses its CD10 expression which is linked to its follicular growth, FL can express CD23. In this case, FL cells are present diffusely in the bone marrow and CD23 is moderately expressed. Note predominant cytoplasmic expression, which could be missed with flow cytometry analysis.

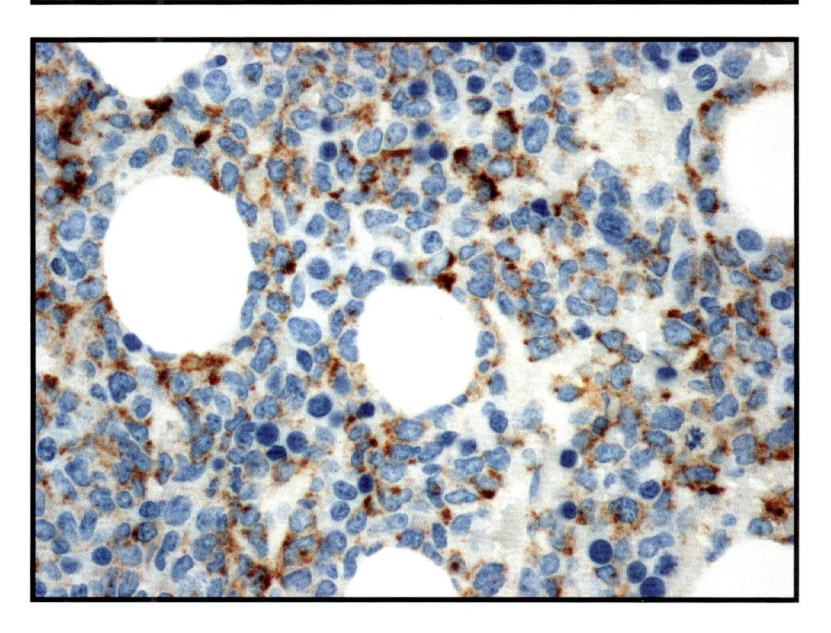

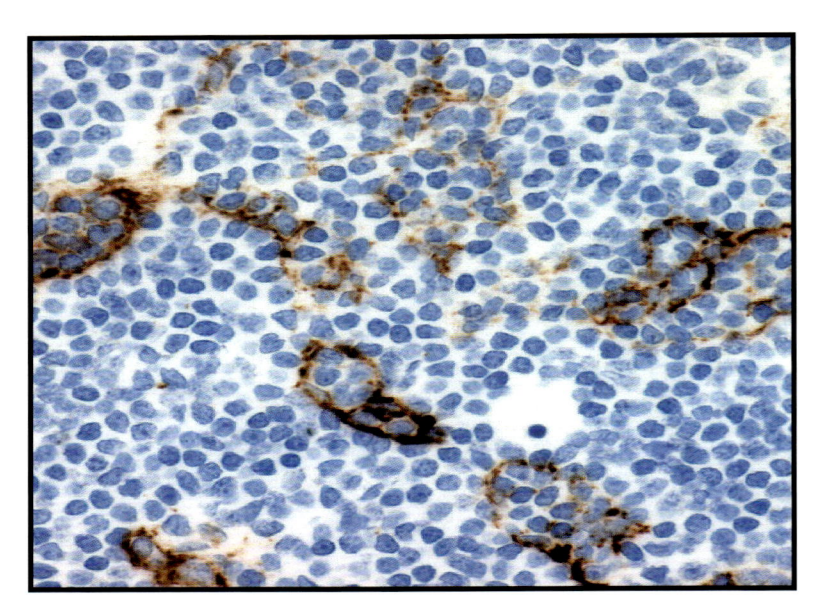

F3.16.7 CD23 in mantle cell lymphoma (MCL)

CD23 is used to distinguish between chronic lymphocytic leukemia, which expresses CD23, and MCL, which can express CD23 only rarely. However, it should be noted that CD23 labels follicular dendritic cells which can be present randomly distributed in MCL in small numbers as shown here. CD23 detection in MCL is method dependent, is typically dim, and generally detected with flow cytometry. Bone marrow and leukemic involvement have been described in CD23+ MCL [Schlette 2003].

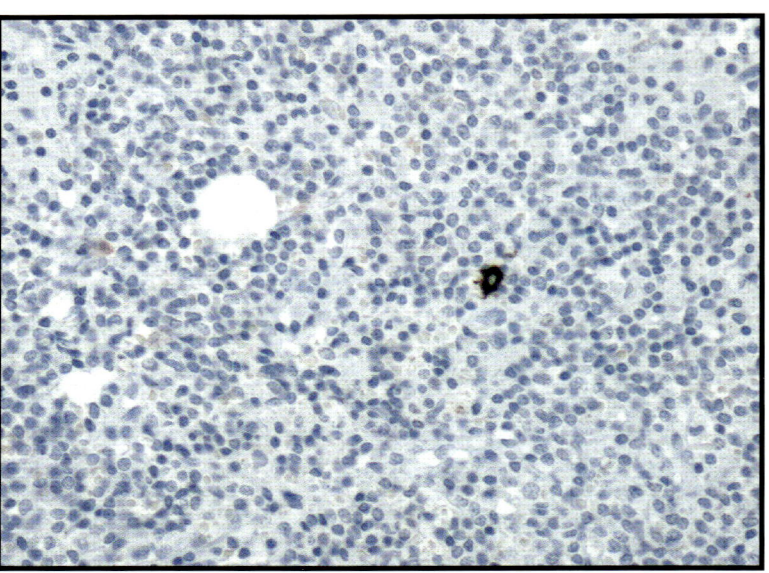

F3.16.8 CD23− CLL

CD23 is positive in the great majority of CLL cases. However, rare cases will not express CD23 as shown here with immunohistochemistry. This case was also negative with flow cytometry. Clinically and morphologically, the features were most compatible with chronic lymphocytic leukemia. Most cells in this field were weakly CD20+ and CD5+. The t(14;19)(q32;q13)-associated CD23− CLL can not be ruled out in this case.

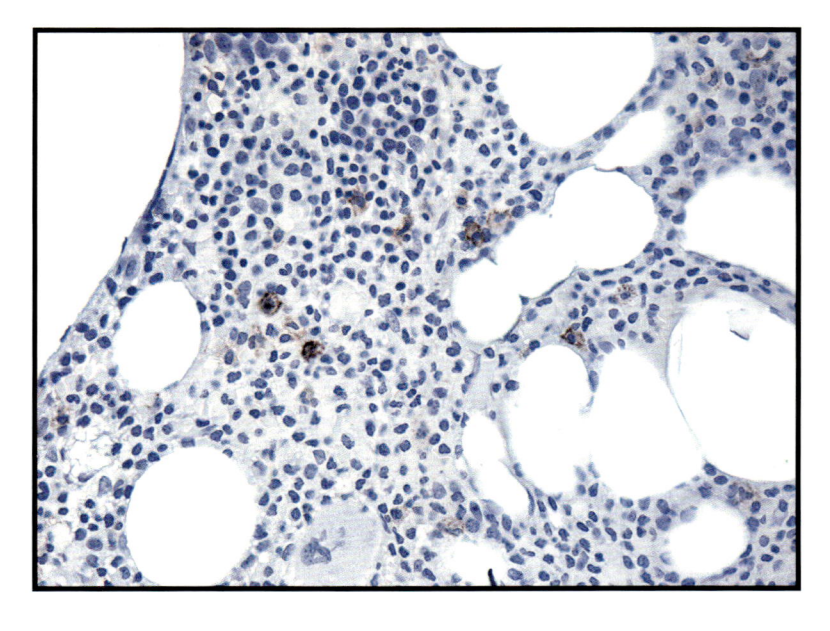

F3.16.9 CD23 in hairy cell leukemia (HCL)

HCL is generally negative for CD23 as illustrated in this case, but CD23 may be expressed in as many as 20% of HCL cases [Chen 2006]. In this case, only rare cells are positive and based on morphologic features, these are most likely not part of the neoplastic population.

3.16   CD23

F3.16.10 CD23 in bone marrow with diffuse involvement by chronic lymphocytic leukemia (CLL)

Despite consistent expression of CD23 in CLL, the level of expression of most cases and in most cells is relatively weak. This is well illustrated in this case where most of the cells are positive, but only weakly. This weak expression is of great diagnostic importance and if not interpreted as "positive," most cases of CD23+ CLL would be missed. Such weak positivity should not be interpreted as background staining.

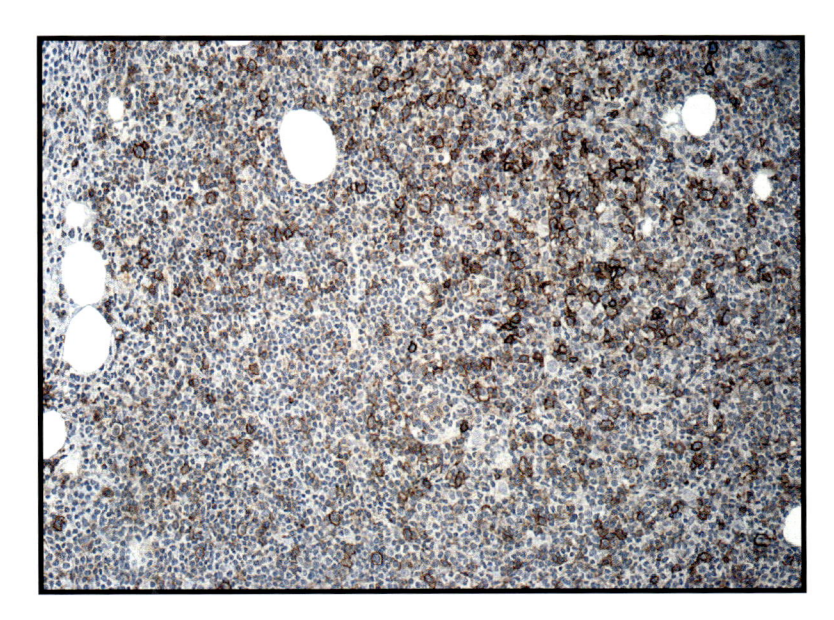

F3.16.11 CD23 in chronic lymphocytic leukemia (CLL) with focal bone marrow involvement

The intensity of CD23 expression may vary from case to case in CLL and there may be some differences between the nodular, interstitial, or diffuse pattern of involvement with immunohistochemistry. This case with focal pattern of BM involvement shows strong expression of CD23.

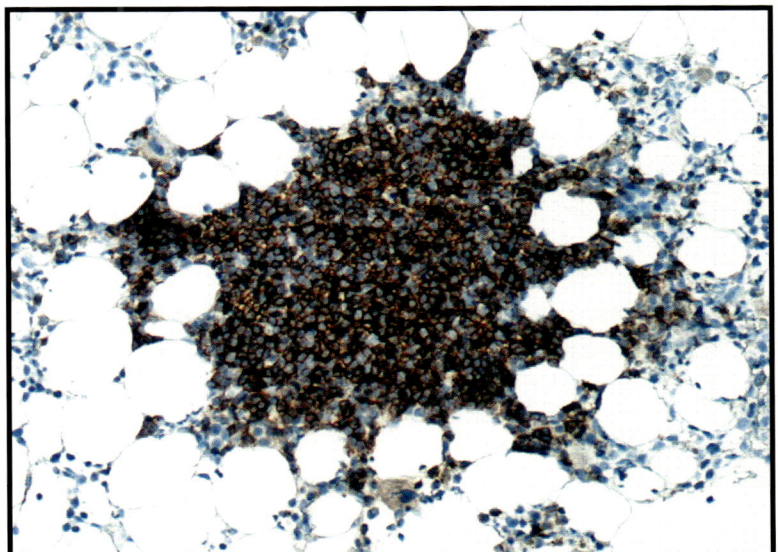

F3.16.12 CD23 in interstitial chronic lymphocytic leukemia (CLL)

Despite its interstitial nature, the largest cells, presumably the prolymphocytes residing in the proliferation centers show the highest levels of CD23 as it is commonly seen in the lymph nodes involved by CLL. Note that in this case the level of expression is in between that illustrated in diffuse CLL (F3.16.10) and nodular CLL (F3.16.11).

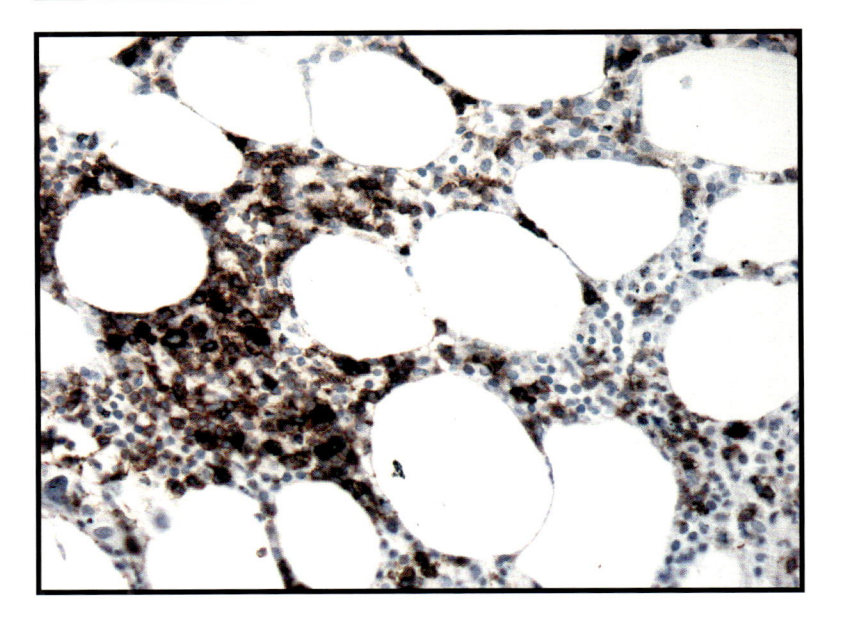

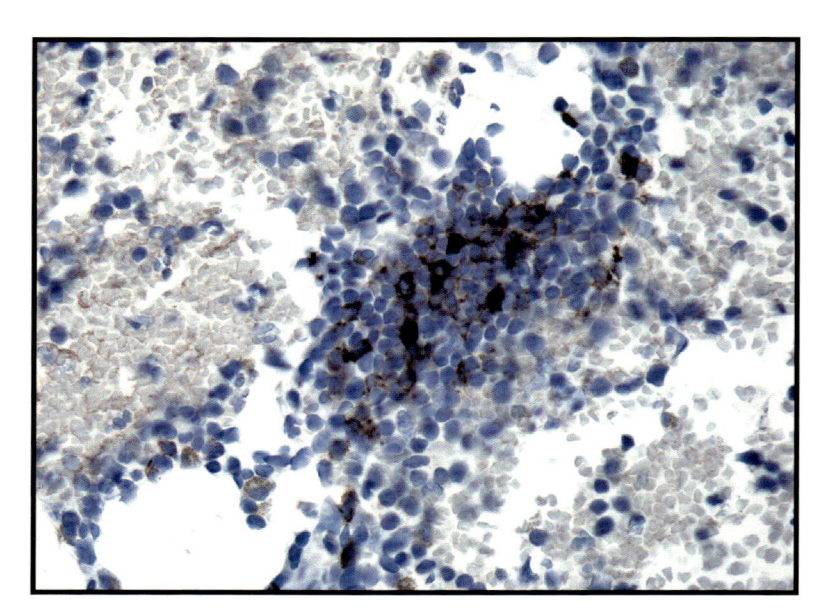

F3.16.13 CD23 in chronic lymphocytic leukemia (CLL; mixed pattern)

In this bone marrow biopsy specimen, the CLL infiltrates were found predominantly in an interstitial pattern. However, in areas with focal involvement, only the large cells, presumably prolymphocytes, show strong expression of CD23, while smaller cells have weak expression as in the predominant interstitial areas in the rest of the BM.

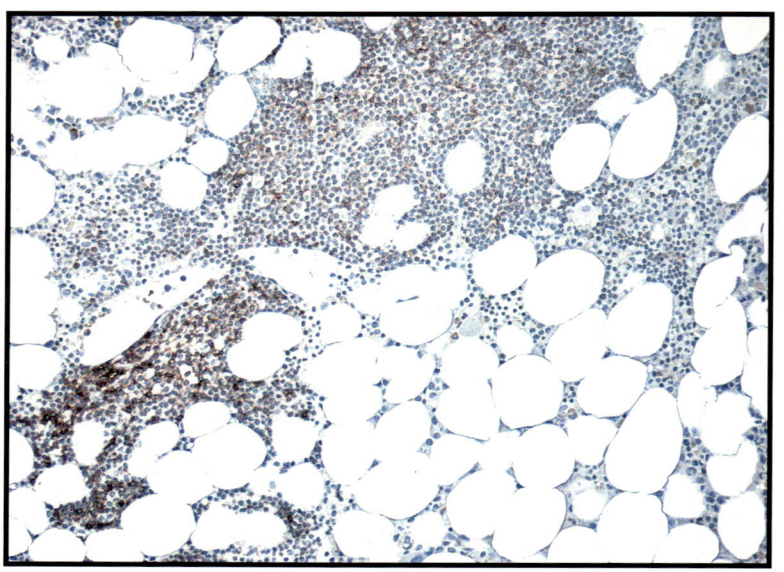

F3.16.14 CD23 in chronic lymphocytic leukemia (CLL) with a predominantly interstitial pattern of bone marrow involvement

Different case than that illustrated in **F3.16.13**. In most areas, the small lymphocytes are very weakly positive for CD23 or negative, and only the larger cells, which are presumably prolymphocytes, show higher expression of CD23. If such weak expression levels of CD23 are not correctly interpreted, many cases of CLL would be considered negative for CD23 with immunohistochemistry.

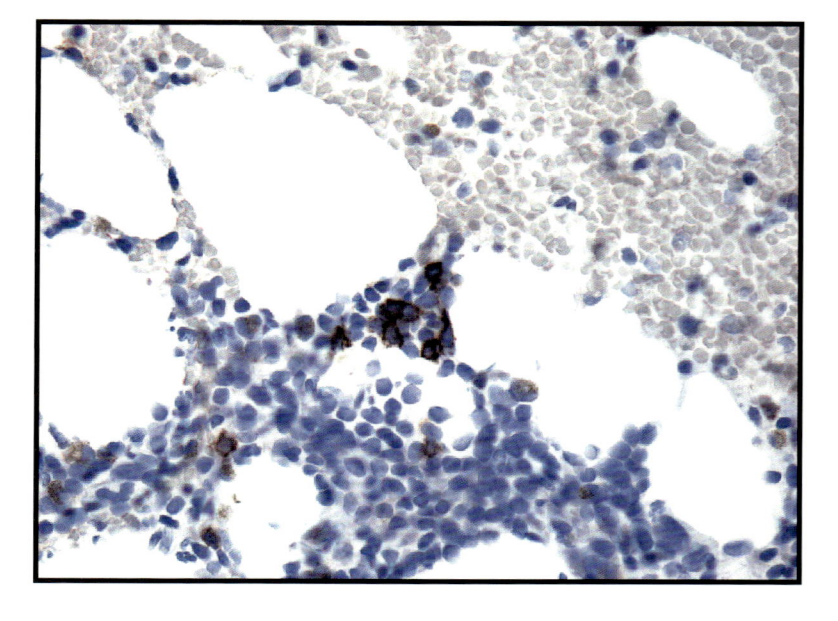

F3.16.15 CD23 expression in small lymphoid clusters

This image illustrates a small cluster of CD23+ lymphocytes. This is always an abnormal finding. Finding only a single cluster of CD23+ of this size would raise the suspicion of chronic lymphocytic leukemia (CLL) involvement. If more than 1 cluster is found and if CD5+, such a finding would be compatible with CLL in a patient evaluated for a lymphoproliferative disorder. It cannot be overemphasized that CD23 is never present in small clusters of benign lymphoid cells in the bone marrow.

3.17 CD25

CD25 is an IL-2 receptor α chain. It is also known as Tac-antigen (PROW). CD25 is a transmembrane molecule expressed by activated (PHA-stimulated) T cells and activated B cells stimulated with anti-IgM antibody, as well as on lipopolysaccharide-stimulated/activated monocytes and macrophages. Virally transformed T cells also express CD25. Human T-lymphotropic virus-1 (HTLV-1)–infected neoplastic cells of HTLV-1-associated T-cell leukemia/lymphoma and HIV-infected T cells express CD25 [Helinski 1988; Gessain 1989; Kobayashi 1989]. Some consistent patterns of reactivity with anti-CD25 Ab are not fully understood or explained, including cytoplasmic positivity in megakaryocytes and very variable cytoplasmic positivity in adipocytes as shown here [Horny 2007a].

Importantly and for diagnostic purposes, CD25 is identified in hairy cell leukemia [Goodman 2003; de Totero 1994]. CD25 is also one of the best markers of neoplastic mast cells because benign mast cells do not express this marker. Studies have described its expression in mastocytosis involving different organs [Pardanani 2005; Castells 2004; Escribano 2002; Escribano 1999; Valent 2001]. The experience with CD25 Ab in BM application is limited to mast cell disorders.

F3.17.1 CD25 in histologically normal bone marrow (slide courtesy of P Horny, MD, Institute of Pathology, Ansbach, Germany)

CD25 is detected in lymphoid cells (red arrow), which may represent either activated T or B cells. Megakaryocytes invariably show cytoplasmic staining with anti-CD25 antibody, but the staining is very variable from cell to cell (blue arrow).

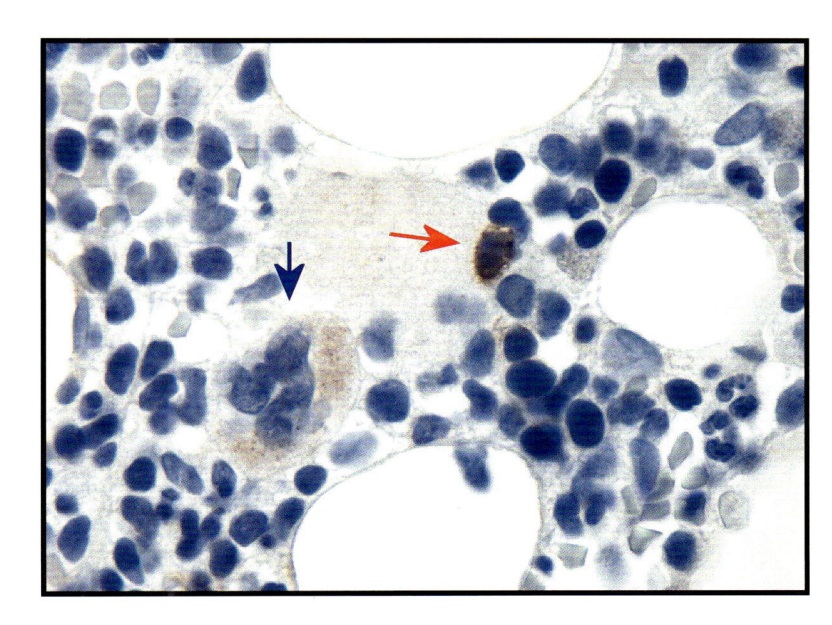

F3.17.2 CD25 in histologically normal bone marrow (slide courtesy of P Horny, MD, Institute of Pathology, Ansbach, Germany)

Activated monocytes also express CD25; this cell with low nuclear-cytoplasmic ratio has morphologic characteristics of a monocyte. Membranous expression and weak Golgi-type staining are detected (red arrow). As usual, megakaryocytes are showing cytoplasmic staining. Neutrophils and precursors appear to show weak staining in this area, but it is not certain that this is a specific reaction.

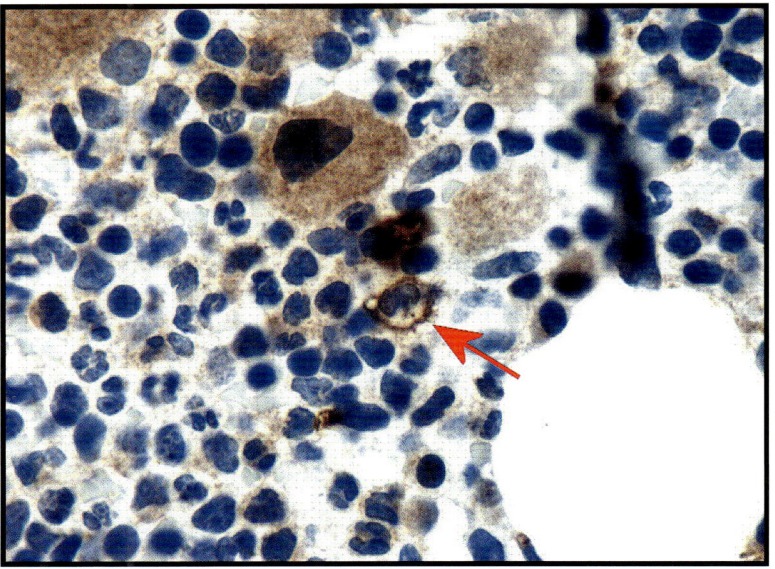

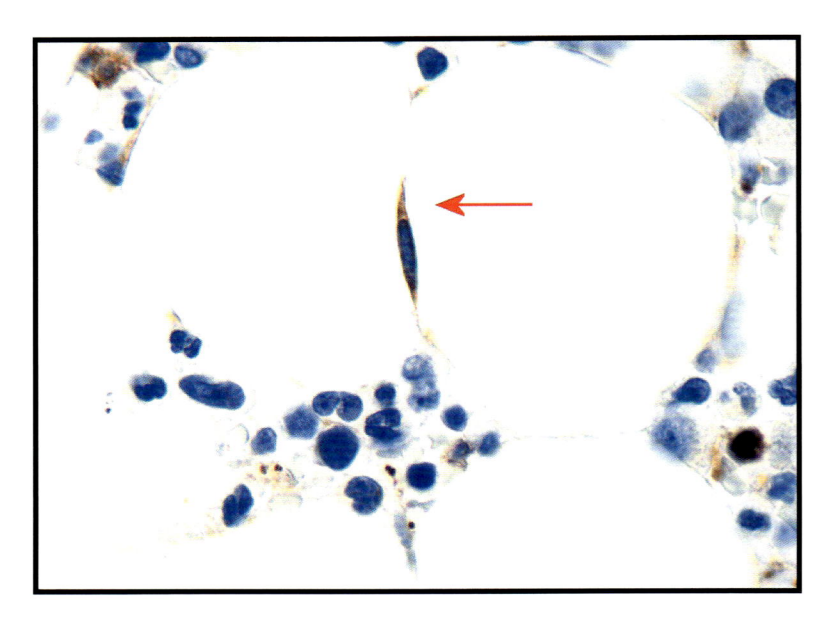

F3.17.3 CD25 in adipocytes (slide courtesy of P Horny, MD, Institute of Pathology, Ansbach, Germany)

In the bone marrow, adipocytes show staining with anti-CD25 antibody. Whether specific or not, this staining can be detected. While weak in many cells, in others the staining may be quite significant. The localization of the signals is reproducibly cytoplasmic, which is similar to cytoplasmic staining in megakaryocytes. Weak cytoplasmic staining in an adipocyte is demonstrated here (arrow).

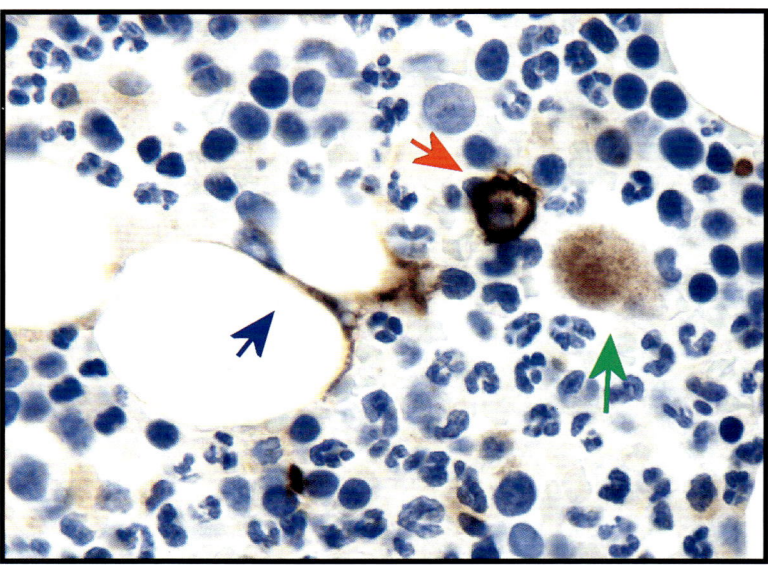

F3.17.4 CD25 in mastocytosis (slide courtesy of P Horny, MD, Institute of Pathology, Ansbach, Germany)

A mast cell with strong expression of CD25 is detected (red arrow). Tangential cut of the megakaryocyte cytoplasm (green arrow) and focal staining in adipocytes (blue arrow) are also present. The intensity of CD25 expression in atypical mast cells appears much higher than in activated benign lymphocytes, monocytes, and other cells.

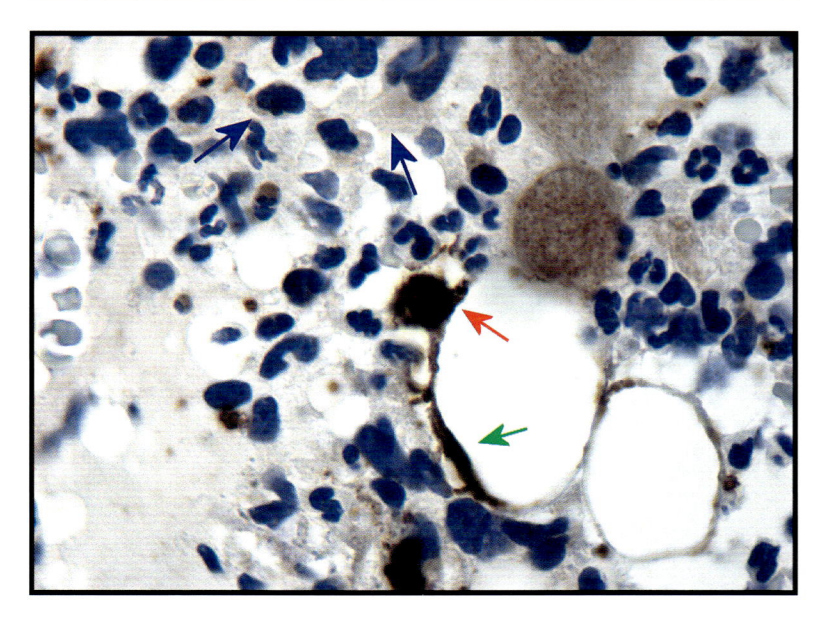

F3.17.5 CD25 in mastocytosis (slide courtesy of P Horny, MD, Institute of Pathology, Ansbach, Germany)

CD25 is strongly expressed by a mononuclear cell adjacent to an adipocyte (red arrow). This could be an atypical mast cell, but it is not always possible to identify the nature of various cells positive for CD25. An adipocyte is strongly stained in this area (green arrow). Few other weakly stained cells are also present (blue arrows). The nature of these cells cannot be identified with certainty.

3.17 CD25

F3.17.6 CD25 in activated lymphocytes (slide courtesy of P Horny, MD, Institute of Pathology, Ansbach, Germany)

Several cells in this field appear to be lymphocytes. They are presumed activated T and B lymphocytes (blue arrows). The expression is manly localized on the surface, but some cytoplasmic expression is also possible. Rare cells have more myeloid morphology and are most likely basophils or basophil precursors, which are known to be CD25 positive (red arrows).

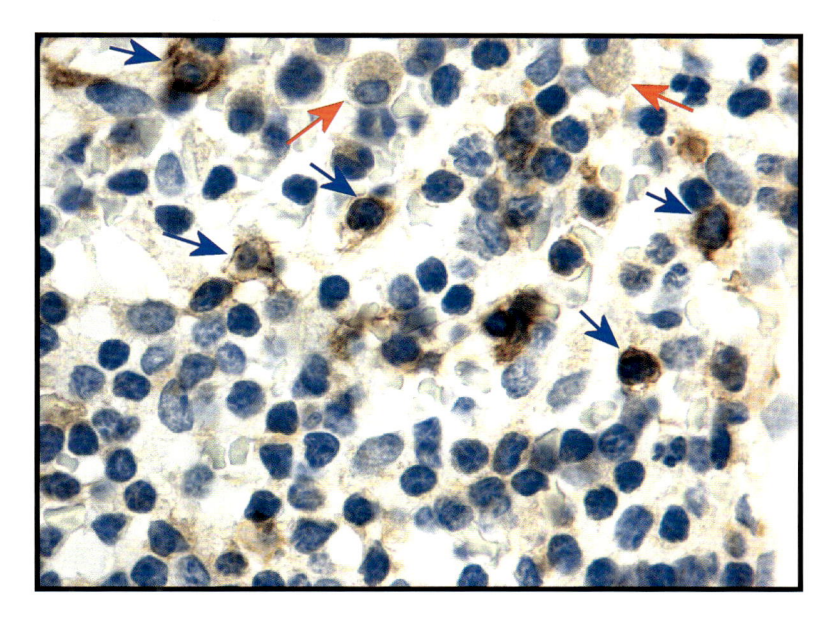

F3.17.7 CD25 in systemic mastocytosis (slide courtesy of P Horny, MD, PhD, Institute of Pathology, Ansbach, Germany)

Atypical mast cells show very strong membranous expression of CD25. This is easily appreciated on low magnification examination. Similarly, even rare atypical mast cells, and especially if they are spindled (atypical morphology), will be easy to detect on low magnification examination.

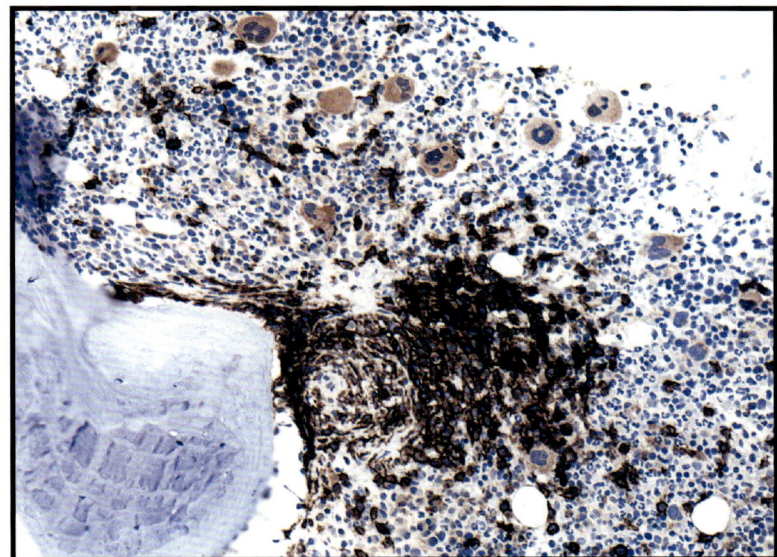

F3.17.8 CD25 in system mastocytosis (slide courtesy of P Horny, MD, Institute of Pathology, Ansbach, Germany)

Strong membranous expression is present in all tumor cells. Occasional malignant mast cell also demonstrates Golgi-type dotlike paranuclear positivity (red arrow). CD25 is an excellent marker of atypical mast cells throughout the body.

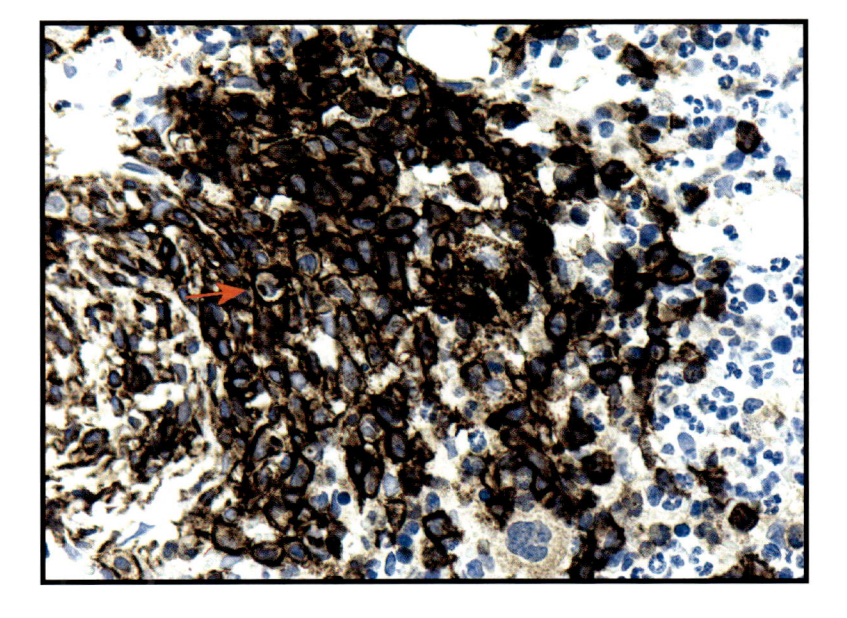

3.18 CD30

CD30 is also known as Ber-H2 antigen and Ki-1 antigen (PROW). It is involved in T-cell–mediated cell death and negative selection of T cells in the thymus. CD30 is a member of the TNFR family of molecules and activates NFkB through interaction with TRAF2 and TRAF5 [Falini 1995; Aizawa 1997]. It is expressed by activated T lymphocytes, activated B lymphocytes, activated NK cells, monocytes, Hodgkin cells in Hodgkin lymphoma, non-Hodgkin lymphomas including anaplastic large cell lymphoma (ALCL), other peripheral T-cell lymphomas, and some DLBCLs (but never together with ALK-1). It is also present in embryonal carcinoma, as well as mixed germ cell tumor [de Bruin 1995]. CD30 is most often used to detect either cHL or ALCL, with the former being a relatively common B-cell malignancy and the latter a relatively uncommon T-cell malignancy. However, its expression in activated lymphocytes is increasingly important with ever more potent and sensitive detection systems, which enhance detection of CD30 in numerous benign cells. Often, in lymph nodes, the benign cells are found in both T-cell zones (paracortex) and B-cell zones (germinal centers). In these benign lymphocytes the expression of CD30 is usually detected as fine membranous staining as well as very fine dotlike Golgi-type expression. In normal BM, there is virtually no expression of CD30. However, some chunky granular extracellular positivity is frequent and it is not clear whether it represents a nonspecific reaction or cross-reactivity to Ag in phagocytic macrophages. In some biopsy specimens, CD30 staining will result in weak dotlike positivity in endothelial cells. Very rarely, some definitely specific-appearing staining is found in rare large cells in some B-cell lymphomas, but caution must be exercised not to interpret this finding as evidence of cHL. cHL may appear in the BM involved by CLL or other conditions, but the diagnosis needs to be based on both morphologic appearance and demonstration of a typical HL phenotype (both CD30 and CD15 or EBV need to be demonstrated) in particular if cells are few and/or dispersed.

F3.18.1 CD30 in histologically normal bone marrow

CD30 is not expressed in the normal BM. On immunohistochemistry, some staining that appears extracellular is frequently detected. It has the appearance of chunky granular or globular staining (arrows). The extent of the detection of these extracellular signals varies from specimen to specimen. Its biological significance, if any, is not known.

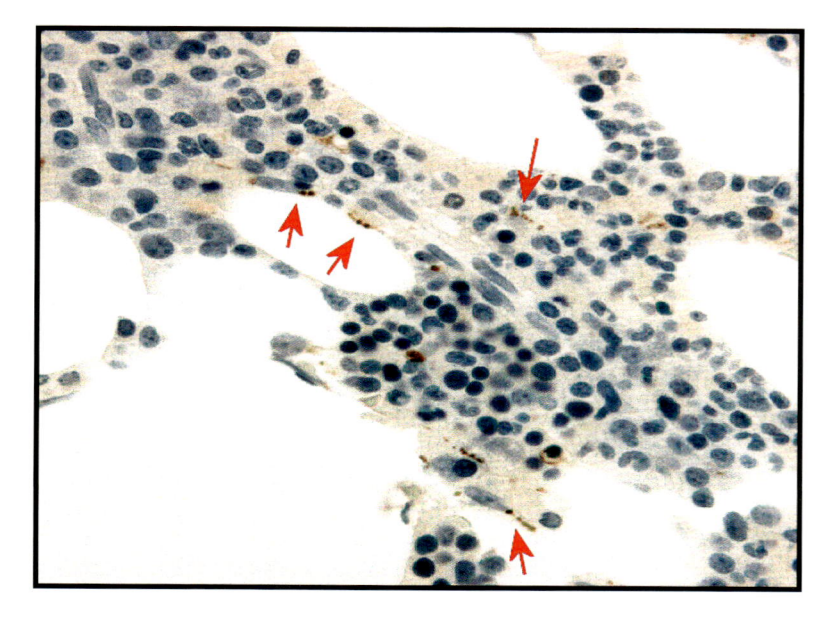

F3.18.2 CD30 in histologically normal bone marrow

In occasional BM biopsy specimens, some spindle cells that are compatible with endothelial cells show dotlike expression; however, this does not appear to be the Golgi-type pattern, because the staining is not always paranuclear, and there are multiple dots per cell (red arrows). The biological significance of this finding, if any, is not clear.

3.18 CD30

F3.18.3 CD30; cytoplasmic expression in rare cells in histologically normal bone marrow

Some apparently histologically normal BM sections will demonstrate globular positivity for CD30 in rare cells, which probably represents an artefact (red arrow). Weak and ill-defined reactivity, which is difficult to localize, is a relatively frequent phenomenon (blue arrows).

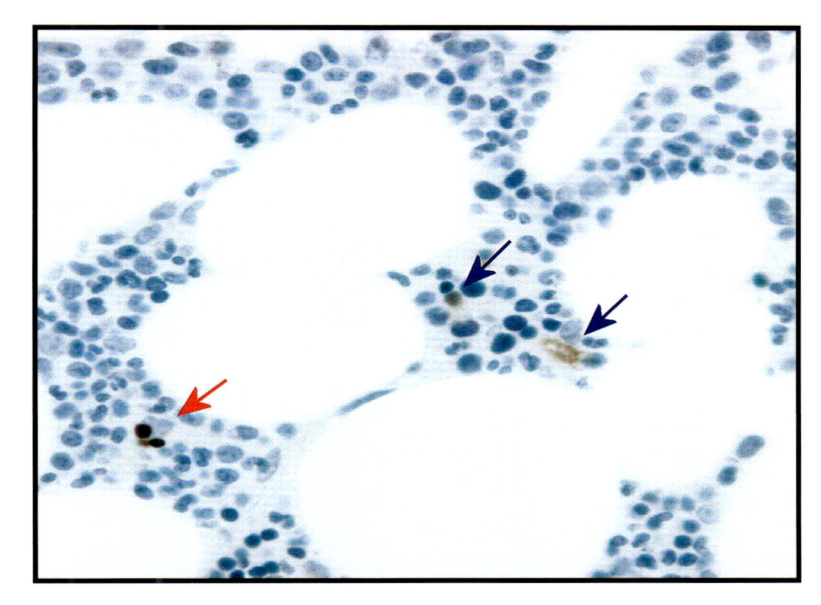

F3.18.4 CD30 in histologically normal bone marrow

Rarely, few large cells show irregular distribution of staining with CD30 antibody (arrows). The morphologic features of these cells are probably not specific enough to determine the cell type.

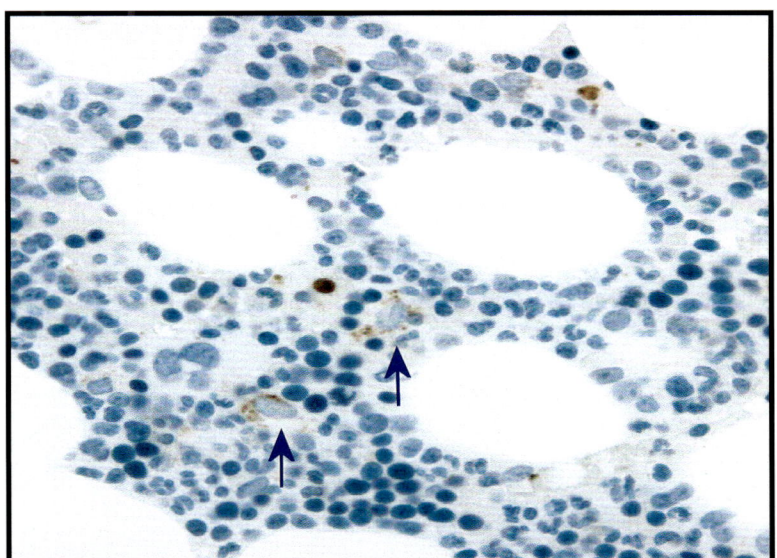

F3.18.5 CD30 in myeloproliferative disease

Many of the cells that appear weakly positive are eosinophils. Eosinophil granules may give a false appearance of weak to moderate positivity on immunohistochemistry. A single spot with what appears to be more specific staining is probably extracellular.

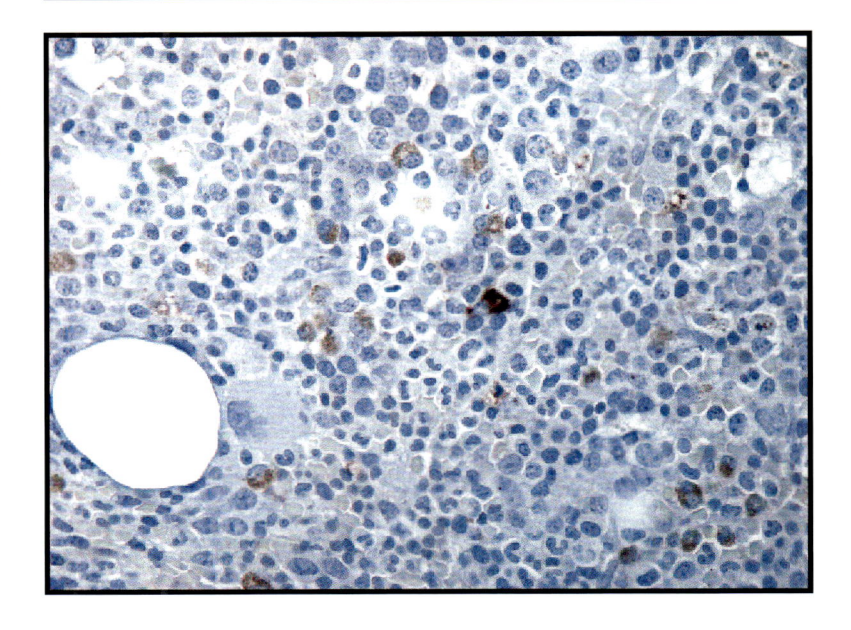

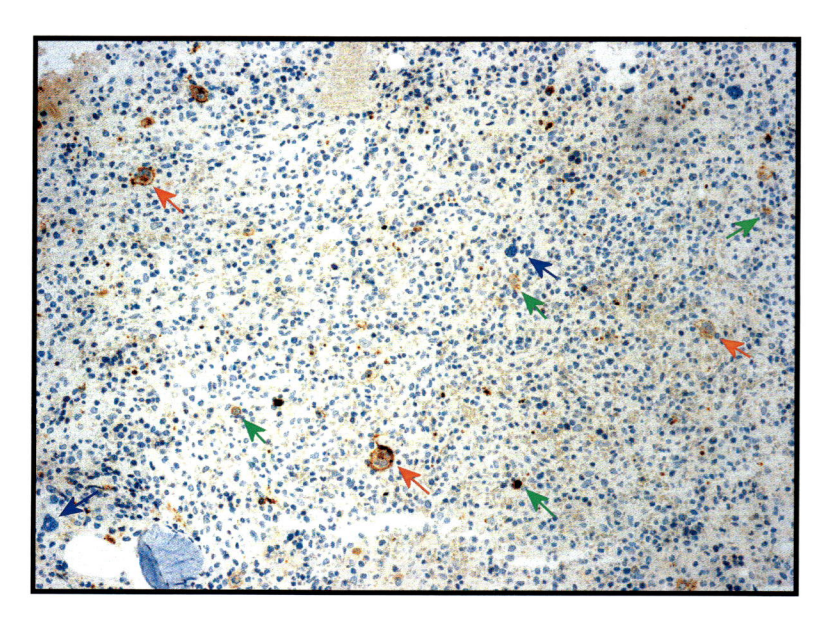

F3.18.6 CD30 in classical Hodgkin lymphoma (cHL)

CD30 is usually easy to demonstrate in cHL. The bone marrow biopsy specimen is hypercellular, at least focally, and also fibrotic and clearly positive for CD30 (red arrows) and in most cases for CD15. The Hodgkin cells do not need to be numerous and not all neoplastic cells are positive in every case. Some large negative cells are megakaryocytes (blue arrows). Green arrows point to extracellular positivity which is difficult to interpret.

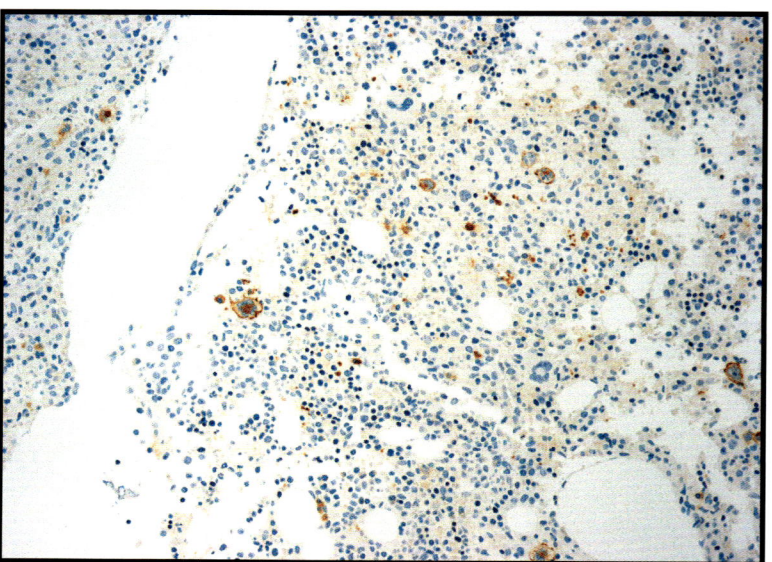

F3.18.7 CD30 in classical Hodgkin lymphoma

Different case than that shown in **F3.18.6**. The Hodgkin cells are clearly positive for CD30. The positivity is membranous, cytoplasmic, dotlike Golgi type or a combination of the three. Some bone marrow biopsy specimens do not show fibrosis (as shown here). In such cases, immunohistochemical demonstration of CD30 (and preferably Pax-5 and/or CD15 positivity in large cells) is required for the diagnosis.

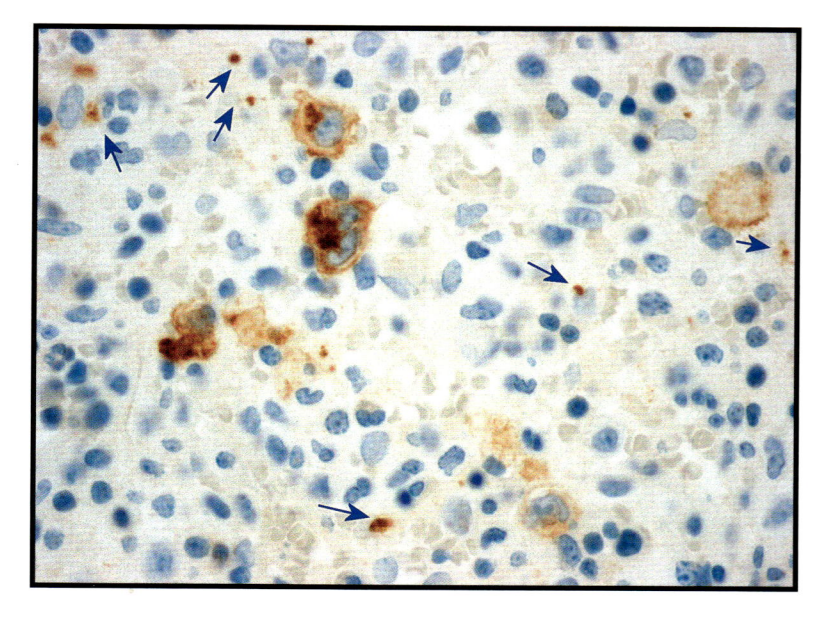

F3.18.8 CD30 in classical Hodgkin lymphoma

The same case as seen in **F3.18.7**. The Hodgkin cells show CD30 in Golgi location as well as variable diffuse cytoplasmic and membranous expression. This varies from cell to cell. As in lymph nodes, the exact pattern of CD30 positivity or consistency from cell to cell is not so important. The neoplastic cells were also clearly CD15+. Some extracellular positivity is also noted (arrows), but it has no diagnostic value.

3.18 CD30

F3.18.9 CD30 in bone marrow with marginal zone lymphoma (MZL)

This BM biopsy specimen is from a 42-year-old man with a history of gastric MZL. Several lymphoid aggregates in the BM were most consistent with MZL. Rare large cells, which are weakly positive for CD30 (but CD15– and EBER–) are present (red arrows). A few smaller lymphocytes also showed possible CD30 weak expression (blue arrows). These findings are of indeterminate diagnostic significance and the diagnosis was unchanged.

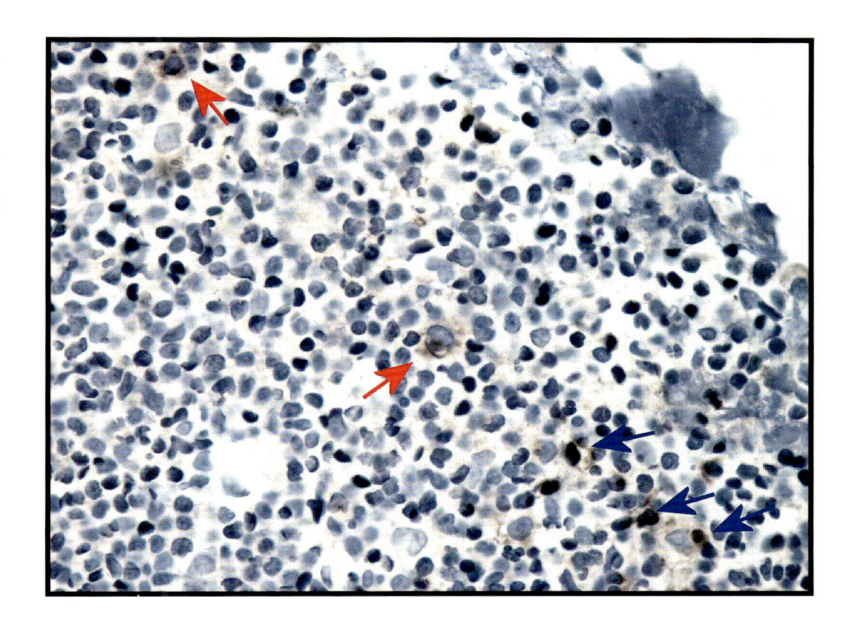

3.19 CD31 (PECAM)

CD31 is primarily an adhesion molecule and is also known as PECAM-1, GPiia', and endocam (PROW). CD31 binds in a homophilic manner (CD31 binds CD31 on the apposing cell), thereby mediating adhesion among endothelial cells and between leukocyte and endothelial cells. CD31 is expressed by leukocytes including monocytes, megakaryocytes (platelets), and granulocytes as well as endothelial cells in the BM. PECAM1 is implicated in several functions, including transendothelial migration of leukocytes, angiogenesis, and integrin activation [Newman 1997]. Many cells will be positive in almost any BM biopsy, and it may be not the best choice as a megakaryocytic marker despite its use in some institutions [Horny 2007b]. In the BM, CD34 marks endothelial cells and megakaryocytes and has similar, but more restricted, distribution than CD31. While CD31 is consistently expressed in normal megakaryocytes and platelets, CD34 is variably expressed in megakaryocytes, but not in platelets. Also, it is not known what determines CD34 expression in megakaryocytes [Calapso 1992; Torlakovic 2002d]. However, CD31 expression may vary significantly in abnormal/dysplastic megakaryocytes. It is seen in a Golgi-type, focal or diffuse cytoplasmic, and membranous pattern of expression or any combination of these. Normal megakaryocytes generally display strong cytoplasmic expression. While CD31 can be used as a megakaryocytic marker, von Willebrand factor (factor VIII–related Ag), CD61, and CD42b are more specific [Chuang 2000; Qiao 1996; Fox 1990]. CD31 is also strongly expressed in extramedullary reactive plasma cells, focally in BM-reactive plasma cells, and occasionally in extramedullary plasmacytomas [Govender 1997].

F3.19.1 CD31 in normal bone marrow

CD31 is expressed in many cells of the BM including monocytes, granulocytes, platelets, and megakaryocytes. Lymphoid subsets and endothelial cells also are clearly demonstrated. With so many different cell types showing CD31 expression, prudent use and interpretation of results obtained with this antibody are recommended.

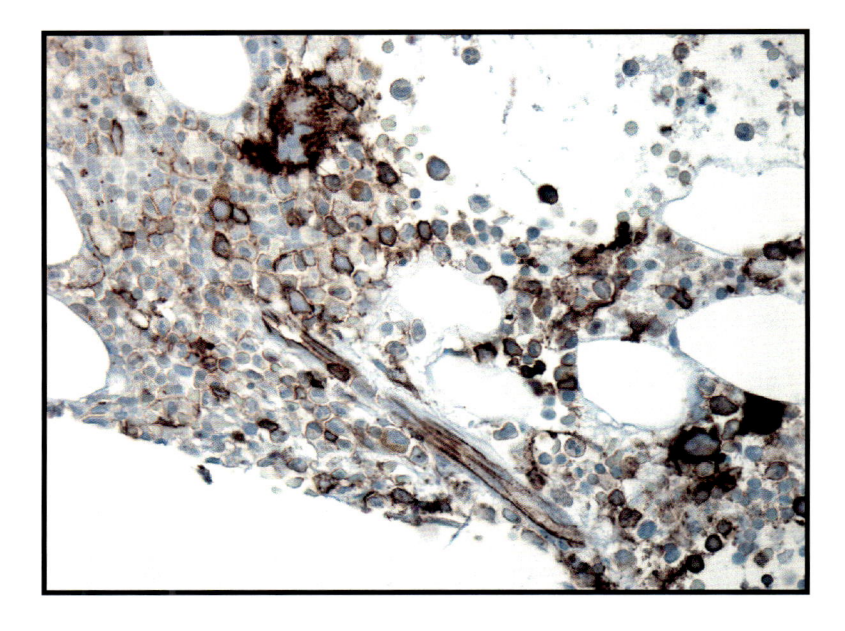

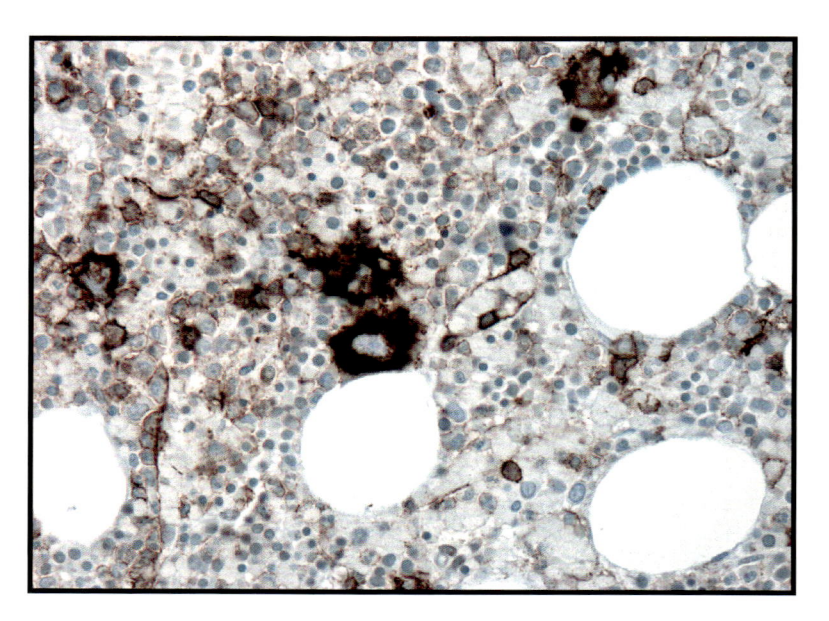

F3.19.2 CD31 in normal bone marrow

While megakaryocytes are the most strongly reacting cells in the histologically normal BM, many other cell types also express CD31, which complicates the interpretation of the results. In this area, it is certain that erythroid precursors are negative, and all other cells appear to be positive to some degree.

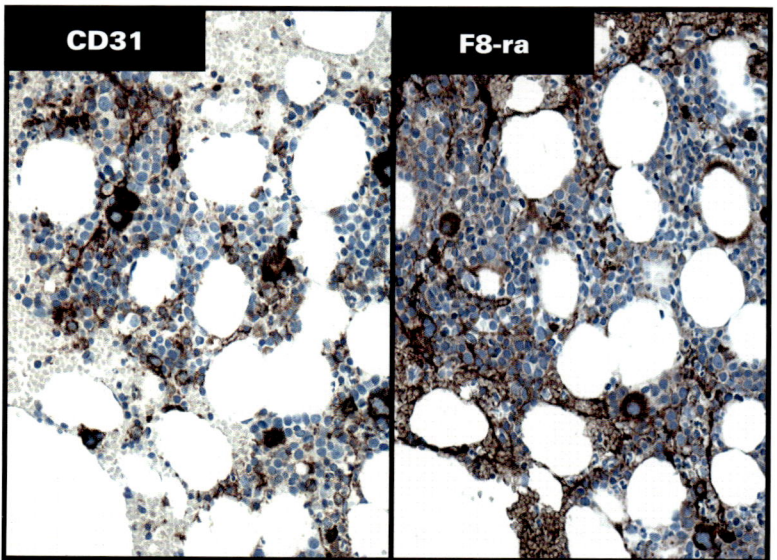

F3.19.3 CD31 compared with von Willebrand factor (F8-related antigen; F8-ra) in myelodysplastic syndrome

In this figure, the CD31 staining may appear to be more selective than that of F8-ra with better signal-noise ratio. While F8-ra is often present in extracellular localization because it also labels platelets, the CD31 actually stains a larger spectrum of different cell types. F8-ra is more specific than CD31 for megakaryocyte differentiation.

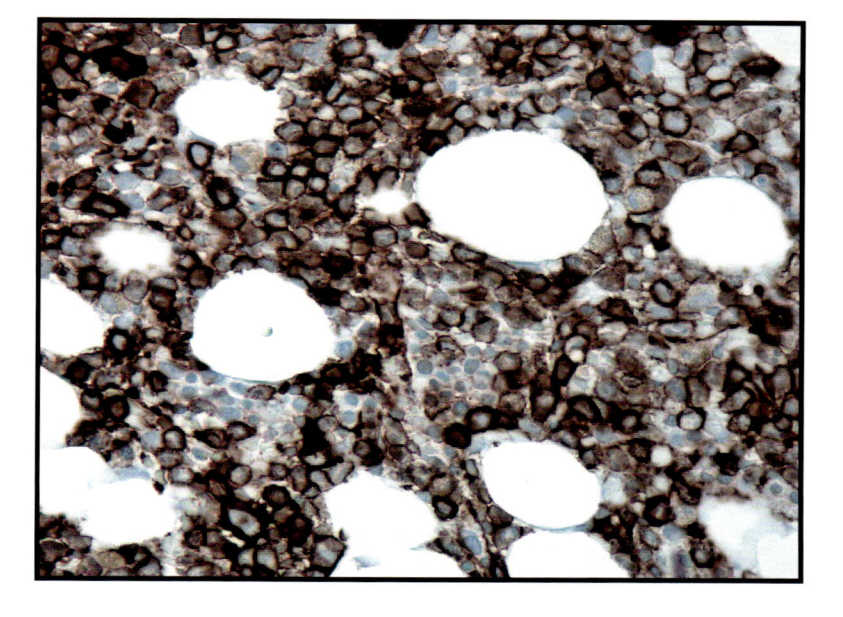

F3.19.4 CD31 in acute myelomonoblastic leukemia

CD31 expression is not unusual in any acute myeloid leukemia and in particular, it is present in acute myelomonoblastic leukemia. This illustrates that CD31 should not be used as a marker for megakaryoblastic differentiation despite its strong expression in megakaryocytes and platelets.

3.19 CD31 (PECAM)

F3.19.5 CD31 in acute megakaryoblastic leukemia

While CD31 is expressed in megakaryoblastic leukemia, it is not uniform or very highly expressed. In many other myeloid leukemias its expression may be more intense (compare with F3.19.4).

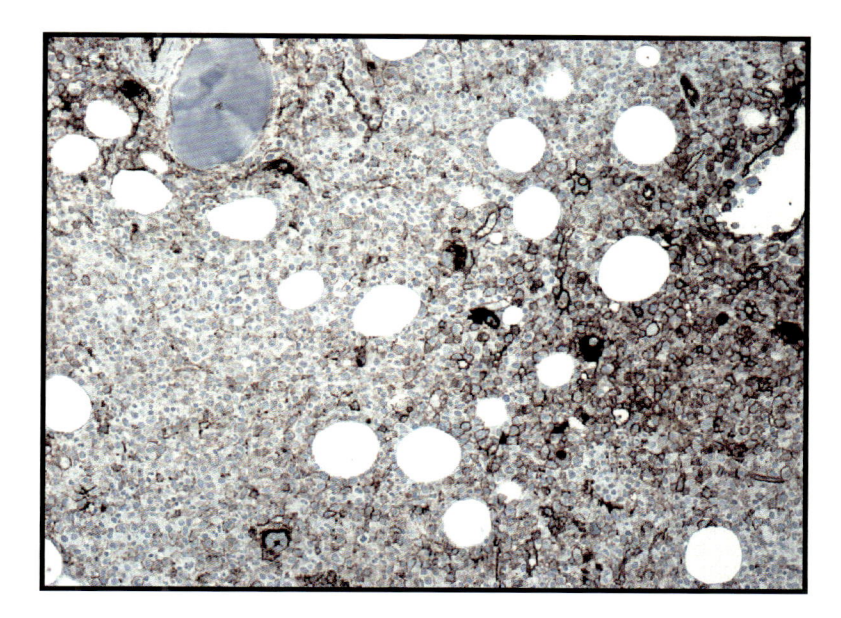

F3.19.6 CD31 in acute myeloid leukemia (AML) with maturation

This AML in a 42-year-old woman was characterized with flow cytometry, cytochemistry, and morphologic analysis as most consistent with an AML with maturation. Immunohistochemistry revealed strong expression of membranous CD31 in most cells. As described before, this finding is not sufficient for the diagnosis of acute megakaryoblastic leukemia.

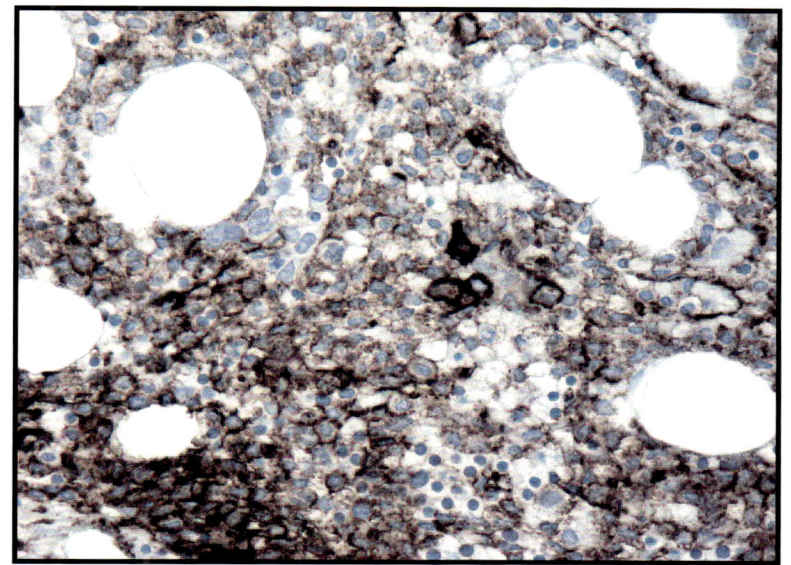

F3.19.7 CD31 in acute myelomonoblastic leukemia

Because CD31 is expressed in both monocytes and neutrophils, myelomonoblastic leukemia is expected to show membranous expression as demonstrated in this 80-year-old man.

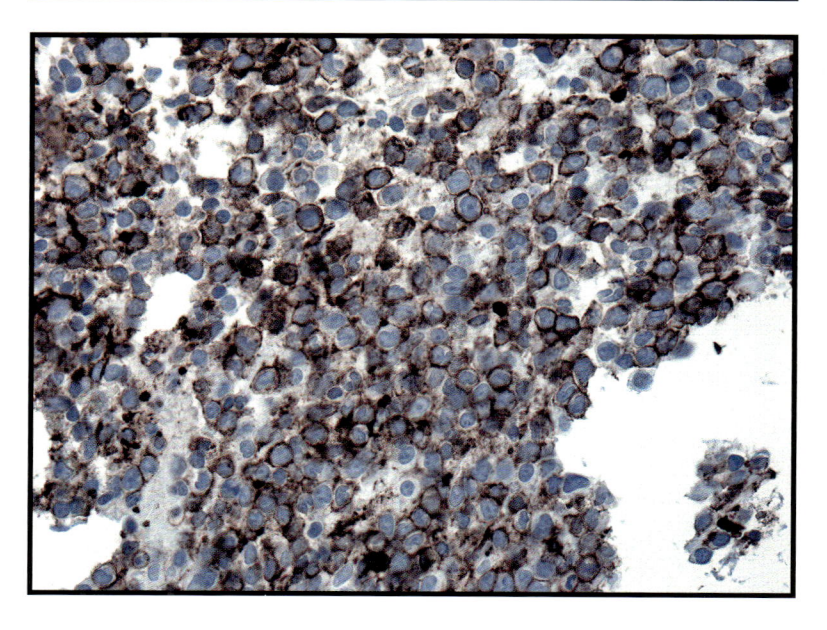

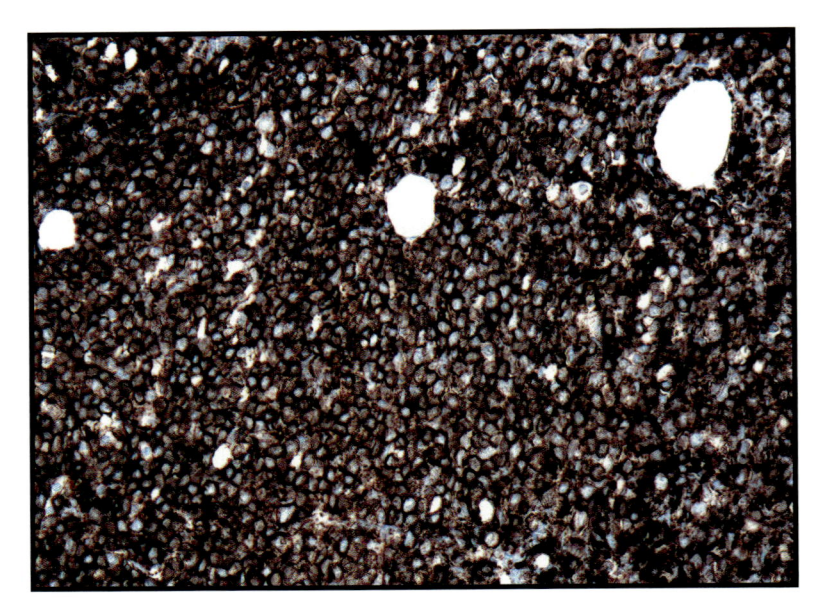

F3.19.8 CD31 in precursor B-cell lymphoblastic leukemia

Very strong expression of CD31 is detected in this case of precursor B-cell lymphoblastic leukemia in a biopsy specimen from a 9-year-old girl. Flow cytometry showed no evidence of aberrant marker expression. Normal cells of B lineage express CD31 and therefore this finding is not unusual.

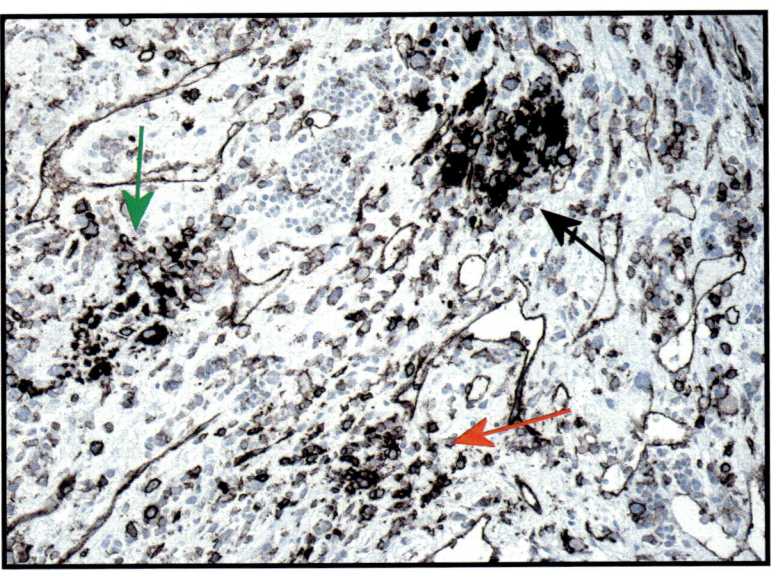

F3.19.9 CD31 in precursor B-cell acute lymphoblastic leukemia after chemotherapy with 30% residual blasts

Note the 3 groups of CD31+ cells: cluster of megakaryocytes (black arrow), cluster of platelets with rare megakaryocytes (green arrow), and cluster of leukemic blasts (red arrow).

3.20 CD33

CD33 is also known as gp67 and p67. The CD33 expression is highly specific to the hematopoietic cells and shows prominent expression on early myeloid cells. The biologic role of CD33 is unknown (PROW). CD33 is expressed by myeloid progenitors including monocytes/macrophages, granulocyte precursors with decreasing expression with maturation. Elizabeth Hyjek, MD, PhD reported CD33 expression in paraffin-embedded tissues on normal/neoplastic myelomonocytic lineage cells, mast cells, and dendritic cells [Bansal 2007]. CD33 detection with IHC may be useful in differentiating the diagnosis of myeloid tumors from their lymphoid mimics and other nonhematopoietic tumors. In particular, it identifies the myeloid nature of myelomonocytic and monoblastic leukemias, which may be difficult or impossible to detect with MPO antibodies [Andrews 1983; Hoyer 2008]. CD33 is also important in differentiating between hematodermic neoplasm and monoblastic leukemia. CD33 is consistently absent from this lesion, while it is readily demonstrated in acute monoblastic leukemia [Yu 2008].

3.20 CD33

F3.20.1 CD33 in histologically normal bone marrow

A large number of cells is positive for CD33. However, only histologically recognizable myeloid precursors and mast cells are positive. This patient appears to have a normal myeloid to erythroid precursor (M-E) ratio, but the signal-to-noise ratio is not optimal and therefore, this may not be the best antibody to be used to determine the M-E ratio. Myeloperoxidase appears to be a better choice for this purpose.

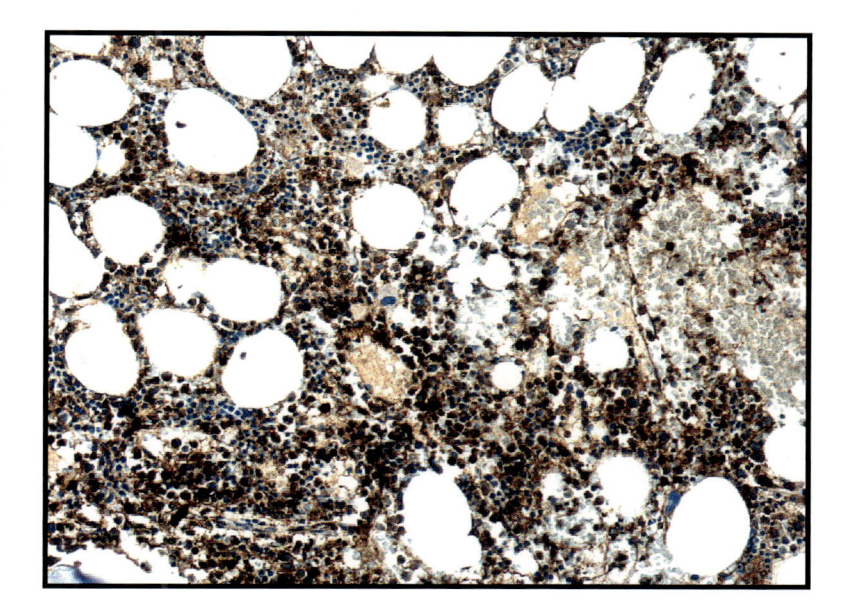

F3.20.2 CD33 in histologically normal bone marrow

Same case as in F3.20.1. Very thick sections are often a problem in the interpretation of signal localization in the BM biopsy. This is clearly illustrated by the fact that it is difficult to focus in a single plane on the nuclei of most cells. Myeloid precursors are variably positive and erythroid precursors should be negative.

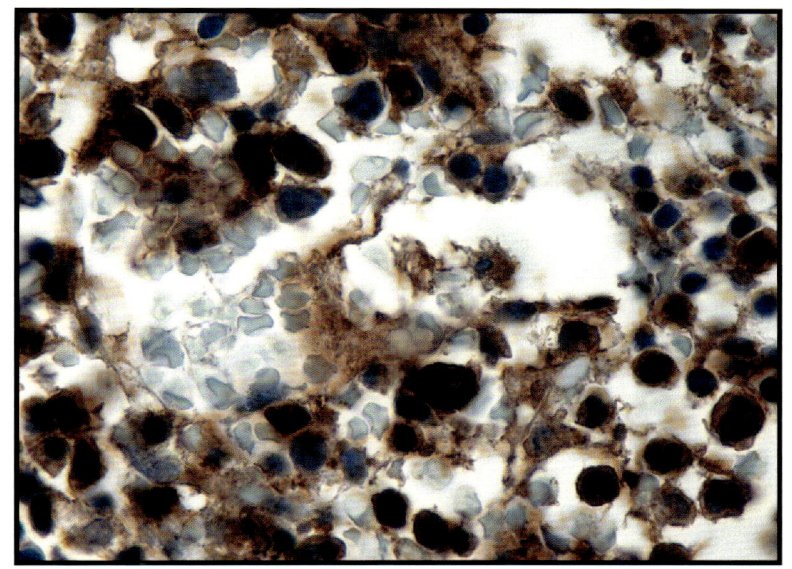

F3.20.3 CD33 in histologically normal bone marrow

Harsh antigen retrieval protocols or even routine protocols, if applied to thick sections or suboptimally pretreated slides with insufficient adhesive properties, will cause lifting of the tissue; this in turn will cause problems focusing as seen in this case. Blue arrow points to phagocytic macrophage and red arrow to a Golgi-type positivity possibly in myeloid precursor or mast cell precursors. It would be prudent to repeat this test. Interpretation of suboptimal material may result in erroneous conclusions.

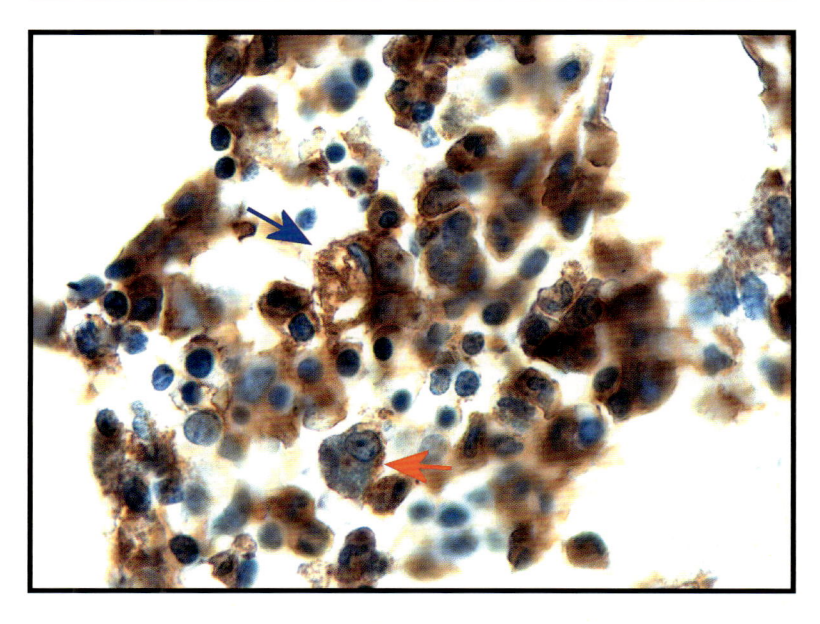

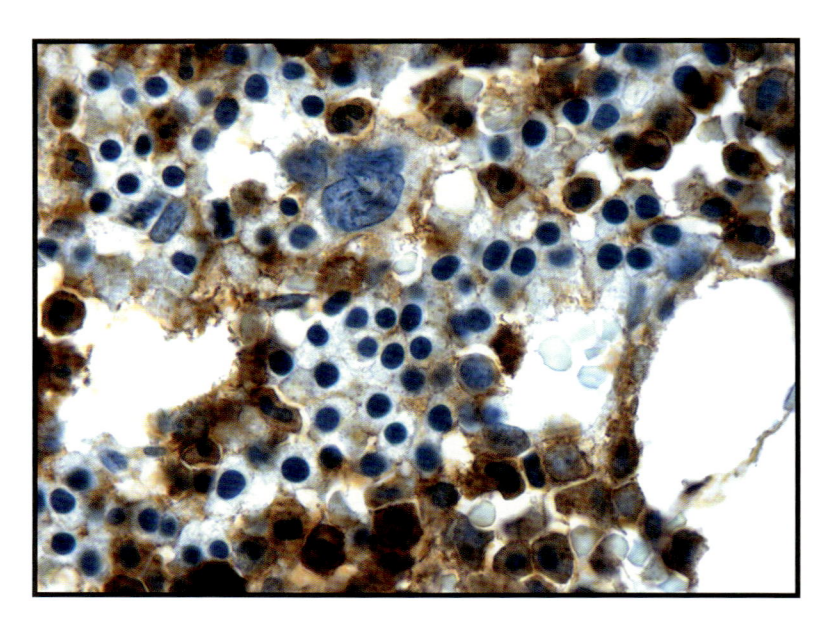

F3.20.4 CD33 in histologically normal bone marrow

CD33 is not expressed by normal erythroid precursors or megakaryocytes. Neutrophils show both membranous and variable cytoplasmic positivity. Despite overall unclear low magnification appearance, signal-to-noise ratio is very good.

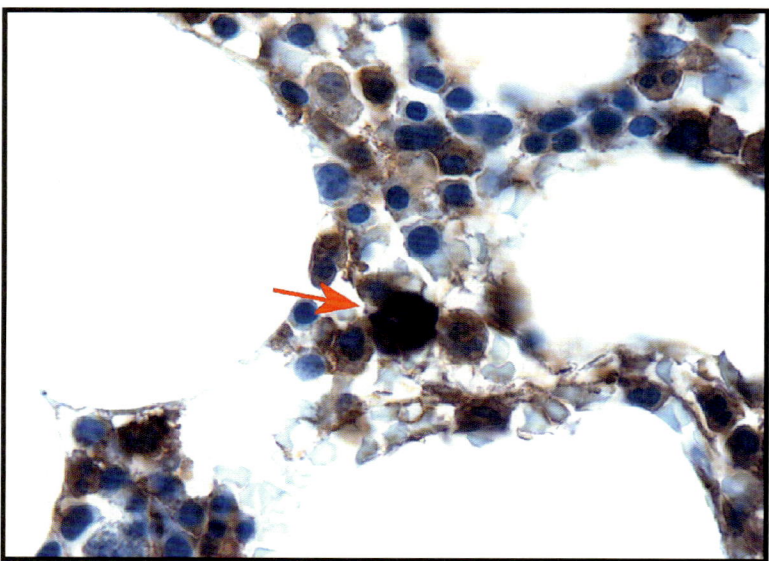

F3.20.5 CD33 in benign mast cells

In a histologically normal bone marrow specimen, very few mast cells can be found. However, they appear to express higher levels of CD33 when evaluated with immunohistochemistry (red arrow). This was a consistent finding throughout the biopsy.

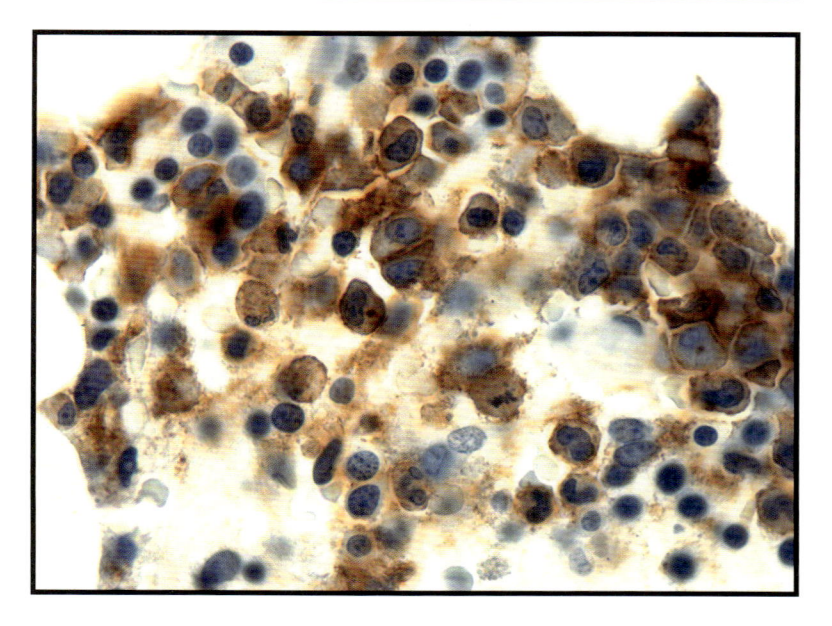

F3.20.6 CD33 in histologically normal bone marrow

Despite more or less clear signal-to-noise ratio, if a primary antibody is further diluted, the interpretation is easier. One can easily appreciate weak, but definite membranous positivity as well as fine Golgi-type positivity in rare myeloid cells. Whether such dilution is clinically useful is questionable, because of the potential false-negative results in neoplastic conditions.

F3.20.7 CD33 in intestinal myeloid sarcoma

The value of CD33 as a myeloid antigen is questionable in myeloid sarcoma, which clearly expresses myeloperoxidase (MPO). In this setting, the CD33 primary antibody does not appear to have any diagnostic usefulness. When MPO is expressed, there is definitive evidence of myeloid differentiation and any other myeloid marker is redundant.

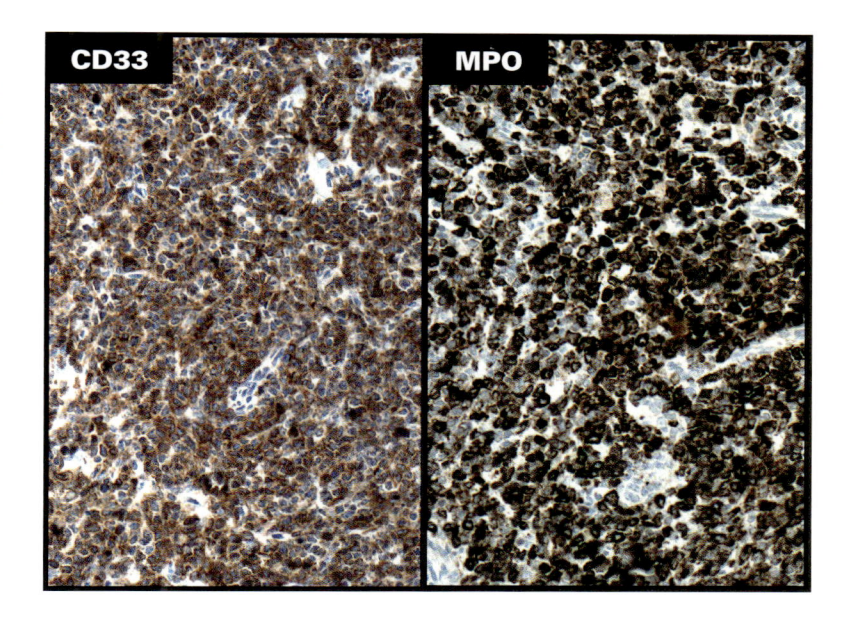

F3.20.8 CD33 in acute monoblastic leukemia

While myeloperoxidase (MPO) was clearly negative in the leukemic cells in this acute monoblastic leukemia, CD33 is strongly positive. Therefore, demonstration of CD33 is useful in the evaluation of MPO− acute myeloid leukemias. CD33 is also expressed in mature monocytes, histiocytes, macrophages, dendritic cells, and mast cells.

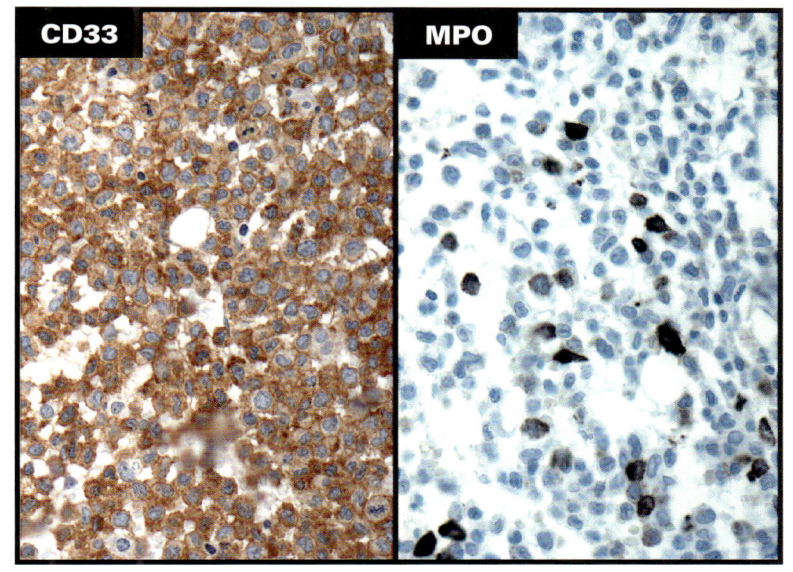

F3.20.9 CD33 in mast cell disease

CD33 is an excellent marker for both benign and malignant mast cells. Myeloperoxidase (MPO) is consistently negative in mast cell disease. CD33 appears to be an excellent marker of myeloid differentiation in MPO− myeloid lesions.

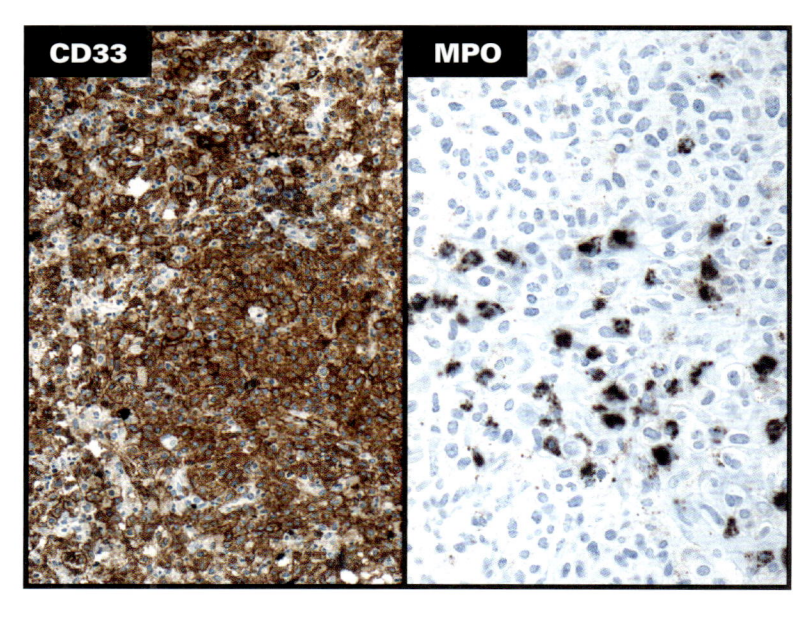

3.21 CD34

CD34 is also known as gp105-120 (PROW). CD34 is a surface glycophosphoprotein expressed on various cells, including early hematopoietic stem cells and progenitor cells, endothelial cells, and embryonic fibroblasts [Krause 1996]. Not all functions of CD34 are known. CD34 has a role in cell adhesion and inhibition of hematopoiesis [Baumheter 1993; Fackler 1992; Charbord 1996; Fackler 1995]. In hematopoiesis, it is rapidly downregulated as soon as the differentiation process begins. In the BM, it is also found in the early and mature megakaryocytes, but the expression is cytoplasmic rather than membranous [Machhi 2001; Torlakovic 2002d]. The immunohistochemical detection of CD34 protein using QBEND10 antibody is a well-established method for the detection of myeloid blasts in myelodysplastic syndrome (MDS) or AML, as well as for the detection of lymphoblasts in acute lymphoblastic leukemia in BM trephine sections [Reddy 2001; Horny 1995; Toth 1999]. The number of CD34+ cells can be evaluated as a percentage of positive cells in a cell count of 500 or detection of rounded aggregates of CD34+ cells with more than 3 or 5 positive cells depending on the author [Torlakovic 2002d; Toth 1999; Min 1995; Soligo 1991; Baur 2000]. Not all neoplastic myeloblasts or lymphoblasts are CD34+. A negative reaction does not exclude the presence of malignant blasts. It may also be used for the evaluation of angiogenesis [Pruneri 1999; Sezer 2000].

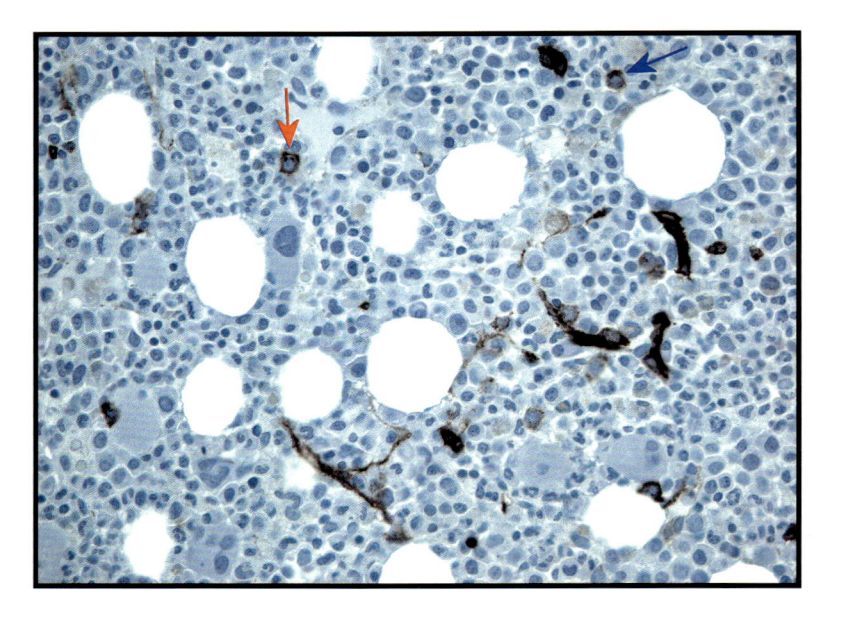

F3.21.1 CD34 in histologically normal bone marrow

This BM biopsy specimen is from an 18-year-old woman with classical Hodgkin lymphoma. The BM was not involved. Endothelial cells are strongly stained. Only 2 small cells with, what appears to be cytoplasmic staining only (blue arrow) and cytoplasmic and membranous staining (red arrow), are identified in this field at 400× magnification. BM aspirate differential count revealed 1.2% blasts.

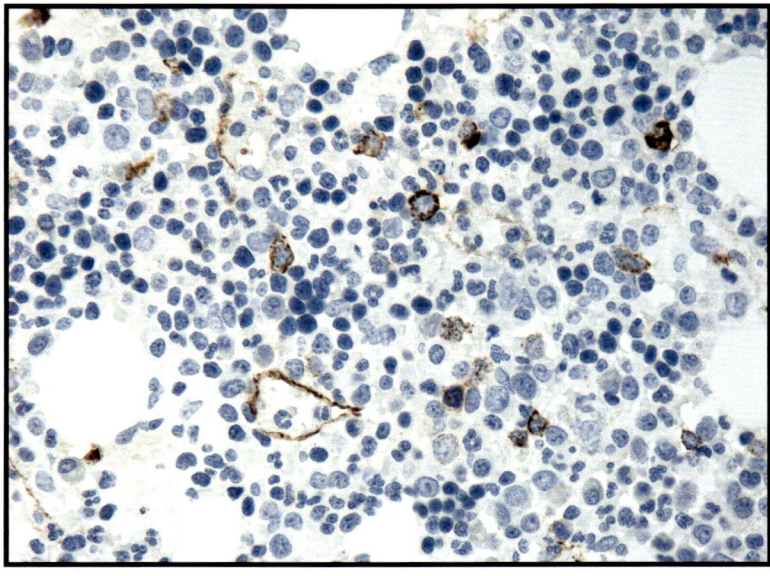

F3.21.2 CD34 in refractory anemia with excess blasts-1 (RAEB-1)

CD34 staining highlights small mononuclear and endothelial cells with cytoplasmic and membranous staining. This illustration shows typical result of immunohistochemistry staining in the bone marrow with slightly increased blasts. There were 7% blasts in the BM aspirate and only minimal evidence of abnormal maturation. Cytogenetic analysis was normal. These findings are interpreted as RAEB-1.

F3.21.3 CD34 in chronic myeloid leukemia (CML) with slightly increased blast count

This patient has CML. Most of the CD34+ cells are small and mononuclear, compatible with CD34+ blasts. Morphologic analysis of the aspirate smears revealed 4.2% blasts, close to the threshold of 5%. A 500-cell count on the CD34-stained sections showed 6% blasts, indicating slightly increased blasts. These findings are compatible with an early accelerated phase. Monitoring for impending blast crisis was recommended.

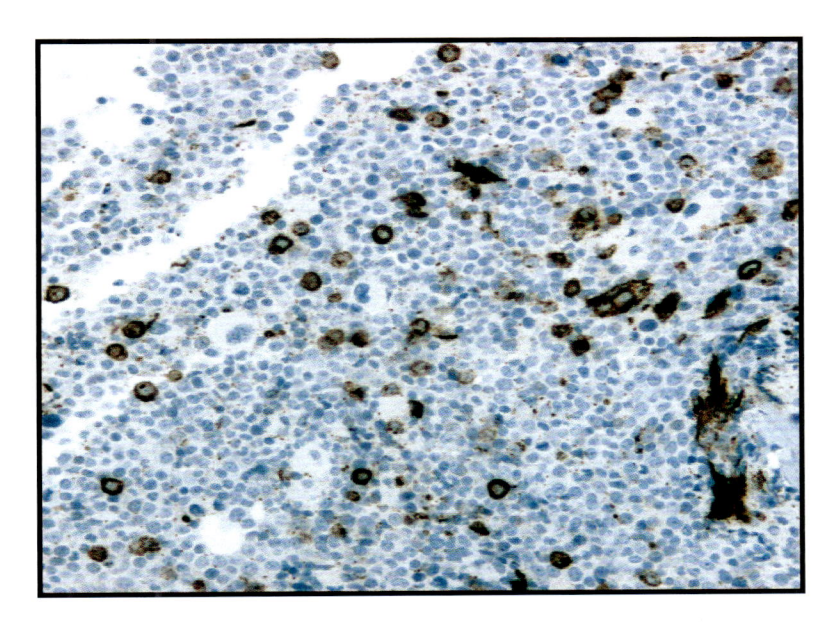

F3.21.4 CD34+ cells in acute myeloid leukemia (AML) with maturation

This specimen was from a patient with AML with maturation. Both blood and BM eosinophilia (blue arrows) were seen. No evidence of monocytic differentiation was found. The BM contained 25% blasts. Endothelial cells were also strongly stained (red arrow). Cytogenetic analysis showed normal karyotype.

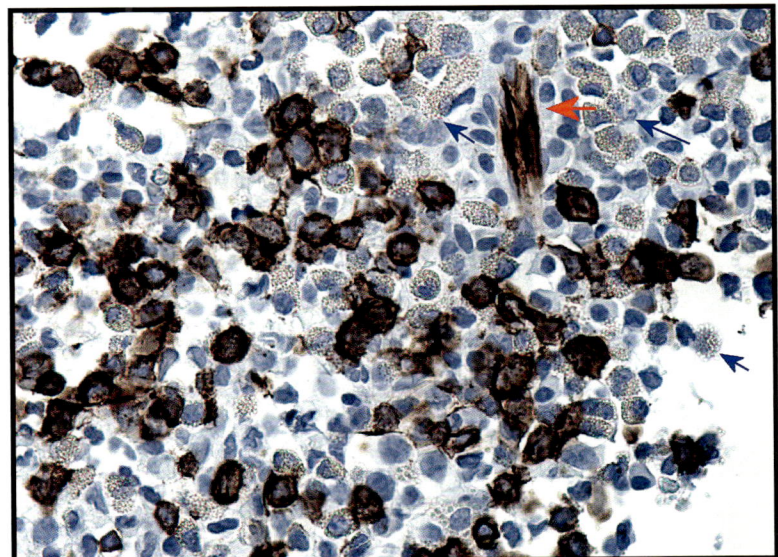

F3.21.5 CD34 in megakaryocytes

CD34 is expressed in a variable number of megakaryocytes in bone marrow biopsy specimens with diverse hematologic disorders and its expression is mainly cytoplasmic. In chronic myeloid leukemia, where large numbers of small megakaryocytes can be found, the CD34 is detected in many megakaryocytes. The biological role of the CD34 in megakaryocytes in myeloproliferative or other disorders, if any, is not known.

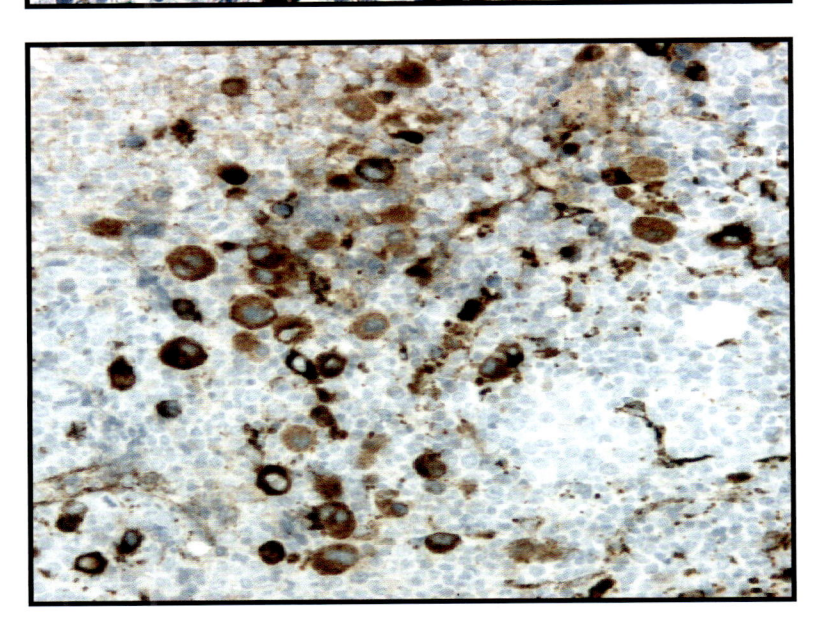

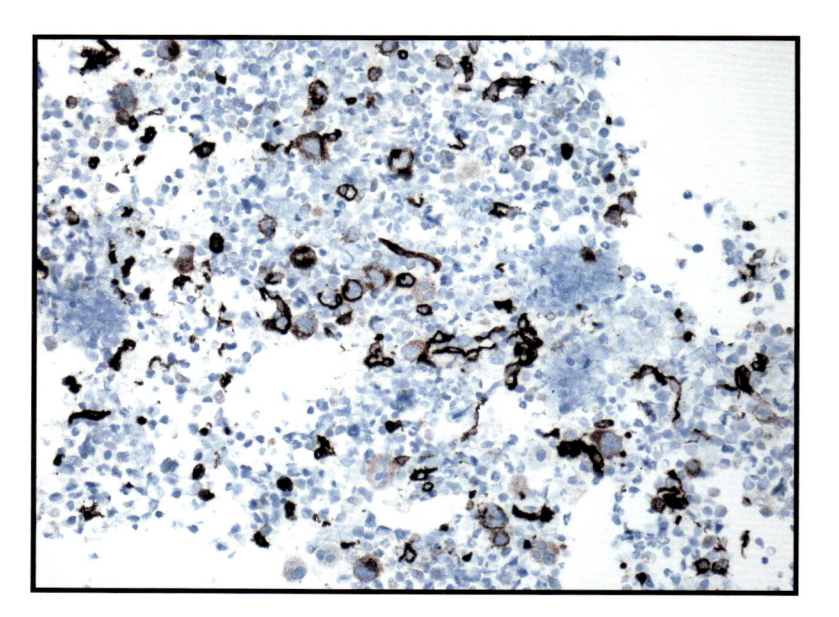

F3.21.6 CD34: Megakaryocytes

In this case of chronic myeloid leukemia (CML), the small megakaryocytes and a few micromegakaryocytes are highlighted by the CD34 immunostaining. While it was once suggested that the CD34 expression in megakaryocytes is more often seen in myelodysplastic syndrome, in our experience, no disease-specific distribution was found. The CD34+ small megakaryocytes are not megakaryoblasts and this phenomenon does not represent transformation to acute megakaryoblastic leukemia.

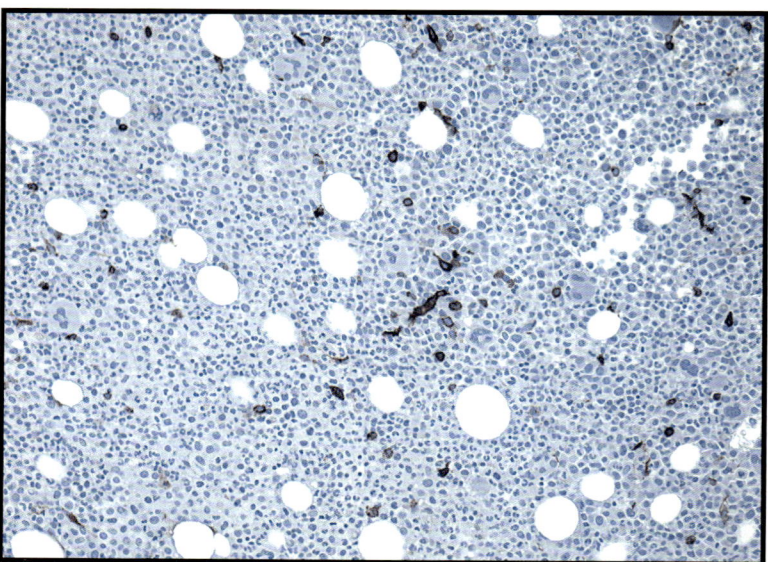

F3.21.7 CD34 in hyperplastic bone marrow

Most non-neoplastic BM biopsy specimens, including those with reactive changes, do not show CD34 expression in megakaryocytes. Also note that a hyperplastic BM shows no evidence of the increased vascularity that is often found in both myeloproliferative and myelodysplastic diseases.

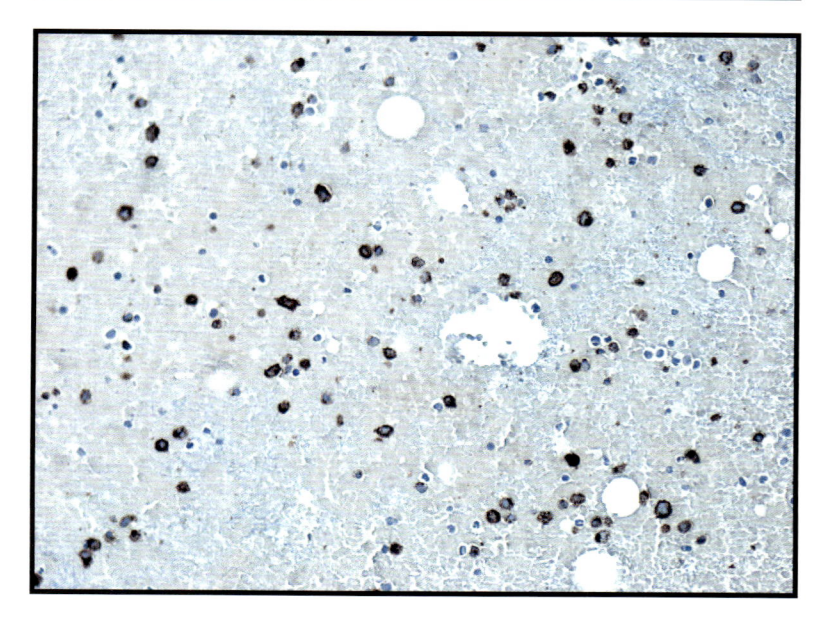

F3.21.8 CD34: in clot section, clotted blood only with no bone marrow particles present

The immunostaining was helpful in this patient because no core biopsy or BM particles were obtained. The exact percentage of the blasts in the BM cannot be determined. However, the combined evidence of pancytopenia with rare circulating blasts and immunophenotyping of the blasts (CD34+, CD117+, MPO+, TdT–, CD3–, Pax-5–, CD79a–) using immunohistochemistry in the clotted aspirate specimen was consistent with the diagnosis of acute myeloid leukemia in this 84-year-old man.

3.21   CD34

F3.21.9 CD34 in hypocellular acute myeloid leukemia; clot section, no bone marrow particles present

While a small number of cells is never exciting to evaluate, paucicellular ("blood only") clot specimens may occasionally be informative because the small number of the CD34+ monoculear cells that are morphologically compatible with blasts and are not endothelial cells, is a very abnormal finding. This is sufficient to suspect significantly increased blasts or acute leukemia even if no other material is available.

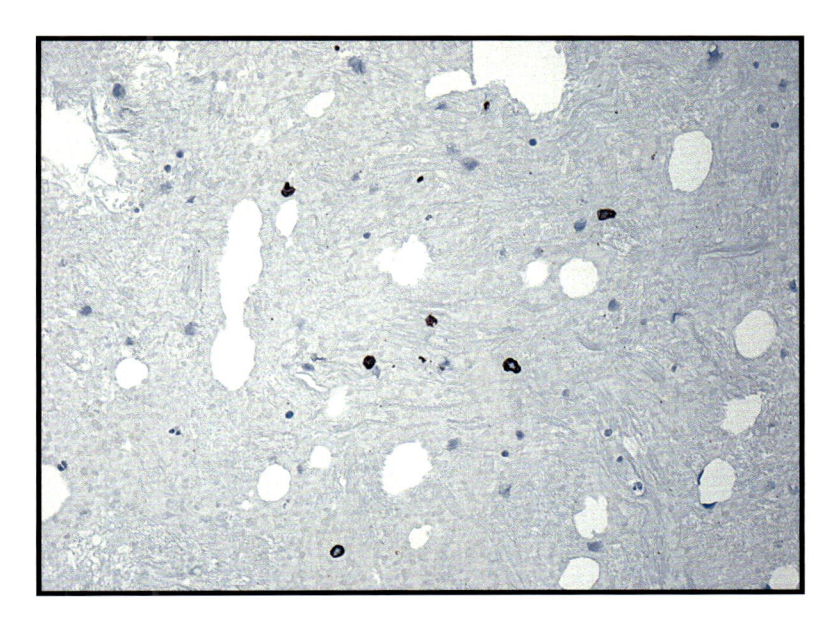

F3.21.10   CD34 in a precursor B-cell acute lymphoblastic leukemia

Approximately 30% of CD34+ cells were detected with flow cytometry. Note predominant cytoplasmic dotlike positivity in many leukemic cells. This type of positivity is not detected on routine flow cytometric analysis because only membranous CD34 is evaluated in acute leukemia panels. On the other hand, a weak surface positivity is difficult to detect on immunohistochemistry in paraffin-embedded tissues.

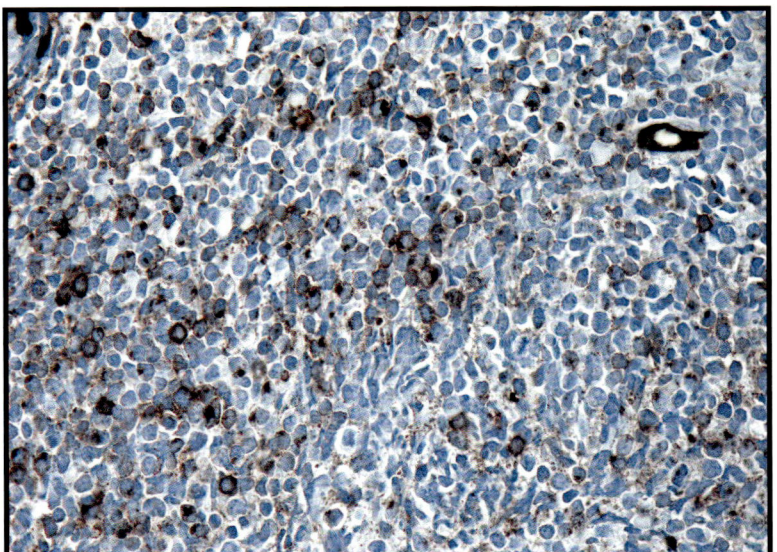

F3.21.11   CD34 in hypocellular acute myeloid leukemia

This bone marrow biopsy specimen was from a 68-year-old woman with pancytopenia and a rare blast in the peripheral blood smear. The BM is less than 30% cellular. CD34 staining reveals more than 30% CD34+ cells, presumably blasts. In good quality BM imprints, this observation can be made without CD34 immunohistochemistry.

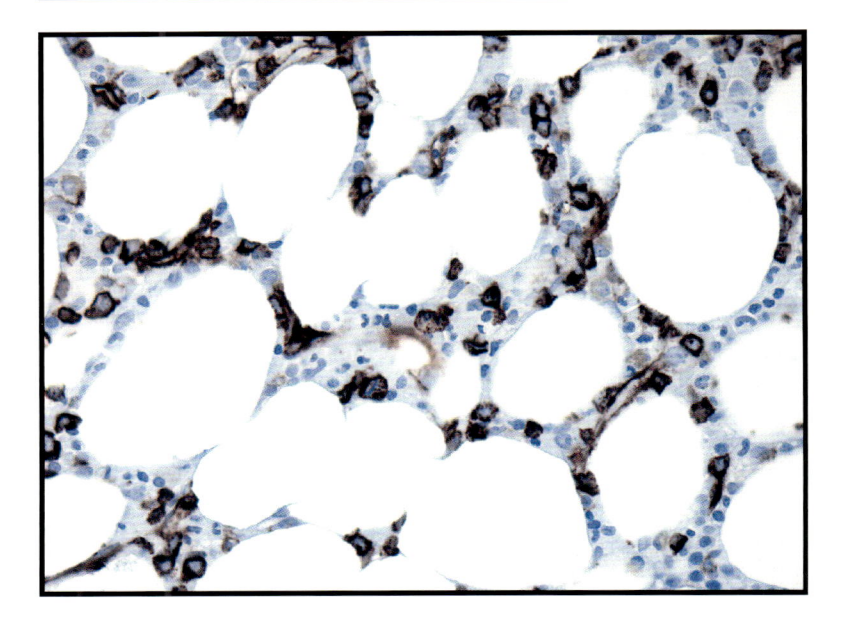

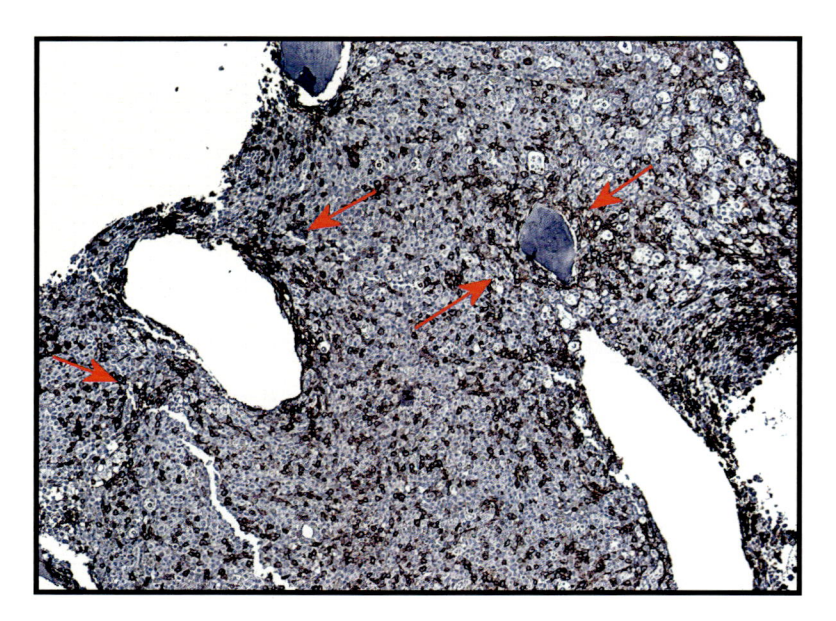

F3.21.12 **CD34 in acute myeloid leukemia with maturation**

The CD34+ cells show a slight tendency for clustering around bony trabeculae and blood vessels (red arrows). In other areas, the blasts are more evenly distributed. It appears that leukemic blasts may mimic normal localization of myeloid precursors.

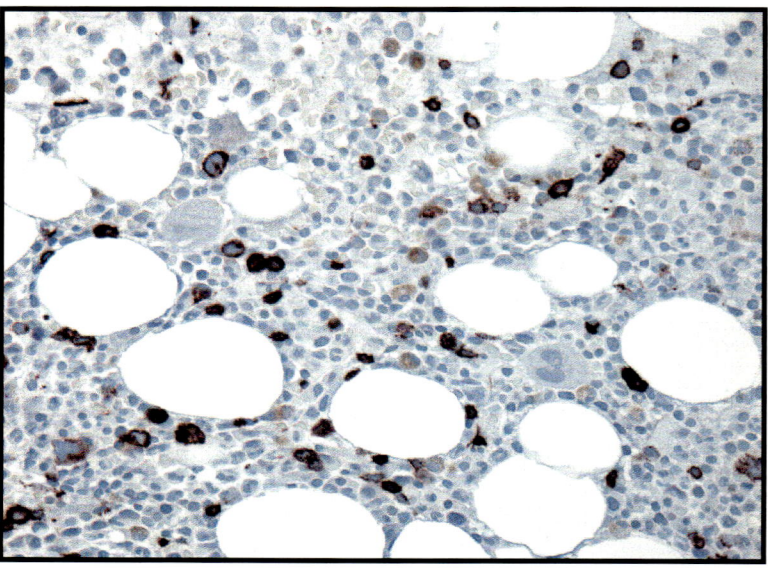

F3.21.13 **CD34 in an acute myelomonocytic leukemia with 47% blasts.**

Occasionally, immunohistochemistry shows that the CD34 counts in the bone marrow biopsy are not representative of the blast count. In this case, the CD34 count revealed 12% positive cells consistent with blasts. However, cytological evaluation clearly showed more than 40% blasts (including promonocytes, monoblasts, and myeloblasts). The highest blast percentage by any method should be used for the diagnosis.

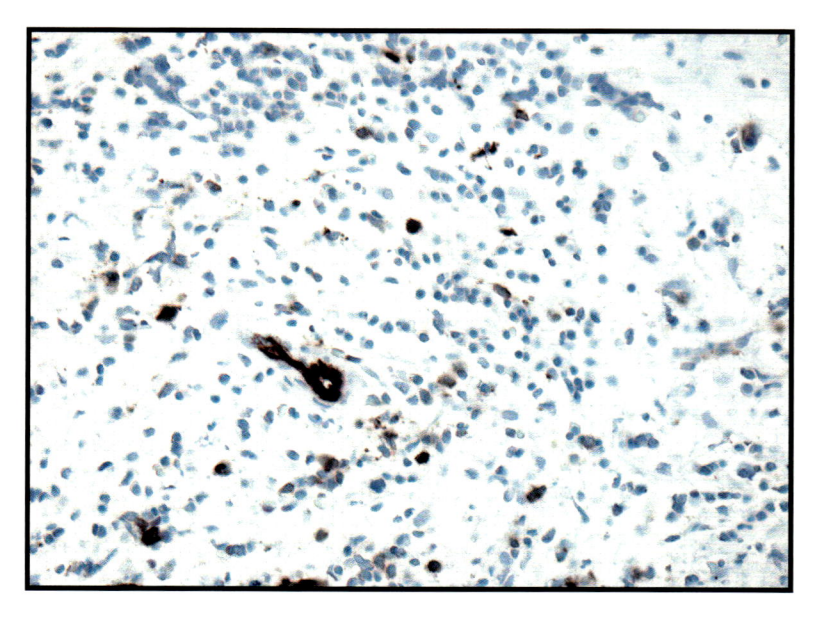

F3.21.14 **CD34 in precursor B-ALL 14 days after induction chemotherapy**

CD34 that was present in almost all blasts at diagnosis; it is not detectable with either immunohistochemistry or flow cytometry 14 days after induction chemotherapy. However, almost all cells illustrated here are blasts. Similarly, the TdT is also negative. CD20 and CD10 were the only 2 markers that could be demonstrated on the blast population at this time. It appears that chemotherapy induced immunophenotypic change in this acute leukemia.

3.21 CD34

F3.21.15 CD34 in serous atrophy

This biopsy specimen with serous atrophy has no CD34+ cells because of the lack of hematopoiesis. There is also no evidence of vascular proliferation, and marrow sinusoids are clearly highlighted.

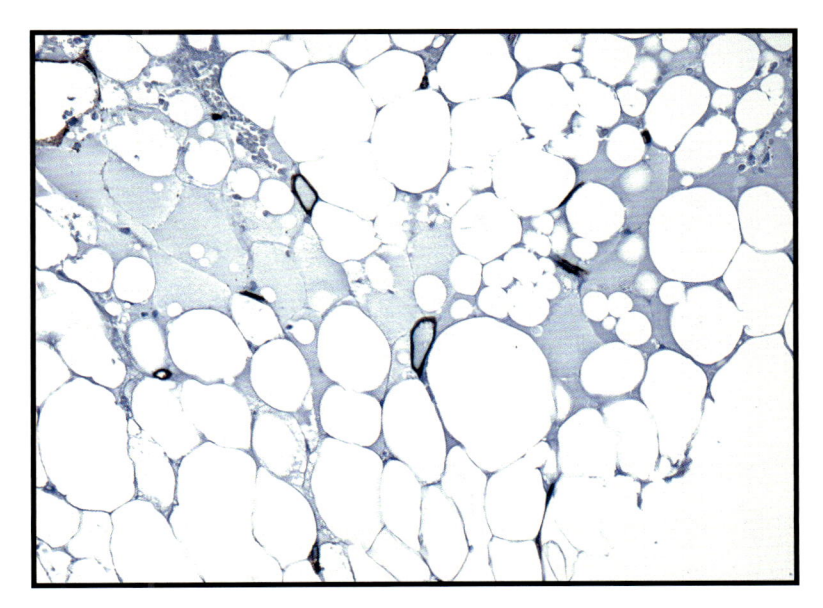

F3.21.16 CD34, day 14 after chemotherapy for acute lymphoblastic leukemia

The CD34 staining highlights dilated sinusoids, which is a common finding after chemotherapy. Variable cellularity was found (normocellular marrow with no evidence of dilated sinusoids in the right lower corner). No morphologic evidence or evidence of increased CD34+ blasts was found. Therefore, the normocellular areas represent bone marrow recovery, rather than residual leukemia.

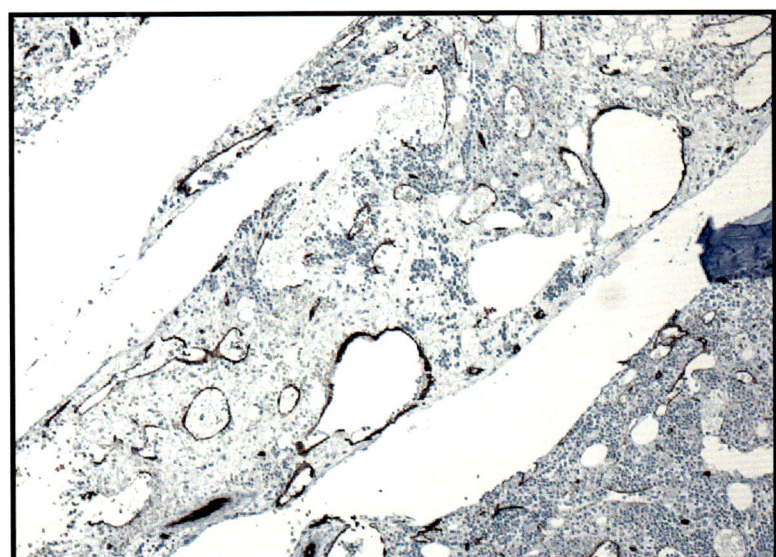

F3.21.17 CD34, day 14 after chemotherapy for acute myeloid leukemia

The patient was a 6-month-old girl. The CD34 staining revealed small foci of CD34+ cells in the vicinity of the large sinusoid. The blast count was not increased in the aspirate smears. However, the CD117+ cells were also found in clusters in this area. This finding is highly suspicious for residual leukemia.

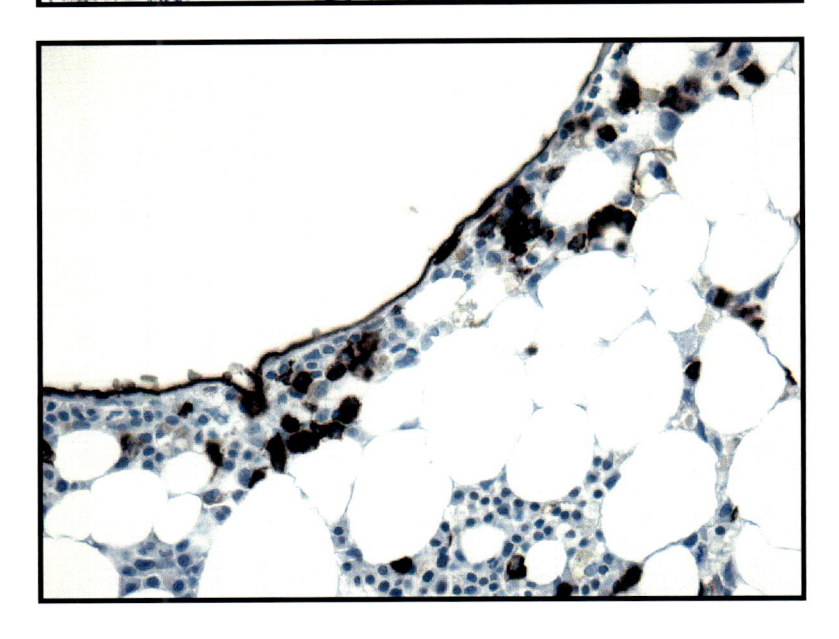

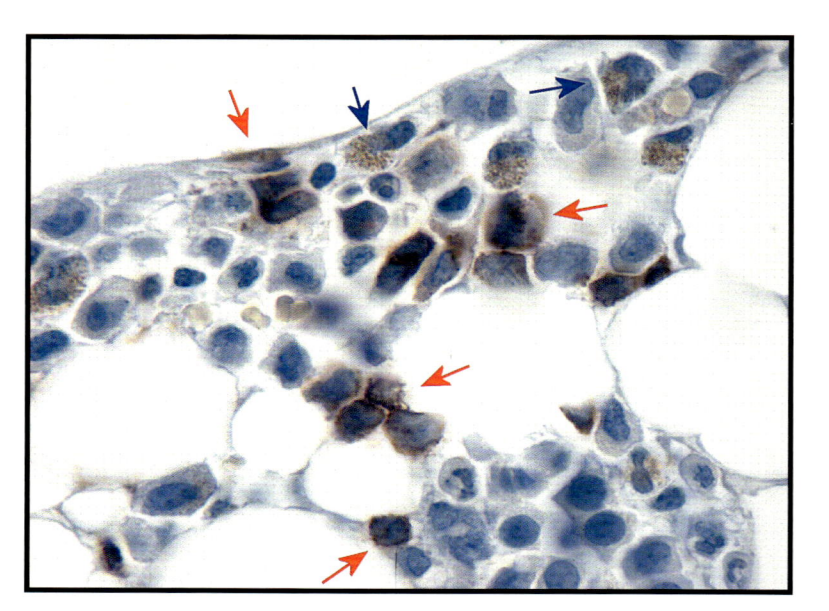

F3.21.18 CD117, day 14 after chemotherapy

The same patient as seen in **F3.21.17**. CD117 staining labeled small clusters of cells in the vicinity of a large sinusoid (same area as in **F3.21.17**), some of which were morphologically consistent with either blasts or early myeloid precursors (red arrows). Eosinophils stand out (blue arrows), too. CD34 and CD117 staining suggest a possible small focus of residual leukemic cells. Clinical significance of such a finding is not clear because the very next biopsy showed no morphologic or immunophenotypic evidence of residual leukemic cells.

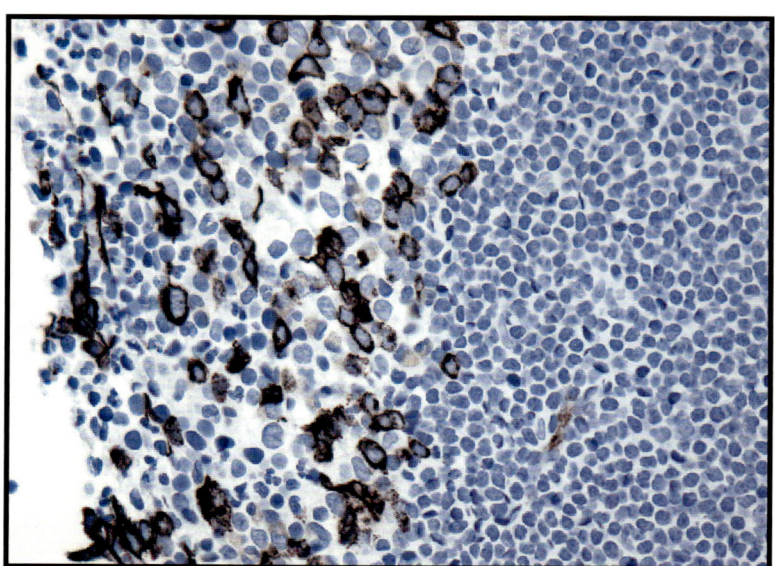

F3.21.19 CD34 in a chronic myelomonocytic leukemia (CMML) with synchronous chronic lymphocytic leukemia (CLL)

This 57-year-old man presented with both CMML and CLL. The most interesting finding was that CD34 and TdT were upregulated in the cells in the vicinity of the lymphoid aggregates of CLL. This image shows CLL aggregate (right) surrounded by bone marrow involved by CMML with increased CD34+ cells in areas close to the lymphoid aggregates.

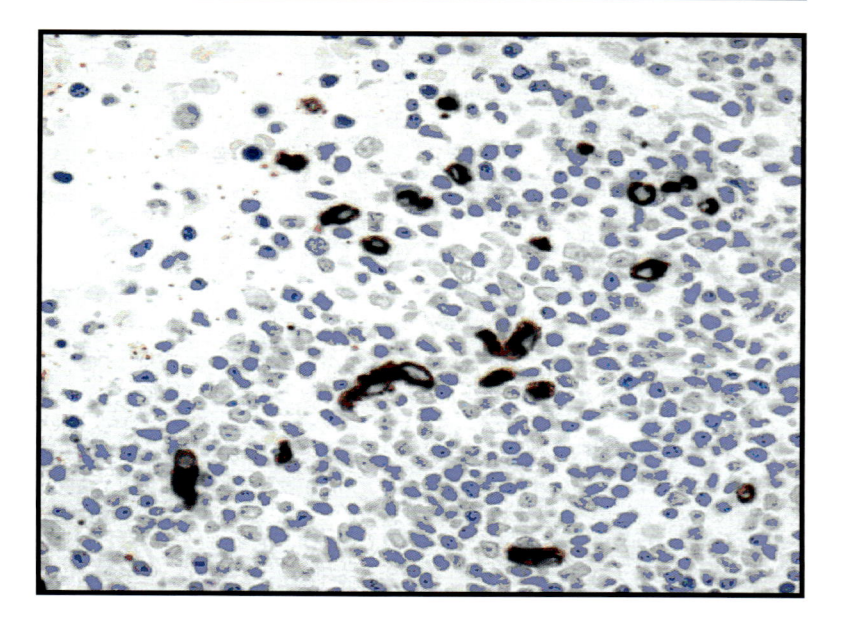

F3.21.20 CD34 in endothelial cells in lymphoid aggregates of mantle cell lymphoma

This bone marrow biopsy specimen was from a 57-year-old man with mantle cell lymphoma with large lymphoid aggregates. Incipient vascular proliferation is detected on CD34 staining. These small, rounded, endothelial cells should not be interpreted as blasts. The intensity of CD34 staining is much higher in endothelial cells and they frequently show, in some shape or form, cytoplasmic "tails" or incipient spindling.

3.21 CD34

F3.21.21 CD34 in megakaryocytes

The CD34 pattern of staining in megakaryocytes may be either cytoplasmic, membranous or both. Membranous expression is mostly limited to small megakaryocytes and is a rare phenomenon on immunohistochemistry. However, the pattern of expression does not show perfect correlation with the size. A small early megakaryocyte with cytoplasmic expression (left) and somewhat larger megakaryocytes with membranous expression only (right) are shown.

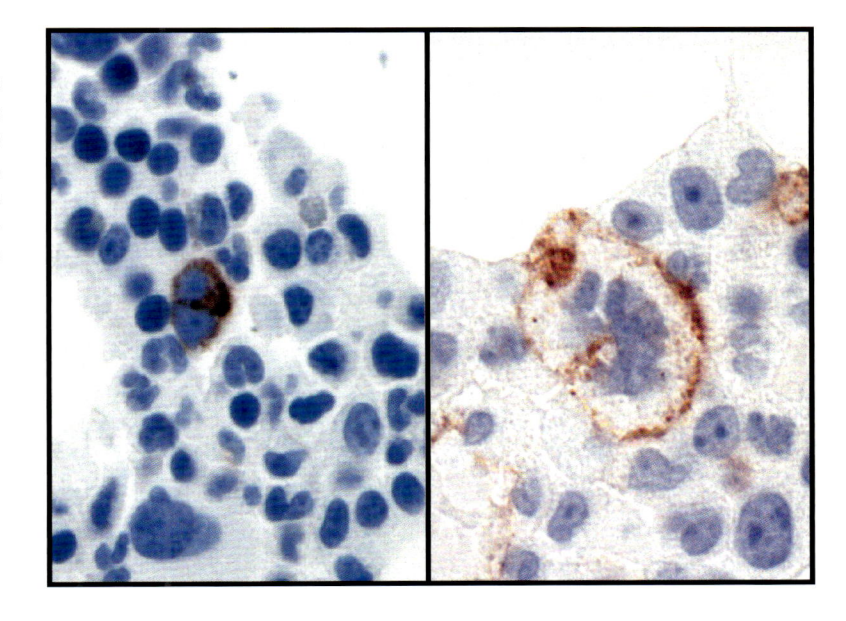

3.22 CD35

CD35 (C3bR; C4bR; CR1; immune adherence receptor which plays a major role in the removal and processing of immune complexes and facilitating their localization to lymphoid follicles) is expressed on erythrocytes, neutrophils, monocytes, eosinophils, B lymphocytes, and 10% to 15% of T-lymphocytes (PROW) [Roozendaal 2007]. It has also been identified on glomerular podocytes, follicular-dendritic cells, and some astrocytes. In diagnostic immunohistochemistry, CD35 detection is used to identify follicular dendritic cells, where it may be present in a more diffuse manner than CD23 or CD21 [Meugé-Moraw 1996; Horny 1994]. Follicular dendritic cells are closely related to BM stromal cell progenitors and to myofibroblasts [Muñoz-Fernández 2006]. Its cytoplasmic expression in granulocytes makes its appearance in the BM biopsy "dirty." CD35 expression is easier to interpret in the germinal centers of the lymphoid follicles in the BM, where it assumes dendritic appearance similar to that in lymph nodes or other tissues with B-cell follicles and with positive cells not intermixed with granulocytes.

F3.22.1 CD35 in normal bone marrow

CD35 is usually used as follicular dendritic cell marker. However, it is expressed by neutrophils, eosinophils, monocytes, and erythrocytes, and on immunohistochemistry, it is usually detected as cytoplasmic rather than surface antigen. Many of the BM cells should be positive. This should not preclude interpretation of the results in the benign or malignant lymphoid follicles. Image shown here demonstrates usual/expected intensity of CD35 expression in normal BM.

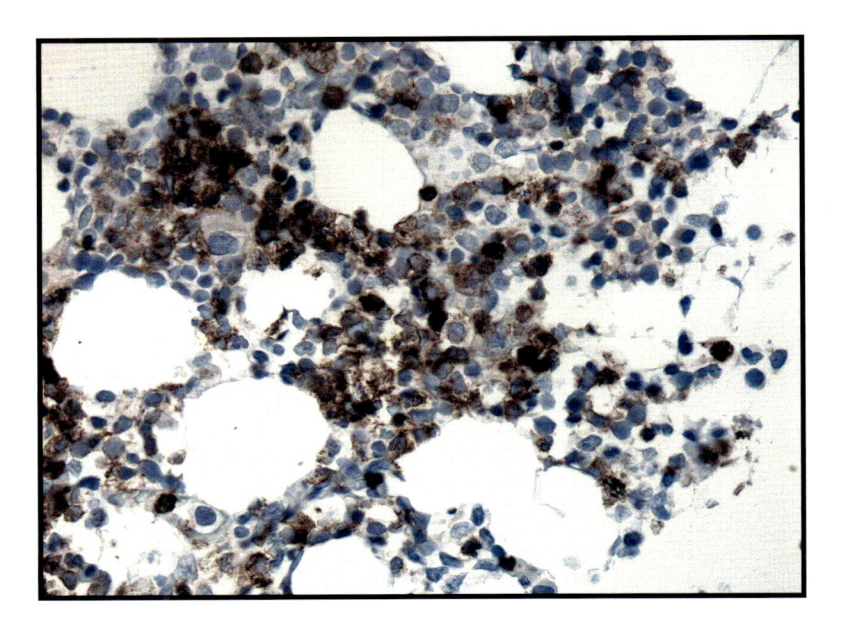

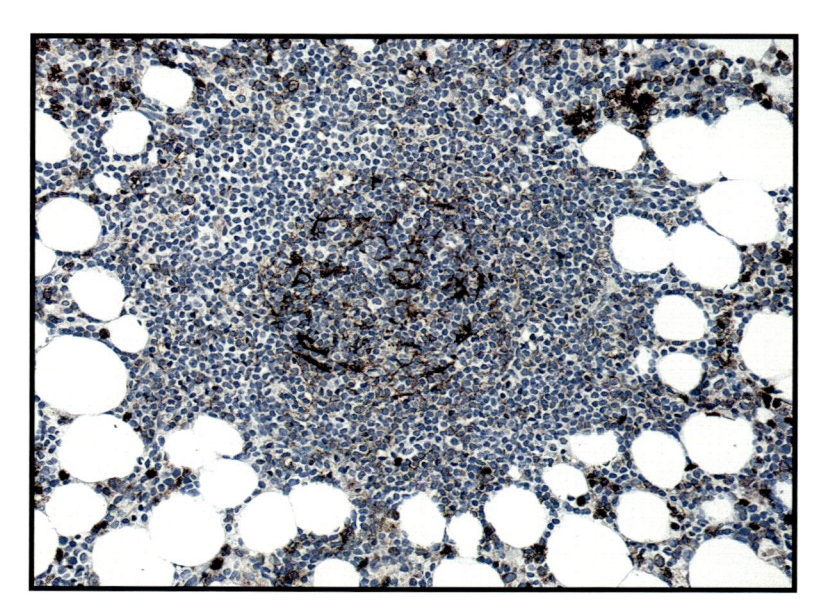

F3.22.2 CD35 in a follicular lymphoma with follicular colonization of benign interstitial lymphoid aggregates

Dendritic cells of the germinal centers are uniformly distributed when marked by CD35. Compare this with CD23 (**F3.22.3**) and CD21 expression in dendritic cells (**F3.22.4**). Importantly, this is an expected result for both benign and malignant germinal centers.

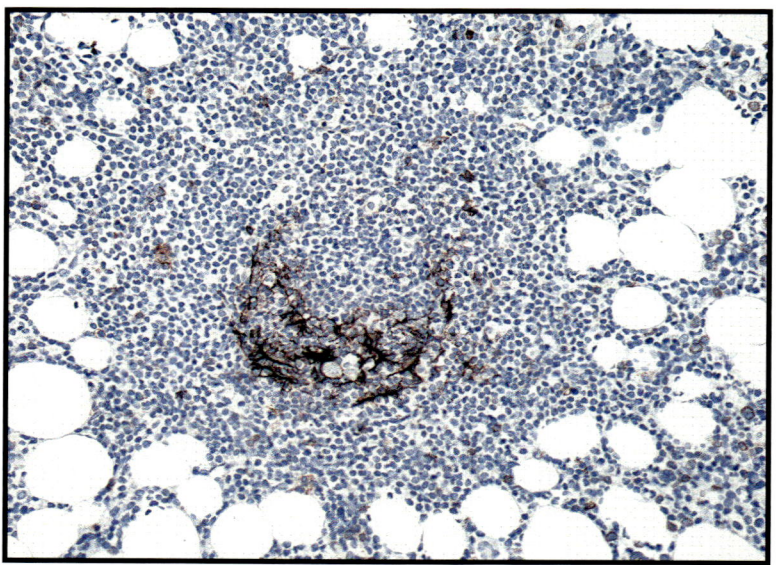

F3.22.3 CD23 for comparison with CD35 staining (see F3.22.2)

There are more CD35+ follicular dendritic cells (FDCs) than CD23+ FDCs (shown here) or CD21+ FDCs (see **F3.22.4**). Such results are common for both benign and malignant germinal centers. Also, there is no polarization of FDCs when they are demonstrated by CD35.

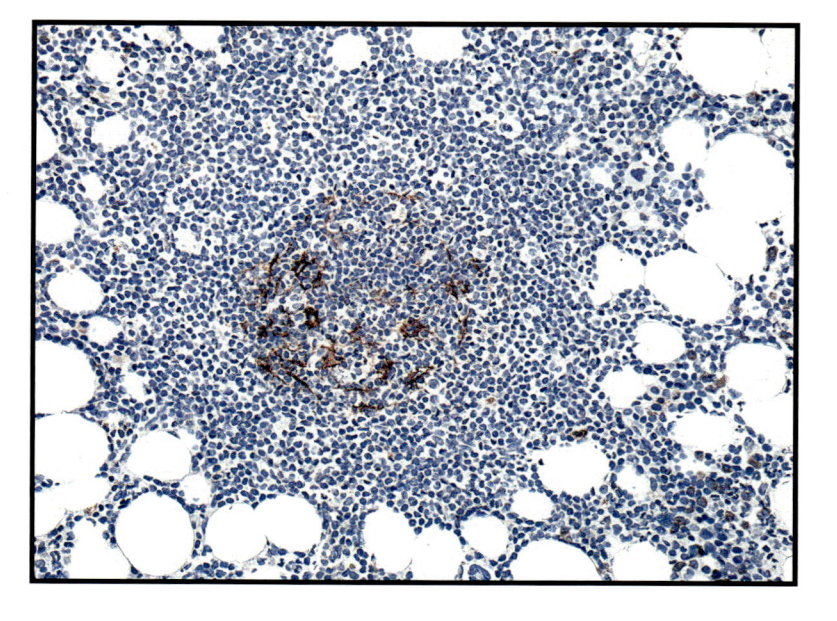

F3.22.4 CD21 for comparison with CD35

CD21 has a distribution similar to that of CD23. In follicular dendritic cells it is polarized in contrast to CD35. It occasionally may be difficult to demonstrate CD21 and CD23 expression in benign mantles of the lymphoid follicles in the bone marrow. However, in this illustration, the mantle is not a true mantle zone, but a "pseudomantle" and contains only CD3+ T-lymphocytes and therefore no expression of CD21 or CD23 is found in small lymphocytes.

F3.22.5 CD35 in follicular dendritic cells in lymphoplasmacytic lymphoma

Only a few CD35+ dendritic cells are demonstrated. This is likely because this follicle contains a predominant population of lymphoplasmacytic lymphoma (very high IgM and plasmacytoid morphology of lymphocytes in the bone marrow [BM]). Because no normal germinal centers are present, the content of the CD35+ follicular dendritic cells may be quite variable. Note the strong expression in granulocytes of the BM.

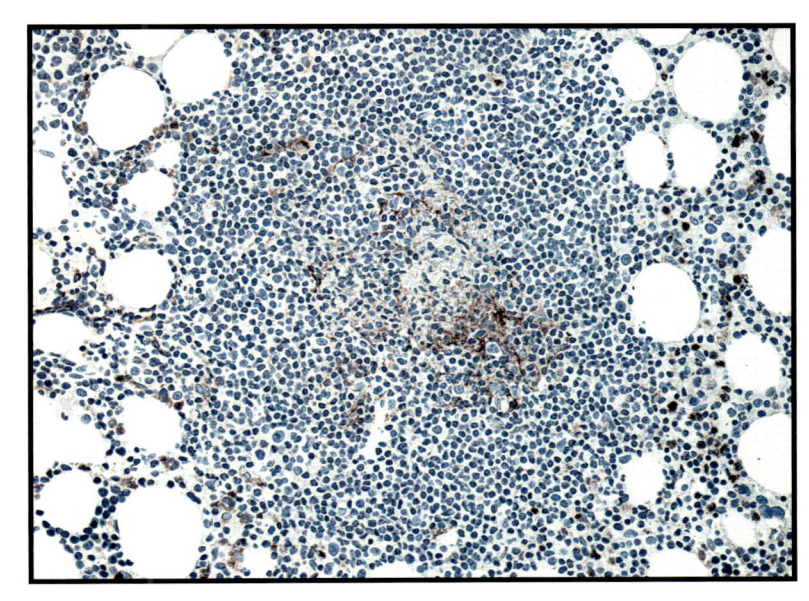

F3.22.6 CD35 in erythroid precursors

CD35 expression on erythroid cells plays a role in controlling inflammatory immunity and innate immune reactions. It is also found on circulating red blood cells where its level of expression may vary in different conditions. When CD35 is detected in the bone marrow on immunohistochemistry, erythroid precursors typically show weak staining compared with that found in neutrophils.

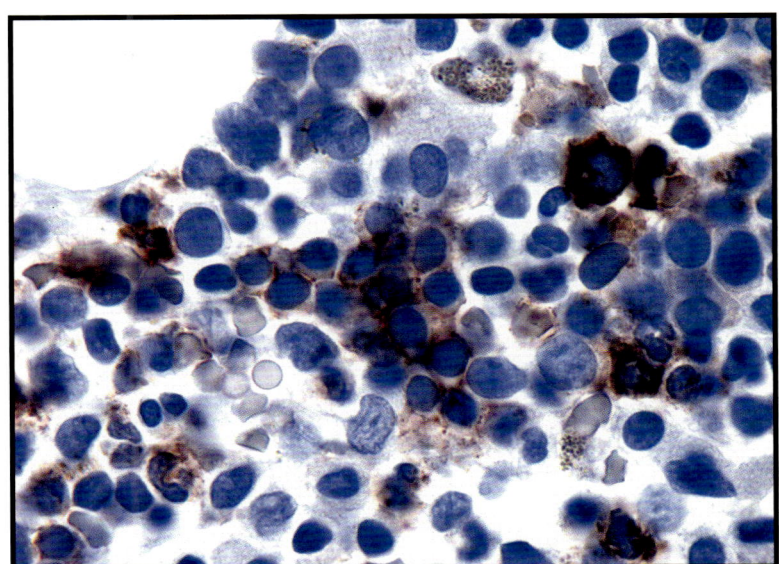

3.23 CD45 (CD45RA)

CD45 is also known as common leukocyte antigen (CLA), B220, EC 3.1.3.4, T200, and Ly5 (PROW). Different isoforms of CD45 are generated by alternative splicing and are expressed in cell type–specific patterns on functional subpopulations of lymphocytes, which include variable splicing of exons 4, 5, and 6, which encode A, B, and C determinants and are recognized by CD45RA, CD45RB, and CD45RC antibodies, respectively. The smallest 180k isoform lacks A, B, and C determinants and is recognized by CD45RO antibodies (PROW). CD45RA isoform, also referred to as just "anti-CD45 Ab" in diagnostic IHC, detects several positive cells in the BM as expected. CD45 is a tyrosine phosphatase, known to be the dominant leukocyte plasma membrane located phosphatase [Tonks 1988]. Its function is not fully understood, but it seems that CD45 is required for T- and B-cell antigen receptor–mediated activation [Trowbridge 1994]. CD45 is one of the most abundant leukocyte cell surface glycoproteins. It is expressed exclusively on the cells of the hematopoietic system. This is a marker of hematopoietic cells and is used in the evaluation of an undifferentiated tumor to rule out lymphoproliferative diseases. However, in the normal BM, most of the cells are negative. Its highest expression is seen in lymphoid cells and monocytes. Early hematopoietic cells including myeloid blasts are weakly positive. Commited megakaryocyte precursors are also positive, but rapidly downregulate CD45 as they mature [Dumon 2006]. As other myeloid cells mature, they either completely lose CD45 expression or show significant downregulation, but the downregulation is not as rapid as in megakaryocyte development. Its diagnostic usefulness is limited in the evaluation of the BM biopsy specimen and very few studies have reported the use of anti-CD45 antibodies [Werner 1992; Petruch 1992].

CD45 was historically considered the only 100% specific hematologic marker [Kurtin 1985; Nandedkar 1998]. However, CD45 was eventually detected in some sarcomas and carcinomas; most recently it was reported in a case of a metastatic undifferentiated carcinoma together with CD5 [Kurtin 1985; Nandedkar 1998]. Therefore, no single marker can be considered 100% specific in diagnostic practice.

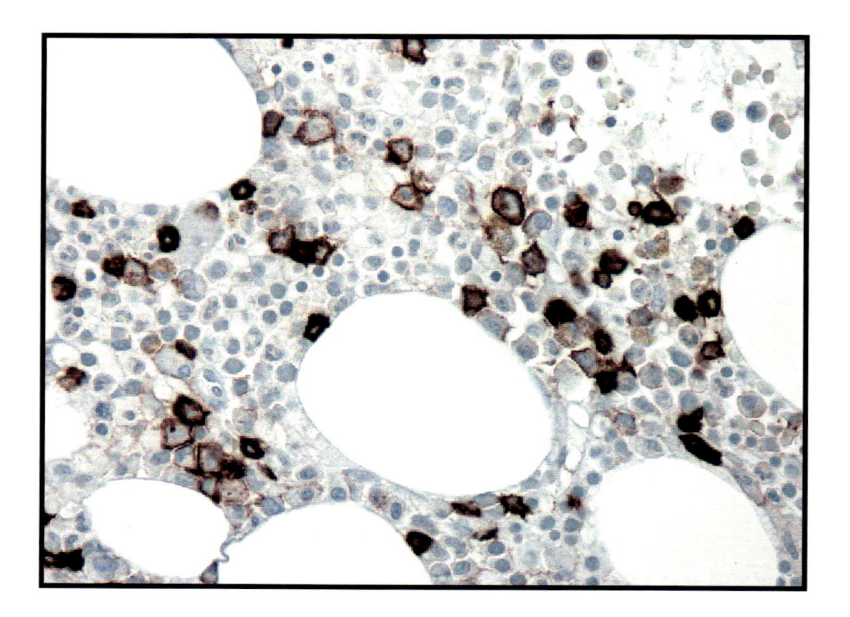

F3.23.1 CD45RA (CD45) in histologically normal bone marrow

Only a small number of hematopoietic cells shows expression of CD45RA. It is found in blasts, monocytes, lymphocytes, and it is decreasingly expressed in maturing neutrophils. A large number of CD45+ cells in the BM almost always points to a pathologic process.

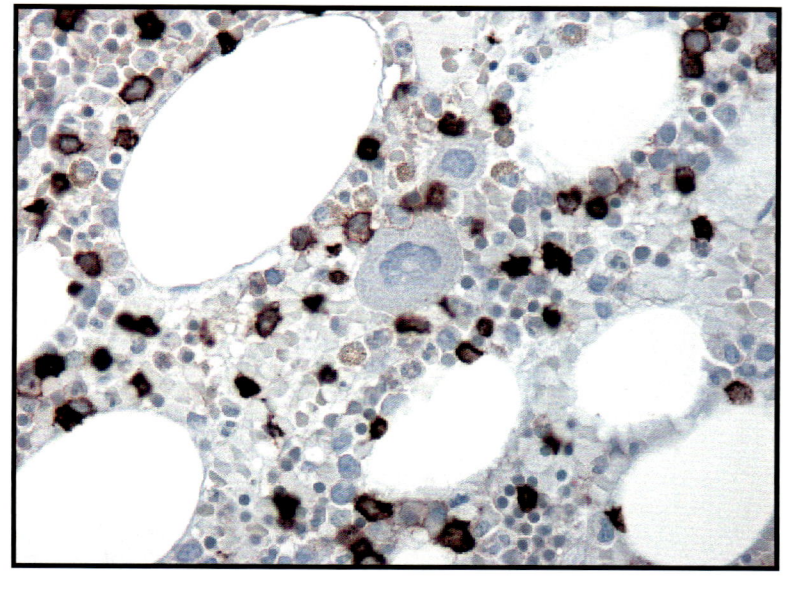

F3.23.2 CD45 in histologically normal bone marrow

Note that all morphologically recognizable megakaryocytes and normal erythroid precursors do not express CD45. This appears to coincide with GATA-1 transcription factor expression, which downregulates PU.1, which is one of the transcription factors involved in regulation of CD45 expression.

F3.23.3 CD45 in histologically normal bone marrow

This 32-year-old patient has classical Hodgkin lymphoma, but no evidence of disease in the BM. Strongly positive CD45 cells are somewhat increased, which is compatible with the mild lymphocytosis and myeloid left shift noted in this biopsy specimen. A cluster of very weakly positive immature neutrophils is also noted (arrows).

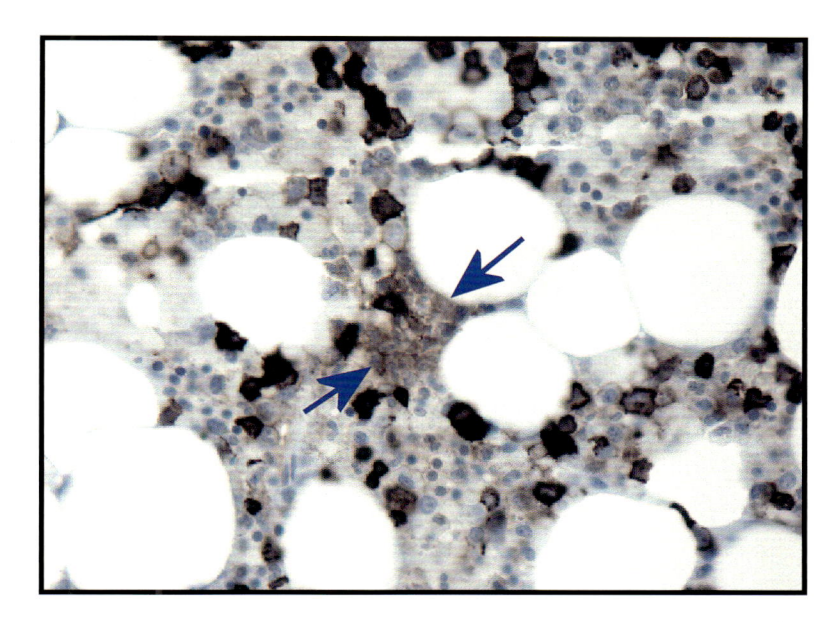

F3.23.4 CD45 in bone marrow negative for classical Hodgkin lymphoma

Same patient as seen in F3.23.3. Compared with normal BM, the number of strongly positive CD45 cells is increased. Some neutrophil precursors also show Golgi-type dotlike positivity (arrow). However, most cells that are positive for CD45 and present in this field are lymphocytes.

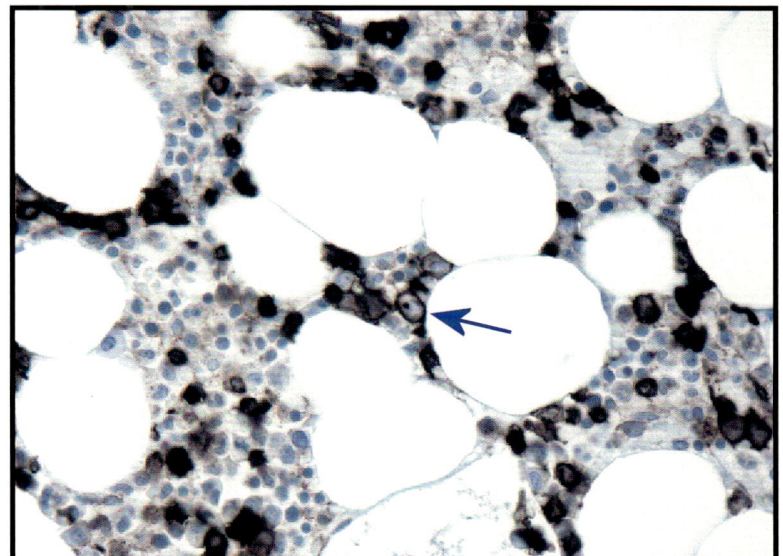

F3.23.5 CD45 in transformed essential thrombocythemia (ET)

Fewer than 5% of patients with ET will develop an acute leukemia, of which most cases occur after cytotoxic therapy. This biopsy specimen is from a 78-year-old woman who received cytotoxic therapy. CD45 is expressed in atypical megakaryocytes and many smaller mononuclear cells, which are blasts. CD45 expression has not been evaluated specifically in myeloproliferative disorders.

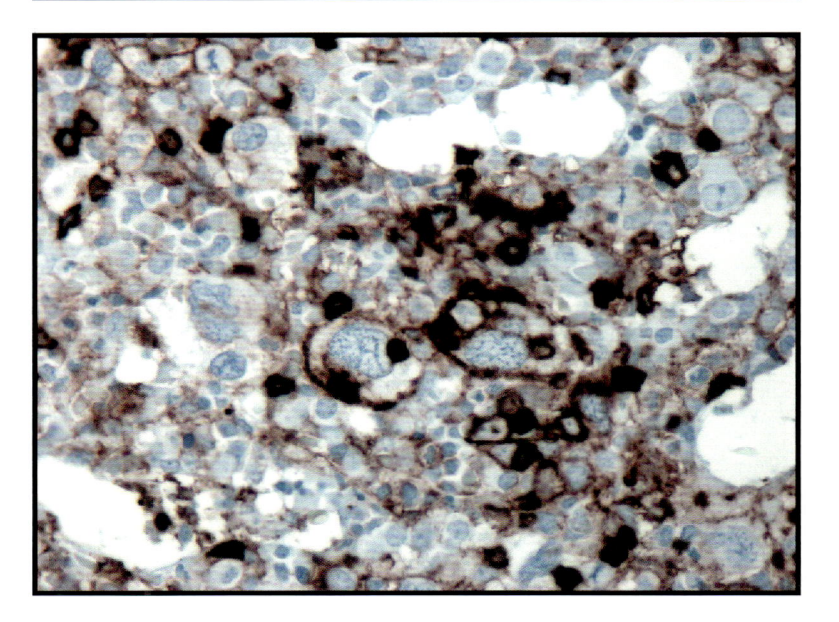

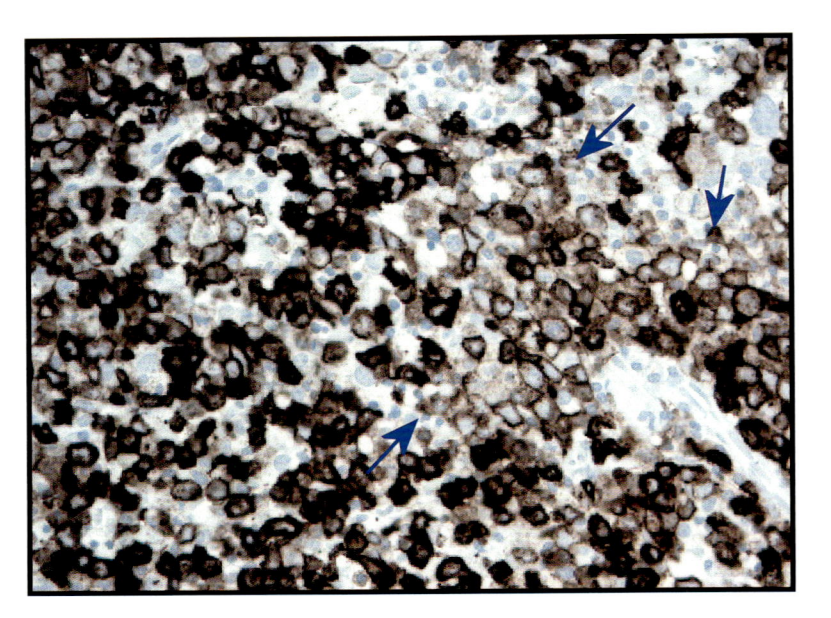

F3.23.6 CD45 in myelomonocytic leukemia

Weakly positive and strongly positive cells are present. Flow cytometry revealed 2 populations; blasts with monocytic differentiation with higher expression of CD45, and blasts with myeloid differentiation with weak CD45 expression. The flow cytometric findings are reflected in similar distribution of CD45+ cells on immunohistochemistry. Arrows point to weakly positive myeloblasts, while strongly positive cells on the left are most likely monocytic.

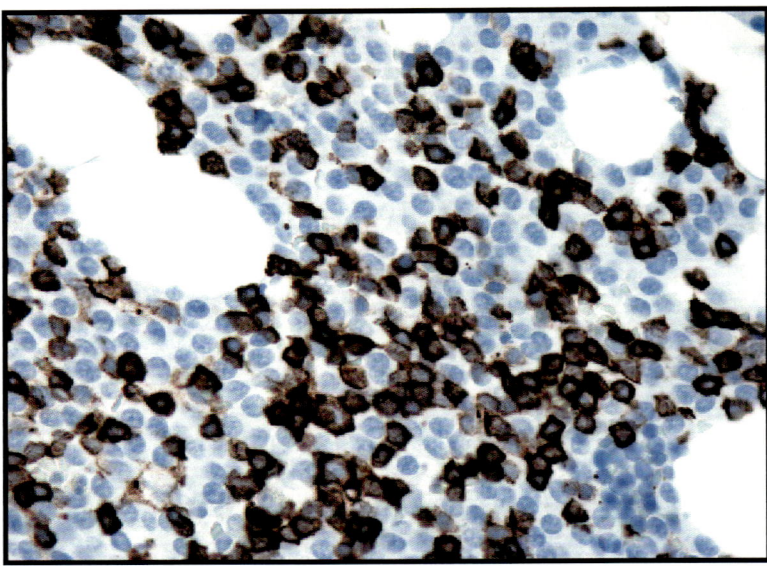

F3.23.7 CD45 in IgA multiple myeloma

In this 55-year-old man with IgA myeloma, most of the CD45+ cells were lymphocytes. The number of CD45+ cells exceeded the number of CD3+ and CD20+ cells combined. This difference was because of increased natural killer cells, which was confirmed with CD56 and CD57 staining.

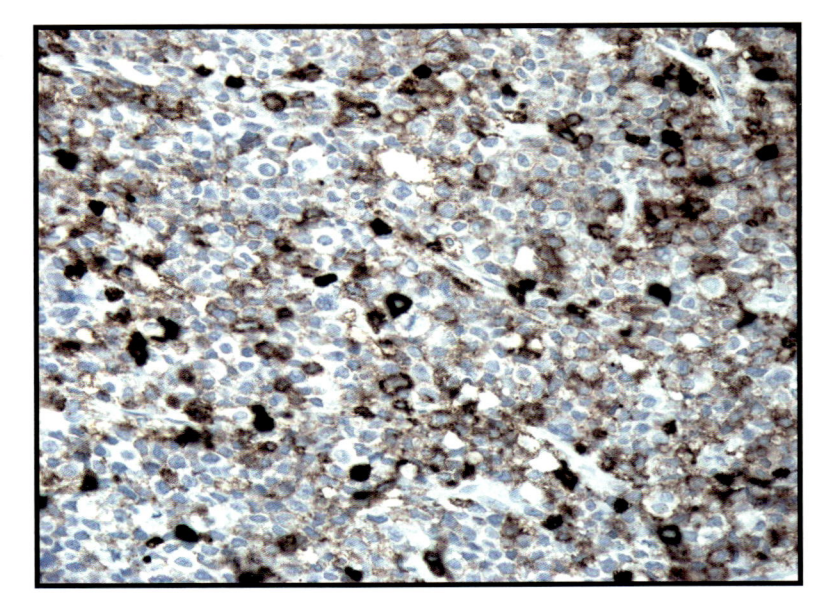

F3.23.8 CD45 in a rare case of well-documented IgM+ myeloma

IgM myeloma is a rare disease. A subpopulation (about 30%) of malignant plasma cells had weak expression of CD45. A slightly higher number was verified with flow cytometric analysis. Rare strongly positive cells are either benign lymphocytes or monocytes. CD45 expression has not been addressed in this rare disease.

3.23 CD45 (CD45RA)

F3.23.9 CD45 in lymphoplasmacytic lymphoma

Many of the malignant lymphocytes do not express CD45. Careful analysis of this specimen showed that CD45 expression was not restricted to cells with small lymphocyte morphology, but was also found in many cells with plasmacytoid morphology, where it appeared to be expressed at the same level of intensity.

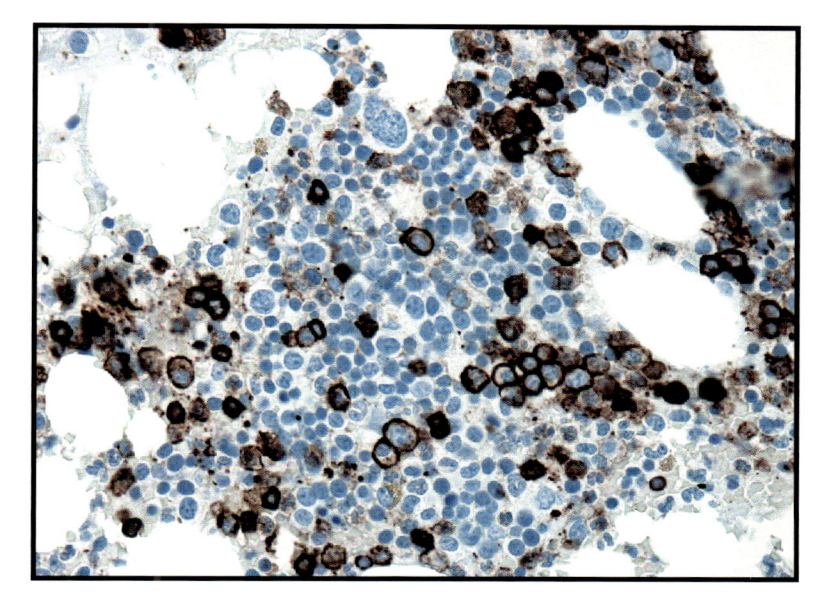

F3.23.10 CD45 in acute monoblastic leukemia

This image illustrates what is meant by "CD45/log side scatter gating," in which CD45dim populations are targeted as potential blasts. The leukemic blasts in both myeloid and lymphoblastic leukemia in most instances express weak surface CD45 as shown in this case of acute monoblastic leukemia in an 83-year-old woman.

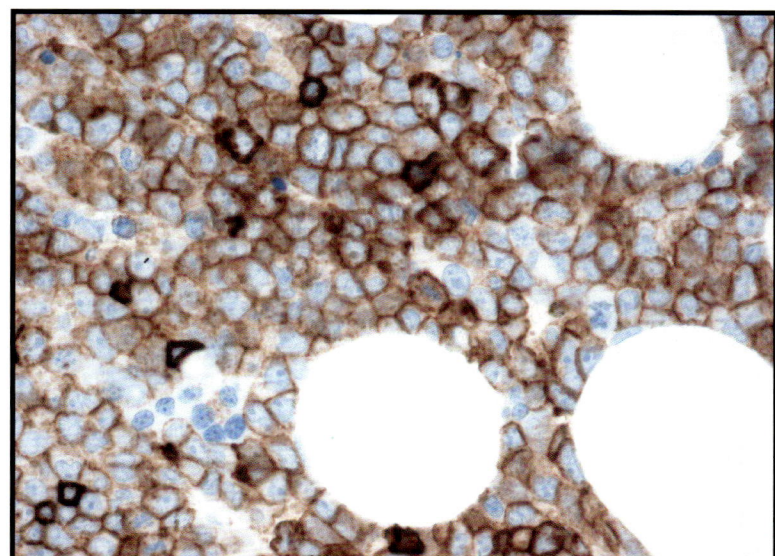

F3.23.11 CD45 in precursor B-cell acute lymphoblastic leukemia

CD45 is usually expressed at low levels in acute leukemias as illustrated in F3.23.10. In many leukemias with lymphoid differentiation, CD45 expression can be significant. Strong expression of CD45 was also demonstrated with flow cytometry. No aberrant expression of T-cell or myeloid antigens was found in this case.

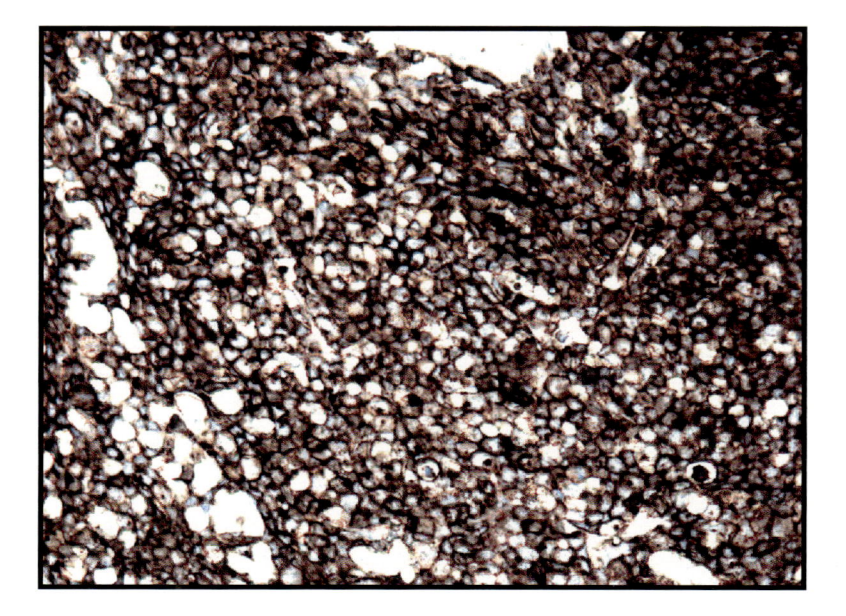

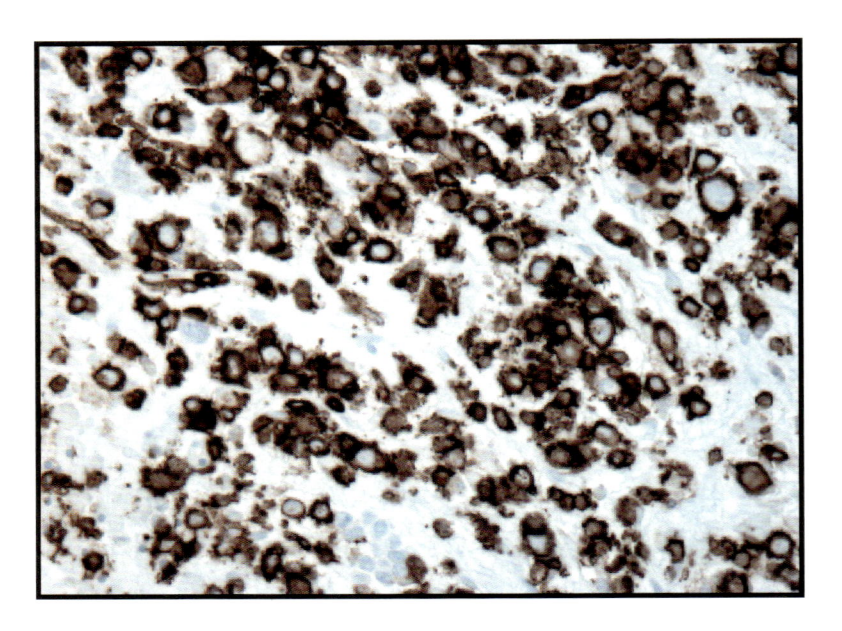

F3.23.12 CD45 expression on day 14 of chemotherapy in a patient with precursor B-cell acute lymphoblastic leukemia

The same case as in F3.23.11. On day 14 of induction chemotherapy, many leukemic cells remain viable. These cells also expressed Pax-5 and CD10. Even though CD45 is a nonspecific marker, it clearly demonstrated the extent of the bone marrow involvement by the residual leukemic population.

3.24 CD45 (CD45RO)

CD45RO antibody detects the smallest CD45 isoform that lacks A, B, and C determinants of the CD45 (PROW). Before anti-CD3 monoclonal Abs were available, CD45RO was used as a "anti-T-cell" Ab, which was not entirely appropriate. Only a subset of T cells shows reactivity with CD45RO (memory T cells), while a subset of B cells and some myeloid cells also can be reactive [Horny 1993; O'Donnell 1995; Loyson 1997; Bluth 1993]. Most human macrophages and granulocytes express Ag detectable with CD45RO [Caldwell 1991]. In contrast to CD45RA, CD45RO detects Ag that is very dimly expressed on immature cells, becoming increasingly brighter beginning at approximately the myelocyte stage. Reactive plasma cells can also show reactivity for CD45RO Ab [Beschorner 1999].

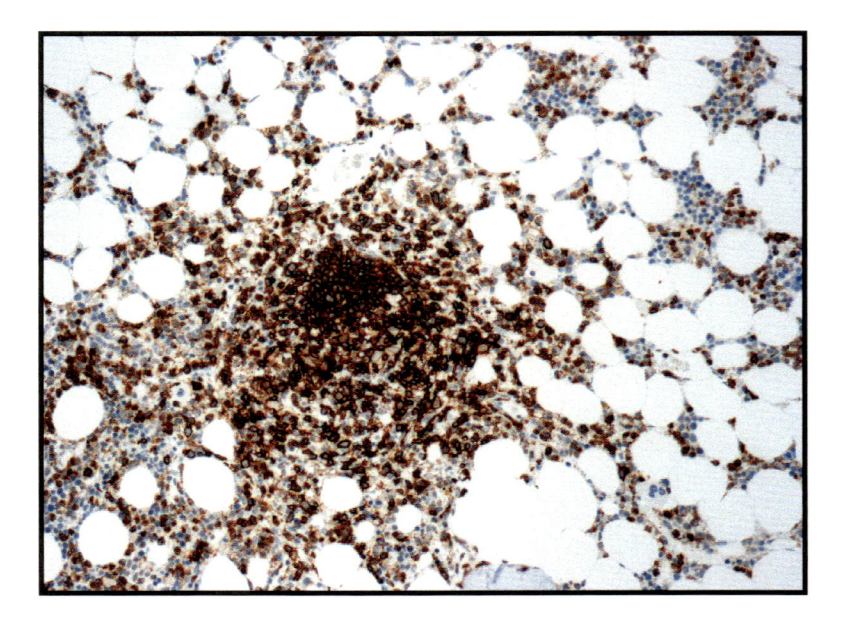

F3.24.1 CD45RO in peripheral T-cell lymphoma (PTCL)

This bone marrow was involved by PTCL. The neoplastic cells were also positive for CD45RO in addition to a series of T cells markers including CD3, CD4, CD2, and CD7. CD45RO designates memory T cells. It is also expressed by a subset of B cells, monocytes, and macrophages.

3.24 CD45 (CD45RO)

F3.24.2 **CD45RO in peripheral T-cell lymphoma (PTCL)**

The higher power clearly demonstrates membranous expression of the CD45RO. Although its diagnostic usefulness is limited, it can be used in the characterization of PTCL. However, its real diagnostic application is in the evaluation of a possible autoimmune lymphoproliferative syndrome (ALPS), where most of the CD4−/CD8− (double negative-cells) are also CD45RO−, which is consistent with the expansion of a naïve T-cell population.

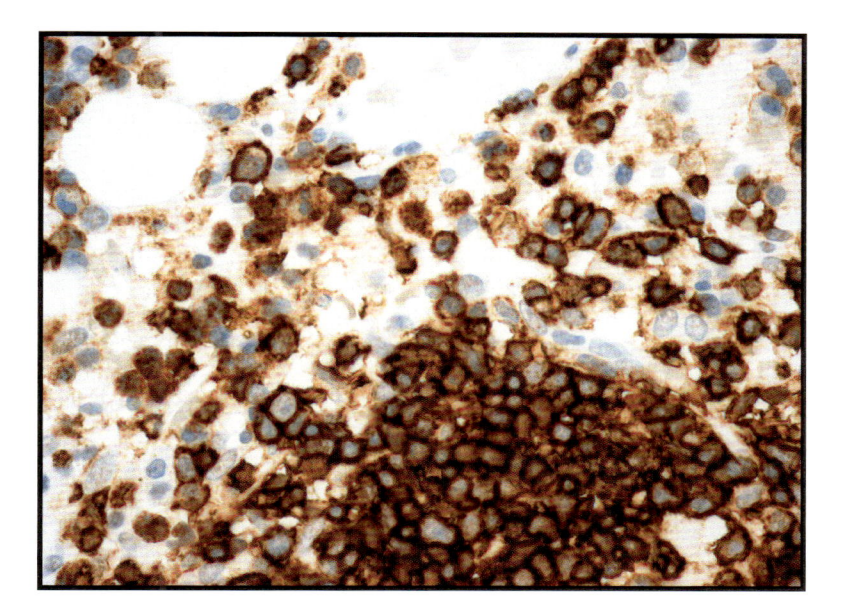

F3.24.3 **CD45RO in myeloid and plasma cells**

CD45RO is expressed in most monocytes and granulocytes with lower expression in immature cells and higher expression at myelocyte stage. This image illustrates numerous neutrophils and precursors and also other segmented granulocytes with CD45RO strong cytoplasmic expression. Rare cell shows exclusive membranous expression of the CD45RO (arrow). They are probably plasma cells [Bluth 1993].

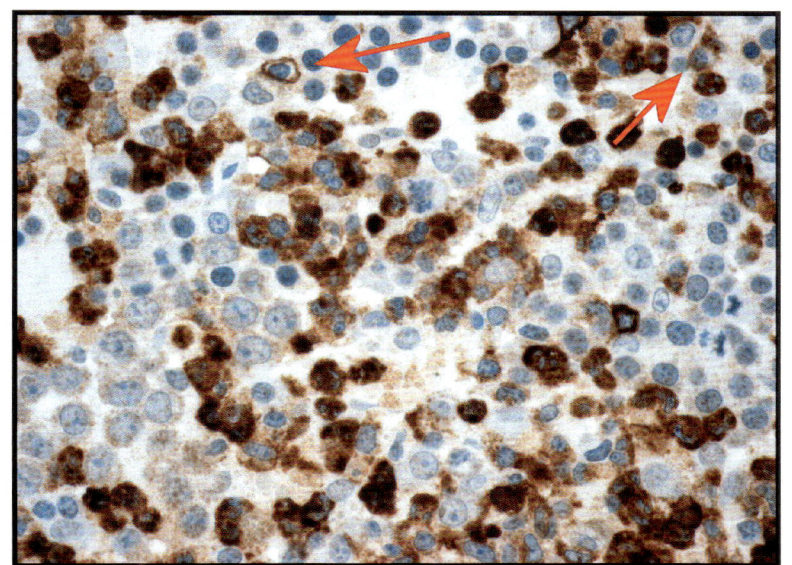

F3.24.4 **CD45RO in acute myeloid leukemia (AML)**

This was a case of an AML without any evidence of maturation. Rare positive cells correspond well with CD3+ cells in this biopsy specimen and therefore leukemic cells are negative. In addition, a relatively frequent artefact of nonspecific nuclear staining with anti-CD45RO antibody is present, which may interfere with interpretation.

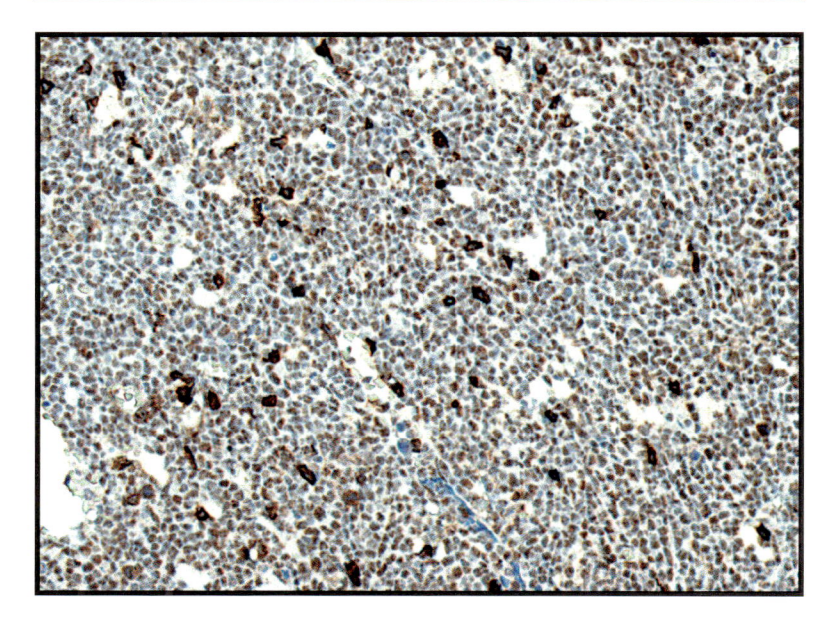

3.25 CD56

CD56 is also known as Leu-19, NKH1, and neural cell adhesion molecule (NCAM) (PROW). In normal BM, only about 1% lymphoid cells presumed to be NK cells express CD56; this is lower than the 2% expression of CD16 seen in NK cells [Shin 1992]. Osteoblasts lining the bone trabeculae also show expression of CD56, which is more intense in inactivated osteoblasts with flattened shape [Ely 2002]. However, there are 2 adjacent stromal cells, subendosteal and endosteal, which play distinct roles in controlling the stem-cell capacity and fate of hematopoietic stem cells (HSC) and probably contribute distinctly to HSC niche formation [Islam 1992; Balduino 2005]. Both subendosteal and endosteal layers appear to express CD56. In acute leukemia, CD56 expression occurs in de novo AML with an overall frequency of 13%, with the highest frequency of 38% in acute monoblastic leukemia. Cases of ALL are consistently CD56− as are promyelocytic, erythroid, and megakaryoblastic acute leukemias [Khanlari 2003]. Very rare benign plasma cells can show weak expression of CD56 in some marrows.

More than 70% of multiple myeloma cases show strong CD56 expression; fewer than 10% of monoclonal gammopathy of undetrmined significance (MGUS) cases are CD56+ A positive association between CD56+ multiple myeloma (MM) and lytic bone lesions has been reported [Kaiser 1996; Hundemer 2007]. Leukemic myelomas and myeloma cell lines tend to lose CD56 expression [Pellat-Deceunynck 1998]. Contrary to some early reports, it appears that the lack of CD56 expression on MM cells is not a prognostic marker in patients treated with high-dose chemotherapy, but is associated with t(11;14) [Hundemer 2007]. Rare CD4+ CD56+ lineage− malignancies are now known to be tumors of plasmacytoid dendritic cells and are also CD123+ [Pilichowska 2007; Jacob 2003]. As expected, in some NK and T-cell lymphoproliferative diseases as well as various neural/neuroendocrine tumors, detection of CD56 by IHC in the BM occasionally may be useful. For example, hepatosplenic T-cell lymphoma is typically found in the sinusoids of the BM and is CD56+/CD57− [Wong 1995].

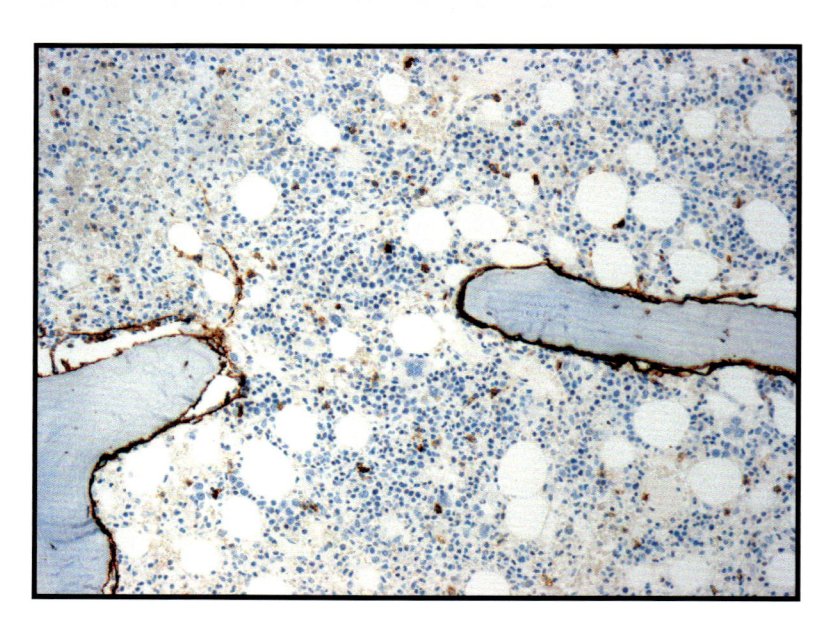

F3.25.1 CD56 in histologically normal bone marrow (ADVANCE)

Bony trabeculae are always lined by CD56+ osteoblasts. ADVANCE is a highly sensitive detection system and it identified in this biopsy some benign plasma cells (unexpected finding) and a larger number of CD56+ lymphoid cells than EnVision+ detecion system (not shown). In addition to osteoblasts, endosteal lining cells also appear to regularly express CD56.

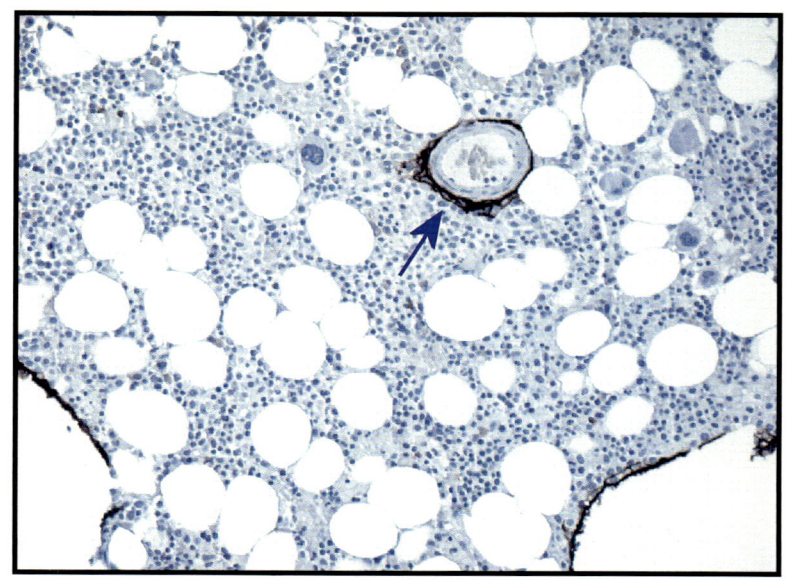

F3.25.2 CD56 in histologically normal bone marrow (EnVision+TM)

Compared with **F3.25.1**, this BM shows excellent signal-to-noise ratio, but no cells in the interstitium were found to express CD56. While the biopsy specimen is not from the same patient as in **F3.25.1**, EnVision+ results were the same (not shown). A population of cells in perivascular localization (arrow) also expressed high levels of CD56 compared with endosteal lining cells. The nature of these cells is not clear, but they may represent pericytes.

F3.25.3 CD56 in rare lymphoid cells

In any bone marrow biopsy, a few small lymphoid cells may be found that show expression of CD56. These cells are most likely natural killer (NK) cells. Most, but not all, NK cells express CD56. NK lymphocytes show not one, but various phenotypes by expressing CD45RA and some combination of surface markers including CD2, CD7, CD8, CD16, CD56, and CD57. CD56 is expressed mainly on NK cells in the peripheral blood. 2 of 4 positive cells show irregular cytoplasmic membranes (arrows).

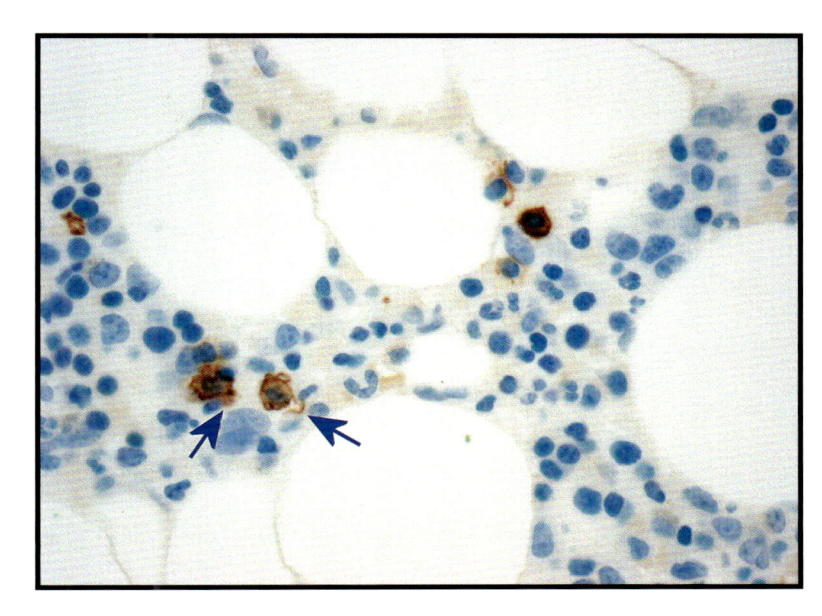

F3.25.4 CD56 in lymphoid cells

This bone marrow biopsy specimen was involved by CD56– peripheral T-cell lymphoma. Only rare benign-appearing cells were identified by CD56 staining. It is presumed that these represent normal natural killer cells. Note distinct membranous staining and very weak cytoplasmic reaction. While membranous localization is expected, weak cytoplasmic reaction is often seen. Specific staining, antigen diffusion, or technical artefacts are possible explanations of this finding.

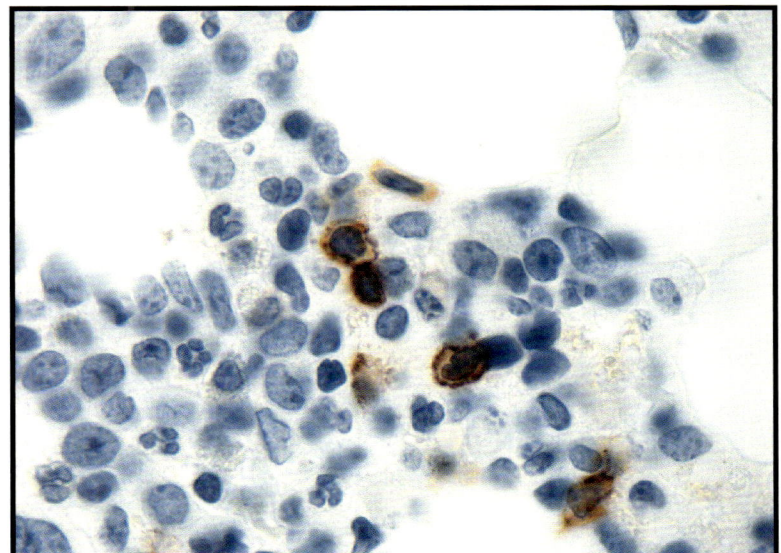

F3.25.5 CD56 in monoclonal gammopathy of undetermined significance (MGUS)

Rare benign plasma cells weakly express CD56. CD56 expression can be detected in fewer than 10% of MGUS cases. Arrows point to weakly positive plasma cells, one of which is binucleated. However, there is no definite cytological atypia in these plasma cells.

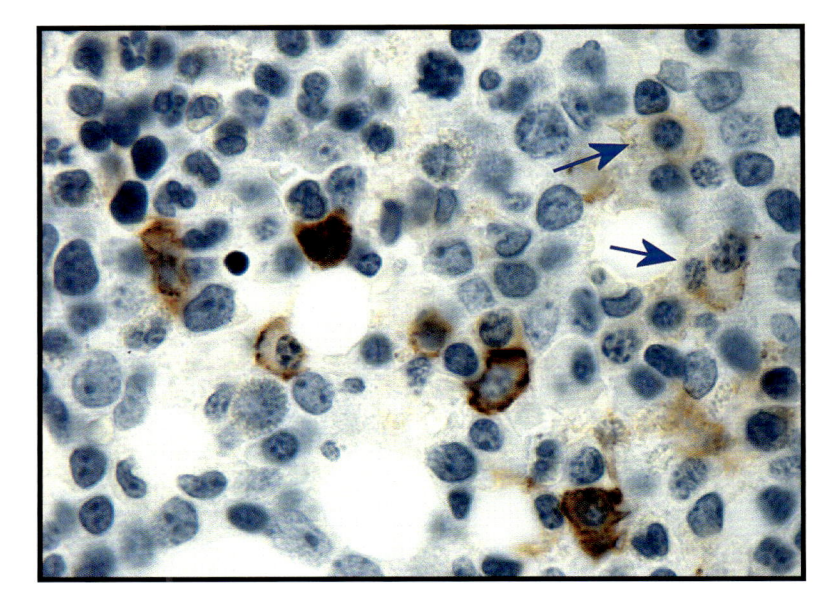

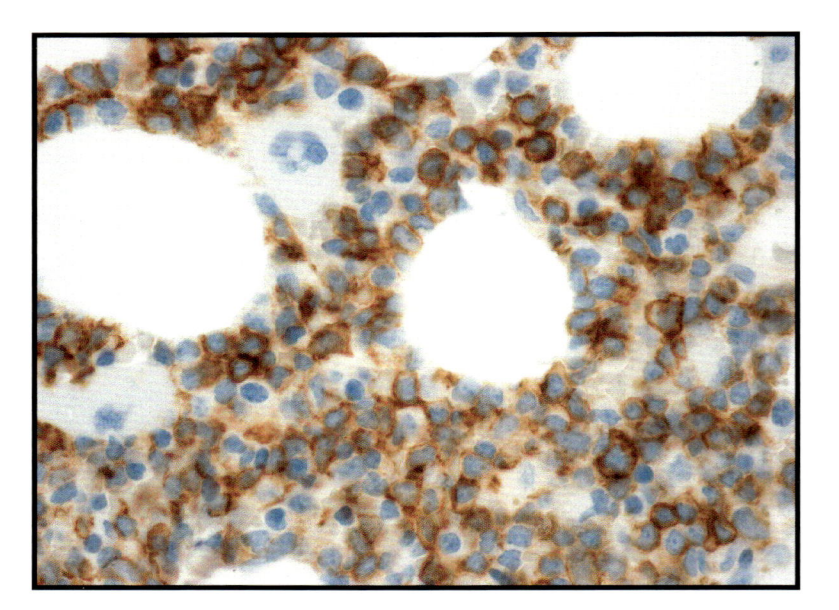

F3.25.6 CD56 in CD56+/CD4+ hematodermic neoplasm

This biopsy specimen from a 45-year-old man shows a neoplasm currently believed to arise from plasmacytoid dendritic cells (CD123high). The bone marrow involvement appeared 12 months after skin lesions were detected. Note the blastic morphology and membranous expression of the CD56. Most cases run an aggressive clinical course.

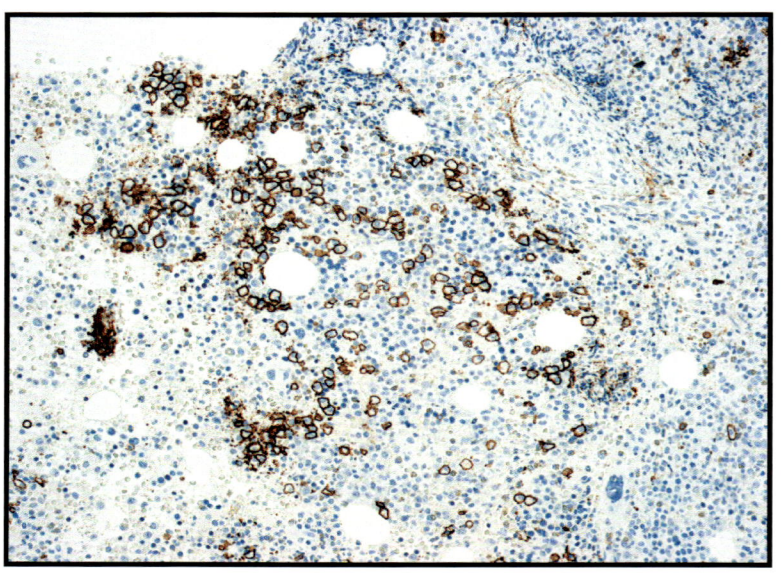

F3.25.7 CD56 in neoplastic plasma cells

This 64-year-old woman had concurrent systemic mastocytosis and plasma cell myeloma. Immunohistochemical staining of this bone marrow biopsy revealed 8% plasma cells with CD56 expression, which were also IgG-κ monotypic. The patient also had lytic bone lesions and serum IgG-κ paraprotein. Plasma cell neoplasia associated with mastocytosis has been previously reported [Horny 2004].

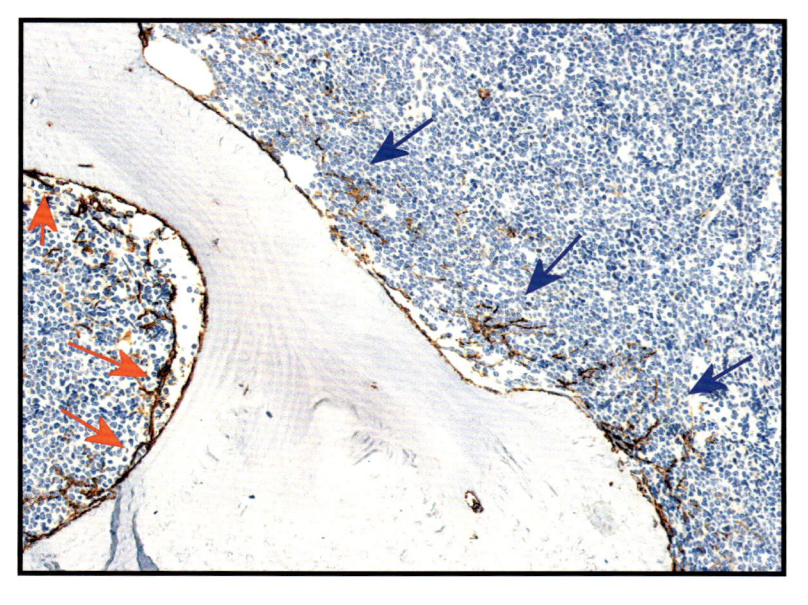

F3.25.8 CD56 in endosteal and paratrabecular localization

Paratrabecular CD56 expression in cells lining the bone in areas appears to split in 2 parts (red arrows). It cannot be determined whether this represents 2 distinct biological strata or a single split layer. In addition to endosteal lining cells, a few stromal dendritic cells also can express CD56 (blue arrows), which is highlighted in F3.25.9.

3.25   CD56

F3.25.9 CD56 in paratrabecular stromal dendritic cells

These dendritic cells appear in a peritrabecular localization. This patient had acute myeloid leukemia without differentiation. Such dendritic cells are not found in histologically normal bone marrow biopsies. Here they are identified in a condition with diffuse involvement of the BM and are localized only in the paratrabecular region. Their biological significance is not clear.

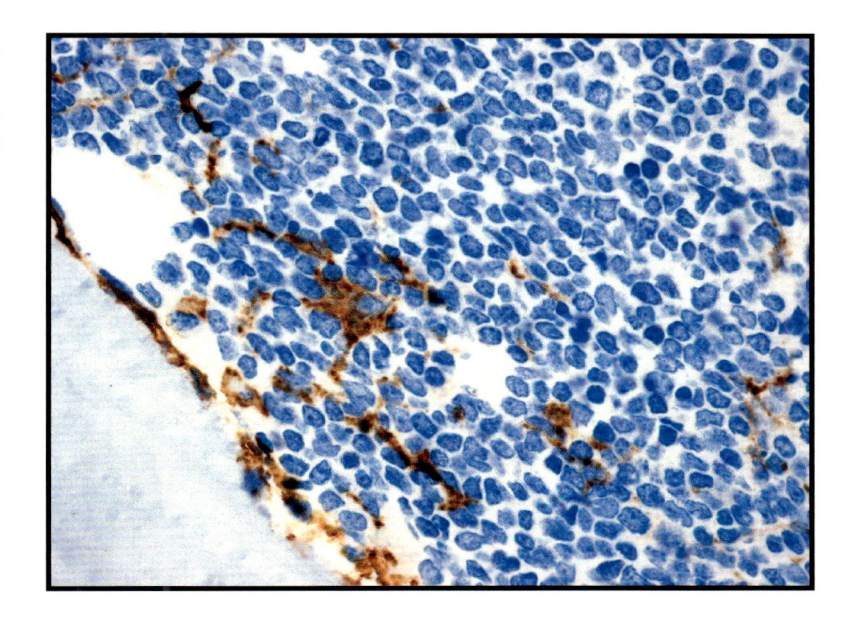

3.26 CD57

CD57 is also known as human natural killer-1 (HNK1) or Leu-7 (OMIM). The latter has been commonly used in the past to designate a marker of neuroendocrine differentiation [Miettinen 1993; Wick 2000]. CD57 staining is used in the evaluation of possible T-cell large granular lymphocytic leukemia, other T-cell disorders as well as NK-cell disorders [Osuji 2007; Morice 2002; Evans 2000]. CD57+ T cells are normally found in germinal centers and localize predominantly in the light zone of the germinal center [Bossaller 2006]. They are also present in follicular lymphoma and can be detected in the BM involved by follicular lymphoma [Alvaro 2006]. CD57 is also a valuable marker in the evaluation of the autoimmune lymphoproliferative syndrome (ALPS). Typically, the aberrant immunophenotype of the proliferating cells is often CD4−, CD8−, CD45RO−, and CD57+ [Lim 1998; Goldman 2002]. This aberrant population of CD3+ cells may form large lymphoid aggregates in the BM, which should not be diagnosed as peripheral T-cell lymphoma.

F3.26.1 CD57 in histologically normal bone marrow (BM; ADVANCE)

This biopsy specimen is from a 43-year-old man with recently diagnosed classical Hodgkin lymphoma and no evidence of disease in the BM. The number of CD57+ cells in histologically normal BM and most BM biopsy specimens is rather low, because of the low number of CD57+ natural killer (NK) cells in the normal BM biopsy. Compared with an entirely normal BM, this biopsy specimen possibly shows a slightly increased number of CD57+ lymphoid cells (presumably NK cells).

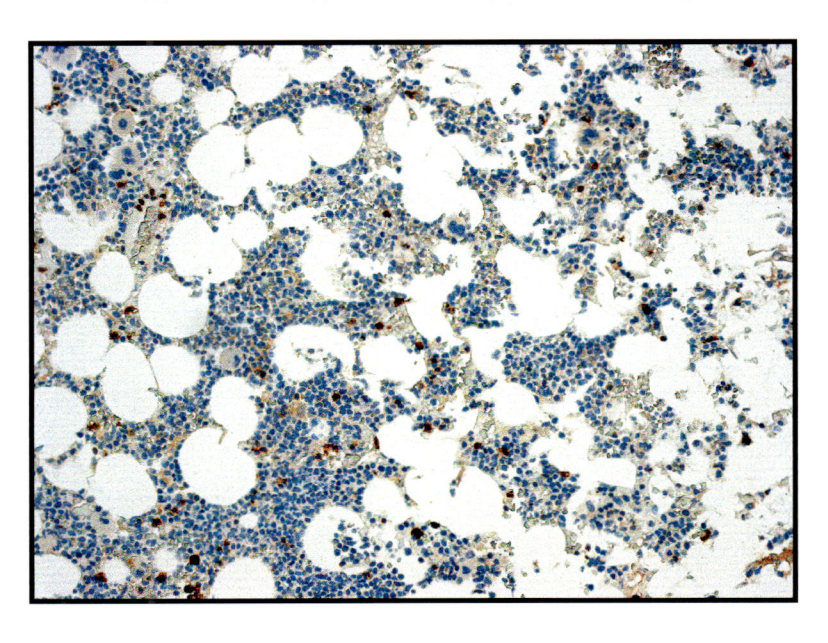

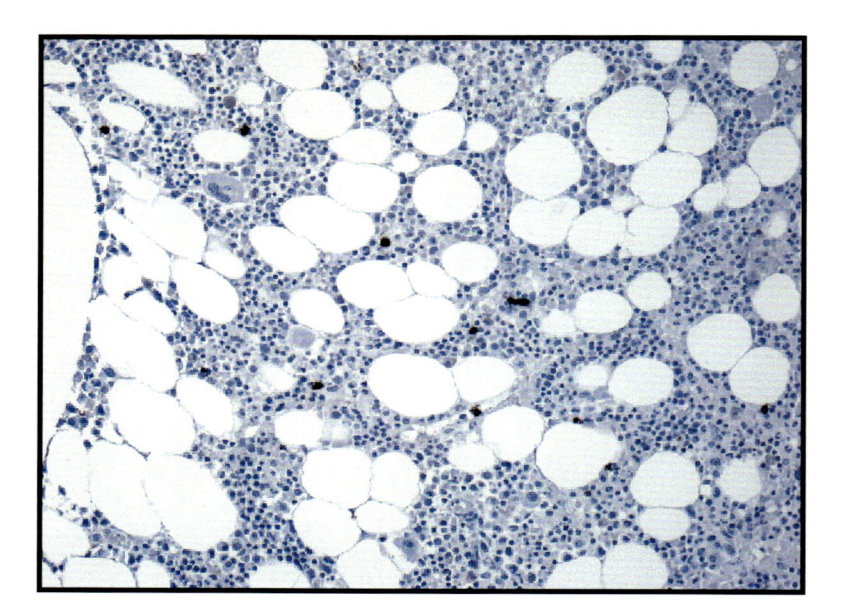

F3.26.2 CD57 in histologically normal bone marrow (EnVision+)

This biopsy specimen is from a 14-year-old girl recently treated for classical Hodgkin lymphoma. Her BM was not involved either at presentation or at this time. Occasional small strongly positive lymphocytes can be observed on low magnification and are presumed to represent natural killer cells.

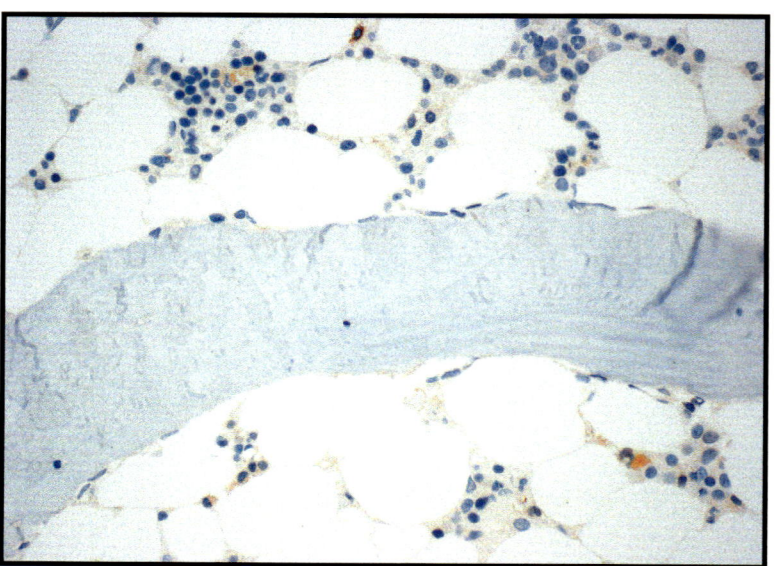

F3.26.3 CD57 in slightly hypocellular bone marrow

This biopsy specimen is from a 68-year-old patient with chronic moderate normochromic normocytic anemia, but no definite pathologic findings in the BM. The overall cellularity was estimated at 20% and cytogenetic analysis showed no abnormal findings. The CD57+ lymphoid cells (natural killer cells) are difficult to find. Note that in contrast to CD56, endosteal lining cells are not positive for CD57.

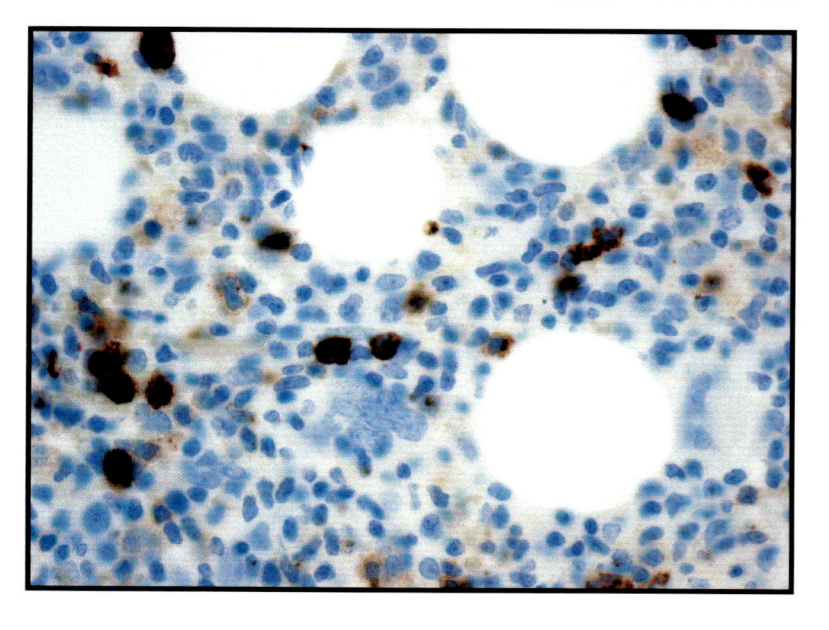

F3.26.4 CD57 in CD57-negative peripheral T-cell lymphoma (PTCL)

This biopsy specimen is from a 43-year-old man with PTCL involving the bone marrow. CD57 was not expressed in this CD8+ primary nodal PTCL (not otherwise specified). The CD57+ lymphoid cells are increased compared with normal BM and appear to represent tumor-infiltrating natural killer cells with strong expression of CD57. These cells can be found increased in the BM in various conditions.

F3.26.5 CD57 possible expression in a small subset of cells in peripheral T-cell lymphoma (PTCL)

This biopsy specimen is from a 61-year-old man with primary nodal CD4+/CD57– PTCL (not otherwise specified). There is a single focus of lymphoma in the bone marrow. A few large cells are positive for CD57 and have atypical morphologic features. Other atypical lymphocytes are clearly negative. Smaller positive cells are most likely tumor-infiltrating natural killer cells. The conventional approach is to call the lesion "negative" for a certain marker if fewer than 10% of the cells are positive.

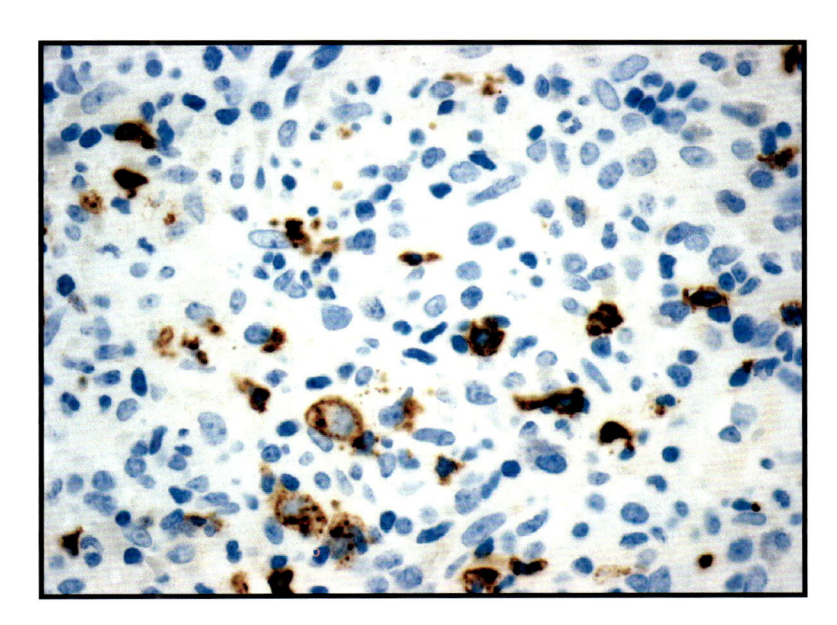

F3.26.6 CD57 in T-cell large granular lymphocytic leukemia (T-LGL)

Two cases of T-LGL are illustrated. Case 1 showed only a slight increase in CD3+ cells. Similarly, the number of CD8+ cells was only slightly increased. However, the number of CD57+ cells is much higher than in normal bone marrow (compare with F3.26.1). Case 2 shows a moderately increased number of CD57+ cells. In both cases, clinical correlation and confirmation of T-cell clonality by molecular analysis are needed for the diagnosis of T-LGL.

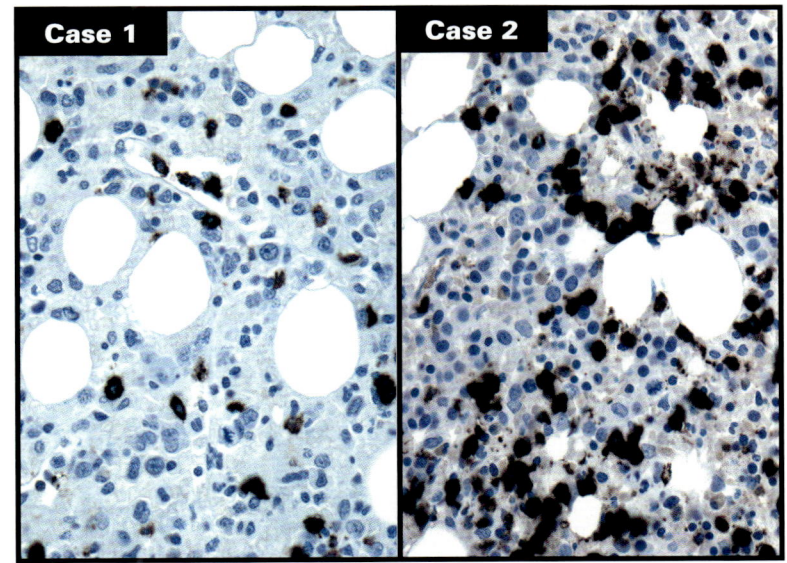

3.27 CD61 and CD42b

CD61 is ITGB3, which stands for integrin, β3. It is also known as platelet glycoprotein IIIa (GP3A) or glycoprotein IIIa (GPIIIa) (OMIM). Integrin β3 is found along with the α IIb chain in platelets [Duperray 1989]. In general, integrins have a role in cell adhesion as well as cell-surface mediated signaling. CD61 reactivity in the BM is the same as that of CD42b, which is also known as GPIbα, GPIba, and glycocalicin, and is an additional megakaryocyte/platelet-specific marker [Deutsch 2006]. CD42b, being the actual binding site for von Willebrand factor (vWF) and thrombin, is not related to CD61 directly (PROW). It appears that CD61 and CD42b give comparable results in immunohistochemistry tests. However, CD41a (GP IIb/IIIa) has been found to be expressed more than CD42b or CD61 in immature megakaryocytes and as such may be more useful in the evaluation of acute leukemia. Unfortunately, the anti-CD41a Abs that are in use in flow cytometry can not be used in paraffin-embedded tissues [Qiao 1996]. It is important to note that blasts in acute panmyelosis with myelofibrosis (APMF) and blasts in acute megakaryoblastic leukemia (AMKL) are immunophenotypically different; in APMF the blasts are generally CD34+ and rarely CD61+ (or other megakaryocytic marker), but in AMKL the blasts are CD34+ only in 60% of cases and by definition, they express some megakaryocytic markers with CD61 being expressed in the great majority of cases [Orazi. 2005; Helleberg 1997]. CD61, however, nicely highlights abnormal megakaryocytic forms in APMF. The blasts in Down syndrome (DS)–related transient myeloproliferative disease are also consistently positive for CD34, while DS-AMKL is less consistently so [Langebrake 2005]. CD61 is expressed in DS-TMD [Girodon 2000]. Because of its biological restriction to DS-TMD and DS-AMKL, it is worth mentioning here that both of these disorders in DS are related to GATA-1 mutations; GATA-1 is an essential transcription factor for megakaryocyte and erythroid differentiation [Mundschau 2003].

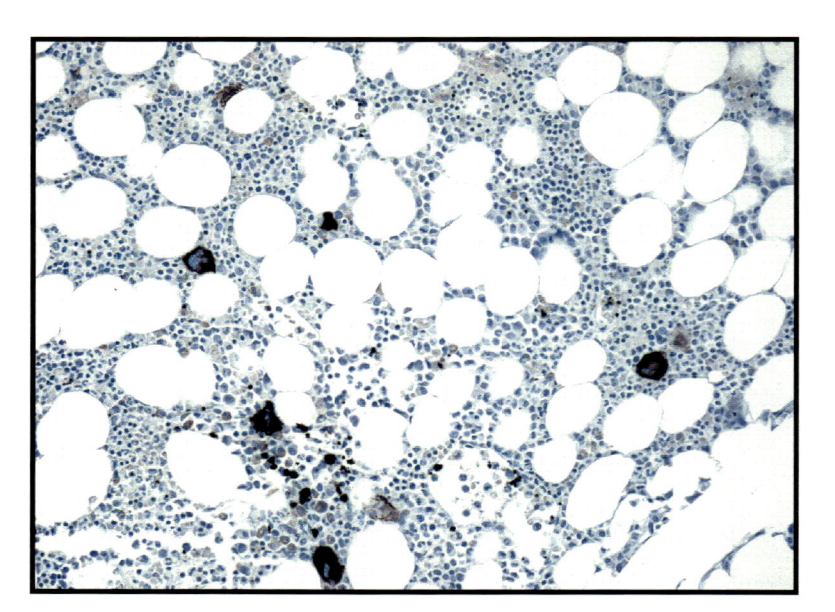

F3.27.1 CD61 in histologically normal bone marrow

In contrast to von Willebrand factor (FVIII-related antigen) or CD31, CD61 is specific for megakaryocytes and platelets and is not detected in the endothelial cells. If the staining in normal megakaryocytes and platelets is not as intense as illustrated here, it may occasionally be difficult to detect CD61 or CD42b expression in megakaryoblastic leukemia.

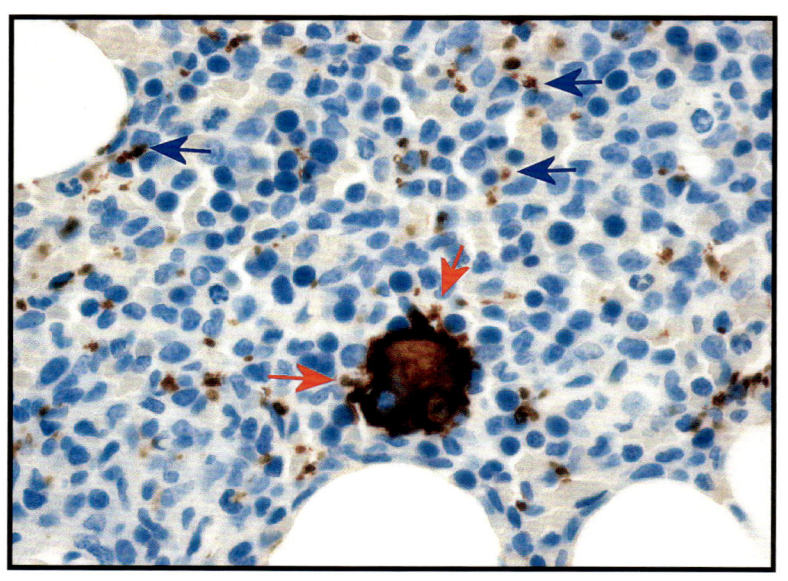

F3.27.2 CD61 in platelets

CD61 is regularly detected in platelets, which are small, extracellular globular structures when detected on immunohistochemistry in the bone marrow. This patient had a myelodysplastic syndrome. Platelet budding is illustrated (red arrows) and numerous platelets can be seen throughout the biopsy specimen (blue arrows pointing to some).

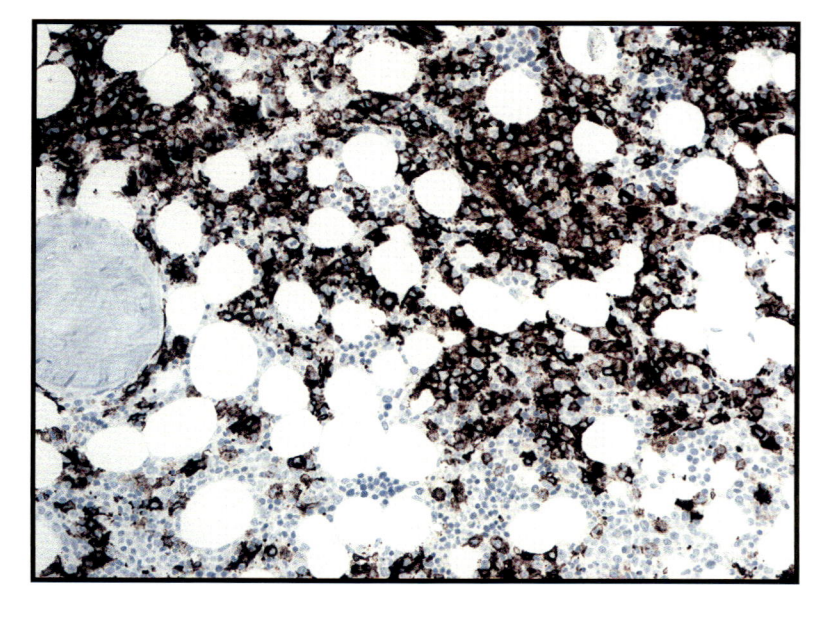

F3.27.3 CD61 in acute megakaryoblastic leukemia

The blasts show very strong cytoplasmic and membranous expression of CD61. While dotlike weak cytoplasmic expression of CD61 or other megakaryocyte markers can occasionally be seen in acute erythroid leukemia, the strong expression, as illustrated here, is seen only in megakaryoblastic leukemia.

3.27   CD61 and CD42b

F3.27.4   CD61 in myelodysplastic syndrome associated with systemic mastocytosis

This biopsy specimen is from a 73-year-old woman with refractory anemia with excess blasts. There is significant trilinear dyshematopoiesis. Dysplastic megakaryocytes are highlighted, but the blasts are negative for CD61. Arrows point to a focal paratrabecular infiltrate of atypical mast cells.

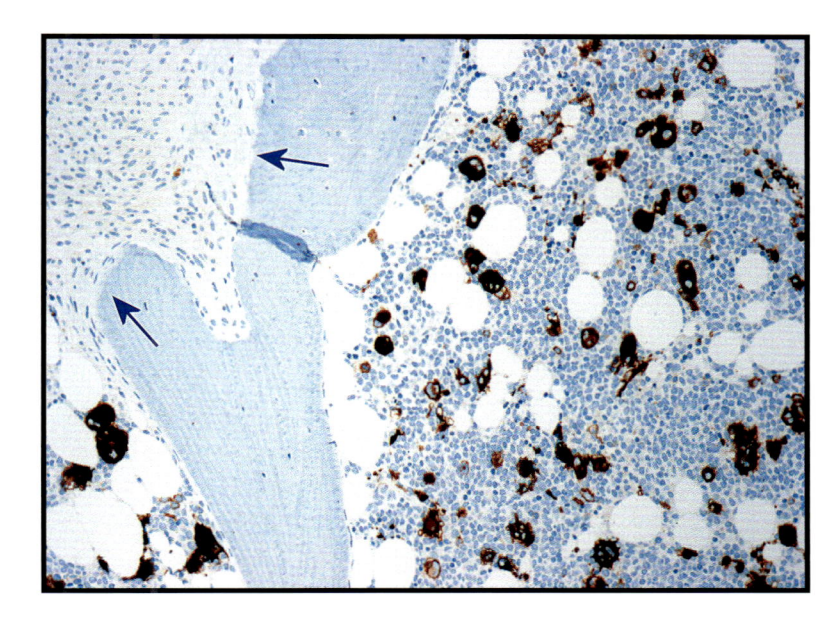

F3.27.5   CD61 in acute panmyelosis with myelofibrosis (APMF)

Occasionally, APMF is a diagnosis of exclusion. This biopsy specimen is from a 47-year-old man who did not have splenomegaly. Trilinear dyshematopoiesis was seen, and very small abnormal megakaryocytes were prominent. All abnormal megakaryocytes were connected to vascular spaces. This unique distribution of megakaryocytes is relatively frequently demonstrated in many conditions showing megakaryocyte abnormalities.

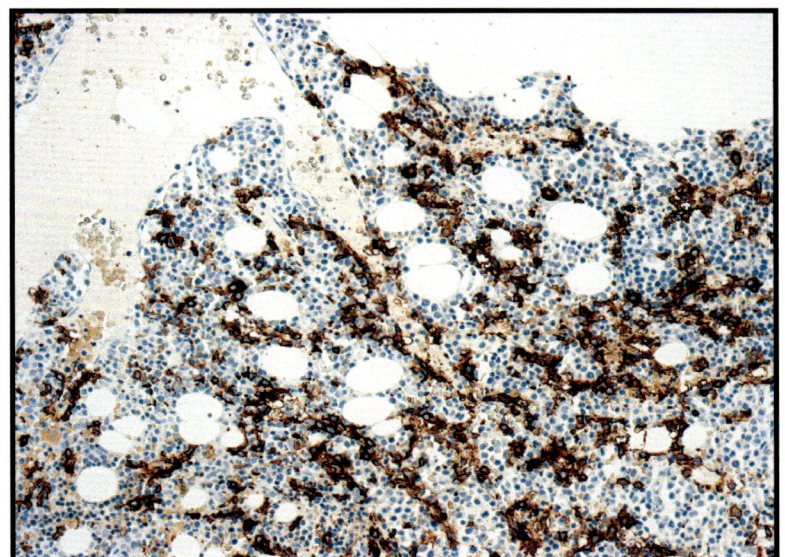

F3.27.6   CD61 in acute panmyelosis with myelofibrosis (APMF)

Same case as in F3.27.5. Rare larger, possibly more mature megakaryocytes show membranous expression of CD61 (red arrow). Most abnormal megakaryocytes have cytoplasmic staining with or without obvious Golgi-type positivity (blue arrows). Very few of the CD61+ cells produce platelets resulting in very low peripheral platelet count (78×10^9/L) and also very few platelets in the bone marrow (green arrows).

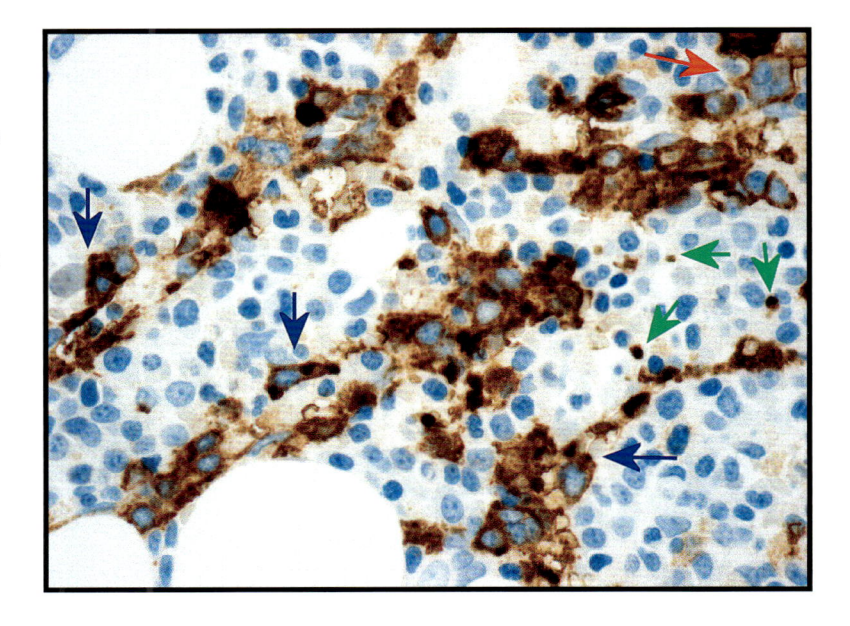

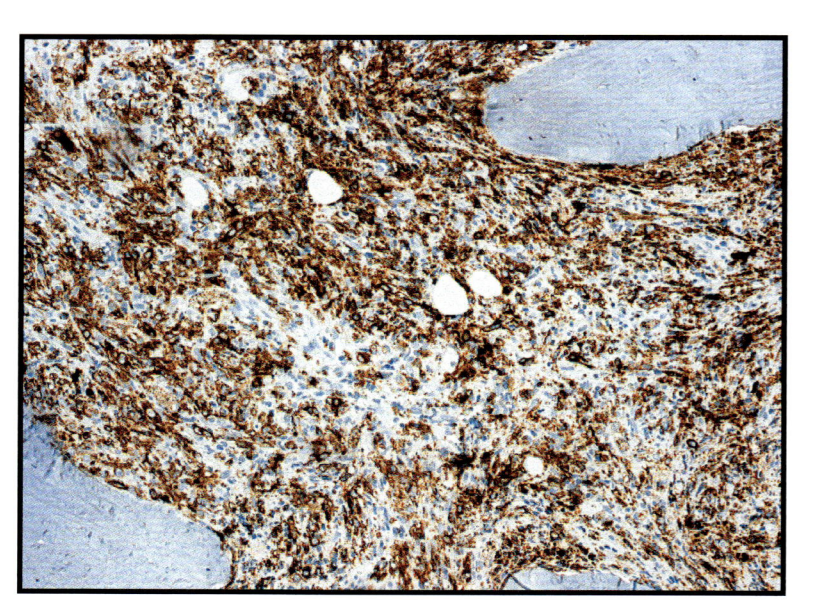

F3.27.7 CD61 in acute megakaryoblastic leukemia

This biopsy specimen is from a 7-year-old boy with bone marrow fibrosis. Extensive fibrosis of the BM is not uncommon in acute megakaryoblastic leukemia; however, it is not always possible to obtain a good specimen for flow cytometric analysis. Hence, immunohistochemistry is important in diagnosing acute megakaryoblastic leukemia. The blasts were also CD34+ and had somewhat spindled appearance probably secondary to fibrosis. Various metastatic sarcomas are in the differential diagnosis. CD61 can be demonstrated in rhabdomyosarcoma (as is CD34 and CD7), therefore this immunophenotype per se does not exclude metastatic rhabdomyosarcoma [Roullet 2007].

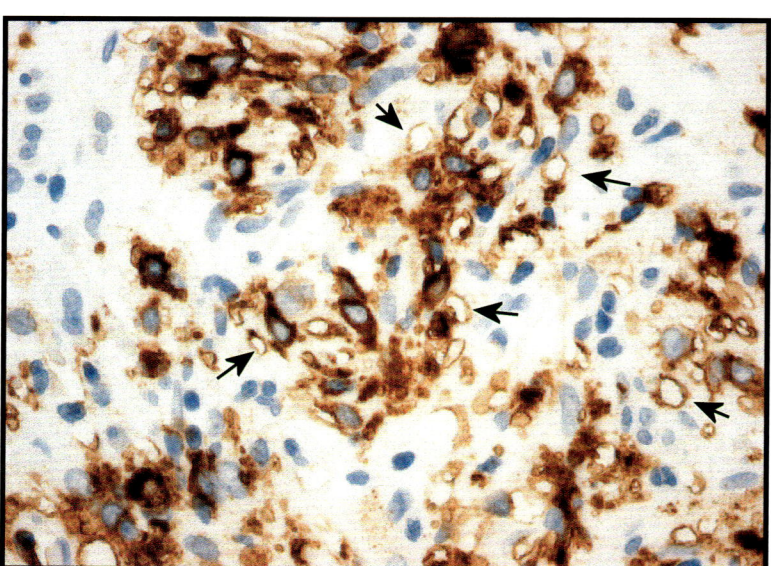

F3.27.8 CD61 in acute megakaryoblastic leukemia

Same case as in F3.27.7. CD61+ blasts are somewhat spindled. Also, bubblelike spaces highlighted by CD61 are present (arrows). This is not von Willebrand factor and no red blood cells were found in the "ruffles"; therefore these are not vascular spaces, but may represent cytoplasmic fragmentation.

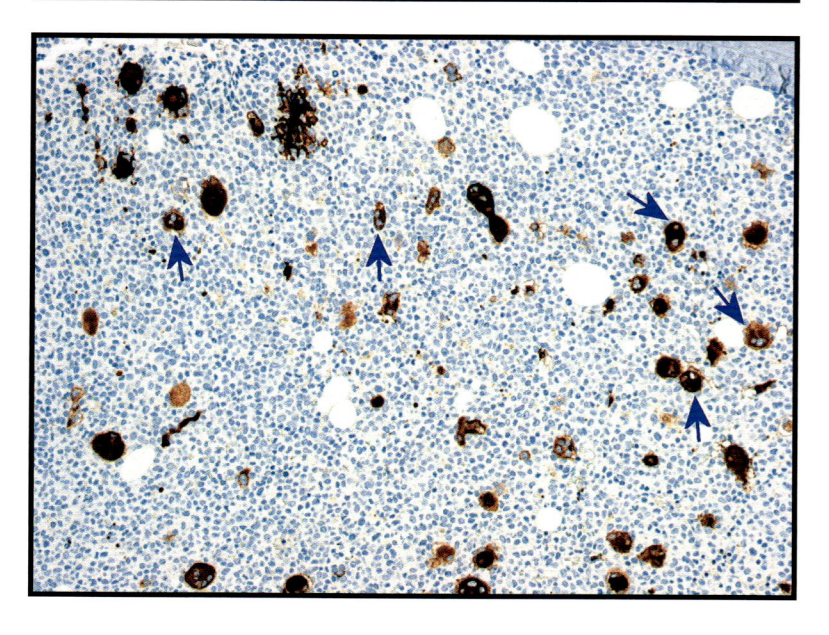

F3.27.9 CD61 in acute myeloid leukemia

This biopsy specimen is from a 65-year-old woman who presented with bone marrow failure. CD61 highlighted many dysplastic megakaryocytes. Many small bilobed forms are present (arrows). Small hypolobated megakaryocytes are often found in the 5q– syndrome. However, cytogenetic analysis showed no evidence of 5q– in this patient.

F3.27.10 CD61 in chronic idiopathic myelofibrosis (CIMF), prefibrotic stage

This biopsy specimen is from a patient with CIMF. Tight clusters of megakaryocytes are present and there is significant cytologic atypia of large megakaryocytes with increased nuclear-cytoplasmic ratio. Neutrophil hyperplasia is also present. This case shows greater variation of the intensity of staining from cell to cell than a normal bone marrow biopsy specimen. This may represent suboptimal tissue processing rather than biological variation in CD61 expression.

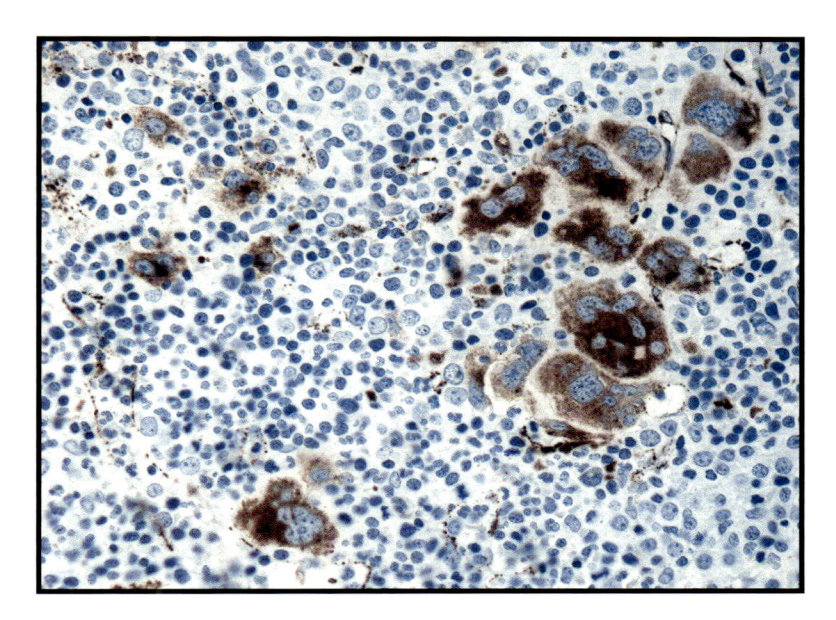

F3.27.11 CD42b in histologically normal bone marrow

Some variation in the intensity of staining is present. This image would look identical with CD61 staining. The selection of the primary antibody currently depends on personal preference; published literature does not report any significant differences between CD42b and CD61 expression. Platelets are seen (blue arrows), and megakaryocytes show some variability in staining intensity (red arrow).

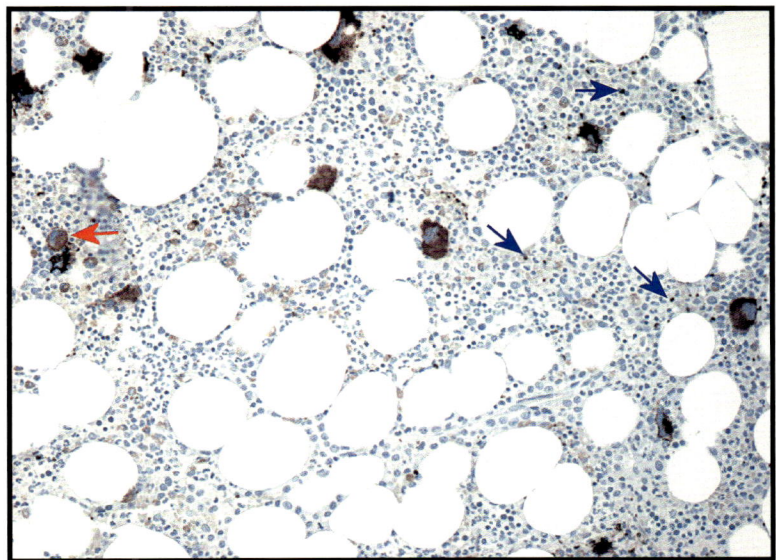

F3.27.12 CD42b in histologically normal bone marrow

Similar to CD61, platelets are also clearly visualized by CD42b (arrows). In our experience, CD42b may show slight tendency for more variation in staining intensity than CD61, which may not be the case if the tissue was fixed with other types of fixatives that favor CD42b epitope preservation.

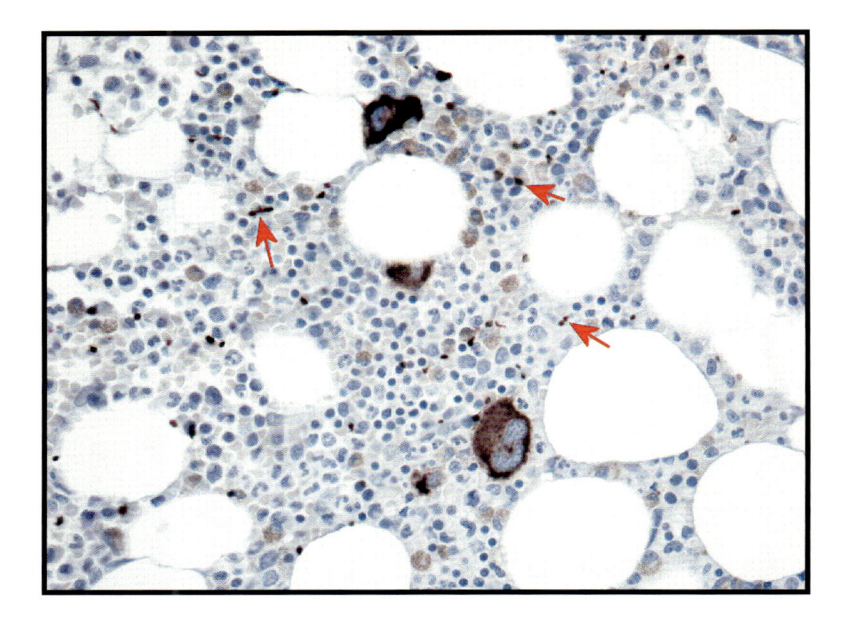

3.28 CD68

CD68 is also known as gp110; macrosialin. CD68 is a 110-kDa heavily glycosylated lysosomal transmembrane glycoprotein (PROW). It is strongly expressed in monocytes and macrophages, but is also expressed in dendritic cells, neutrophils, basophils, mast cells, myelid progenitor cells, a subset of CD34+ hemopoietic BM progenitor cells, activated T cells, approximately 40% of peripheral blood B cells, and weakly in about half of precursor B lymphoblastic leukemia cases (PROW). In addition to the aforementioned cell types, CD68+ stromal cells have been reported to have a role in fetal development of the BM, by being instrumental in chondrolysis process [Charbord 1996]. IHC will demonstrate CD68 mainly in the cytoplasm, and the pattern of staining is granular because of its localization in the lysosomes [Holness 1993]. Its function is not known at this time (OMIM). CD68 molecules are also weakly expressed on the surface of mature CD14+ monocytes. CD68 expression appears to start very early during granulomonopoietic differentiation [Strobl 1995; Knapp 1994]. Virtually all MPO+ BM cells coexpress CD68. CD68 expression is strongly upregulated in early MPO+ precursor cells, which lack lactoferrin (LF) and CD14 molecules. However, mature BM and peripheral blood granulocytes express considerably lower levels of CD68. Accordingly, it is expected that acute myeloid leukemia cases express CD68. CD68 expression is, however, not restricted to cells of myeloid origin; a subset of CD19+ peripheral blood B lymphocytes and 50% of B-ALL are also weakly positive. CD68 is not considered a myeloid lineage marker and is not included in the EGIL scoring system. T cells generally do not express CD68 and CD56+ NK cells express CD68 only rarely [Scheinecker 1995; Helin 2008; Manaloor 2000]. Despite its low specificity, CD68 continues to be used in diagnostic pathology with significant applications in BM pathology.

In follicular lymphoma, the pattern of CD68high+ macrophages, high content of CD8+/TIA-1+ T cells, and CD123+ cells were found to be positively correlated with indolent behavior [Alvaro 2006]. The appearance of the peculiar BM CD68+/lysozyme–/CD123var/Ki-67– monocytic nodules, which are most likely dendritic cells, have been suggested to be associated with more advanced disease and worse outcome in patients with MDS and CMML [Chen 2003; Orazi 2006]. Detection of CD68 by either PG-M1 or KP-1 clones or of CD163 is not useful for discriminating between CML and CMML [Orazi 2006; Manaloor 2000; Lau 2004; Nguyen 2005].

Most of the images here show results with PG-M1 clone for detection of CD68 because it is somewhat more specific for monocytic differentiation than KP-1, the other widely used monoclonal Ab for detection of CD68 [Helin 2008]. Ki-M6, Ki-M7, and EBM11 are also in use [Helin 2008]. It appears that PG-M1 gives a better signal-to-noise ratio than KP-1 and stains a narrower spectrum of cells. For example, in acute myeloid leukemia, KP-1 also stains nonmonocytic subtypes that are not stained with PG-M1 or CD14 [Helin 2008]. However, if CD68 is used as a myeloid marker, the KP-1 clone should be used. In the evaluation of hematologic processes, both KP-1 and PG-M1 could be used with a different purpose.

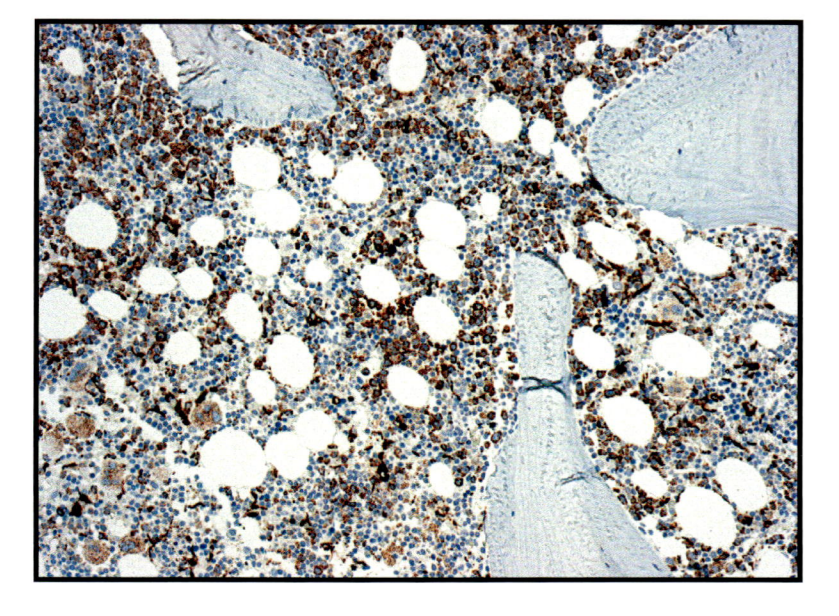

F3.28.1 CD68 (KP-1) in histologically normal bone marrow (ADVANCE)

This overview illustrates that many cells in the normal BM are positive. Because CD68 is a lysosomal membrane marker, all cells with significant content of lysosomes should be detected. The staining is strongest in macrophages/monocytes and stromal dendritic cells, moderate in neutrophils, and weak in megakaryocytes.

F3.28.2 CD68 (PG-M1) in histologically normal bone marrow (EnVision+)

PG-M1 antibody shows more selective reactivity with the macrophage/monocyte CD68 molecule; it is less sensitive than KP-1 in detection of the CD68 as a component of the lysosomal membrane and it is also less sensitive than naphthyl butyrate esterase in detecting monocytes in chronic myelomonocytic leukemia [Strobl 1995].

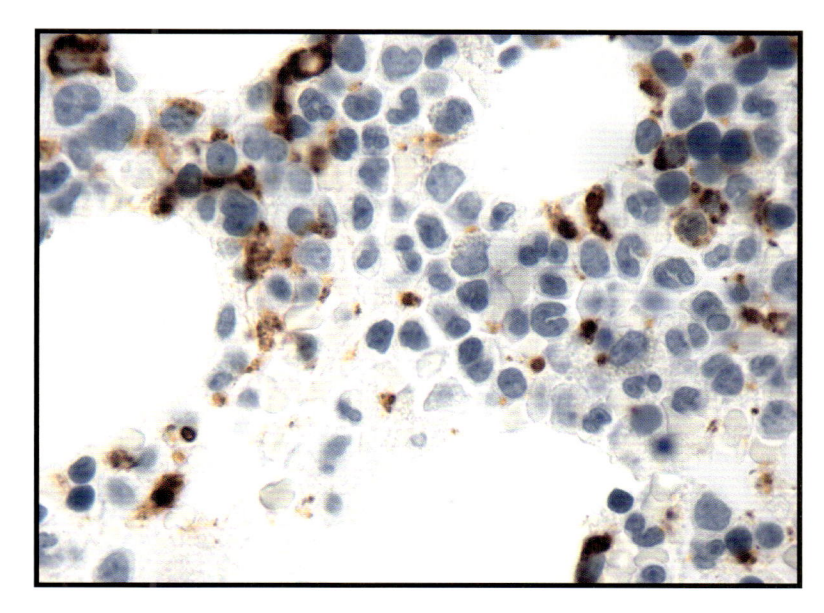

F3.28.3 CD68 in histologically normal bone marrow (KP-1, EnVision+)

KP-1 monoclonal antibody detects CD68 in various cell types including neutrophil precursors. Segmented neutrophils are very weakly stained or negative (green arrows), while eosinophils and their precursors do not express CD68 (red arrow).

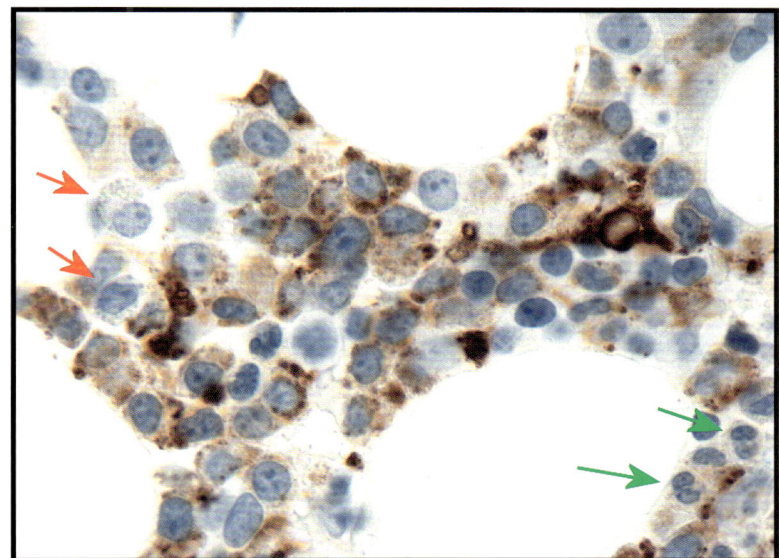

F3.28.4 PG-M1 in marginal zone lymphoma

CD68 may often be detected as weak cytoplasmic staining in normal marginal zone B cells and it is also detected in some marginal zone lymphomas. As illustrated here, the expression is identified as small cytoplasmic dots that vary in number (arrows) and most of which correlate with scant lysosomes rather than Golgi-type dotlike expression.

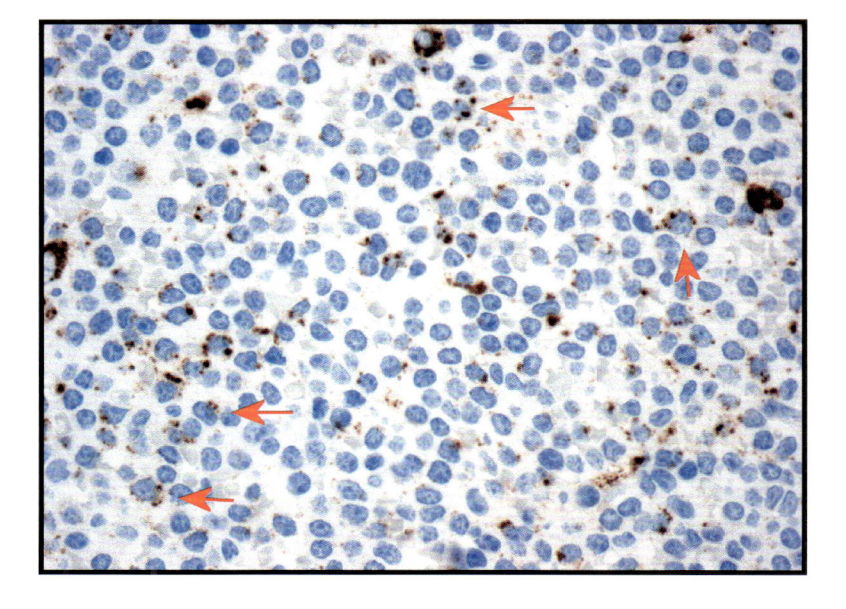

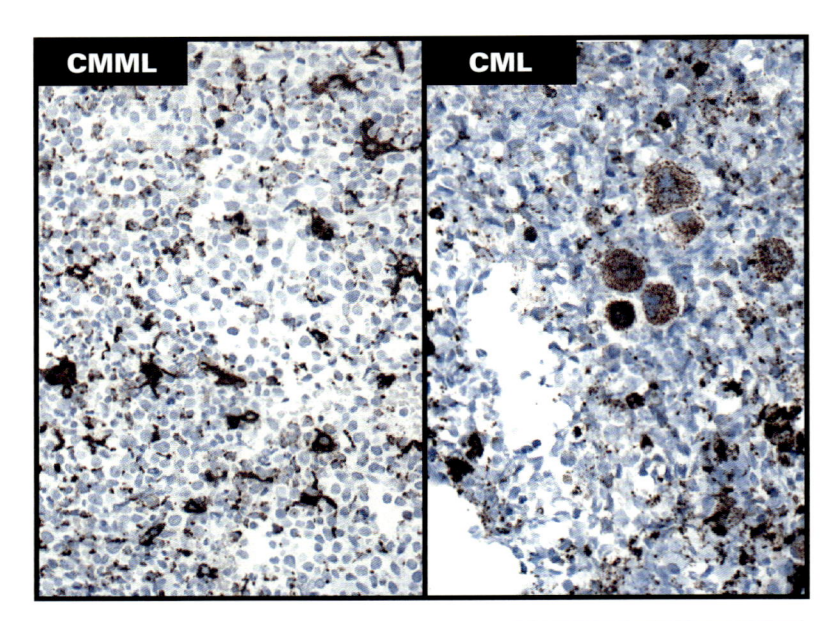

F3.28.5 PG-M1 in chronic myelomonocytic leukemia (CMML) and chronic myeloid leukemia

This clone does not detect neutrophils, and it is an insensitive marker for the monocytic component of CMML. Therefore, it is not recommended to use this antibody to distinguish between these 2 entities.

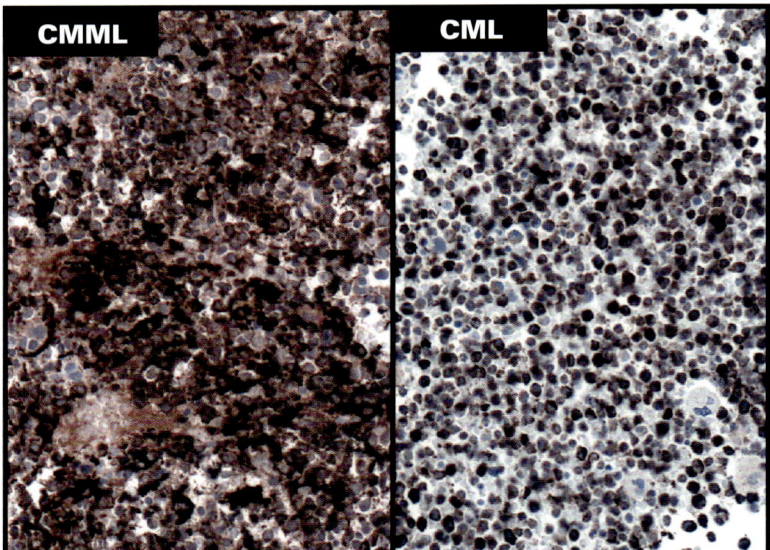

F3.28.6 KP-1 in chronic myelomonocytic leukemia (CMML) and chronic myeloid leukemia (CML)

In both CMML and CML the KP-1 antibody marks neutrophils and precursors as well as monocytic cells; megakaryocytes are variably stained. This antibody is not useful in distinguishing these 2 disorders.

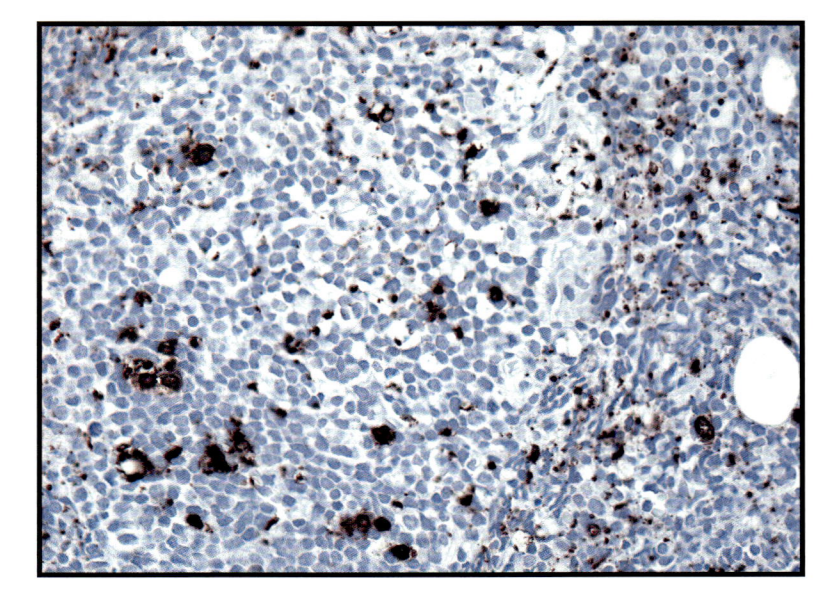

F3.28.7 PG-M1 in precursor B-cell lymphoblastic leukemia at presentation

Lymphoblasts are CD68−. This contrasts to the frequent expression of CD68 in acute myeloid leukemia, particularly myelomonocytic and monoblastic/monocytic leukemias. Dendritic CD68+ cells that are present in normal bone marrow are not present. Only rare macrophages/monocytes are strongly positive.

F3.28.8 PG-M1 and lysozyme in precursor B-cell lymphoblastic leukemia on day 14 after chemotherapy

CD68+ dendritic cells/macrophages are slightly increased compared with a prechemotherapy biopsy specimen (F3.28.7). Arrow points to a small megakaryocyte that is positive for CD68 as expected. Lysozyme (LZ) also identifies a similar dendritic population, but does not identify the lysosomal membrane like CD68, rather a content of the lysosomal vesicles, and therefore the intensity and distribution are somewhat different.

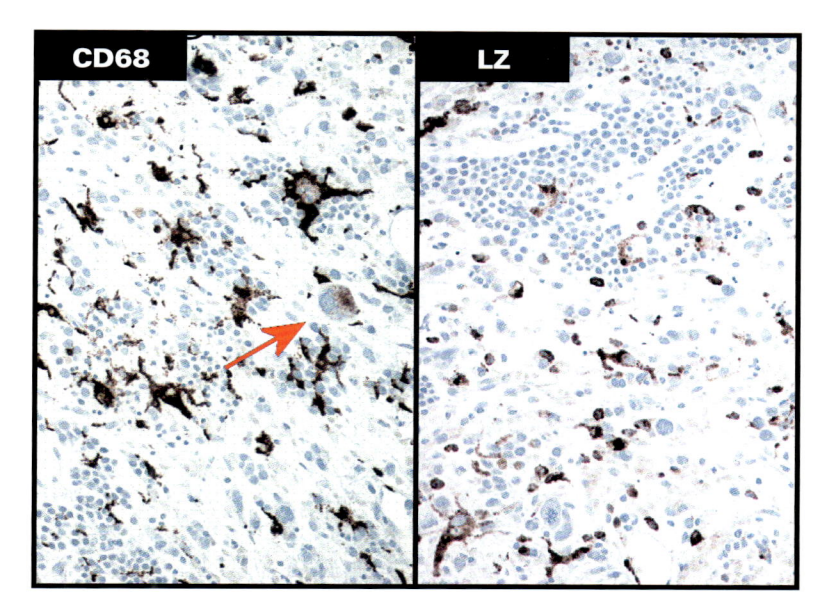

F3.28.9 PG-M1 and CD10 in precursor B-cell acute lymphoblastic leukemia (B-ALL) on day 14 after chemotherapy

CD10 also identifies a dendritic cell population (right). This is a different stromal population than the one identified by CD68, but it is also somewhat increased compared with normal bone marrow. One of the functions of the CD10+ population is to support B-cell maturation. Their possible role in the biology of precursor B-ALL is not known.

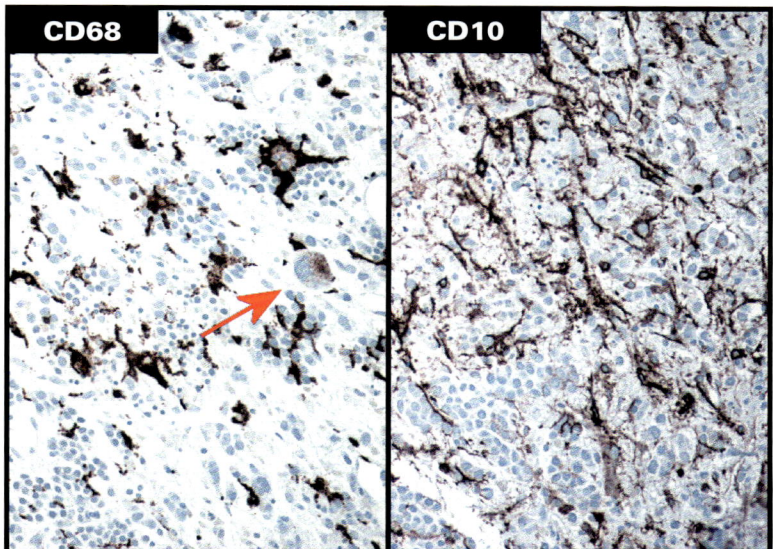

F3.28.10 PG-M1 in a hemophagocytic syndrome

This biopsy specimen is from a young adult with a hemophagocytic syndrome associated with a peripheral T-cell lymphoma. CD68+ cells are markedly increased, which probably reflects a reaction to involvement by peripheral T-cell lymphoma as well as a systemic response and increase in the hemophagocytic cells.

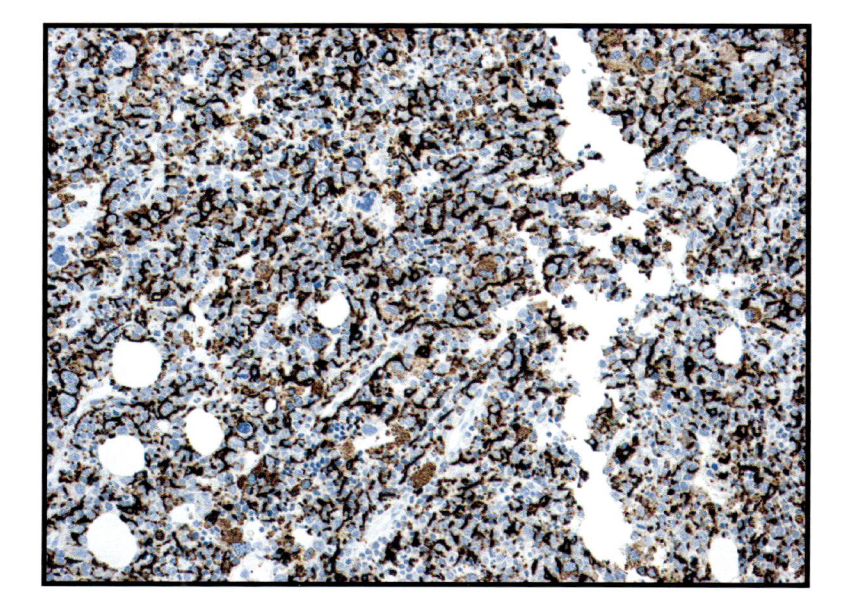

3: Cluster of Differentiation Markers

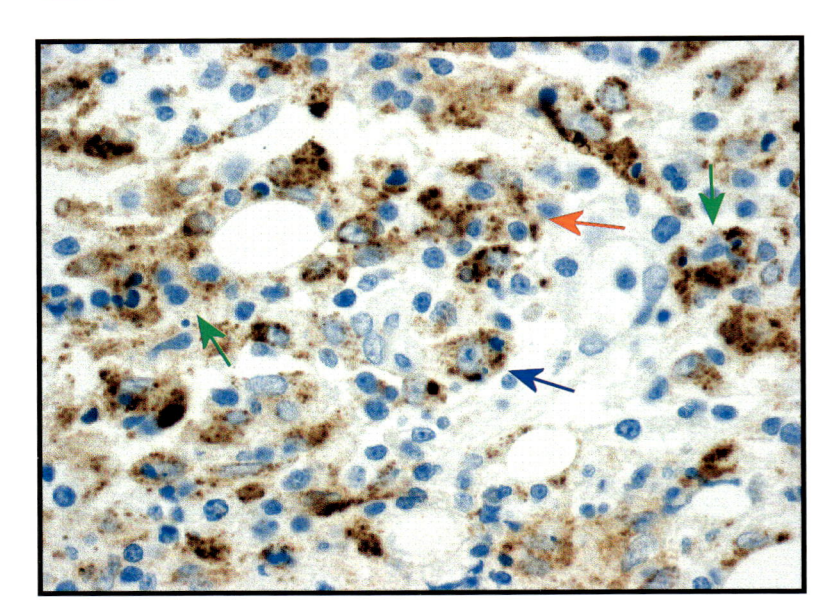

F3.28.11 PG-M1 in hemophagocytic syndrome

The same specimen as above (see F3.28.10). Hemophagocytic macrophages are illustrated. Most positive cells contain fragments of phagocytosed cells. Some phagocytosed cells appear viable (red arrow) or as cellular debris (blue arrow) or both (green arrows).

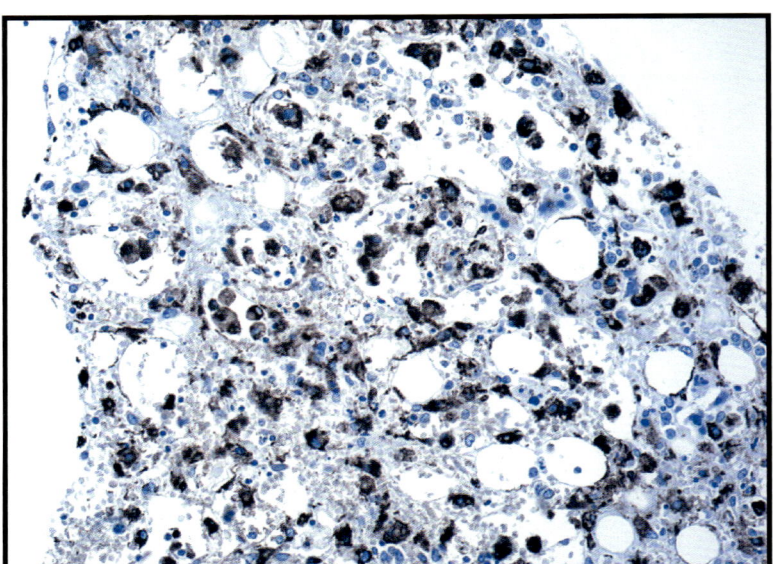

F3.28.12 CD68 (PG-M1) in a postmortem specimen from a 9-year-old girl with hemophagocytic syndrome after a presumed viral infection

The child died of systemic mycosis after receiving corticosteroid therapy. There is a total lack of hematopoietic cells, partly because of hemophagocytic syndrome and possibly suppression secondary to systemic mycosis. The patient was HIV–. Positive cells are more rounded than in those seen in F3.28.11.

3.29 CD79a

CD79a is also known as Ig-α or MB1. CD79a is a part of the B lymphocyte antigen receptor (OMIM). The B-cell receptor consists of Ig and 2 other proteins, Ig-α (CD79a) and Ig-β (CD79b) [Ha 1992]. A study comparing 5 different clones for detecting CD79a in routinely processed tissues identified a JCB117 clone as the most specific [Bhargava 2007]. IHC of the BM is widely used to detect CD79a. IHC is particularly useful in the detection of both benign and malignant precursor B cells and terminally differentiated B cells, in contrast to CD20, whose expression is more or less limited to mature B-cell phenotype [Arber 1996a; Arber 1996b; Chetty 1995; Mason 1995; Chuang 1997; Pezzella 2000; Toth 1999; Nowicki 1999; Pileri 1999; Pilozzi 1998; Hashimoto 2002]. Pax-5 is not expressed in the terminal B-cell stage, so CD79a is the most widely detectable B-cell Ag even though it is not entirely specific [Torlakovic 2002c]. Because it continues to be expressed in terminal B-cell differentiation, CD79a is the best marker of lymphoplasmacytic lymphoma in the BM. A variable percentage of malignant cells in LPL shows some degree of terminal B-cell differentiation, which will invariably affect the number of CD20+ and Pax-5+ cells with decreased expression usually proportional to plasma cell differentiation. CD79a is typically found in both malignant and benign plasma cells in addition to all mature B cells. Therefore, CD79a will be present in all cells of LPL, as illustrated in **F3.29.9**. Although CD79a is expressed in all mature B-cell disorders, CD20 is the marker of choice for the detection of most mature B cells because it is more specific. CD79a is very weakly expressed at the germinal center stage of development, and may also be a very poor marker of hairy cell leukemia (see **F3.29.8**). CD79a is found in 79% of precursor B-ALL, where it is coexpressed with Pax-5+ [Arber 1996]. CD79a is detected in 84% of CD20− B-cell neoplasias treated with rituximab, which were strongly positive for CD20 before therapy [Arber 1996]. Together with Pax-5, CD79a is a useful marker of neoplastic cells after rituximab therapy. CD79a expression is present in all cases of precursor B-ALL before therapy. However, in acute leukemia, it is not limited to precursor B-ALL. In particular, it has been reported to be expressed in up to 50% of precursor T-ALL cases [Pilozzi 1998; Hashimoto 2002; Tiacci 2004]. It is also typically found in AML with t(8;21), which may also show expression of other B-cell markers including CD19, CD20, and TdT [Tiacci 2004].

F3.29.1 CD79a bone marrow biopsy with reactive features

This biopsy specimen is from a patient with classical Hodgkin lymphoma with no involvement of the BM. The BM may show increased hematogones, which results in increased expression of several early B-cell markers including CD79a. While Pax-5 often demonstrates linear arrangement of B-cell precursors, this is also sometimes observed with CD79a as shown here. Similar or larger number of cells are highlighted by Pax-5 because this transcription factor upregulates CD79a.

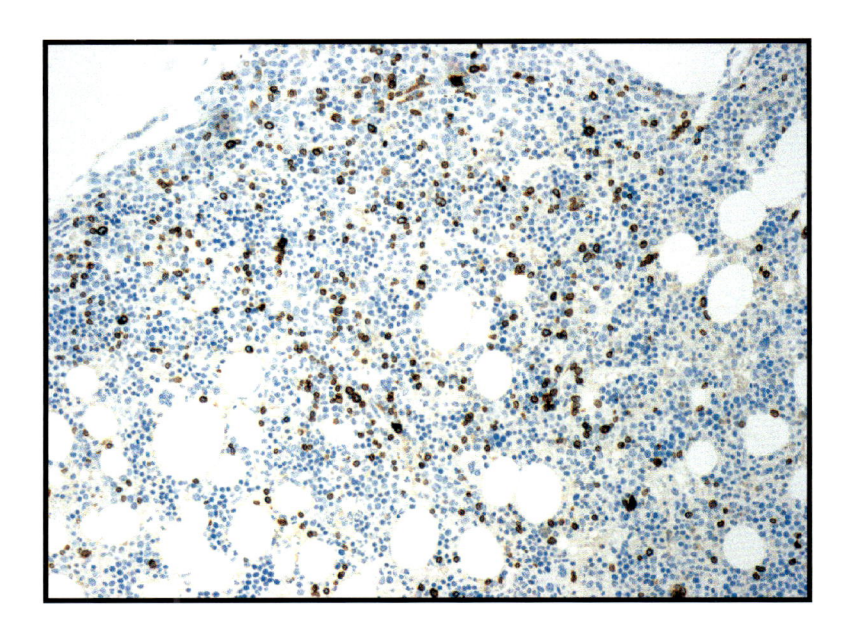

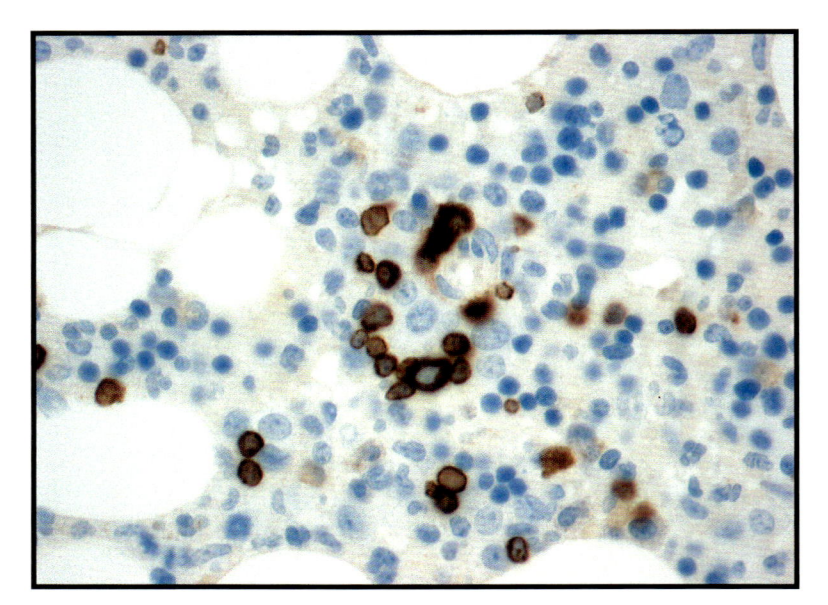

F3.29.2 CD79a in hematogones

This row of CD79a+ hematogones includes about 7 cells. It is more likely that there are 2 closely located rows including 3 and 4 cells each. Pax-5 may occasionally demonstrate large number of hematogones in rows; however, CD79a+ rows typically contain about 3 cells.

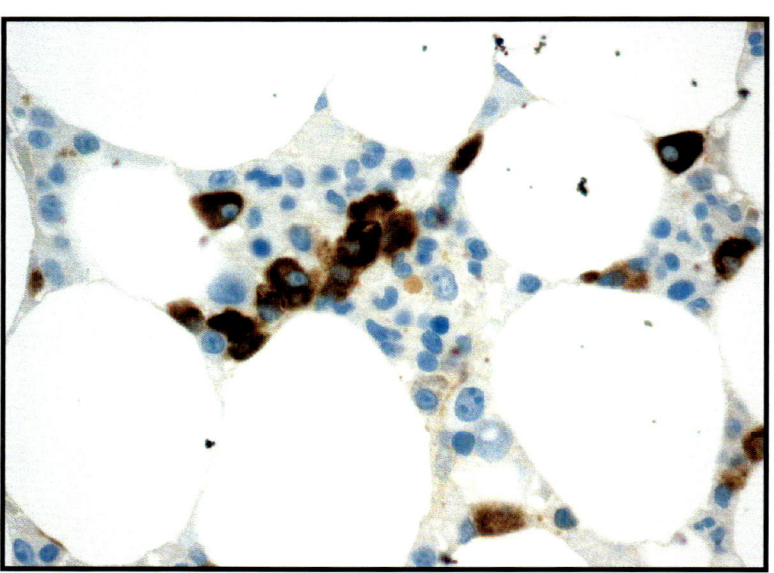

F3.29.3 CD79a in plasma cells

Despite Pax-5 downregulation at terminal B-cell differentiation, CD79a continues to be detected in plasma cells in the cytoplasmic compartment. Therefore, CD79a is found in cells before and after they express CD20. CD79a is detected in both benign and malignant plasma cells.

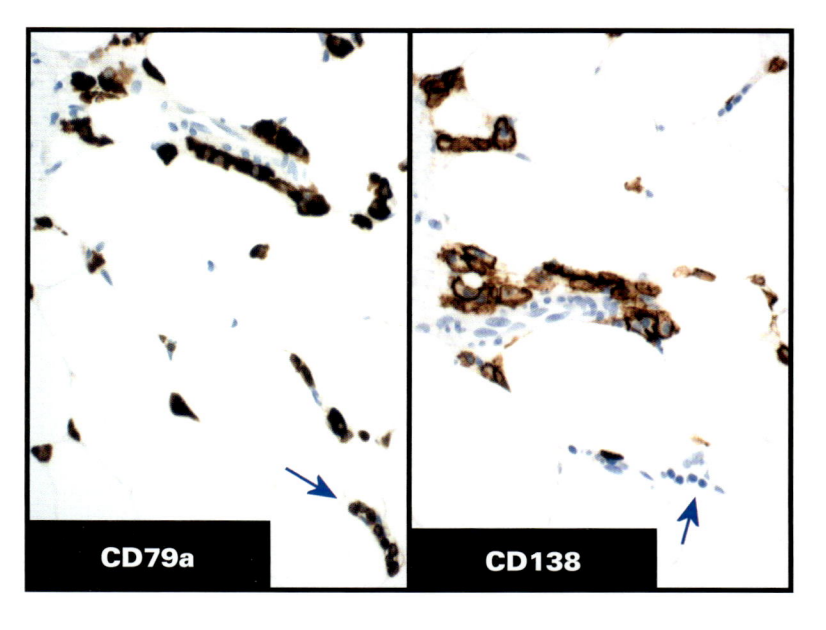

F3.29.4 CD79a in focally hypocellular bone marrow with follicular lymphoma (FL)

This biopsy specimen is from a 64-year-old woman with stage IV FL. Here, FL was found in paratrabecular localization and focally interstitially in hypocellular areas. In this area, the relatively high CD79a expression is because of the plasma cell content, which is confirmed by their CD138 expression. Only a small number of lymphoma cells is present and highlighted by CD79a (arrows). CD20 is a better marker for demonstration of total tumor volume in this biopsy specimen.

F3.29.5 **CD79a; intrasinusoidal localization of follicular lymphoma**

In contrast to the more usual paratrabecular localization seen in follicular lymphona (FL), this specimen illustrates multifocal intrasinusoidal localization by FL. This is uncommon. Intrasinusoidal small B-cell lymphomas are often, but not always, splenic marginal zone lymphoma.

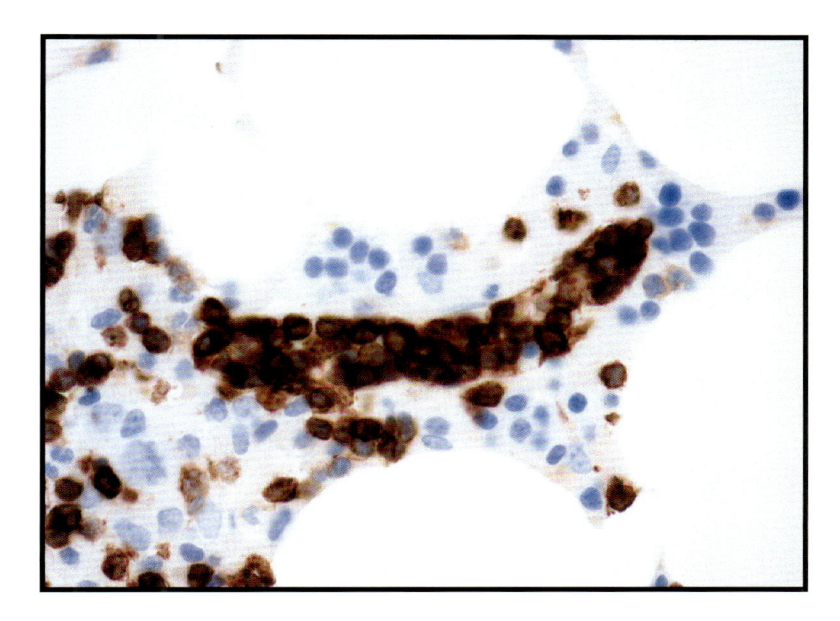

F3.29.6 **CD79a in plasma cell myeloma**

This biopsy specimen is from a 52-year-old woman with multiple myeloma. Bone marrow aspirate smears showed 35% plasma cells. CD79a is expressed by malignant plasma cells, but its expression varies widely from case to case and from cell to cell. CD138 and Ig light chains are much better choices for detection of malignant plasma cells in BM biopsy.

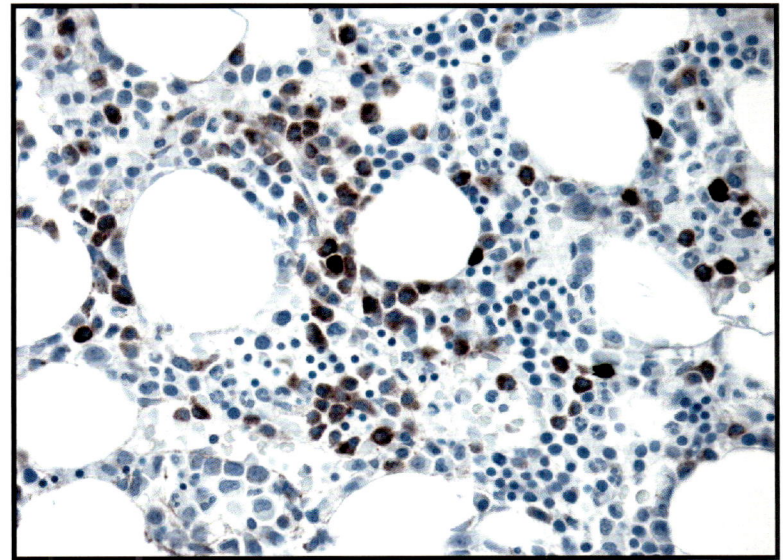

F3.29.7 **CD79a in hematogones after rituximab therapy**

This bone marrow was previously involved by follicular lymphoma. In the current biopsy specimen, CD20 was negative. CD79a staining revealed a few positive randomly distributed cells, while Pax-5 and TdT were slightly increased. In patients treated with rituximab, CD20 may be entirely negative when hematogones are increased. However, markers that detect immature B cells including Pax-5 and TdT will be increased (with typical ratio of Pax-5>TdT>CD34).

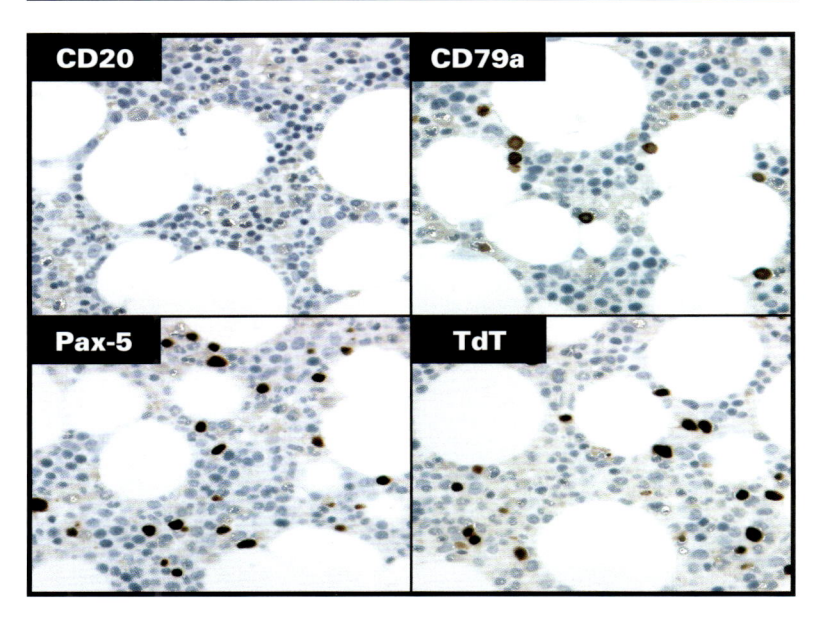

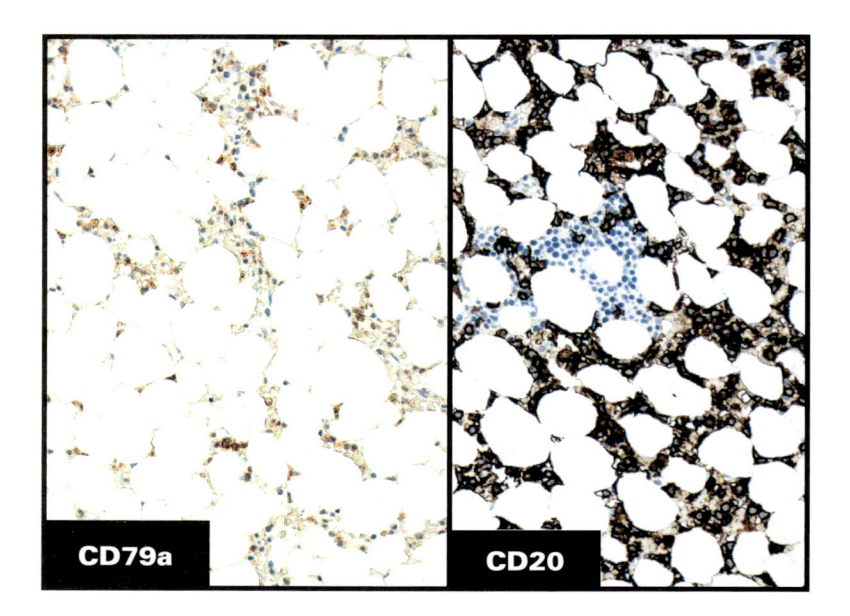

F3.29.8 CD79a in hairy cell leukemia (HCL)

In contrast to CD20, which is known to be most strongly expressed in HCL, CD79a may be a very weakly expressed B-cell marker in this disease. CD79a should not be used instead of CD20, but rather as an adjunct to CD20, in the evaluation of B-cell lymphoproliferative disorders.

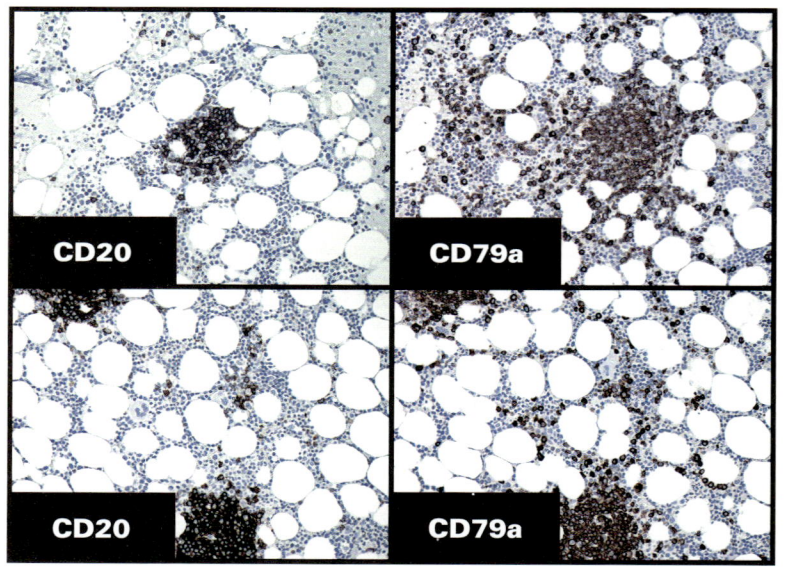

F3.29.9 CD79a is the optimal marker of lymphoplasmacytic lymphoma (LPL)

CD79a invariably detects all cells of LPL, while CD20 and Pax-5 may be rather weak or negative in a significant population of malignant cells with variation in the intensity and the percentage of positive cells. In many cases, CD20+ cells form interstitial lymphoid aggregates (left) and CD20− plasmacytoid lymphocytes and plasma cells are found interstitially as shown here.

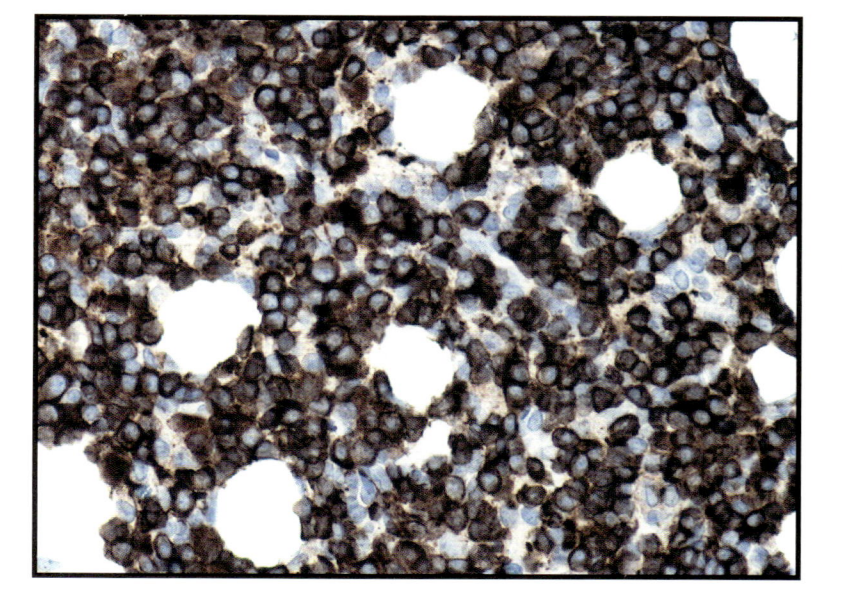

F3.29.10 CD79a in precursor B-cell acute lymphoblastic leukemia (B-ALL)

This biopsy specimen is from a 22-month-old child with precursor B-ALL. Most such cases are characterized by high Pax-5 and high CD79a expression. While CD79a is not entirely specific, it is invariably found in precursor B-ALL. In the European Group for the Immunologic Classification of Leukemia scoring system, cytoplasmic CD79a expression is scored as "2" as strong evidence of B-cell differentiation.

3.29 CD79a

F3.29.11 CD79a in precursor B-cell acute lymphoblastic leukemia (B-ALL)

In contrast to the case illustrated in F3.29.10, this biopsy specimen showed precursor B-ALL at presentation with unusually low expression of CD79a (blue arrow). Only occasional cells had strong expression (red arrow). Pax-5 and PU.1, the 2 transcription factors essential for B-cell development were also found to be very weakly expressed. There was no evidence of myeloid or T-cell differentiation. The biological significance of this finding is not clear.

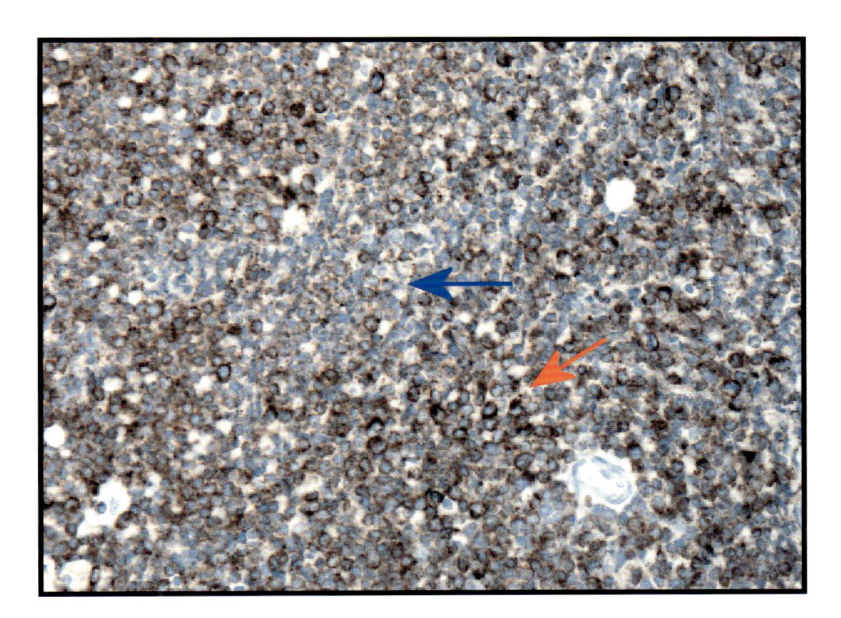

F3.29.12 CD79a in pure erythroid acute leukemia

CD79a is expressed by a subpopulation of blasts. CD79a is not a B-cell lineage restricted marker. It is expressed in as many as 25% or more precursor T-cell lymphoblastic leukemia cases and in several acute myeloid leukemia cases. Pure erythroid acute leukemia is a rare disease and it is not known how frequently CD79a can be detected in this disease with immunohistochemistry.

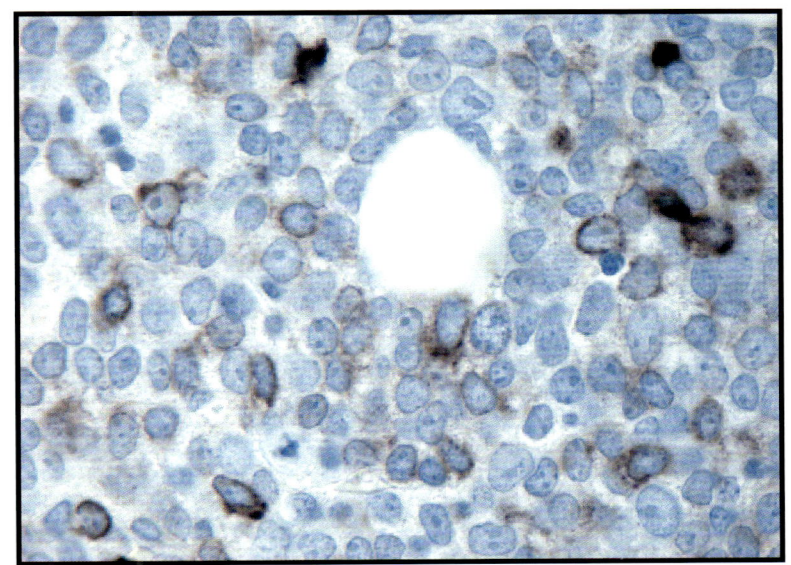

3.30 CD99

CD99 is also known as MIC2, MIC2X, MIC2Y, CD99R, and E2 (PROW, OMIM). This protein is expressed on all human tissues tested, with the possible exception of spermatozoa [Stevenson 1994]. This transmembrane glycoprotein p30 is a product of the MIC2 gene located on the pseudoautosomal region of X and Y chromosomes (OMIM). The function of CD99 is not fully elucidated. However, it was demonstrated that it enhances apoptosis in T cells [Jung 2003; Pettersen 2001]. Also, CD99 regulates sequential steps in the transendothelial migration of neutrophils and monocytes during inflammation as well as transendothelial migration of human mobilized peripheral blood CD34+ cells [Lou 2007; Imbert 2006; Schenkel 2001]. CD99 is a T-cell surface glycoprotein involved in spontaneous rosette formation with erythrocytes [Hamilton 1988]. Clinical usefulness of the CD99 detection in the bone marrow biopsy with IHC is very limited. However, it can be demonstrated as overexpressed in ALL and AML as well as metastatic Ewing sarcoma [Gelin 1989]. Other cells that show significant expression are Sertoli cells, granulosa cells, ependymal cells, pancreas, and adenohypophysis, which are almost never in consideration in the BM biopsy [Hamilton 1988].

It appears that all TdT+ AMLs are also CD99+, but not all CD99+ cases are TdT+ because CD99 is more often expressed than TdT in AMLs, including the M3, M6, and M7 FAB subtypes [Zhang 2000; Kang 2006]. Despite a previous report that CD99 is not expressed in monoblastic leukemia [Zhang 2000], we have encountered 1 monoblastic TdT+ case, which is illustrated here (**F3.31.1**). The higher the sensitivity of the CD99 test, the higher the probability that clinically irrelevant expression will be detected. Ideally and similar to optimization of the HER2/*neu* in breast carcinoma, the CD99 protocol would need to be optimized to detect only overexpression as significant staining. In the BM, moderately strong staining with CD99 needs to be detected in CD34+ cells of BM and in immature lymphocytes and granulocytes [Robertson 1997; Dworzak 1994]. Furthermore, very strong staining should be demonstrated in the BM involved by Ewing sarcoma, lymphoblastic lymphoma, and AML. ALK+ anaplastic large cell lymphoma was reported to express CD99 in about 70% of cases and overall 50% of ALCL and occasional DLBCL cases also do so [Sung 2005].

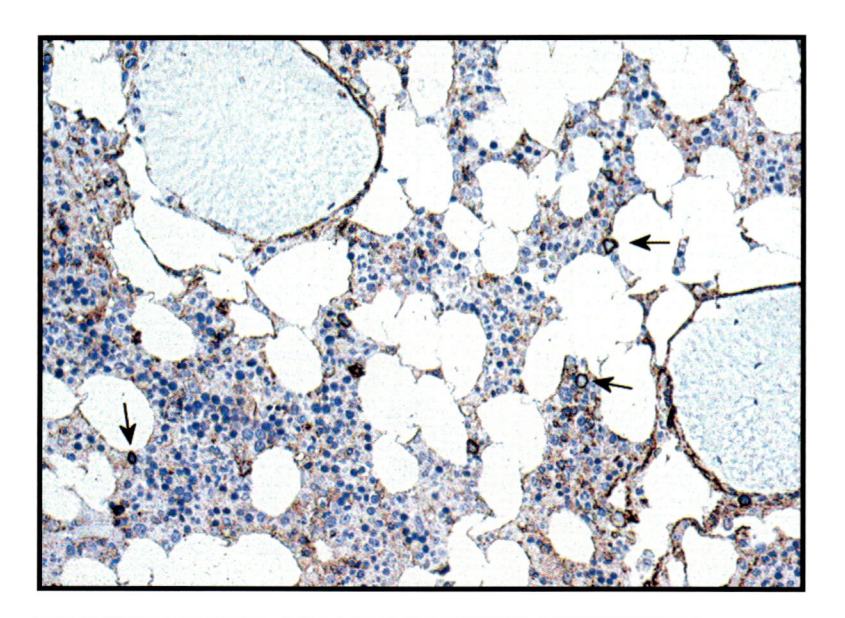

F3.30.1 CD99 in histologically normal bone marrow

While numerous cells express CD99 at variable intensity, only bone lining cells and presumed hematopoietic precursors show strong and distinct expression noticeable at low magnification.

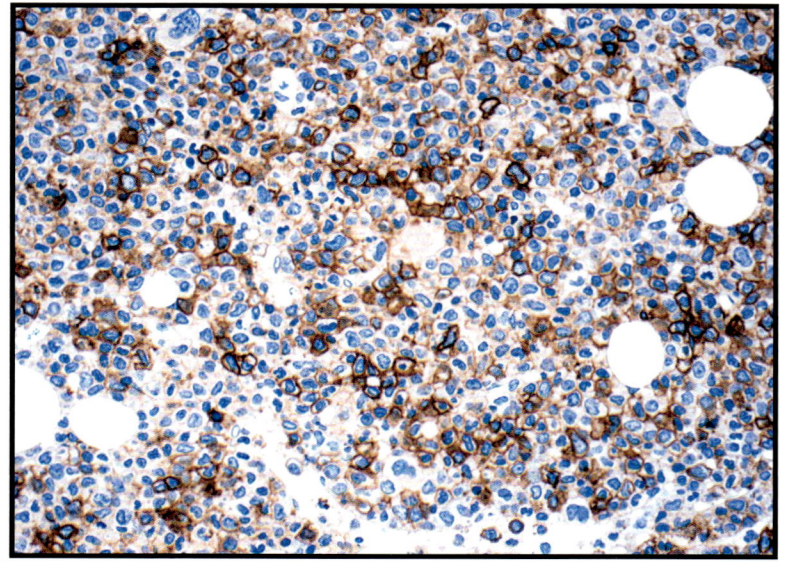

F3.30.2 CD99 in acute monoblastic leukemia

This biopsy specimen is from a 65-year-old man with acute monoblastic leukemia. Strong CD99 expression is illustrated. CD99 is traditionally considered a marker of a lymphoblastic leukemia/lymphoma and Ewing sarcoma. However, CD99 is expressed to some degree in most tissues. No TdT or other lineage-specific lymphoid markers were detected in this case.

F3.30.3 CD99 in acute myelomonoblastic leukemia

This biopsy is from an 80-year-old man who presented with pancytopenia. A small population of blastlike cells is strongly positive. Myeloid luekemias vary widely in CD99 expression, but no systematic studies have been published.

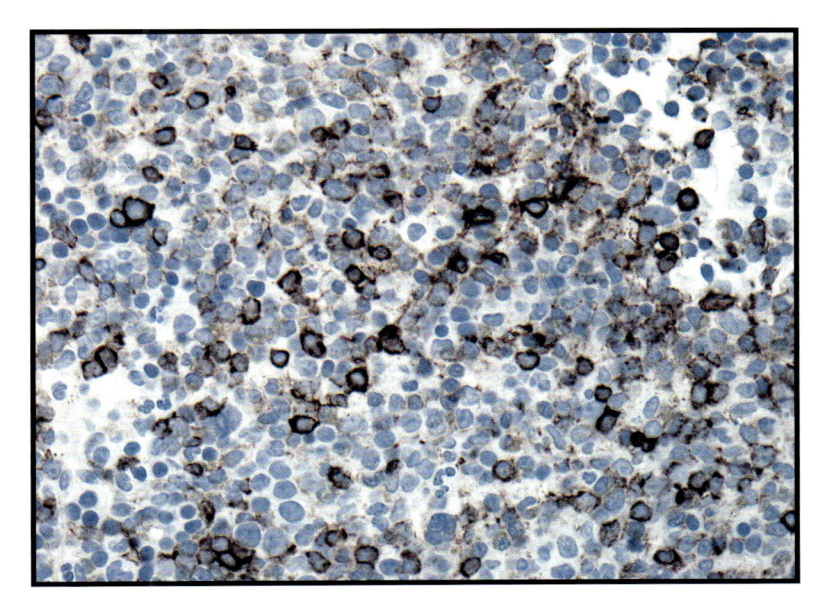

F3.30.4 Weak expression of CD99 in sinusoidal endothelial cells (ADVANCE)

The expression of CD99 appears variable in endothelial cells lining bone marrow sinusoids (arrows). Compare with the consistently strong expression in a hematopoietic precursor cell (dashed arrow). The lining of adipocytes is also weakly positive but inconsistent, which is presumed to be a specific staining. Monocytes consistently express high levels of CD99 with flow cytometry [Kang 2006] and 3 are seen here in the lumen of the sinusoid.

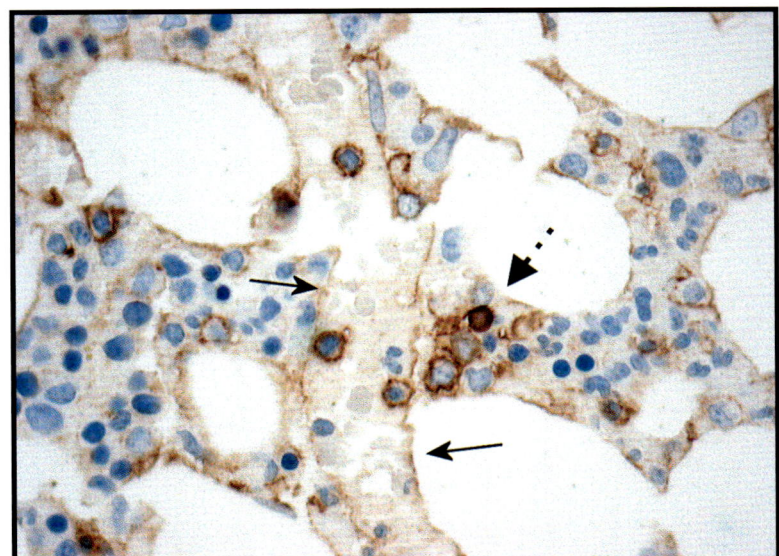

F3.30.5 CD99 in osteoblasts (ADVANCE)

CD99 is expressed in osteoblasts and in osteosarcoma cells. CD99 has been described to act as an oncosuppressor in osteosarcoma [Manara 2006]. A seam of osteoblasts shows membranous expression of CD99. Note that endothelial cells of the paratrabecular sinusoid are also positive for CD99 (arrow).

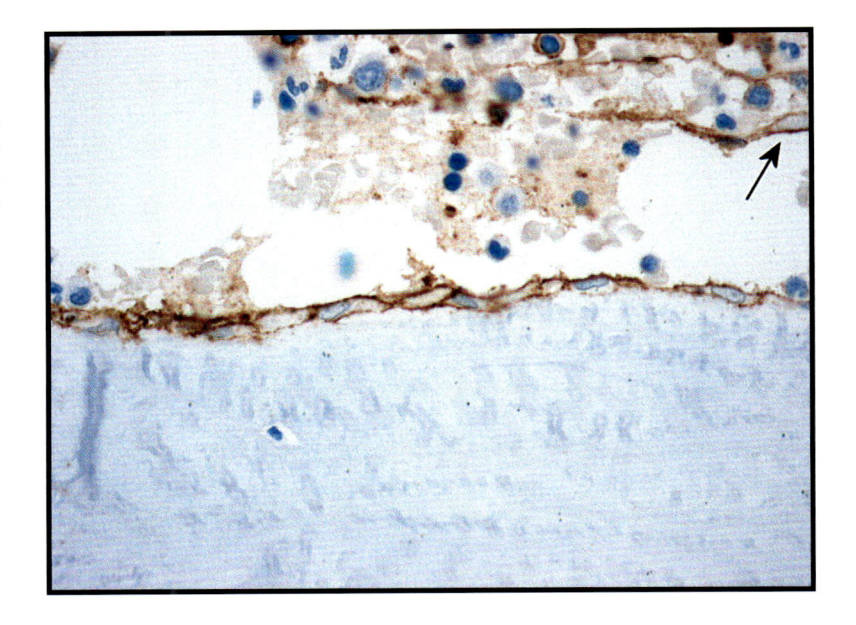

3: Cluster of Differentiation Markers

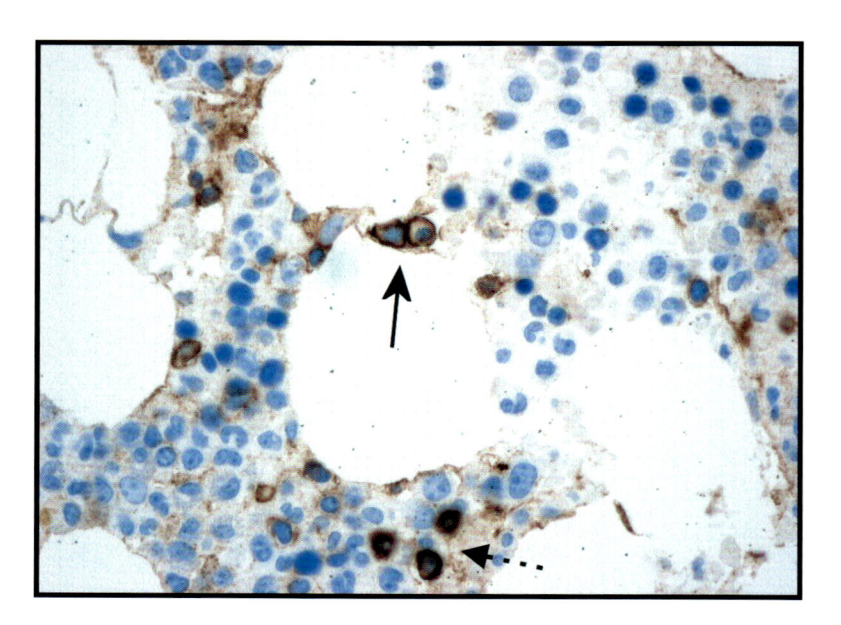

F3.30.6 CD99 in benign plasma cells

CD99 expression in benign plasma cells in the bone marrow is illustrated (arrow). This 37-year-old woman had nodular sclerosis Hodgkin lymphoma and only reactive changes in the BM. 3 presumed lymphoid precursors show strong expression of CD99 (dashed arrow). Several other cells show much weaker expression.

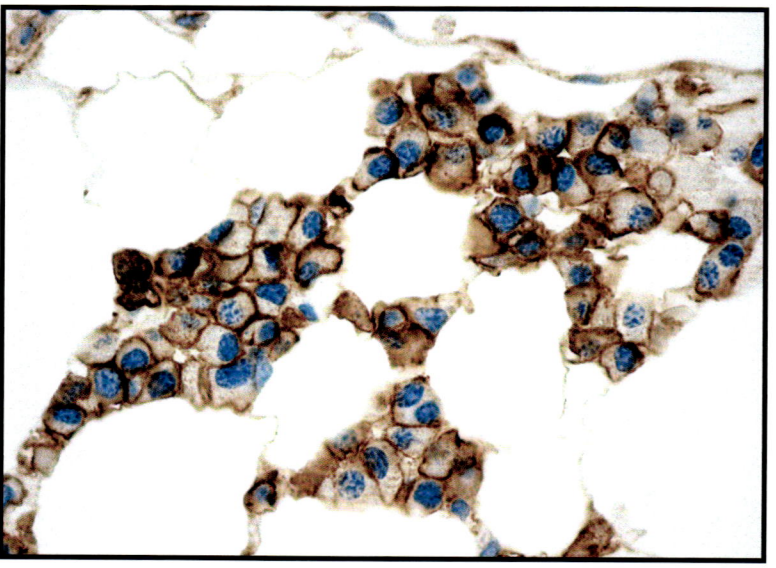

F3.30.7 CD99 in multiple myeloma

CD99 is generally not considered to be a marker of myeloma. However, CD99 can be found expressed by both benign plasma cells and multiple myeloma. Only membranous positivity may be considered specific in such cases.

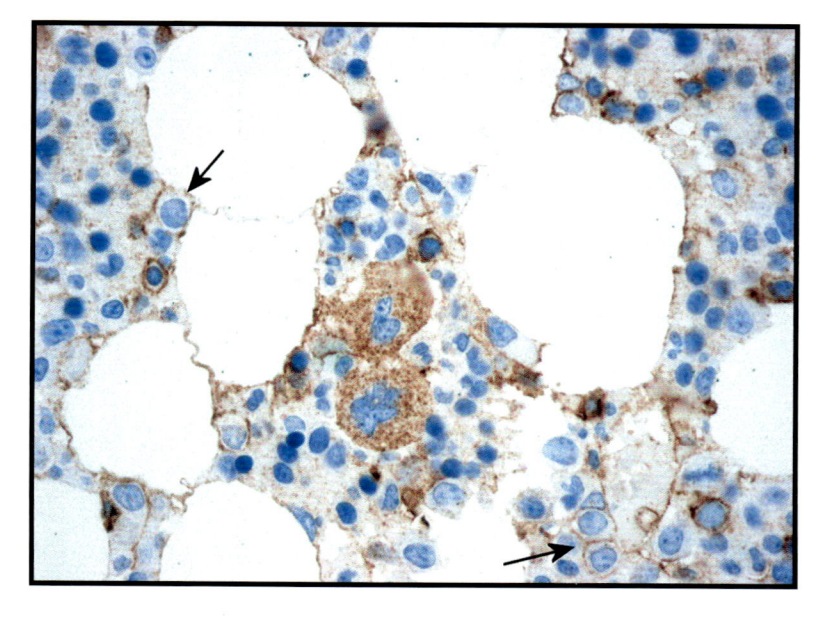

F3.30.8 CD99 in megakaryocytes (ADVANCE)

It is difficult to find any description of CD99 in megakaryocytes. However, as CD34 and CD99 are consistently coexpressed in the bone marrow and knowing that some megakaryocytes express CD34, it is likely that this image illustrates specific expression of the CD99 in megakaryocytes. Arrows point to maturing myeloid precursors, which show declining expression of CD99 as maturation progresses.

F3.30.9 CD99 is consistently negative in erythroid precursors and mature granulocytes (ADVANCE)

Even with very sensitive detection systems and optimized conditions, CD99 was found consistently negative in erythroid precursors (arrows) and more mature forms of neutrophils (dashed arrow). The strongest positivity is always seen in the most immature cells and intravascular monocytes. This figure illustrates difficulty in applying CD99 immunohistochemistry to screen for rare cells of metastatic Ewing sarcoma.

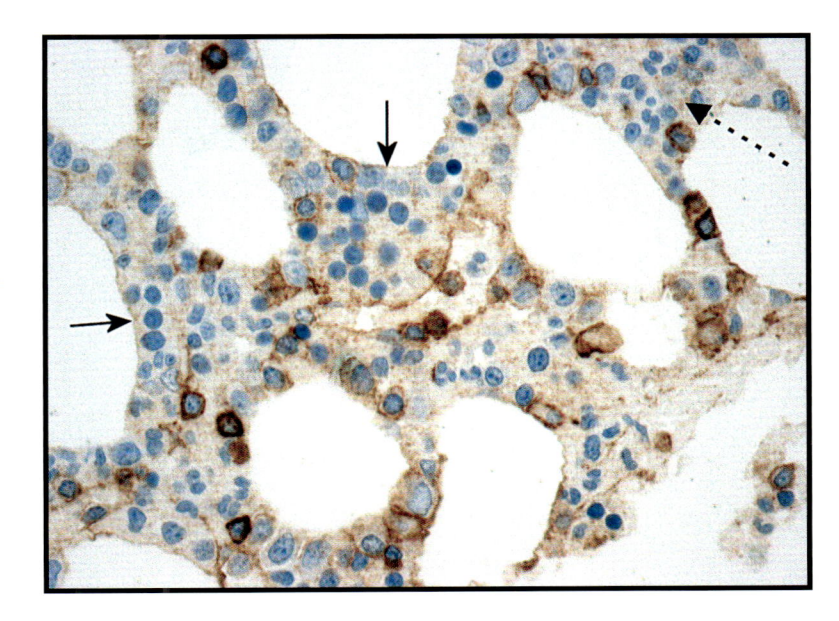

F3.30.10 CD99 in precursor T-cell acute lymphoblastic leukemia (T-ALL)

CD99 is very frequently and strongly expressed in precursor T-ALL. However, it lacks specificity. It is less often (about 25%) expressed in precursor B-cell ALL, but it appears regularly expressed early in B-cell development. In this case of precursor B-ALL, the CD99 antigen is clearly expressed.

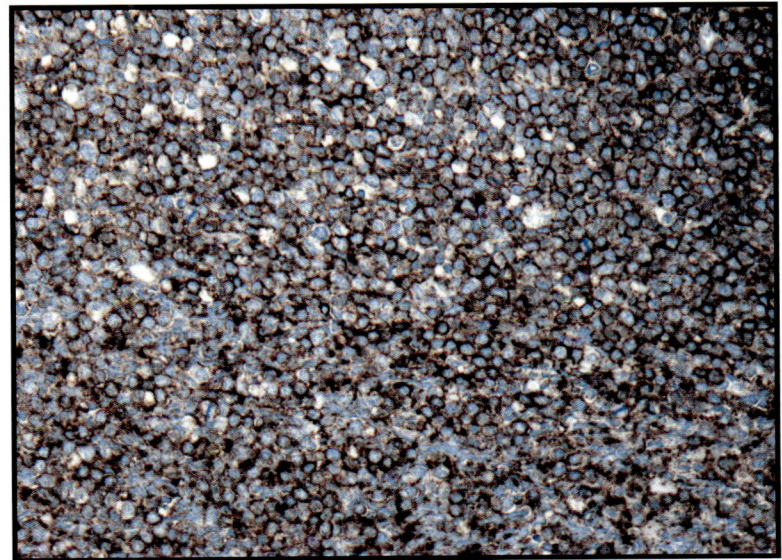

F3.30.11 CD99 is strongly expressed in stromal cells and also in large blastlike cells in postchemotherapy precursor B-cell acute lymphoblastic leukemia (ALL)

In addition to a weak CD99 expression in blastic cells of residual ALL cells, there is an unusually intense CD99 expression in large and numerous stromal cells. This illustration suggests that CD99 could be upregulated in stromal cells in bone marrow injury. However, no studies on this biological phenomenon have been published and its clinical significance, if any, is not known.

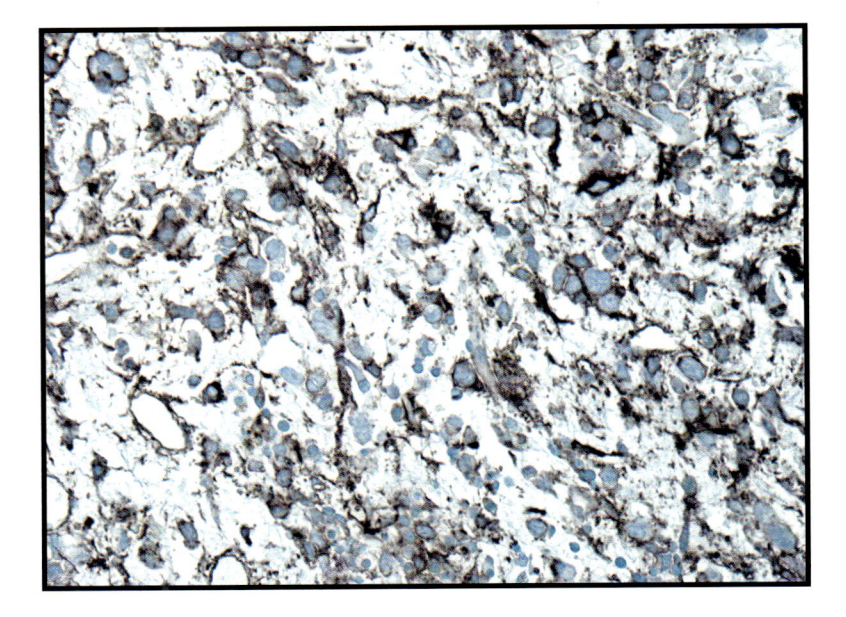

3.31 CD117

CD117 is also known as c-KIT or stem cell factor receptor (SCFR) (PROW). It is a tyrosine kinase receptor, which is mutated in systemic mastocytosis [Galli 1994; Nagata 1995]. In the BM, CD117 is expressed by approximately 70% of CD34+ cells in normal BM [Ashman 1991]. Benign mast cells in the BM and other tissues also express CD117 [Mayrhofer 1987]. As a myeloid marker, it is expressed in most myeloid leukemias, but its significance is highlighted because CD117 is expressed early in myeloid differentiation when other myeloid markers are not yet expressed. It is less expressed in more differentiated forms of AML, including only 75% of acute promyelocytic leukemias and in almost none of the promonocytic types (FAB M5b is generally negative) [Cascavilla 1998]. In erythroid leukemia, CD117 is usually negative [Nomdedéu 1999]. In contrast, in megakaryoblastic leukemia, CD117 appears to be expressed in most cases [Hans 2002]. However, the discrepancies between BM aspirate blast count and CD117+ and CD34+ blast count in 500 cells are significant and account for 60% of cases recently reported which had either higher blast count on IHC (19% cases) or lower blast count (about 40% cases) [Bataille 2007]. CD117 is also a marker of neoplastic/atypical plasma cells just like CD56 [Bataille 2006; Kraj 2004; Ocqueteau 1996; Dunphy 2007b]. However, CD117 and CD56 are not expressed in most cases of IgM myeloma [Feyler 2008].

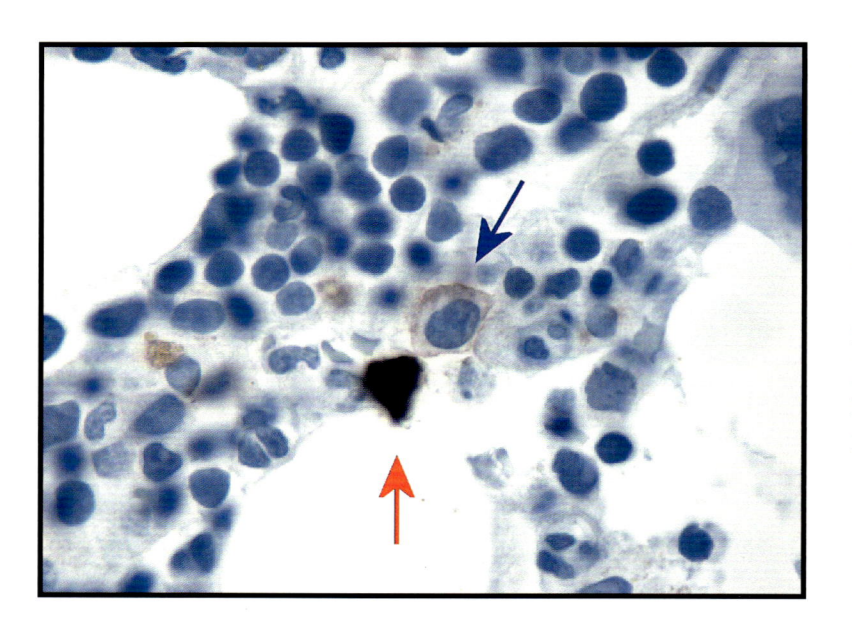

F3.31.1 CD117 in histologically normal bone marrow

It is likely that most myeloid blasts and possibly some promyelocytes can be detected using immunohistochemistry demonstrating weak membranous staining for CD117 (blue arrow). The optimization of the CD117 test should aim to convicingly detect the normal myeloid blast population. The detection of benign mast cells is not a sufficient endpoint since there is a great difference in CD117 expression in myeloid leukemia blasts and mast cell disorders, but both need to be identified with this test. Mast cells also express CD117 on the cellular membrane, but due to very high expression levels, the expression may appear to be present also in the cytoplasm (red arrow).

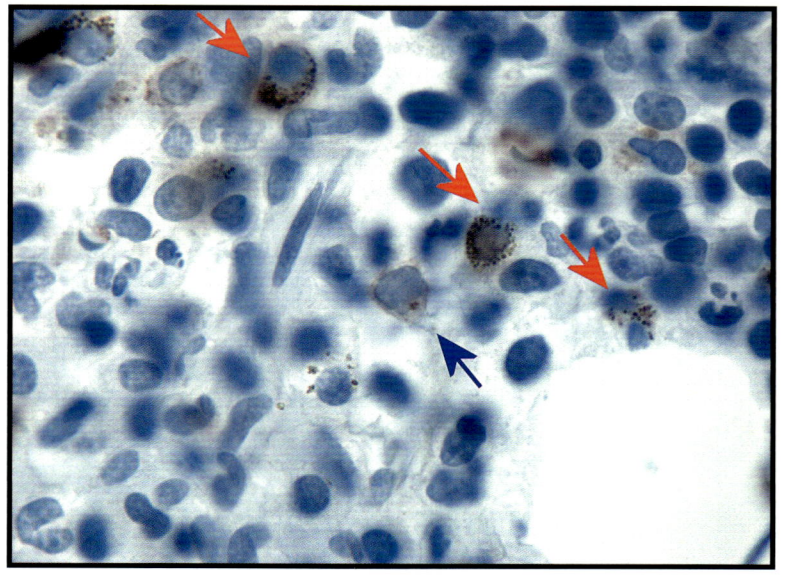

F3.31.2 CD117 in histologically normal bone marrow

Some cells show very weak expression of CD117, mainly as dotlike Golgi-type positivity (blue arrow). Note that many eosinophils and their precursors have cytoplasmic granulation that appears vaguely brown in immunohistochemistry slides (red arrows). This should be recognized and not interpreted as positive staining.

F3.31.3 CD117 in bone marrow with reactive changes

BM blasts, including normal CD117+ blasts, are not increased in BM biopsies with reactive changes. In this 2.5-cm long biopsy specimen, only a few plasma cells were found and only one CD117+ blast was detected (not shown).

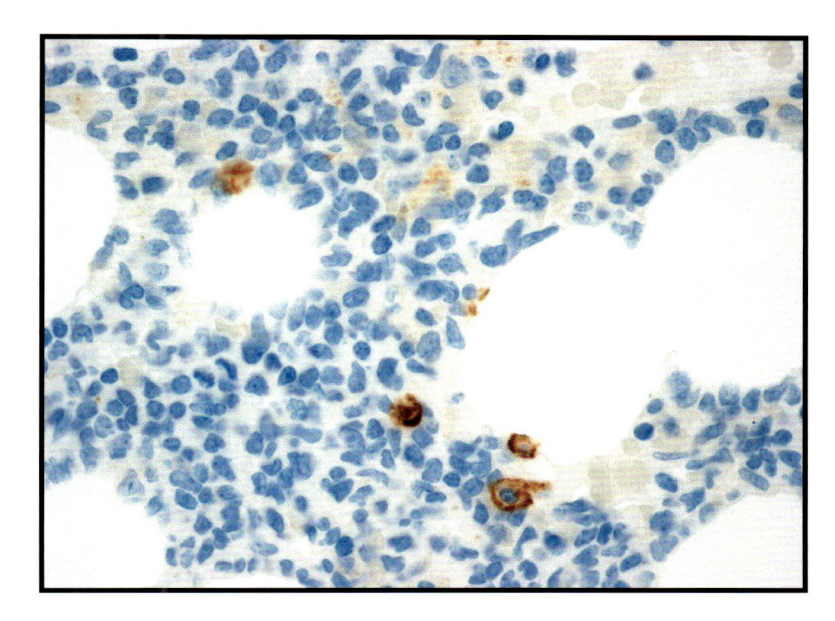

F3.31.4 CD117 in acute biphenotypic leukemia (acute myeloid leukemia/precursor B-cell lymphoblastic leukemia)

This specimen is from a 69-year-old man who presented with pancytopenia. There was no evidence of a Ph chromosome. Note that CD117 is detected as predominantly weak cytoplasmic and membrane expression, which is commonly seen in myeloid leukemias positive for CD117.

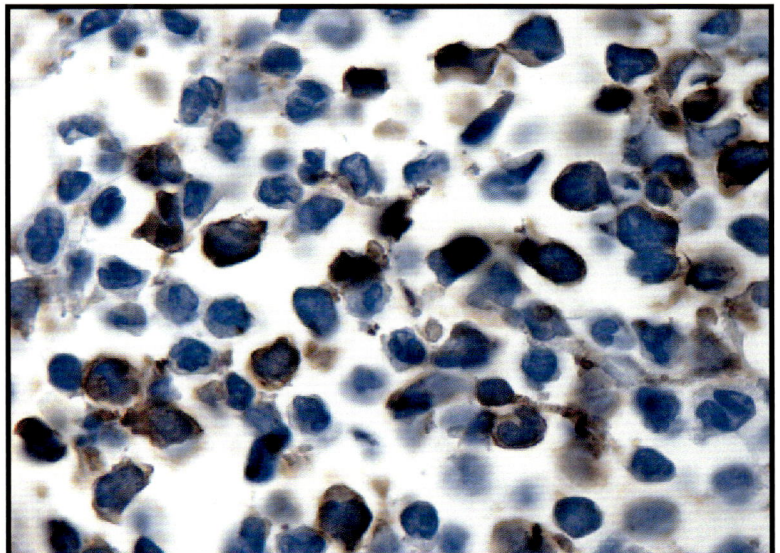

F3.31.5 CD117 in acute myeloid leukemia (AML), minimally differentiated

CD117 is a good marker of AML, minimally differentiated, without maturation, with maturation, promyelocytic leukemia, and also monoblastic and megakaryoblastic leukemias. Only acute erythroid leukemia and acute monocytic leukemia are typically negative.

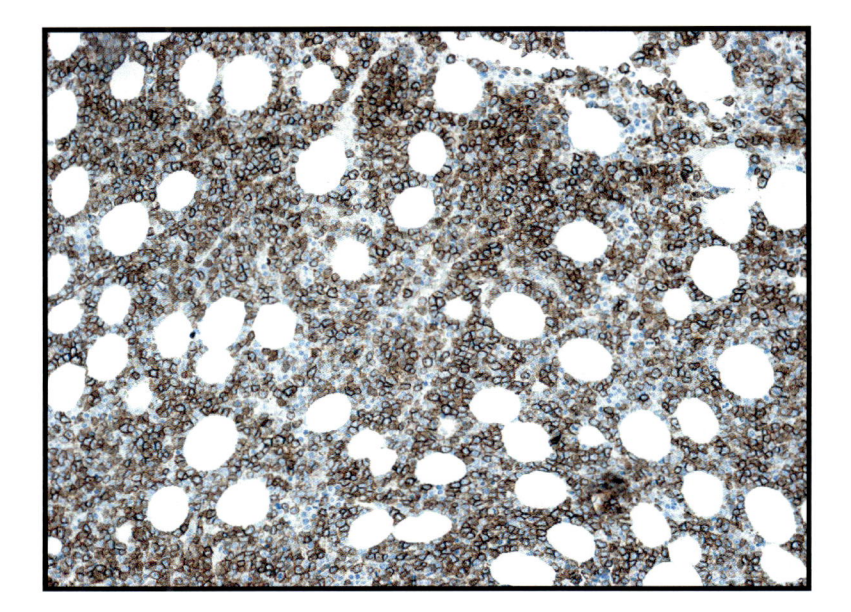

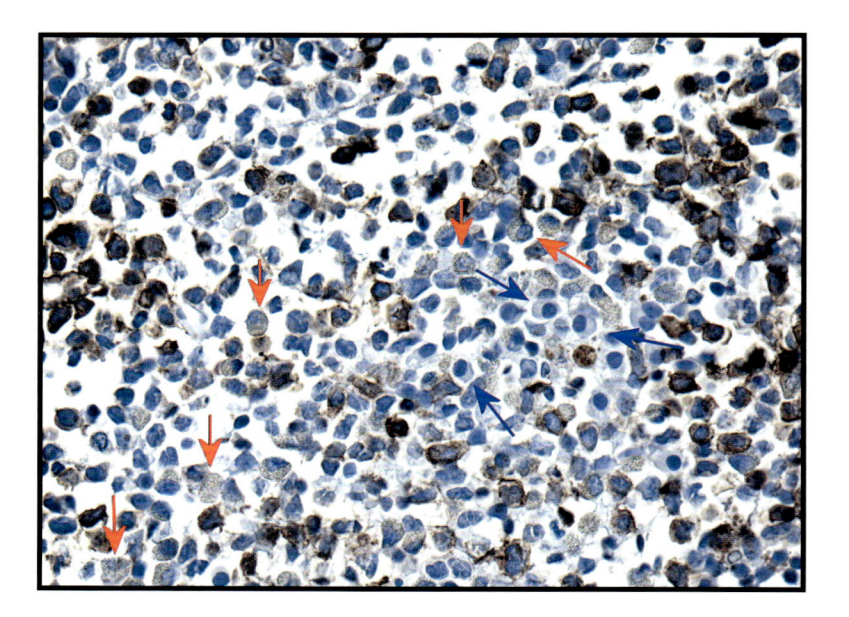

F3.31.6 CD117 in acute myeloid leukemia (AML) with maturation

In contrast to myeloperoxidase (MPO), CD117 is not expressed in eosinophils (red arrows) despite being a myeloid marker, because its expression is limited to the earliest stages of neutrophil maturation. This difference between MPO and CD117 is common in AML with maturation, but rarely seen in AML-M0 or AML-M1. In this field some plasma cells are also negative (blue arrows).

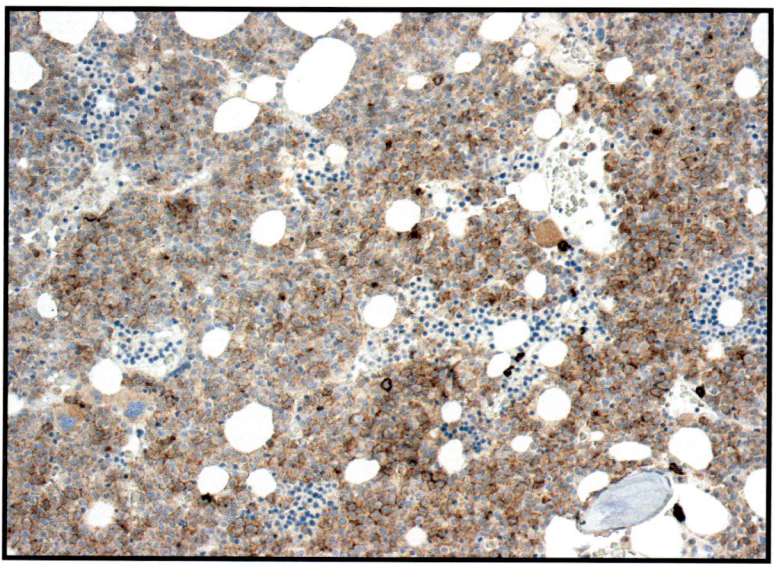

F3.31.7 CD117 in acute promyelocytic leukemia (APL)

CD117 is expressed in most myeloid leukemias including promyelocytic subtype (about 70% cases). In this case of APL, the CD117 antigen was expressed at lower levels than in usual undifferentiatiated myeloid leukemias or those with minimal myeloid maturation. The expression was weak cytoplasmic and moderate membranous.

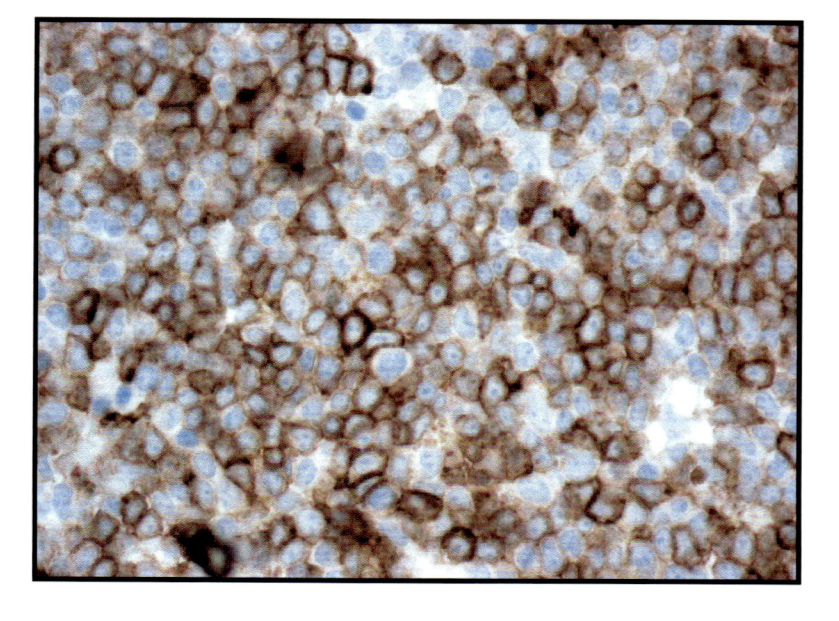

F3.31.8 CD117 in acute myelomonoblastc leukemia

In this case of acute myelomonoblastic leukemia, the blast cells in both the monocytic and neutrophil lineages express CD117. Despite the 2 different cell lines of differentiation, both were found to express CD117. Acute monoblastic leukemias are also readily positive, but CD117 is rarely expressed in acute monocytic leukemia.

F3.31.9 CD117 in acute erythroid leukemia

Only mast cells are positive (strongly) for CD117. None of the potential blasts expressed CD117. Therefore, in this erythroid leukemia, CD117 was negative. This was confirmed with flow cytometric analysis.

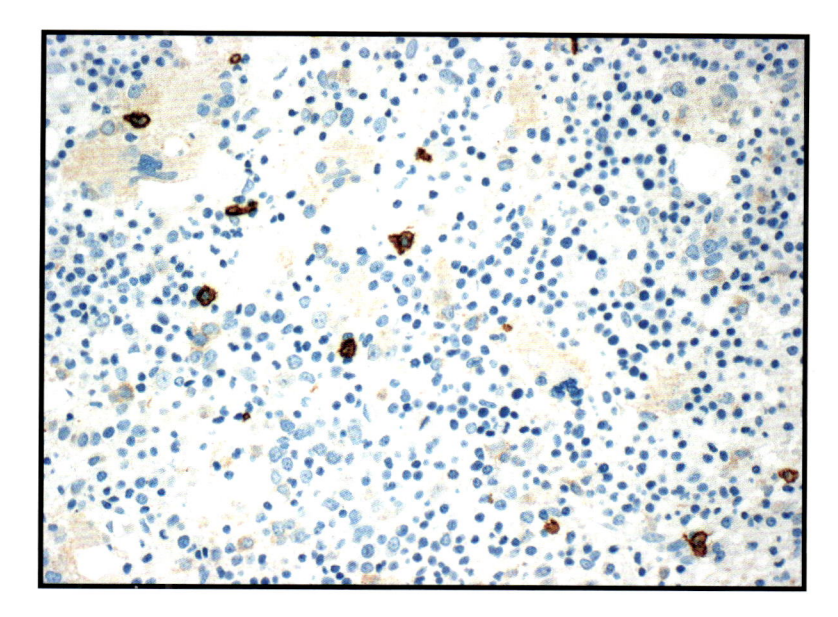

F3.31.10 CD117 in acute erythroid/myeloid leukemia

This biopsy specimen is from a 68-year-old woman with pancytopenia. High magnification reveals a large number of blasts that are positive for CD117. In weakly positive or "negative" cases, it is critical to evaluate the cells under high magnification (at least at 200× magnification). When evaluating many target antigens, "weak," "focal," and/or "dotlike only" forms of expression are critical to note for correct interpretation of the results.

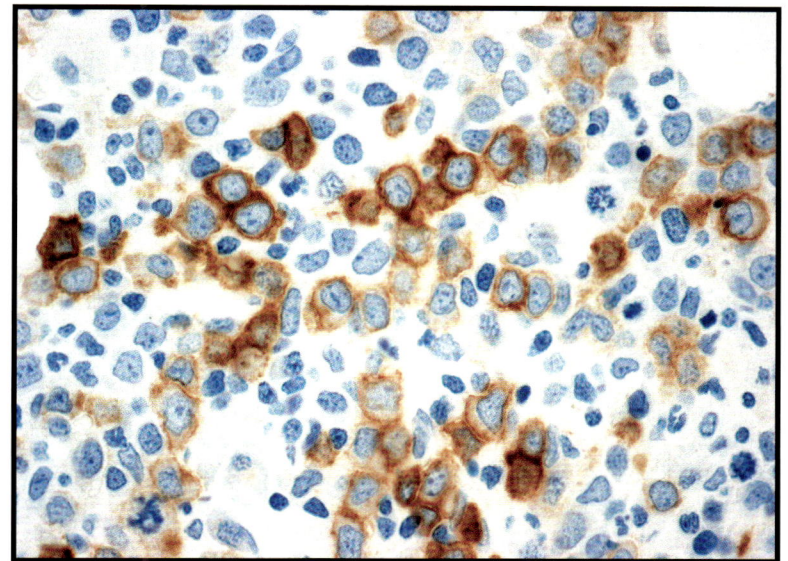

F3.31.11 CD117 in chronic myeloid leukemia (CML) blast crisis

This specimen is from a patient with a 2-year history of CML. Blastic transformation resulted in 80% von Willebrand factor+ and CD61+ blasts with only partial (about 45%), but definite expression of CD117, which is illustrated here. Most of the megakaryoblastic leukemias express CD117. Blasts in acute myelofibrosis also express CD117.

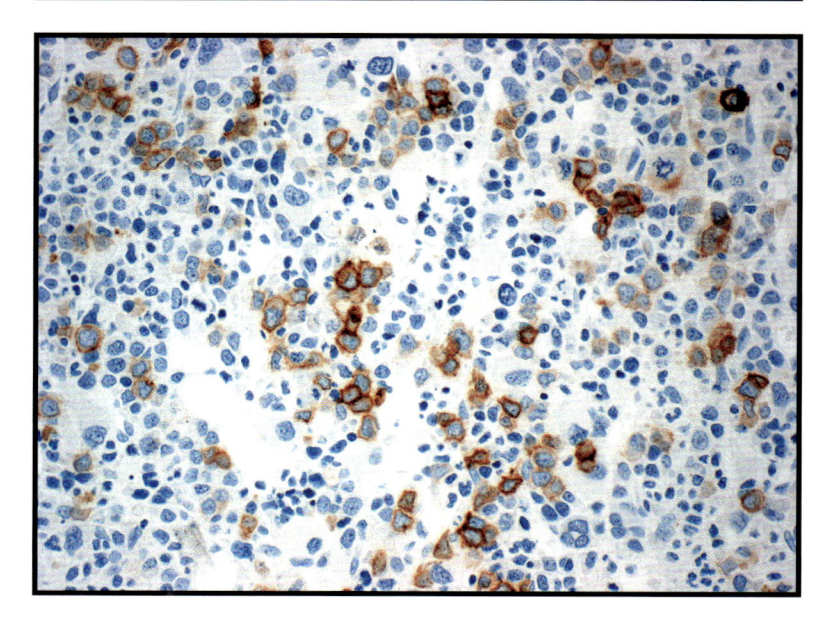

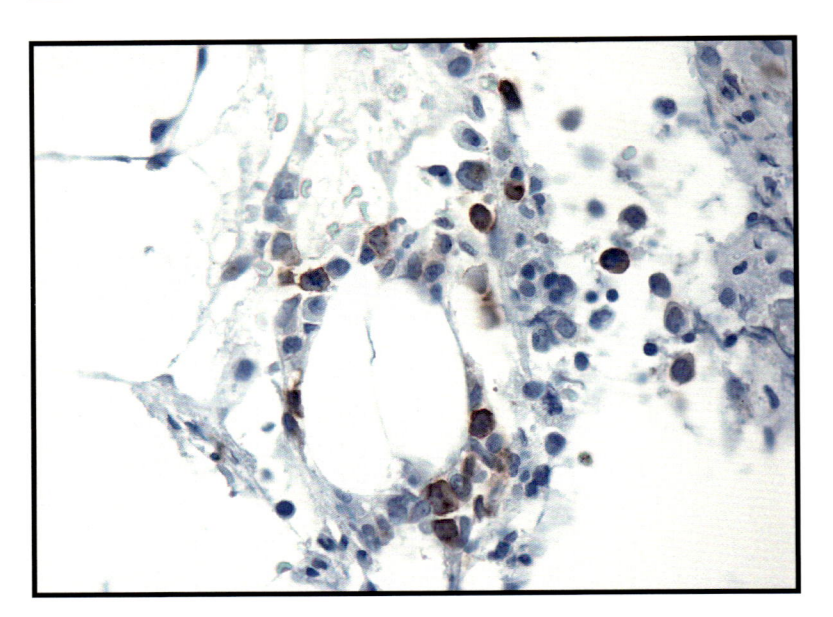

F3.31.12 CD117 in hypocellular acute myeloid leukemia

The blast population may be difficult to demonstrate with immunohistochemistry or flow cytometry in hypocellular acute leukemia. In this specimen, CD34 staining highlighted about 30% of cells. Because of the weak CD117 expression, the blasts are difficult to identify. Therefore, high magnification is often necessary to evaluate CD117 immunostaining.

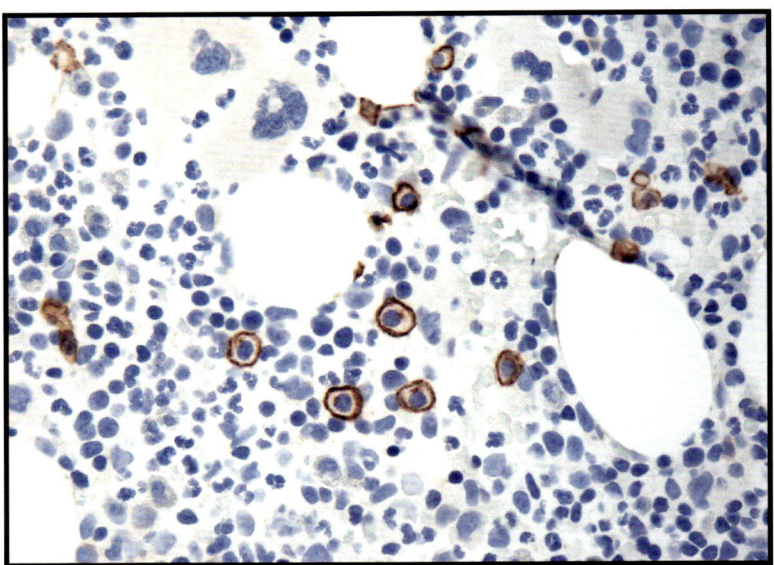

F3.31.13 CD117 in indolent systemic mastocytosis (ISM; slide courtesy of P Horny, MD, Institute of Pathology, Ansbach, Germany)

There is a good demonstration of membranous CD117 in mast cells. Cytoplasmic expression is not present. The variation of detection of membranous expression of CD117 in mast cells and in myeloid blasts may also partly depend on various technical parameters and therefore will vary among laboratories.

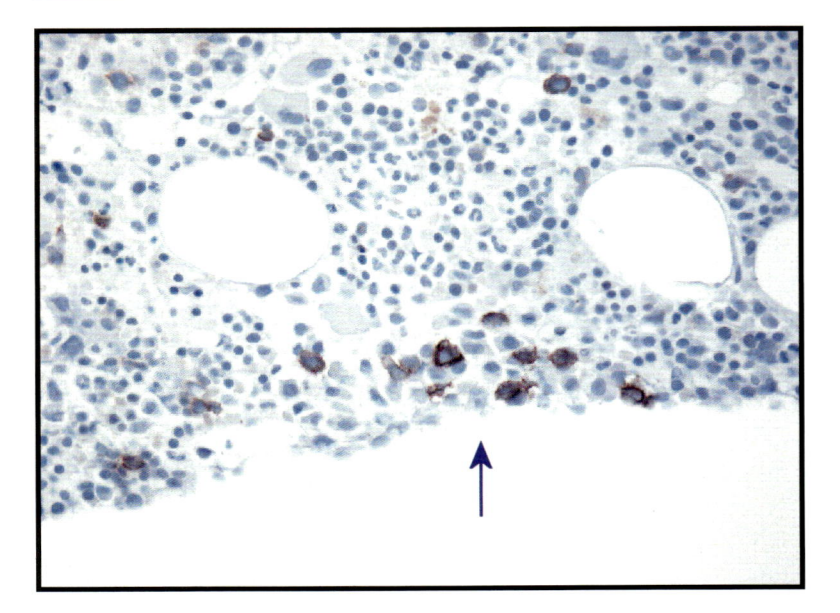

F3.31.14 CD117 after chemotherapy

In this patient with acute myeloid leukemia and CD34+/CD117+ blasts seen on flow cytometry, only ill-defined small clusters of variably CD34−/CD117+ cells were identified after induction chemotherapy in a paratrabecular position. This may be consistent with myeloid reconstitution and should not be interpreted as evidence of focal residual leukemic blasts. At the time of this writing, one year later, the patient remains well with no evidence of leukemia.

3.31   CD117

F3.31.15 CD117 in myeloproliferative disease

This biopsy specimen is from a patient with clinical evidence of polycythemia vera. The bone marrow was hypercellular and loose aggregates of megakaryocytes were noted. CD117+ cells were increased and present in ill-defined clusters. The significance of this finding remains unclear because the patient was well without aggressive chemotherapy 4 years later. The CD34 cell count was not increased. Some of the CD117+ cells could be early erythroid precursors.

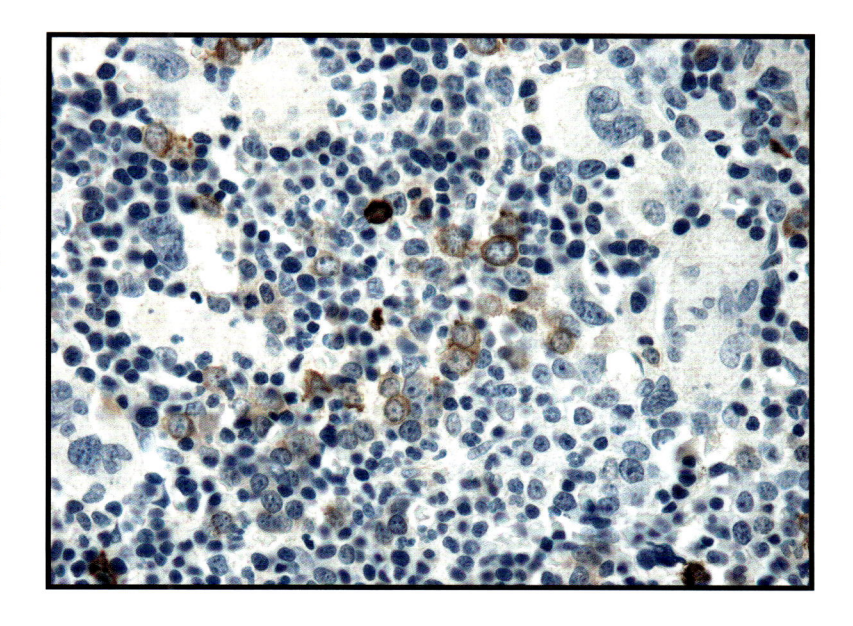

3.32 CD123

CD123 is an interleukin 3 receptor, α (low affinity) also known as IL3RA (OMIM). It is a regulatory glycoprotein and supports survival, proliferation, and development of progenitor cells [Dzionek 2000]. IHC applications are used mainly to demonstrate plasmacytoid dendritic cells [Sorg 1999]. However, it is widely expressed by myeloid leukemias, precursor B-lymphoblastic leukemia, and regularly in hairy cell leukemia. It can also be detected in other mature B-cell lymphoproliferative diseases [Muñoz 2001; Riccioni 2004]. The presence of CD123+ small interstitial nodules in the BM reinforces the diagnosis of CMML, because these are not found in other myeloproliferative diseases [Orazi 2006].

F3.32.1 CD123 in histologically normal bone marrow

This specimen is from a 17-year-old girl with newly diagnosed classical Hodgkin lymphoma. The BM was not involved and only showed mild reactive changes. CD123 was identified in very rare and very small ill-defined clusters of mononuclear cells with high nuclear-cytoplasmic ratio. These are compatible with plasmacytoid dendritic cells. The small nodules of plasmacytoid dendritic cells are more typical of chronic myelomonocytic leukemia [Muñoz 2001], but can also be observed in other conditions including reactive BM.

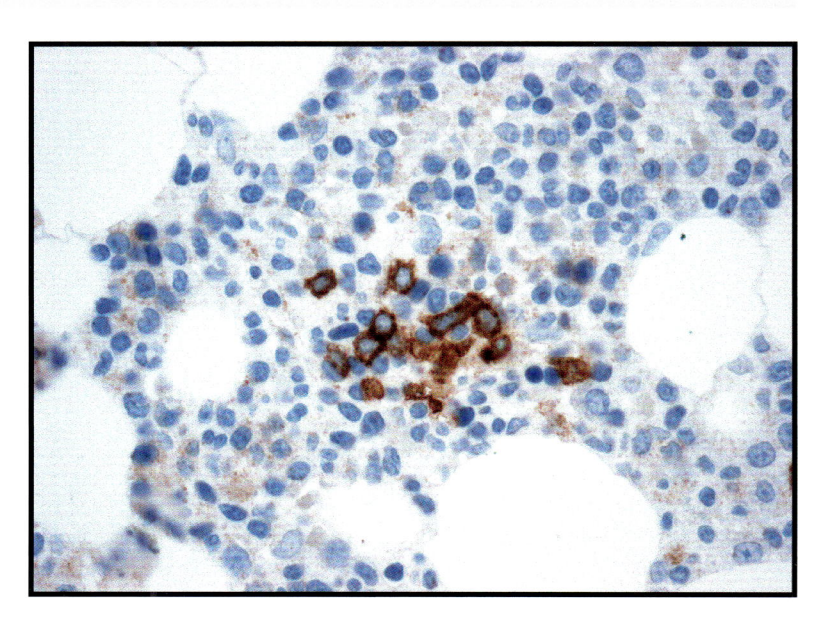

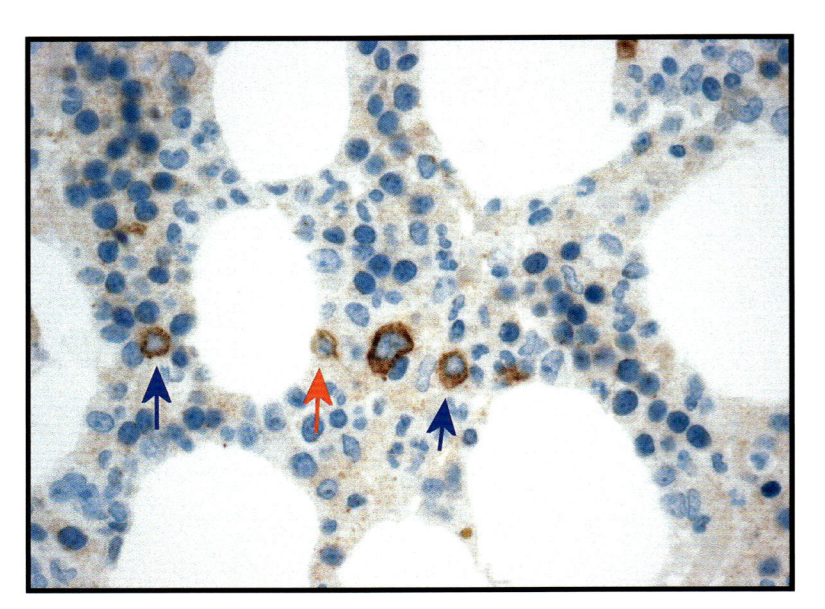

F3.32.2 CD123 in histologically normal bone marrow

The same specimen as seen in **F3.32.1**. Four cells show CD123 expression in this area. Of note, the size and nuclear features vary somewhat from cell to cell. Blue arrows point to cells with what appears to be cytoplasmic expression and the red arrow shows a cell with possible membranous expression. The largest cell (center) has both cytoplasmic and membranous reactivity.

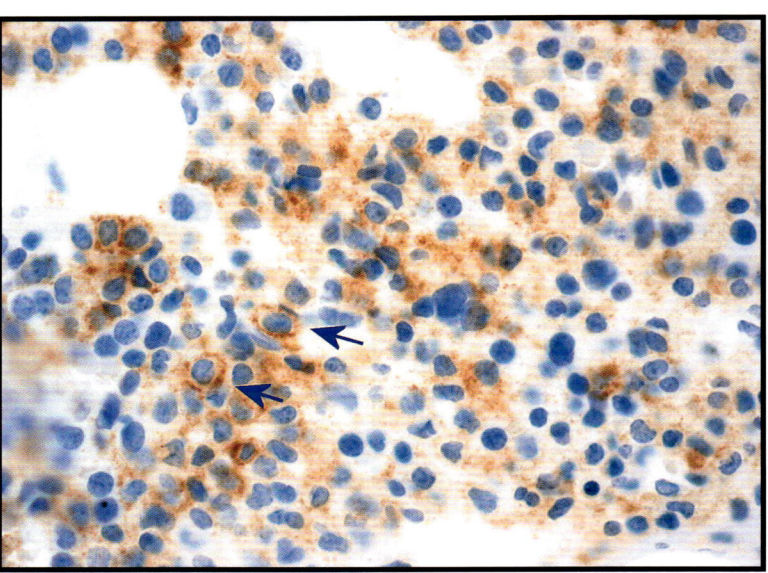

F3.32.3 CD123 in hairy cell leukemia (HCL)

This biopsy specimen is from a 62-year-old man with pancytopenia, splenomegaly, and dry tap at bone marrow aspiration. Flow cytometric analysis revealed usual hairy cell leukemia immunophenotype. Peripheral blood smear showed occasional typical hairy cells. CD123 is variably expressed in this case of HCL, and hairy cellular borders are causing irregular appearance of this membranous positivity (arrows).

3.33 CD138

CD138 is a heparin sulfate proteoglycan also known as syndecan-1 (OMIM). During development, syndecan-1 is expressed in epithelial and mesenchymal cells, but in adult tissues its expression is predominantly localized to the epithelium [O'Connell 2004]. In mature epithelial tissues, syndecan-1 facilitates the interactions of epithelial cells with the extracellular matrix and modulates growth factor responses [Carey 1997]. Therefore, the CD138 can be detected in various metastatic carcinomas in the BM. In the hematolymphoid system, CD138 expression is present only when and where B lymphocytes associate with extracellular matrix, namely as B-cell precursors in BM and as immobilized plasma cells in interstitial matrices. Expression is lost immediately before maturation and release of B lymphocytes into the circulation, and is absent on circulating and mature peripheral B lymphocytes [Sanderson 1989]. In normal BM, only a small number of CD138+ plasma cells is present. CD138 is considered the best marker of plasma cells and is widely used in the BM evaluation for multiple myeloma [Joshi 2007; Dunphy 2007a]. CD138 is also expressed variably in LPL, DLBCL including plasmablastic lymphoma, and DLBCL with secretory differentiation [Sebestyén 1999]. Angioimmunoblastic T-cell lymphoma is a condition that causes a significant increase in the number/percentage of plasma cells in the BM (as high as >50%), does not represent a primary plasma cell disorder, and is not a primary B-cell disorder [Grogg 2007]. The plasma cells in this disorder will be polyclonal. Similarly, we have seen a case of AML, which in relapse, showed 80% cellularity of the BM with at least 50% of plasma cells being polytypic and polyclonal. Therefore, the WHO criteria for the diagnosis of myeloma should be strictly adhered to [Jaffe 2001]. CD138 was also described in benign and malignant myeloid cells [Seftalioglu 2003a; Seftalioglu 2003b]. Reactive plasma cells are frequently seen in a perivascular distribution. This is a nonspecific feature, but it is stated to favor the diagnosis of secondary erythrocytosis rather than polycythemia vera [Kass 2001; Kreft 2007; Thiele 2005].

3.33   CD138

F3.33.1 CD138 in bone marrow with no pathologic features

The biopsy specimen was obtained from a 38-year-old woman with history of acute myeloid leukemia whose disease is now in remission 24 months after chemotherapy. There is a slight tendency of CD138+ plasma cells to group in a perivascular location or to be associated with adipocytes.

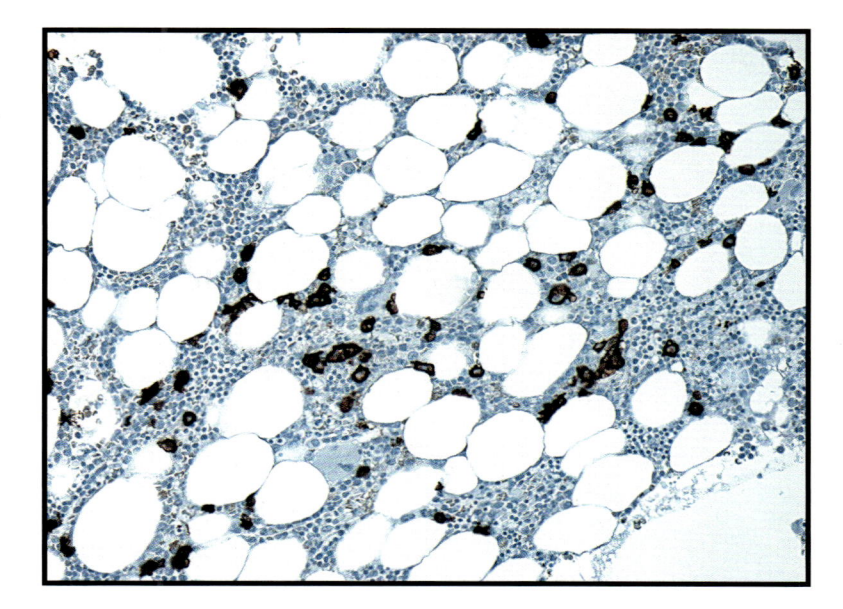

F3.33.2 CD138 highlighting reactive plasma cells

The bone marrow biopsy specimen is from a 56-year-old woman with a history of acute myeloid leukemia. The BM is hypercellular, but there was no evidence of leukemic cells. This image illustrates almost exclusive perivascular arrangement of reactive plasma cells. This is a common phenomenon, but in itself does not exclude plasma cell neoplasia.

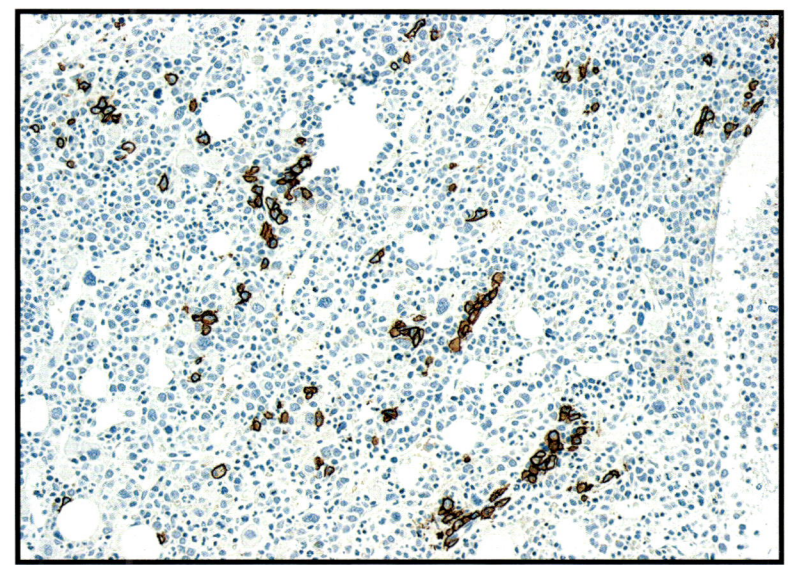

F3.33.3 CD138 in perivascular distribution in IgA myeloma

Perivascular distribution is usually seen in reactive plasmacytosis, but in itself does not have diagnostic value because the perivascular distribution can also be seen in plasma cell malignancies as seen in this case of IgA myeloma. All perivascular plasma cells expressed IgA-κ.

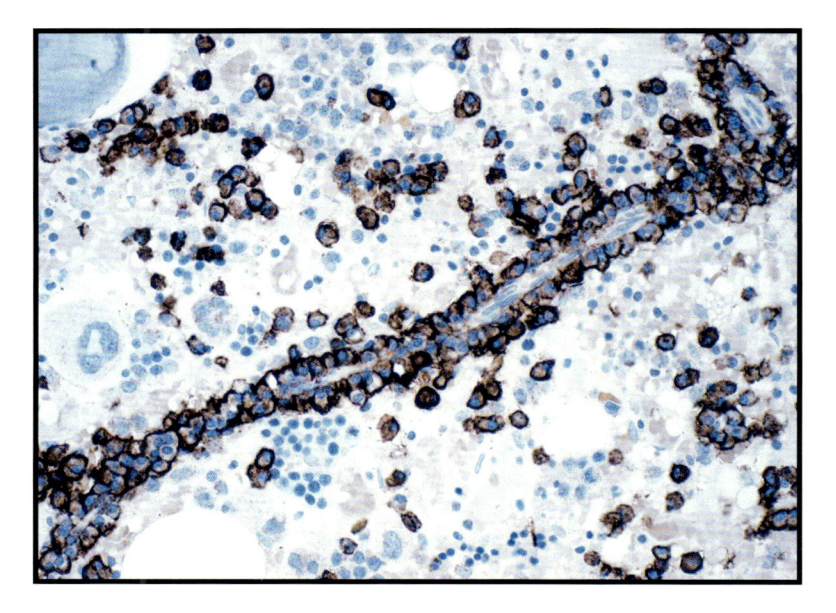

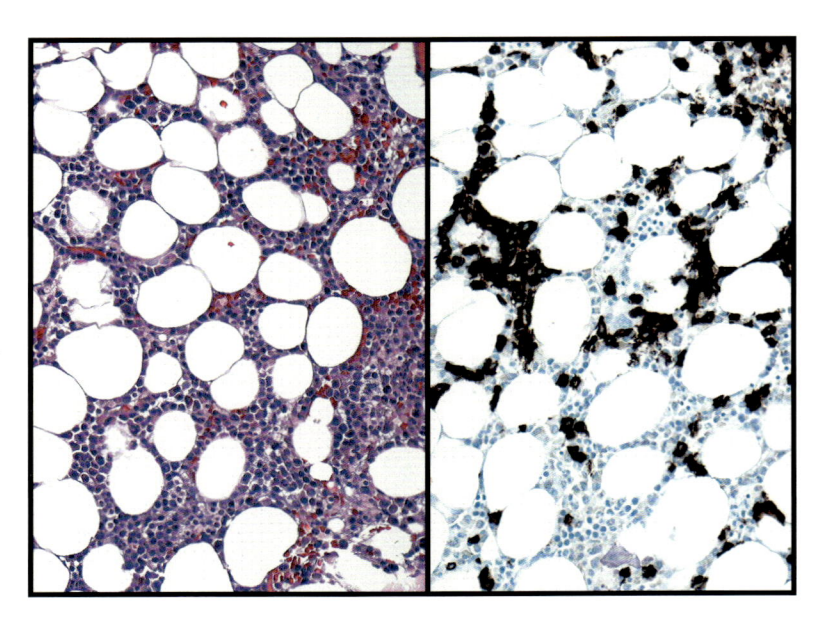

F3.33.4 CD138 in multiple myeloma (MM)

This specimen illustrates interstitial type of bone marrow involvement by MM. Morphologic analysis alone is not always sufficient (left) to accurately determine the extent of BM involvement. Malignant plasma cells may be confused with maturing myeloid cells; in this case higher magnification revealed extensive interstitial involvement. Immunostaining for CD138 clearly determined the extent of BM involvement.

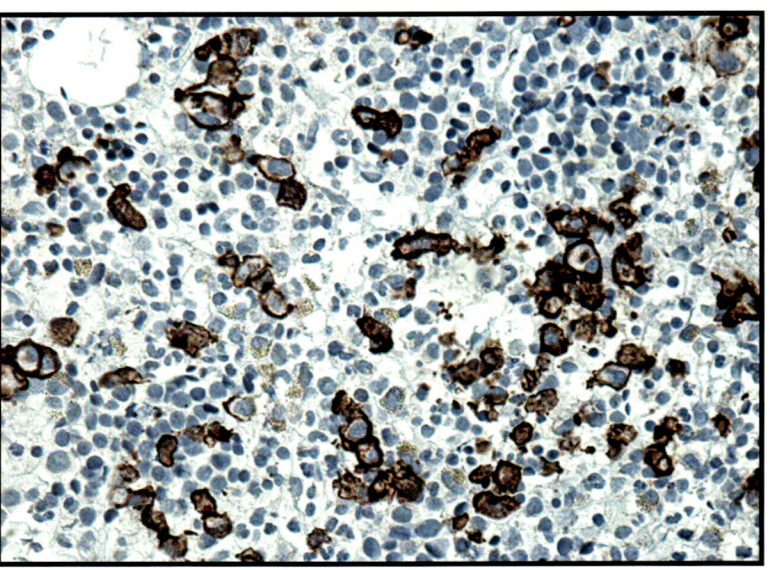

F3.33.5 CD138 in multiple myeloma

The quantitative analysis of the bone marrow tumor burden is much more accurate when myeloma cells are stained by anti-CD138 antibody. This is particularly relevant when plasma cells are difficult to recognize morphologically, as in this specimen where they do not form solid sheets and the nuclear morphology is nonspecific. The CD138 expression is generally membranous, but some Golgi-type and focal cytoplasmic positivity are frequent.

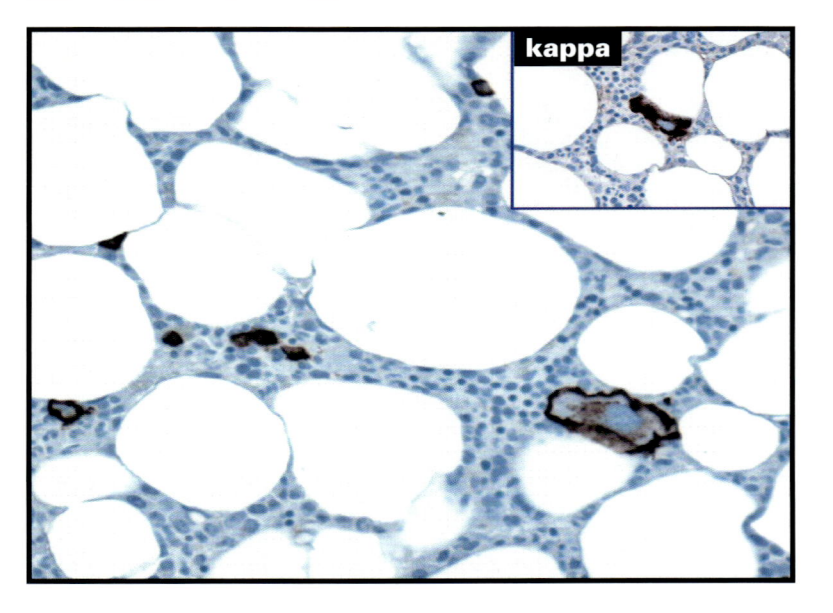

F3.33.6 CD138 in multiple myeloma

This bone marrow biopsy specimen is from a patient with multiple myeloma after chemotherapy. The number of positive cells is very small, but the positive cells are gigantic, with clearly atypical nuclei and monotypic Ig light chain κ expression indicating residual tumor cells. Smaller positive cells may represent either normal plasma cells or smaller myeloma cells.

F3.33.7 CD138 in bone marrow with diffuse involvement by multiple myeloma

This biopsy specimen was from a 47-year-old man with diffuse involvement of the BM at presentation. CD138 immunostaining is usually not contributory in such cases, but may be necessary if malignant plasma cells have anaplastic morphologic features to confirm their plasma cell phenotype.

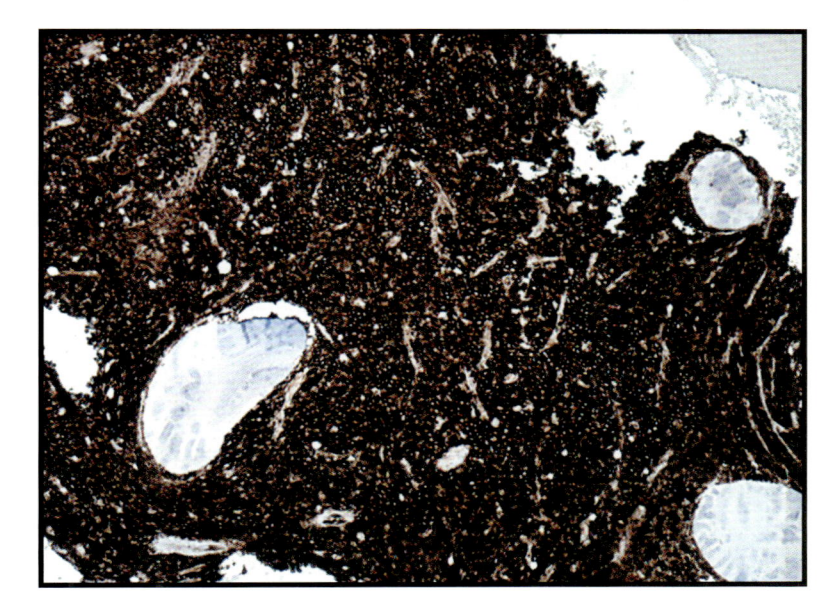

F3.33.8 CD138/MUM-1 double staining in multiple myeloma

Myeloma cells express both CD138 and MUM1 as shown here with brown staining of the cytoplasmic membrane (CD138) and of the nuclei (MUM1). An antibody cocktail was used. Myeloid precursors are not staining.

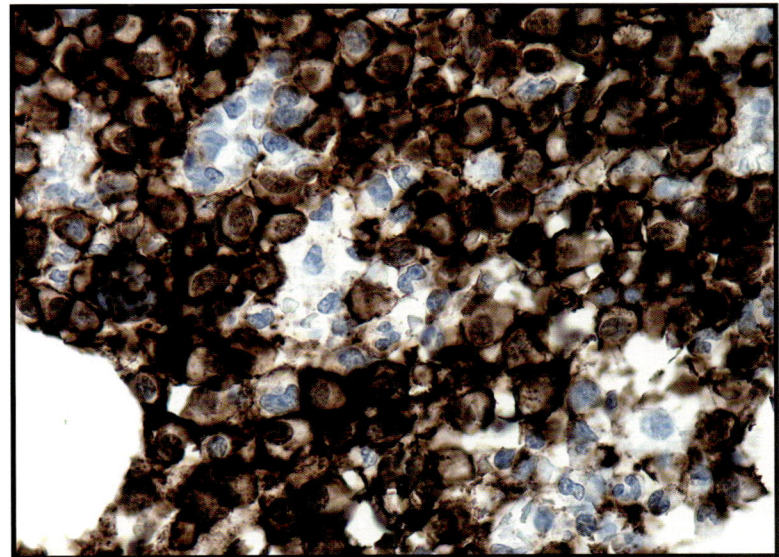

F3.33.9 CD138 variable expression in multiple myeloma (MM)

CD138 antigen is not always strongly and/or diffusely expressed in MM even though it is currently viewed as the best marker for the demonstration of plasma cells. This biopsy specimen from a 56-year-old man was obtained at presentation and therefore the variable level of CD138 expression does not represent therapy-associated phenomenon.

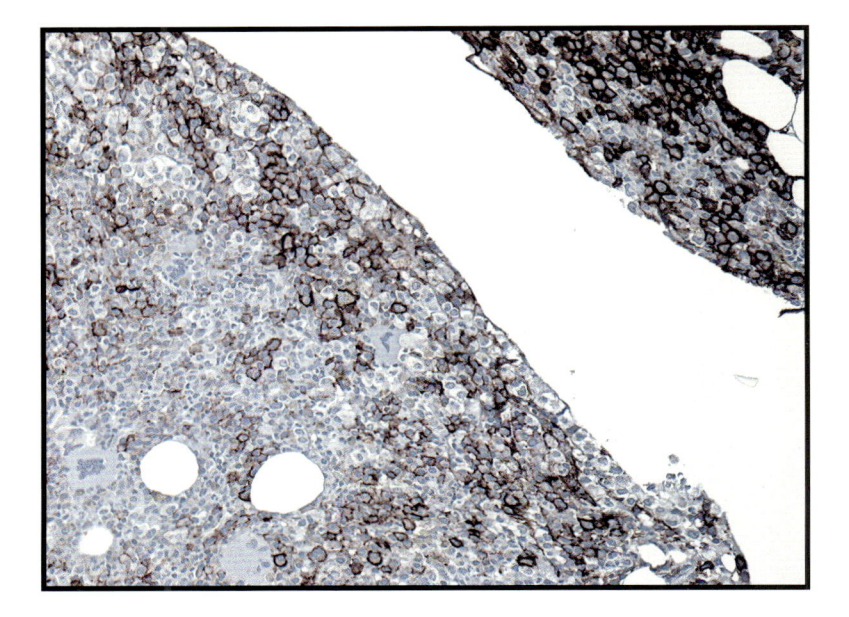

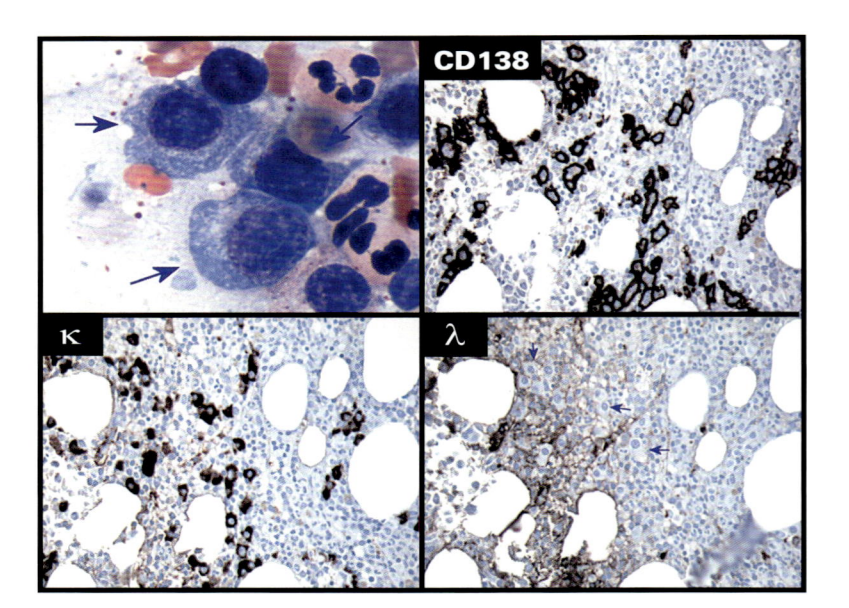

F3.33.10 CD138 demonstrating borderline increase in plasma cells

This biopsy specimen is from a 55-year-old man after stem cell transplantation for myeloma. Plasma cells comprise approximately 10% of the cellularity in this core section and about 7% in the aspirate smears. The tumor cells can be identified with confidence by using morphology (plasma cells with macronucleoli), CD138 to estimate the total tumor volume. Monoclonality is supported by demonstrating light chain restriction (κ in this example).

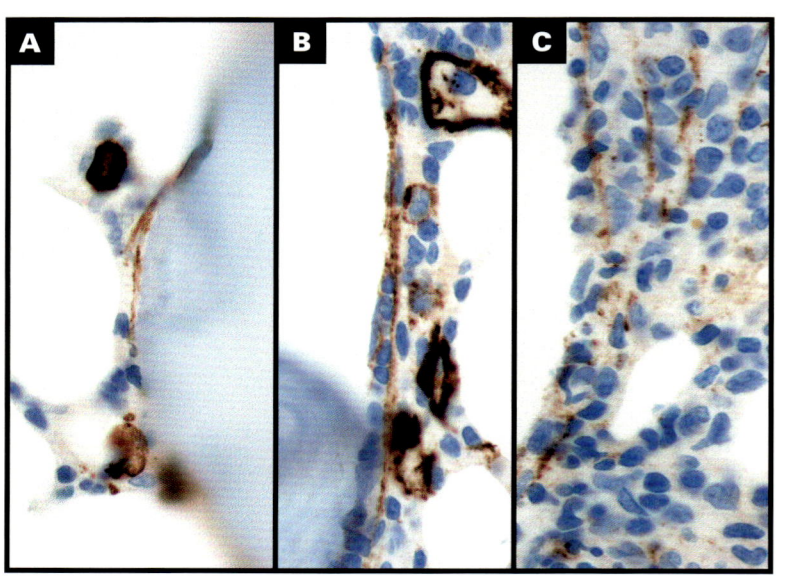

F3.33.11 Stromal expression of CD138

Single layer of paratrabecular linear positivity in (presumably) fibrocytes close to the bony trabeculae **A, B**, while parallel layers of similar cells are present in a patient with acute myeloid leukemia **C**. The biology or potential pathophysiological significance of these CD138+ stromal cells is not known. It appears to be similar to the induced CD138 in breast and head and neck carcinoma stroma, rather than shedding of CD138 in fibrotic areas of multiple myeloma [O'Connell 2004; Bayer-Garner 2001].

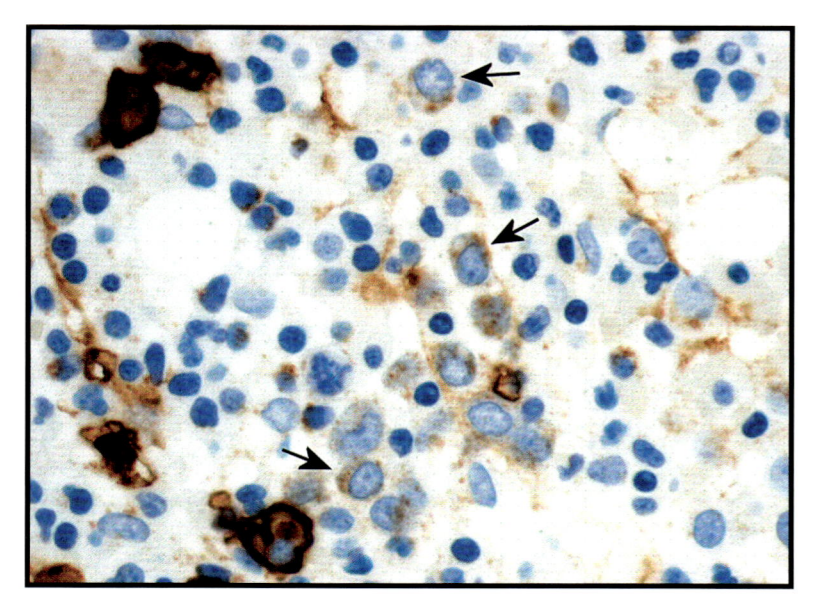

F3.33.12 CD138 weak expression in blasts

This patient has acute erythroid/myeloid leukemia. In addition to occasional strongly stained plasma cells, a weak cytoplasmic expression of CD138 was noted in blastic appearing cells. CD138 is known to be expressed in pre-B cells and also in normal and neoplastic myeloblasts.

F3.33.13 CD138 in reactive cells in CLL

This hypercellular biopsy specimen was from a 67-year-old man who also had well-characterized chronic myelomonocytic leukemia. Chronic lymphocytic leukemia lymphocytes showed no evidence of CD138 expression, but many neoplastic lymphoid aggregates were surrounded with a polytypic plasma cell population as demonstrated by a κ/λ ratio of 4:1 (not shown).

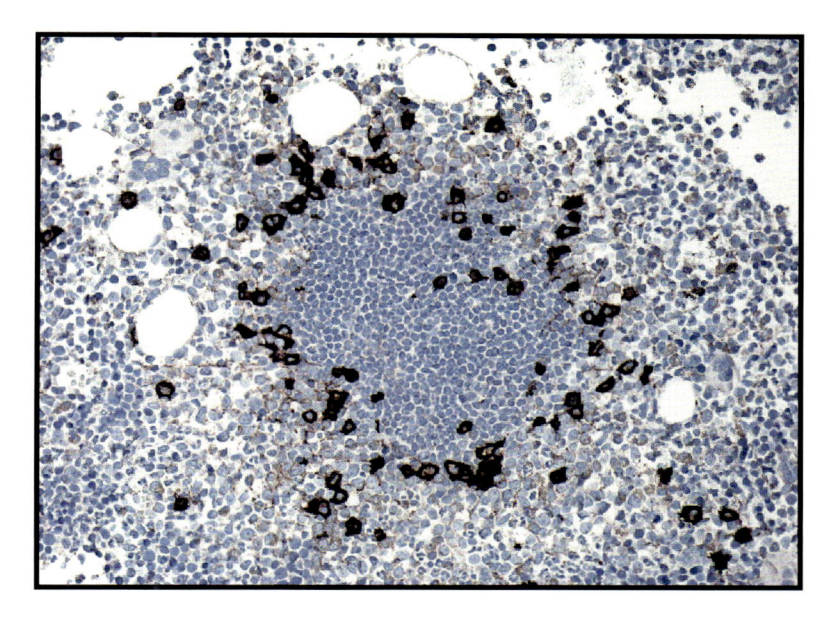

F3.33.14 CD138 in marginal zone or lymphoplasmacytic lymphoma

This biopsy specimen is from a 54-year-old woman with a history of a diffuse large B-cell lymphoma. Current biopsy was performed for restaging after chemotherapy. The plasma cells are present in perivascular lymphoplasmacytic aggregates and are surrounded with CD20−/+, CD79a+++, CD3− small lymphocytes. Despite unremarkable plasma cell morphology and perivascular distribution, they were monotypic as demonstrated by a very high κ/λ ratio (>30, not shown). Serum IgM paraprotein was 15 g/L.

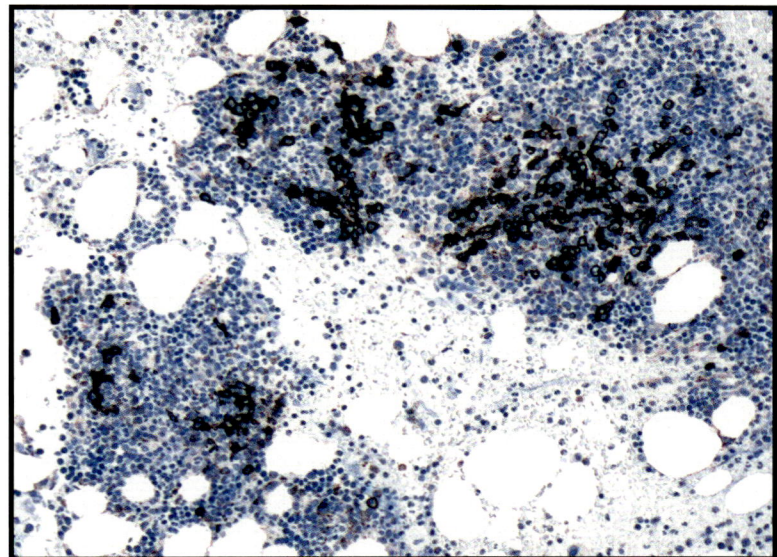

F3.33.15 CD138 in lymphoplasmacytic lymphoma

Multiple lymphoid aggregates are present in this specimen and have a cuff of plasma cells and plasmacytoid lymphocytes. Note variable CD138 expression. This variation probably reflects various stages in terminal B-cell maturation. These cells also expressed IgM-κ. Serum IgM paraprotein was 37 g/L.

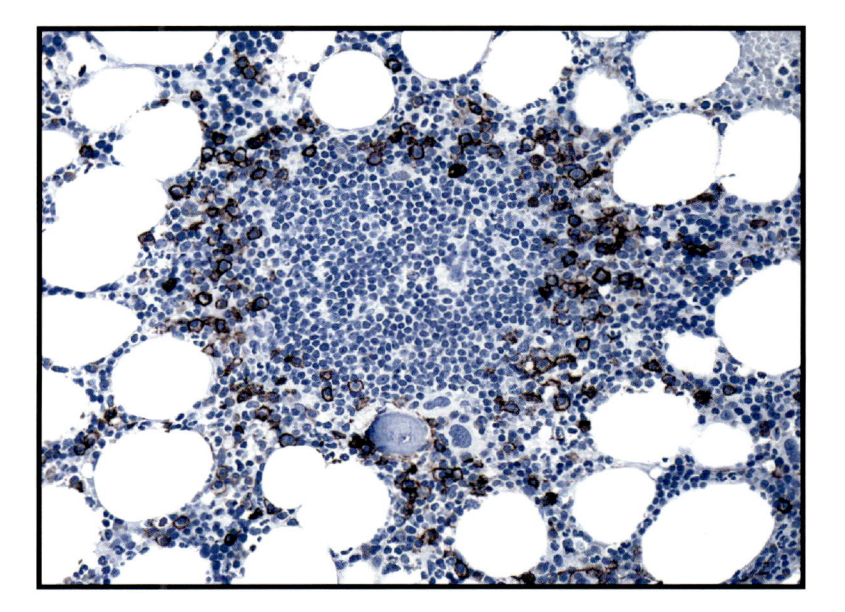

3.34 CD235a (Glycophorin A)

Glycophorins A (GYPA) and B (GYPB) are 2 major sialoglycoproteins present on human erythrocyte membrane (OMIM). They bear the antigenic determinants for the MN and Ss blood groups. Glycophorins are also receptors for erythrocyte invasion by the malarial parasite *Plasmodium falciparum* [Baum 2002]. Glycophorin A is a red blood cell marker. It is frequently used in flow cytometric applications and IHC and therefore it is one of the more important markers for BM pathology [Ngo 2008; Dunphy 2007b; McCloskey 2004; Sadahira 2001; Chang 2000; Sadahira 1999; Pileri 1999; Oertel 1996; Wilkins 1994; Thiele 1993; Tupitsyn 1989; van der Valk 1989; Mullink 1985]. It is generally considered to be a very good marker because its expression is limited to red blood cells. Even though it is a good quality primary Ab and has a high specificity, glycophorin A is not a perfect marker of erythroid differentiation. Its sensitivity is lower than specificity and it is a poor marker of the early stages of normal erythroid maturation. It can also be absent in some cases of erythroid leukemia. However, non-nucleated red blood cells are strongly stained, which may interefere with interpretation of the results, in particular in the estimation of the myeloid-erythroid ratio. For best practice, both glycophorin A and hemoglobin A are recommended for diagnostic BM IHC. However, in contrast to glycophorin A (clone JC 159), glycophorin C (clone Ret49f) and spectrin may be superior for demonstration of early erythroid cells and probably even more useful than hemoglobin A [Ngo 2008; Sadahira 1999]. Glycophorin C is illustrated in **F2.2**. Immunohistochemical staining for spectrin shows cytoplasmic staining in early erythroid precursors, while in later stages membranous pattern is detected (not shown) [Sadahira 1999].

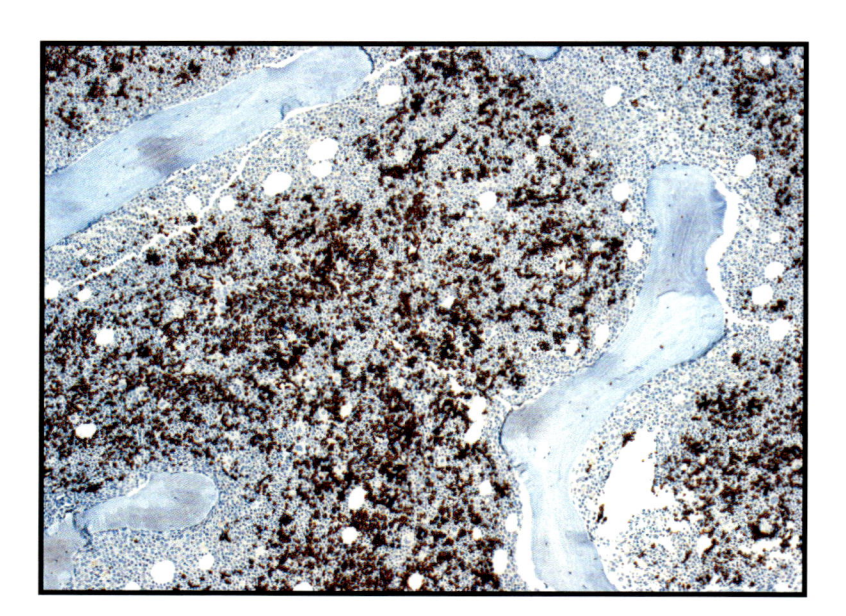

F3.34.1 Glycophorin A in adult bone marrow with myelodysplastic syndrome (MDS)

Demonstration of glycophorin with immunohistochemistry is usually nonproblematic and good signal-to-noise ratio is easy to develop (as shown here). It appears that this would be an optimal antibody for evaluating the myeloid-erythroid ratio on low magnification. A band of myeloid precursors (no staining) is seen in its usual paratrabecular position.

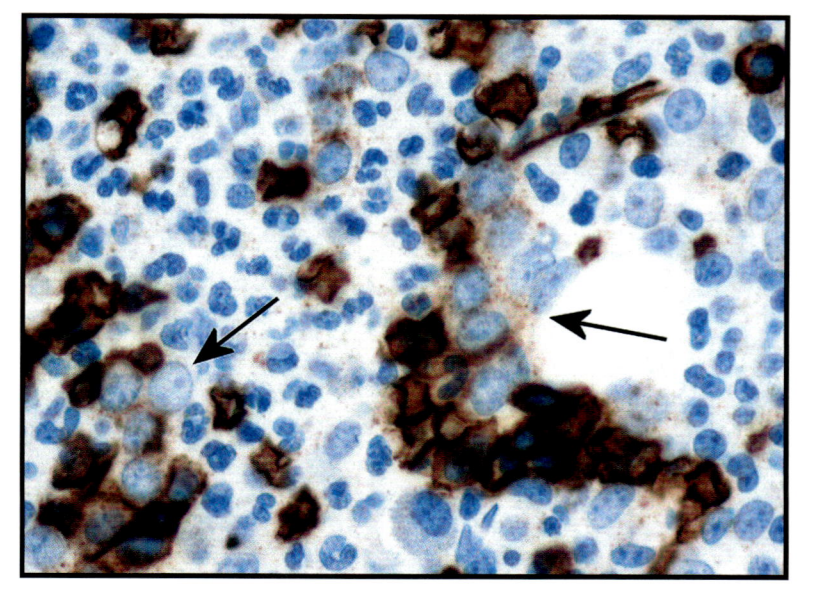

F3.34.2 Glycophorin A in early red blood cell precursors

While the majority of stages in erythroid development show strong expression, it is important to note that the early erythroid precursors show weak or no reactivity (arrows), while mature red blood cells regularly express glycophorin. In flow cytometry, mature red blood cells are excluded from the analysis by gating. This "exclusion" may be more difficult with immunohistochemistry and creates a difficulty in establishing the myeloid-erythroid ratio.

F3.34.3 Glycophorin A (CD235a) in adult bone marrow with myelodysplastic syndrome (MDS)

Close inspection reveals that many of the non-nucleated red blood cells in the vascular spaces (black arrows) strongly express glycophorin. Notably, some of the nucleated red blood cells are not stained strongly (red arrow). See also **F3.34.2**.

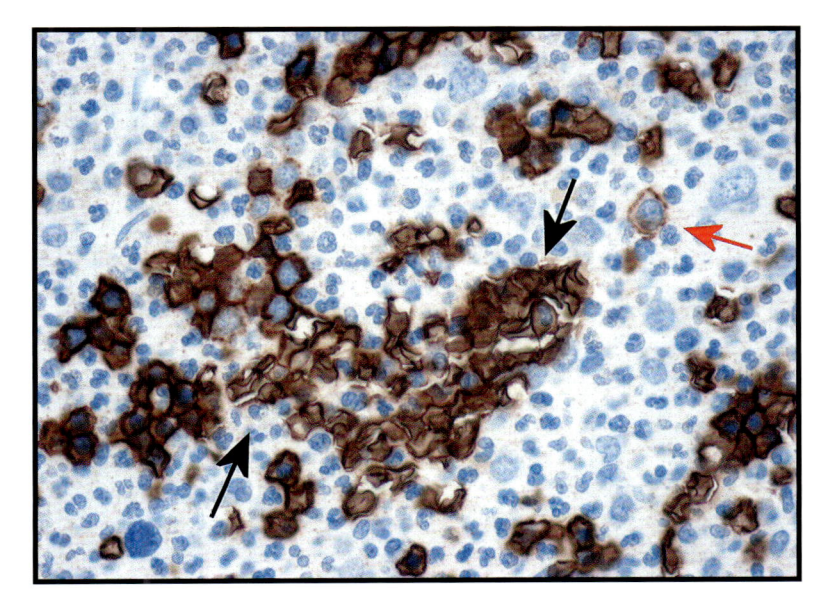

F3.34.4 Glycophorin A in acute myeloid/erythroid leukemia

This biopsy specimen shows great predominance of erythroid precursors with abnormal maturation. When cells are present in sheets or large groups and the staining is uniform and intense, the interpretation of results is not difficult.

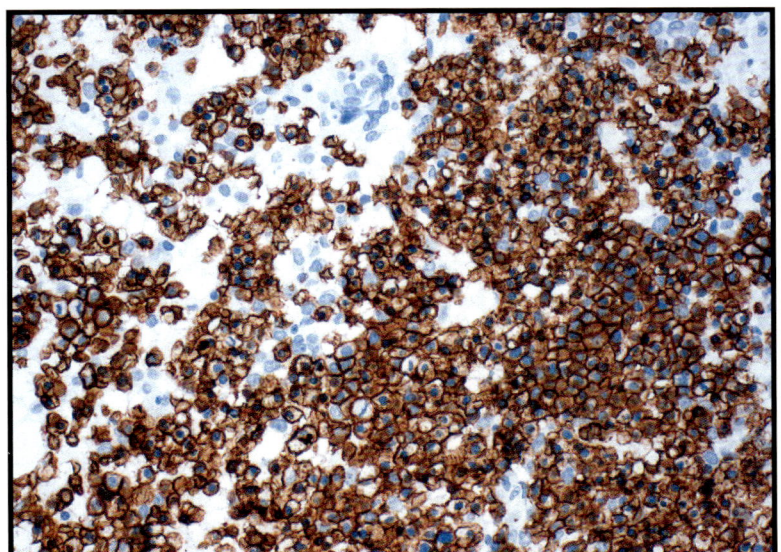

F3.34.5 Glycophorin A in acute myeloid/erythroid leukemia

Different case than that seen in **F3.34.4**. In some cases of acute myeloid/erythroid leukemia, the staining is more variable in the erythroid component. Some erythroid cells are probably negative (red arrows), some are very weakly positive (blue arrow), while most show moderate to strong expression of glycophorin A.

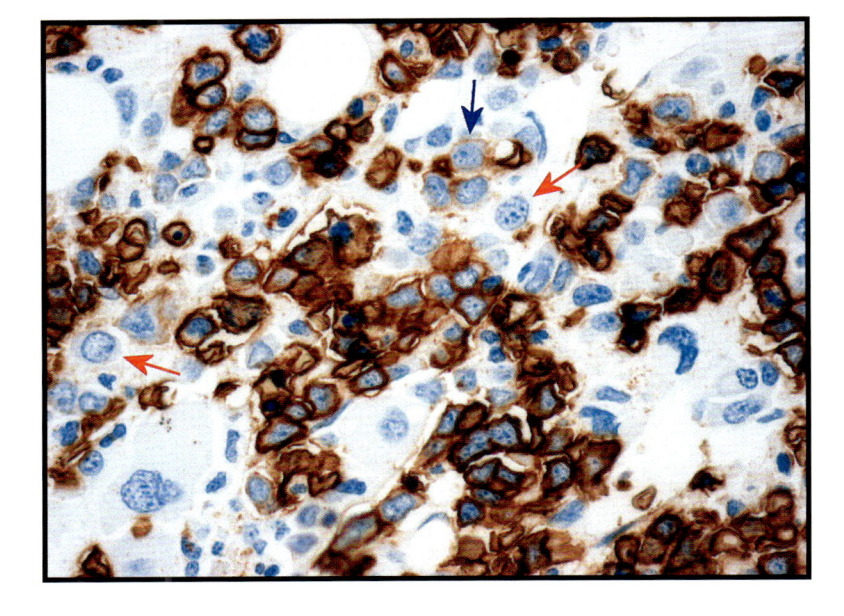

References

Aizawa S, Nakano H, Ishida T, et al. Tumor necrosis factor receptor-associated factor (TRAF) 5 and TRAF2 are involved in CD30-mediated NFκB activation. *J Biol Chem* 1997;272(4):2042-5.

Alvaro T, Lejeune M, Salvadó MT, et al. Immunohistochemical patterns of reactive microenvironment are associated with clinicobiologic behavior in follicular lymphoma patients. *J Clin Oncol* 2006;24(34):5350-7.

Andrásfalvy M, Prechl J, Hardy T, Erdei A, Bajtay Z. Mucosal type mast cells express complement receptor type 2 (CD21). *Immunol Lett* 2002;82(1-2):29-34.

Andrews RG, Torok-Storb B, Bernstein ID. Myeloid-associated differentiation antigens on stem cells and their progeny identified by monoclonal antibodies. *Blood* 1983;62(1):124-32.

Arber DA, Jenkins KA, Slovak ML. CD79 α expression in acute myeloid leukemia: high frequency of expression in acute promyelocytic leukemia. *Am J Pathol* 1996a;149(4):1105-10.

Arber DA, Jenkins KA. Paraffin section immunophenotyping of acute leukemias in bone marrow specimens. *Am J Clin Pathol* 1996b;106(4):462-8.

Ashman LK, Cambareri AC, To LB, Levinsky RJ, Juttner CA. Expression of the YB5.B8 antigen (c-kit proto-oncogene product) in normal human bone marrow. *Blood* 1991;78(1):30-7.

Attygalle A, Al-Jehani R, Diss TC, et al. Neoplastic T cells in angioimmunoblastic T-cell lymphoma express CD10. *Blood* 2002;99(2):627-33.

Aubry JP, Pochon S, Graber P, Jansen KU, Bonnefoy JY. CD21 is a ligand for CD23 and regulates IgE production. *Nature* 1992;358(6386):505-7.

Azuma Y, Kurusu Y, Sato H, Higai K, Matsumoto K. Increased expression of Lewis X and Y antigens on the cell surface and FUT 4 mRNA during granzyme B-induced JurkaT-cell apoptosis. *Biol Pharm Bull* 2007;30(4):655-60.

Balduino A, Hurtado SP, Frazão P, et al. Bone marrow subendosteal microenvironment harbours functionally distinct haemosupportive stromal cell populations. *Cell Tissue Res* 2005;319(2):255-66.

Baldus SE, Wickenhauser C, Stefanovic A, Schmitz B, Thiele J, Fischer R. Enrichment of human bone marrow mononuclear phagocytes and characterization of macrophage subpopulations by immunoenzymatic double staining. *Histochem J* 1998;30(4):285-91.

Bansal I, Flintoft EL, Piggott NH, et al. CD33 antigen detection with a new monoclonal antibody PWS44 reactive in paraffin tissue sections: pattern of reactivity and potential diagnostic utility. *Lab Invest* 2007;87(suppl 1):233A.

Barekman CL, Aguilera NS, Abbondanzo SL. Low-grade B-cell lymphoma with coexpression of both CD5 and CD10: a report of 3 cases. *Arch Pathol Lab Med* 2001;125(7):951-3.

Barrena S, Almeida J, Yunta M, et al. Aberrant expression of tetraspanin molecules in B-cell chronic lymphoproliferative disorders and its correlation with normal B-cell maturation. *Leukemia* 2005;19(8):1376-83.

Basch RS, Kouri YH, Karpatkin S. Expression of CD4 by human megakaryocytes. *Proc Natl Acad Sci U S A* 1990;87(20):8085-9.

Bass RD, Pullarkat V, Feinstein DI, Kaul A, Winberg CD, Brynes RK. Pathology of autoimmune myelofibrosis: a report of three cases and a review of the literature [review]. *Am J Clin Pathol* 2001;116(2):211-6.

Bataille R, Pellat-Deceunynck C, Robillard N, Avet-Loiseau H, Harousseau JL, Moreau P. CD117 (c-kit) is aberrantly expressed in a subset of MGUS and multiple myeloma with unexpectedly good prognosis. *Leuk Res* 2007;32(3):379-82.

Bataille R, Jégo G, Robillard N, et al. The phenotype of normal, reactive and malignant plasma cells. Identification of "many and multiple myelomas" and of new targets for myeloma therapy [review]. *Haematologica* 2006;91(9):1234-40.

Baum J, Ward RH, Conway DJ. Natural selection on the erythrocyte surface. *Mol Biol Evol* 2002;19(3):223-9.

Baumheter S, Singer MS, Henzel W, et al. Binding of L-selectin to the vascular sialomucin CD34. *Science* 1993;262(5132):436-8.

Baur AS, Meugé-Moraw C, Schmidt PM, Parlier V, Jotterand M, Delacrétaz F. CD34/QBEND10 immunostaining in bone marrow biopsies: an additional parameter for the diagnosis and classification of myelodysplastic syndromes. *Eur J Haematol* 2000;64(2):71-9.

Bavikatty NR, Ross CW, Finn WG, Schnitzer B, Singleton TP. Anti-CD10 immunoperoxidase staining of paraffin-embedded acute leukemias: comparison with flow cytometric immunophenotyping. *Hum Pathol* 2000;31(9):1051-4.

Bayer-Garner IB, Sanderson RD, Dhodapkar MV, Owens RB, Wilson CS. Syndecan-1 (CD138) immunoreactivity in bone marrow biopsies of multiple myeloma: shed syndecan-1 accumulates in fibrotic regions. *Mod Pathol* 2001;14(10):1052-8.

Bene MC, Castoldi G, Knapp W, et al. Proposals for the immunological classification of acute leukemias. European Group for the Immunological Characterization of Leukemias (EGIL). *Leukemia* 1995;9(10):1783-6.

Berditchevski F, Zutter MM, Hemler ME. Characterization of novel complexes on the cell surface between integrins and proteins with 4 transmembrane domains (TM4 proteins). *Mol Biol Cell* 1996;7(2):193-207.

Beschorner R, Horny HP, Petruch UR, Kaiserling E. Frequent expression of haemopoietic and non-haemopoietic antigens by reactive plasma cells: an immunohistochemical study using formalin-fixed, paraffin-embedded tissue. *Histol Histopathol* 1999;14(3):805-12.

References

Beyers AD, Spruyt LL, Williams AF. Molecular associations between the T-lymphocyte antigen receptor complex and the surface antigens CD2, CD4, or CD8 and CD5. *Proc Natl Acad Sci U S A* 1992;89(7):2945-9.

Bhargava P, Kallakury BV, Ross JS, Azumi N, Bagg A. CD79a is heterogeneously expressed in neoplastic and normal myeloid precursors and megakaryocytes in an antibody clone-dependent manner. *Am J Clin Pathol* 2007;128(2):306-13.

Biassoni R, Ferrini S, Prigione I, Moretta A, Long EO. CD3− lymphokine-activated cytotoxic cells express the CD3 ε gene. *J Immunol* 1988;140(5):1685-9.

Bierer BE, Burakoff SJ, Smith BR. A large proportion of T lymphocytes lack CD5 expression after bone marrow transplantation. *Blood* 1989a;73(5):1359-66.

Bierer BE, Sleckman BP, Ratnofsky SE, Burakoff SJ. The biologic roles of CD2, CD4, and CD8 in T-cell activation [review]. *Annu Rev Immunol* 1989b;7:579-99.

Blom B, Spits H. Development of human lymphoid cells [review]. *Annu Rev Immunol* 2006;24:287-320.

Blom B, Verschuren MC, Heemskerk MH, et al. TCR gene rearrangements and expression of the pre-T-cell receptor complex during human T-cell differentiation. *Blood* 1999;93(9):3033-43.

Bluth RF, Casey TT, McCurley TL. Differentiation of reactive from neoplastic small-cell lymphoid aggregates in paraffin-embedded marrow particle preparations using L-26 (CD20) and UCHL-1 (CD45RO) monoclonal antibodies. *Am J Clin Pathol* 1993;99(2):150-6.

Bossaller L, Burger J, Draeger R, et al. ICOS deficiency is associated with a severe reduction of CXCR5+CD4 germinal center Th cells. *J Immunol* 2006;177(7):4927-32.

Braylan RC, Orfao A, Borowitz MJ, Davis BH. Optimal number of reagents required to evaluate hematolymphoid neoplasias: results of an international consensus meeting [review]. *Cytometry* 2001;46(1):23-7.

Cabezudo E, Carrara P, Morilla R, Matutes E. Quantitative analysis of CD79b, CD5 and CD19 in mature B-cell lymphoproliferative disorders. *Haematologica* 1999;84(5):413-8.

Calabi F, Belt KT, Yu CY, Bradbury A, Mandy WJ, Milstein C. The rabbit CD1 and the evolutionary conservation of the CD1 gene family. *Immunogenetics* 1989;30(5):370-7.

Caldwell CW, Patterson WP, Toalson BD, Yesus YW. Surface and cytoplasmic expression of CD45 antigen isoforms in normal and malignant myeloid cell differentiation. *Am J Clin Pathol* 1991;95(2):180-7.

Campana D, Janossy G, Coustan-Smith E, et al. The expression of T-cell receptor-associated proteins during T-cell ontogeny in man. *J Immunol* 1989;142(1):57-66.

Carey DJ. Syndecans: multifunctional cell-surface co-receptors [review]. *Biochem J* 1997;327(Pt 1):1-16.

Cascavilla N, Musto P, D'Arena G, et al. CD117 (c-kit) is a restricted antigen of acute myeloid leukemia and characterizes early differentiative levels of M5 FAB subtype. *Haematologica* 1998;83(5):392-7.

Castells MC. Mastocytosis: classification, diagnosis, and clinical presentation [review]. *Allergy Asthma Proc* 2004;25(1):33-6.

Ceredig R. The ontogeny of B-cells in the thymus of normal, CD3 ε knockout (KO), RAG-2 KO and IL-7 transgenic mice. *Int Immunol* 2002;14(1):87-99.

Chadburn A, Knowles DM. Paraffin-resistant antigens detectable by antibodies L26 and polyclonal CD3 predict the B- or T-cell lineage of 95% of diffuse aggressive non-Hodgkin's lymphomas. *Am J Clin Pathol* 1994;102(3):284-91.

Chang H, Yeung J, Brandwein J, Yi QL. CD7 expression predicts poor disease free survival and post-remission survival in patients with acute myeloid leukemia and normal karyotype. *Leuk Res* 2007;31(2):157-62.

Chang H, Yi QL. Acute myeloid leukemia with pseudo-Chèdiak-Higashi anomaly exhibits a specific immunophenotype with CD2 expression. *Am J Clin Pathol* 2006;125(5):791-4.

Chang CC, Eshoa C, Kampalath B, Shidham VB, Perkins S. Immunophenotypic profile of myeloid cells in granulocytic sarcoma by immunohistochemistry. Correlation with blast differentiation in bone marrow. *Am J Clin Pathol* 2000;114(5):807-11.

Chapple MR, MacLennan IC, Johnson GD. A phenotypic study of B lymphocyte subpopulations in human bone marrow. *Clin Exp Immunol* 1990;81(1):166-72.

Charbord P, Tavian M, Humeau L, Péault B. Early ontogeny of the human marrow from long bones: an immunohistochemical study of hematopoiesis and its microenvironment. *Blood* 1996;87(10):4109-19.

Chen YH, Tallman MS, Goolsby C, Peterson L. Immunophenotypic variations in hairy cell leukemia. *Am J Clin Pathol* 2006;125(2):251-9.

Chen YC, Chou JM, Ketterling RP, Letendre L, Li CY. Histologic and immunohistochemical study of bone marrow monocytic nodules in 21 cases with myelodysplasia. *Am J Clin Pathol* 2003;120(6):874-81.

Chen CC, Raikow RB, Sonmez-Alpan E, Swerdlow SH. Classification of small B-cell lymphoid neoplasms using a paraffin section immunohistochemical panel. *Appl Immunohistochem Mol Morphol* 2000;8(1):1-11.

Chetty R, Echezarreta G, Comley M, Gatter K. Immunohistochemistry in apparently normal bone marrow trephine specimens from patients with nodal follicular lymphoma. *J Clin Pathol* 1995;48(11):1035-8.

Chuang SS, Li CY. Useful panel of antibodies for the classification of acute leukemia by immunohistochemical methods in bone marrow trephine biopsy specimens. *Am J Clin Pathol* 1997;107(4):410-8.

Cines DB, Pollak ES, Buck CA, et al. Endothelial cells in physiology and in the pathophysiology of vascular isorders. *Blood* 1998;91(10):3527-61.

Couvelard A, Scoazec JY, Dauge MC, Bringuier AF, Potet F, Feldmann G. Structural and functional differentiation of sinusoidal endothelial cells during liver organogenesis in humans. *Blood* 1996;87(11):4568-80.

Cruse JM, Lewis RE, Sanders CM, et al. Diminished CD10, CD13, and CD15 expression in a differentiated granulocyte population in CML. *Exp Mol Pathol* 2007;83(2):274-6.

Davis RE, Longacre TA, Cornbleet PJ. Hematogones in the bone marrow of adults: immunophenotypic features, clinical settings, and differential diagnosis. *Am J Clin Pathol* 1994;102(2):202-11.

Davoine F, Labonté I, Ferland C, Mazer B, Chakir J, Laviolette M. Role and modulation of CD16 expression on eosinophils by cytokines and immune complexes. *Int Arch Allergy Immunol* 2004;134(2):165-72.

de Bruin PC, Gruss HJ, van der Valk P, Willemze R, Meijer CJ. CD30 expression in normal and neoplastic lymphoid tissue: biological aspects and clinical implications [review]. *Leukemia* 1995;9(10):1620-7.

de Totero D, Carbone A, Tazzari PL, et al. Expression of the IL2 receptor α, β and γ chains in hairy cell leukemia [review]. *Leuk Lymphoma* 1994;14(suppl 1):27-32.

Delibrias CC, Mouhoub A, Fischer E, Kazatchkine MD. CR1(CD35) and CR2(CD21) complement C3 receptors are expressed on normal human thymocytes and mediate infection of thymocytes with opsonized human immunodeficiency virus. *Eur J Immunol* 1994;24(11):2784-8.

Deutsch VR, Tomer A. Megakaryocyte development and platelet production [review]. *Br J Haematol* 2006;134(5):453-66.

Dogan A, Morice WG. Bone marrow histopathology in peripheral T-cell lymphomas [review]. *Br J Haematol* 2004 Oct;127(2):140-54

Duan B, Morel L. Role of B-1a cells in autoimmunity. *Autoimmun Rev* 2006;5(6):403-8.

Dumon S, Heath VL, Tomlinson MG, Göttgens B, Frampton J. Differentiation of murine committed megakaryocytic progenitors isolated by a novel strategy reveals the complexity of GATA and Ets factor involvement in megakaryocytopoiesis and an unexpected potential role for GATA-6. *Exp Hematol* 2006;34(5):654-63.

Dunphy CH, Nies MK, Gabriel DA. Correlation of plasma cell percentages by CD138 immunohistochemistry, cyclin D1 status, and CD56 expression with clinical parameters and overall survival in plasma cell myeloma. *Appl Immunohistochem Mol Morphol* 2007a;15(3):248-54.

Dunphy CH, O'Malley DP, Perkins SL, Chang CC. Analysis of immunohistochemical markers in bone marrow sections to evaluate for myelodysplastic syndromes and acute myeloid leukemias. *Appl Immunohistochem Mol Morphol* 2007b;15(2):154-9.

Dunphy CH, Orton SO, Mantell J. Relative contributions of enzyme cytochemistry and flow cytometric immunophenotyping to the evaluation of acute myeloid leukemias with a monocytic component and of flow cytometric immunophenotyping to the evaluation of absolute monocytoses. *Am J Clin Pathol* 2004;122(6):865-74.

Dunphy CH, Polski JM, Evans HL, Gardner LJ. Evaluation of BM specimens with acute myelogenous leukemia for CD34, CD15, CD117, and myeloperoxidase. *Arch Pathol Lab Med* 2001;125(8):1063-9.

Duperray A, Troesch A, Berthier R, Chagnon E, Frachet P, Uzan G, Marguerie G. Biosynthesis and assembly of platelet GPIIb-IIIa in human megakaryocytes: evidence that assembly between pro-GPIIb and GPIIIa is a prerequisite for expression of the complex on the cell surface. *Blood* 1989 Oct;74(5):1603-11.

Duperray C, Boiron JM, Boucheix C, et al. The CD24 antigen discriminates between pre-B and B-cells in human bone marrow. *J Immunol* 1990;145(11):3678-83.

Dworzak MN, Fritsch G, Buchinger P, et al. Flow cytometric assessment of human MIC2 expression in BM, thymus, and peripheral blood. *Blood* 1994;83(2):415-25.

Dzionek A, Fuchs A, Schmidt P, et al. BDCA-2, BDCA-3, and BDCA-4: three markers for distinct subsets of dendritic cells in human peripheral blood. *J Immunol* 2000;165(11):6037-46.

Elghetany MT. Surface antigen changes during normal neutrophilic development: a critical review. *Blood Cells Mol Dis* 2002;28(2):260-74.

Ely SA, Knowles DM. Expression of CD56/neural cell adhesion molecule correlates with the presence of lytic bone lesions in multiple myeloma and distinguishes myeloma from monoclonal gammopathy of undetermined significance and lymphomas with plasmacytoid differentiation. *Am J Pathol* 2002;160(4):1293-9.

Escribano L, Díaz-Agustín B, Núñez R, Prados A, Rodríguez R, Orfao A. Abnormal expression of CD antigens in mastocytosis [review]. *Int Arch Allergy Immunol* 2002;127(2):127-32.

Escribano L, Díaz Agustín Beatriz, Bravo P, Navalón R, Almeida J, Orfao A. Immunophenotype of BM mast cells in indolent systemic mast cell disease in adults [review]. *Leuk Lymphoma* 1999;35(3-4):227-35.

Escribano L, Orfao A, Villarrubia J, et al. Immunophenotypic characterization of human bone marrow mast cells: a flow cytometric study of normal and pathological BM samples. *Anal Cell Pathol* 1998;16(3):151-9.

Escribano L, Orfao A, Villarrubia J, et al. Expression of lymphoid-associated antigens in mast cells: report of a case of systemic mast cell disease. *Br J Haematol* 1995;91(4):941-3.

Eshoa C, Perkins S, Kampalath B, Shidham V, Juckett M, Chang CC. Decreased CD10 expression in grade III and in interfollicular infiltrates of follicular lymphomas [review]. *Am J Clin Pathol* 2001;115(6):862-7.

References

Eshoa C, Shidham V, Kouzova M, et al. CD14 expression and nonspecific esterase staining in acute myeloid leukemia, AMLM4 and AML-M5 [abstract]. *Am J Clin Pathol* 1999;112:562. Abstract 88.

Estalilla OC, Koo CH, Brynes RK, Medeiros LJ. Intravascular large B-cell lymphoma: a report of five cases initially diagnosed by bone marrow biopsy. *Am J Clin Pathol* 1999;112(2):248-55.

Evans HL, Burks E, Viswanatha D, Larson RS. Utility of immunohistochemistry in bone marrow evaluation of T-lineage large granular lymphocyte leukemia. *Hum Pathol* 2000;31(10):1266-73.

Fackler MJ, Krause DS, Smith OM, Civin CI, May WS. Full-length but not truncated CD34 inhibits hematopoietic cell differentiation of M1 cells. *Blood* 1995;85(11):3040-7.

Fackler MJ, Civin CI, May WS. Up-regulation of surface CD34 is associated with protein kinase C-mediated hyperphosphorylation of CD34. *J Biol Chem* 1992;267(25):17540-6.

Falini B, Pileri S, Pizzolo G, et al. CD30 (Ki-1) molecule: a new cytokine receptor of the tumor necrosis factor receptor superfamily as a tool for diagnosis and immunotherapy [review]. *Blood* 1995;85(1):1-14.

Fend F, Kremer M. Diagnosis and classification of malignant lymphoma and related entities in the BM trephine biopsy [review]. *Pathobiology* 2007;74(2):133-43.

Ferry JA, Yang WI, Zukerberg LR, Wotherspoon AC, Arnold A, Harris NL. CD5+ extranodal marginal zone B-cell (MALT) lymphoma: a low grade neoplasm with a propensity for bone marrow involvement and relapse. *Am J Clin Pathol* 1996;105(1):31-7.

Feugier P, De March AK, Lesesve JF, et al. Intravascular bone marrow accumulation in persistent polyclonal lymphocytosis: a misleading feature for B-cell neoplasm. *Mod Pathol* 2004;17(9):1087-96.

Feyler S, O'Connor SJ, Rawstron AC, et al. IgM myeloma: a rare entity characterized by a CD20− CD56−CD117− immunophenotype and the t(11;14). *Br J Haematol* 2008;140(5):547-51.

Fischer E, Delibrias C, Kazatchkine MD. Expression of CR2 (the C3dg/EBV receptor, CD21) on normal human peripheral blood T lymphocytes. *J Immunol* 1991;146(3):865-9.

Font P, Subirá D. Expression of CD7 in myelodysplastic syndromes (MDS): is this a truly prognostic factor? *Leuk Res* 2008;32(1):185-6.

Font P, Subirá D, Mtnez-Chamorro C, et al. Evaluation of CD7 and terminal deoxynucleotidyl transferase (TdT) expression in CD34+ myeloblasts from patients with myelodysplastic syndrome [published online ahead of print January 18, 2006]. *Leuk Res* 2006;30(8):957-63.

Foran JM, Norton AJ, Micallef IN, et al. Loss of CD20 expression following treatment with Rituximab (chimaeric monoclonal anti-CD20): a retrospective cohort analysis. *Br J Haematol* 2001;114(4):881-3.

Fox N, Damjanov I, Knowles BB, Solter D. Immunohistochemical localization of the mouse stage-specific embryonic antigen 1 in human tissues and tumors. *Cancer Res*. 1983;43(2):669-78.

Gaal K, Sun NC, Hernandez AM, Arber DA. Sinonasal NK/T-cell lymphomas in the United States. *Am J Surg Pathol* 2000;24(11):1511-7.

Gagro A, Dasić G, Sabioncello A, et al. Phenotypic analysis of receptor-ligand pairs on B-cells in B-chronic lymphocytic leukemia. *Leuk Lymphoma* 1997;25(3-4):301-11.

Galli SJ, Zsebo KM, Geissler EN. The kit ligand, stem cell factor [review]. *Adv Immunol* 1994;55:1-96.

Garcia DP, Rooney MT, Ahmad E, Davis BH. Diagnostic usefulness of CD23 and FMC-7 antigen expression patterns in B-cell lymphoma classification. *Am J Clin Pathol* 2001;115(2):258-65.

Gelin C, Aubrit F, Phalipon A, et al. The E2 antigen, a 32 kd glycoprotein involved in T-cell adhesion processes, is the MIC2 gene product. *EMBO J* 1989;8(11):3253-9.

Gessain A, Saal F, Morozov V, et al. Characterization of HTLV-I isolates and T lymphoid cell lines derived from French West Indian patients with tropical spastic paraparesis. *Int J Cancer* 1989;43(2):327-33.

Girodon F, Favre B, Couillaud G, Carli PM, Parmeland C, Maynadié M. Immunophenotype of a transient myeloproliferative disorder in a newborn with trisomy 21. *Cytometry* 2000;42(2):118-22.

Goldman FD, Vibhakar R, Puck JM, et al. Aberrant T-cell antigen receptor-mediated responses in autoimmune lymphoproliferative syndrome. *Clin Immunol* 2002;104(1):31-9.

Goodman GR, Bethel KJ, Saven A. Hairy cell leukemia: an update [review]. *Curr Opin Hematol* 2003;10(4):258-66.

Gore SD, Kastan MB, Civin CI. Normal human bone marrow precursors that express terminal deoxynucleotidyl transferase include T-cell precursors and possible lymphoid stem cells. *Blood* 1991;77(8):1681-90.

Grogg KL, Morice WG, Macon WR. Spectrum of BM findings in patients with angioimmunoblastic T-cell lymphoma. *Br J Haematol* 2007;137(5):416-22.

Gronthos S, Franklin DM, Leddy HA, Robey PG, Storms RW, Gimble JM. Surface protein characterization of human adipose tissue-derived stromal cells. *J Cell Physiol* 2001;189(1):54-63.

Grube M, Moritz S, Obermann EC, et al. CD8+ T cells reactive to survivin antigen in patients with multiple myeloma. *Clin Cancer Res* 2007;13(3):1053-60.

Ha HJ, Kubagawa H, Burrows PD. Molecular cloning and expression pattern of a human gene homologous to the murine mb-1 gene. *J Immunol* 1992;148(5):1526-31.

Haidar JH, Shamseddine A, Salem Z, et al. Loss of CD20 expression in relapsed lymphomas after Rituximab therapy. *Eur J Haematol* 2003;70(5):330-2.

Hamilton G, Fellinger EJ, Schratter I, Fritsch A. Characterization of a human endocrine tissue and tumor-associated Ewing's sarcoma antigen. *Cancer Res* 1988;48(21):6127-31.

Hans CP, Finn WG, Singleton TP, Schnitzer B, Ross CW. Usefulness of anti-CD117 in the flow cytometric analysis of acute leukemia. *Am J Clin Pathol* 2002;117(2):301-5.

Hashimoto M, Yamashita Y, Mori N. Immunohistochemical detection of CD79a expression in precursor T-cell lymphoblastic lymphoma/leukaemias. *J Pathol* 2002;197(3):341-7.

Haynes BF, Heinly CS. Early human T-cell development: analysis of the human thymus at the time of initial entry of hematopoietic stem cells into the fetal thymic microenvironment. *J Exp Med* 1995;181(4):1445-58.

Helin H, Vyberg M, Steensgaard A. CD68. Available at: http://www.nordiqc.org/Epitopes/CD68/CD68.htm. Accessed April 16, 2008.

Helinski EH, Bielat KL, Ovak GM, Meenaghan MA, Wirth JE, Pauly JL. Identification of the interleukin-2 receptor (IL-2R) on human leukemic T cells using colloidal gold and scanning electron microscopy. *J Med* 1988;19(5-6):353-68.

Helleberg C, Knudsen H, Hansen PB, et al. CD34+ megakaryoblastic leukaemic cells are CD38−, but CD61+ and glycophorin A+: improved criteria for diagnosis of AML-M7? *Leukemia* 1997;11(6):830-4.

Hirji N, Lin TJ, Befus AD. Promiscuous CD8: expression and function of CD8 on macrophages, mast cells and dendritic cells. *Mod Asp Immunobiol* 2000;1:140-3.

Hirji NS, Lin TJ, Gilchrist M, et al. Novel CD8 molecule on macrophages and mast cells: expression, function and signaling. *Int Arch Allergy Immunol* 1999;118(2-4):180-2.

Holness CL, Simmons DL. Molecular cloning of CD68, a human macrophage marker related to lysosomal glycoproteins. *Blood* 1993;81(6):1607-13.

Horny HP, Sotlar K, Valent P. Mastocytosis: state of the art [review]. *Pathobiology* 2007a;74(2):121-32.

Horny HP, Sotlar K, Valent P. Diagnostic value of histology and immunohistochemistry in myelodysplastic syndromes [published online ahead of print July 2, 2007]. *Leuk Res* 2007b;31(12):1609-16.

Horny HP, Sotlar K, Sperr WR, Valent P. Systemic mastocytosis with associated clonal haematological non mast cell lineage diseases: a histopathological challenge. *J Clin Pathol* 2004;57(6):604-8.

Horny HP, Wehrmann M, Schlicker HU, Eichstaedt A, Clemens MR, Kaiserling E. QBEND10 for the diagnosis of myelodysplastic syndromes in routinely processed bone marrow biopsy specimens. *J Clin Pathol* 1995;48(4):291-4.

Horny HP, Wehrmann M, Steinke B, Kaiserling E. Assessment of the value of immunohistochemistry in the subtyping of acute leukemia on routinely processed bone marrow biopsy specimens with particular reference to macrophage-associated antibodies. *Hum Pathol* 1994;25(8):810-4.

Horny HP, Wehrmann M, Griesser H, Tiemann M, Bültmann B, Kaiserling E. Investigation of bone marrow lymphocyte subsets in normal, reactive, and neoplastic states using paraffin-embedded biopsy specimens. *Am J Clin Pathol* 1993;99(2):142-9.

Hoyer JD, Grogg KL, Hanson CA, Gamez JD, Dogan A. CD33 Detection by immunohistochemistry in paraffin-embedded tissues: a new antibody shows excellent specificity and sensitivity for cells of myelomonocytic lineage. *Am J Clin Pathol* 2008;129(2):316-23.

Hsu SM, Jaffe ES. Leu M1 and peanut agglutinin stain the neoplastic cells of Hodgkin's disease. *Am J Clin Pathol* 1984;82(1):29-32.

Hudock J, Chatten J, Miettinen M. Immunohistochemical evaluation of myeloid leukemia infiltrates (granulocytic sarcomas) in formaldehyde-fixed, paraffin-embedded tissue. *Am J Clin Pathol* 1994;102(1):55-60.

Human Cell Differentiation Molecules Web site. http://www.hcdm.org/, last accessed June 12, 2008.

Hundemer M, Klein U, Hose D, et al. Lack of CD56 expression on myeloma cells is not a marker for poor prognosis in patients treated by high-dose chemotherapy and is associated with translocation t(11;14). *BM Transplant* 2007;40(11):1033-7.

Hunter ZR, Branagan AR, Manning R, et al. CD5, CD10, and CD23 expression in Waldenstrom's macroglobulinemia. *Clin Lymphoma* 2005;5(4):246-9.

Imbert AM, Belaaloui G, Bardin F, Tonnelle C, Lopez M, Chabannon C. CD99 expressed on human mobilized peripheral blood CD34+ cells is involved in transendothelial migration [published online ahead of print July 6, 2006]. *Blood* 2006;108(8):2578-86.

Islam A, Glomski C, Henderson ES. Endothelial cells and hematopoiesis: a light microscopic study of fetal, normal, and pathologic human bone marrow in plastic-embedded sections. *Anat Rec* 1992;233(3):440-52.

Jacob MC, Chaperot L, Mossuz P, et al. CD4+ CD56+ lineage negative malignancies: a new entity developed from malignant early plasmacytoid dendritic cells. *Haematologica* 2003;88(8):941-55.

Jaffe ES, Harris NL, Stein H, Vardiman JW. *WHO Pathology & Genetics: Tumours of Haematopoietic and Lymphoid Tissues* Lyon, France: IARC Press; 2001.

References

Jiang L, Admirand JH, Moran C, Ford RJ, Bueso-Ramos CE. Mediastinal follicular dendritic cell sarcoma involving bone marrow: a case report and review of the literature. *Ann Diagn Pathol* 2006;10(6):357-62.

Joshi R, Horncastle D, Elderfield K, Lampert I, Rahemtulla A, Naresh KN. Bone marrow trephine combined with immunohistochemistry is superior to bone marrow aspirate in follow-up of myeloma patients. *J Clin Pathol* 2007;61:213-6.

Jung KC, Kim NH, Park WS, Park SH, Bae Y. The CD99 signal enhances Fas-mediated apoptosis in the human leukemic cell line, Jurkat. *FEBS Lett* 2003;554(3):478-84.

Kaiser U, Auerbach B, Oldenburg M. The neural cell adhesion molecule NCAM in multiple myeloma [review]. *Leuk Lymphoma* 1996;20(5-6):389-95.

Kang LC, Dunphy CH. Immunoreactivity of MIC2 (CD99) and terminal deoxynucleotidyl transferase in bone marrow clot and core specimens of acute myeloid leukemias and myelodysplastic syndromes. *Arch Pathol Lab Med* 2006;130(2):153-7.

Kass L, Kapadia IH. Perivascular plasmacytosis: a light-microscopic and Immunohistochemical study of 93 BM biopsies. *Acta Haematol* 2001;105(2):57-63.

Kato N, Yasukawa K, Kimura K, et al. CD2− CD4+ CD56+ hematodermic/hematolymphoid malignancy [review]. *J Am Acad Dermatol* 2001;44(2):231-8.

Kaufmann O, Flath B, Späth-Schwalbe E, Possinger K, Dietel M. Immunohistochemical detection of CD10 with monoclonal antibody 56C6 on paraffin sections. *Am J Clin Pathol* 1999;111(1):117-22.

Keren DF, McCoy JP, Carey JL. Flow cytometry in clinical diagnosis. Chicago, Ill: ASCP Press; 2001:704.

Khanlari B, Buser A, Lugli A, Tichelli A, Dirnhofer S. The expression pattern of CD56 (N-CAM) in human bone marrow biopsies infiltrated by acute leukemia. *Leuk Lymphoma* 2003;44(12):2055-9.

Knapp W, Strobl H, Majdic O. Flow cytometric analysis of cell-surface and intracellular antigens in leukemia diagnosis. *Cytometry* 1994;18(4):187-98.

Kobayashi T, Miwa H, Uchida T, Matsuoka N, Kita K, Shirakawa S. Surface and cytoplasmic expression of CD2, CD13, and CD25 antigens in human T lymphotropic virus type I infected cell line: an immuno-electron microscopic study. *Lab Invest* 1989;60(3):370-4.

Köller M, Willheim M, Krugluger W, et al. Immunophenotyping of human bone marrow -derived macrophages. *Scand J Immunol* 1996;43(6):626-32.

Kraj M, Pogłód R, Kopeć-Szlęzak J, Sokołowska U, Woźniak J, Kruk B. C-kit receptor (CD117) expression on plasma cells in monoclonal gammopathies. *Leuk Lymphoma* 2004;45(11):2281-9.

Krause DS, Fackler MJ, Civin CI, May WS. CD34: structure, biology, and clinical utility [review]. *Blood* 1996;87(1):1-13.

Kreft A, Weber A, Springer E, Hess G, Kirkpatrick CJ. Bone marrow findings in multicentric Castleman disease in HIV− patients. *Am J Surg Pathol* 2007;31(3):398-402.

Kröber SM, Greschniok A, Kaiserling E, Horny HP. Acute lymphoblastic leukaemia: correlation between morphological/immunohistochemical and molecular biological findings in bone marrow biopsy specimens. *Mol Pathol* 2000;53(2):83-7.

Kurtin PJ, Pinkus GS. Leukocyte common antigen: a diagnostic discriminant between hematopoietic and nonhematopoietic neoplasms in paraffin sections using monoclonal antibodies: correlation with immunologic studies and ultrastructural localization. *Hum Pathol* 1985;16(4):353-65.

Lampert IA, Wotherspoon A, Van Noorden S, Hasserjian RP. High expression of CD23 in the proliferation centers of chronic lymphocytic leukemia in lymph nodes and spleen. *Hum Pathol* 1999;30(6):648-54.

Langebrake C, Creutzig U, Reinhardt D. Immunophenotype of Down syndrome acute myeloid leukemia and transient myeloproliferative disease differs significantly from other diseases with morphologically identical or similar blasts. *Klin Padiatr* 2005;217(3):126-34.

Lau SK, Chu PG, Weiss LM. CD163: a specific marker of macrophages in paraffin-embedded tissue samples. *Am J Clin Pathol* 2004;122(5):794-801.

Lee SH. Phenotypic analysis of human bone marrow macrophages. *Blood Cells* 1991;17(1):45-54; discussion 54-8.

Lee SH, Crocker PR, Westaby S, et al. Isolation and immunocytochemical characterization of human bone marrow stromal macrophages in hemopoietic clusters. *J Exp Med* 1988;168(3):1193-8.

Lee ST, Kim HJ, Kim SH. Defining an optimal number of immunophenotypic markers for lineage assignment of acute leukemias based on the EGIL scoring system. *Korean J Lab Med* 2006;26(6):393-9.

Lim MS, Straus SE, Dale JK, et al. Pathological findings in human autoimmune lymphoproliferative syndrome. *Am J Pathol* 1998;153(5):1541-50.

Loken MR, Shah VO, Hollander Z, Civin CI. Flow cytometric analysis of normal B lymphoid development. *Pathol Immunopathol Res* 1988;7(5):357-70.

Loken MR, Shah VO, Dattilio KL, Civin CI. Flow cytometric analysis of human bone marrow. II. Normal B lymphocyte development. *Blood* 1987;70(5):1316-24.

Longacre TA, Foucar K, Crago S, et al. Hematogones: a multiparameter analysis of bone marrow precursor cells. *Blood* 1989;73(2):543-52.

Lopez-Matas M, Rodriguez-Justo M, Morilla R, Catovsky D, Matutes E. Quantitative expression of CD23 and its ligand CD21 in chronic lymphocytic leukemia. *Haematologica* 2000;85(11):1140-5.

Lou O, Alcaide P, Luscinskas FW, Muller WA. CD99 is a key mediator of the transendothelial migration of neutrophils. *J Immunol* 2007;178(2):1136-43.

Loyson SA, Rademakers LH, Joling P, Vroom TM, van den Tweel JG. Immunohistochemical analysis of decalcified paraffin-embedded human bone marrow biopsies with emphasis on MHC class I and CD34 expression. *Histopathology* 1997;31(5):412-9.

Machhi J, Bunyi-Teopengco E, Chang C, et al. CD34 expression in megakaryocytes favors myelodysplasia [abstract]. *Mod Pathol.* 2001;14:171.

Manaloor EJ, Neiman RS, Heilman DK, et al. Immunohistochemistry can be used to subtype acute myeloid leukemia in routinely processed bone marrow biopsy specimens: comparison with flow cytometry. *Am J Clin Pathol* 2000;113(6):814-22.

Manara MC, Bernard G, Lollini PL, et al. CD99 acts as an oncosuppressor in osteosarcoma. *Mol Biol Cell* 2006;17(4):1910-21.

Mason DY, Cordell JL, Brown MH, et al. CD79a: a novel marker for B-cell neoplasms in routinely processed tissue samples. *Blood* 1995;86(4):1453-9.

Mason DY, Gatter KC. The role of immunocytochemistry in diagnostic pathology [review]. *J Clin Pathol* 1987;40(9):1042-54.

Matsue K, Asada N, Takeuchi M, et al. A clinicopathological study of 13 cases of intravascular lymphoma: experience in a single institution over a 9-yr period. *Eur J Haematol* 2008;80(3):236-44.

Matthias P, Rolink AG. Transcriptional networks in developing and mature B-cells [review]. *Nat Rev Immunol* 2005;5(6):497-508.

Mayrhofer G, Gadd SJ, Spargo LD, Ashman LK. Specificity of a mouse monoclonal antibody raised against acute myeloid leukaemia cells for mast cells in human mucosal and connective tissues. *Immunol Cell Biol* 1987;65(Pt 3):241-50.

McClain KL, Natkunam Y, Swerdlow SH. Atypical cellular disorders [review]. *Hematology Am Soc Hematol Educ Program* 2004;283-96.

McCloskey SM, McMullin MF, Morris TC, Markey GM. Bone marrow architecture in acute myeloid/erythroid leukaemia. *Br J Haematol* 2004;126(1):1.

McCormack RT, Nelson RD, Solem LD, LeBien TW. Decreased expression of the common acute lymphoblastic leukaemia antigen (CALLA/CD10) on neutrophils from patients with thermal injury. *Br J Haematol* 1988;69(2):189-95.

McKenna RW, Washington LT, Aquino DB, Picker LJ, Kroft SH. Immunophenotypic analysis of hematogones (B-lymphocyte precursors) in 662 consecutive bone marrow specimens by 4-color flow cytometry. *Blood* 2001;98(8):2498-507.

McMichael AJ, Pilch JR, Galfré G, Mason DY, Fabre JW, Milstein C. A human thymocyte antigen defined by a hybrid myeloma monoclonal antibody. *Eur J Immunol* 1979;9(3):205-10.

Mellstedt H, Choudhury A. T and B-cells in B-chronic lymphocytic leukaemia: Faust, Mephistopheles and the pact with the Devil [review] [published online ahead of print May 19, 2005]. *Cancer Immunol Immunother* 2006;55(2):210-20.

Meugé-Moraw C, Delacretaz F, Baur AS. Follicular dendritic cells in bone marrow lymphoproliferative diseases: an immunohistochemical study including a new paraffin-resistant monoclonal antibody, DR53. *Histopathology* 1996;28(4):341-7.

Miettinen M. Immunohistochemistry in tumour diagnosis [review]. *Ann Med* 1993 Jun;25(3):221-33.

Min YH, Lee ST, Min DW, et al. CD34 immunohistochemical staining of bone marrow biopsies in myelodysplastic syndromes. *Yonsei Med J* 1995;36(1):1-8.

Moreau EJ, Matutes E, A'Hern RP, et al. Improvement of the chronic lymphocytic leukemia scoring system with the monoclonal antibody SN8 (CD79b). *Am J Clin Pathol* 1997;108(4):378-82.

Morice WG, Kurtin PJ, Tefferi A, Hanson CA. Distinct bone marrow findings in T-cell granular lymphocytic leukemia revealed by paraffin section immunoperoxidase stains for CD8, TIA-1, and granzyme B. *Blood* 2002;99(1):268-74.

Muehleck SD, McKenna RW, Gale PF, Brunning RD. Terminal deoxynucleotidyl transferase (TdT)+ cells in bone marrow in the absence of hematologic malignancy. *Am J Clin Pathol* 1983;79(3):277-84.

Mullink H, Henzen-Logmans SC, Tadema TM, Mol JJ, Meijer CJ. Influence of fixation and decalcification on the immunohistochemical staining of cell-specific markers in paraffin-embedded human bone biopsies. *J Histochem Cytochem* 1985;33(11):1103-9.

Mundschau G, Gurbuxani S, Gamis AS, Greene ME, Arceci RJ, Crispino JD. Mutagenesis of GATA1 is an initiating event in Down syndrome leukemogenesis. *Blood* 2003;101(11):4298-300.

Muñoz L, Nomdedéu JF, López O, et al. Interleukin-3 receptor α chain (CD123) is widely expressed in hematologic malignancies. *Haematologica* 2001;86(12):1261-9.

Muñoz-Fernández R, Blanco FJ, et al. Follicular dendritic cells are related to bone marrow stromal cell progenitors and to myofibroblasts. *J Immunol* 2006;177(1):280-9.

References

Nagata H, Worobec AS, Oh CK, et al. Identification of a point mutation in the catalytic domain of the protooncogene c-kit in peripheral blood mononuclear cells of patients who have mastocytosis with an associated hematologic disorder. *Proc Natl Acad Sci U S A* 1995;92(23):10560-4.

Nakayama F, Nishihara S, Iwasaki H, et al. CD15 expression in mature granulocytes is determined by α 1,3-fucosyltransferase IX, but in promyelocytes and monocytes by α 1,3-fucosyltransferase IV. *J Biol Chem*. 2001;276(19):16100-6.

Nandedkar MA, Palazzo J, Abbondanzo SL, Lasota J, Miettinen M. CD45 (leukocyte common antigen) immunoreactivity in metastatic undifferentiated and neuroendocrine carcinoma: a potential diagnostic pitfall. *Mod Pathol* 1998;11(12):1204-10.

Navone R, Valpreda M, Pich A. Lymphoid nodules and nodular lymphoid hyperplasia in bone marrow biopsies. *Acta Haematol* 1985;74(1):19-22.

Ngo N, Lampert IA, Naresh KN. Bone marrow trephine findings in acute myeloid leukaemia with multilineage dysplasia [published online ahead of print October 31, 2007]. *Br J Haematol* 2008;140(3):279-86.

Ngo N, Patel K, Isaacson PG, Naresh KN. Leucocyte common antigen (CD45) and CD5 positivity in an 'undifferentiated' carcinoma: a potential diagnostic pitfall. *J Clin Pathol* 2007;60(8):936-8.

Nguyen TT, Schwartz EJ, West RB, Warnke RA, Arber DA, Natkunam Y. Expression of CD163 (hemoglobin scavenger receptor) in normal tissues, lymphomas, carcinomas, and sarcomas is largely restricted to the monocyte/macrophage lineage. *Am J Surg Pathol* 2005;29(5):617-24.

Nishimura M, Takanashi M, Okazaki H, Satake M, Nakajima K. Role of CD7 expressed in lung microvascular endothelial cells as Fc receptor for immunoglobulin M. *Endothelium* 2006;13(4):287-92.

Nomdedéu JF, Mateu R, Altès A, et al. Enhanced myeloid specificity of CD117 compared with CD13 and CD33. *Leuk Res* 1999;23(4):341-7.

Nowicki M, Miśkowiak B, Konwerska A. Expression of CD79a antigen in acute lymphoblastic leukaemias in children. *Folia Histochem Cytobiol* 1999;37(2):149-50.

O'Connell FP, Pinkus JL, Pinkus GS. CD138 (syndecan-1), a plasma cell marker immunohistochemical profile in hematopoietic and nonhematopoietic neoplasms. *Am J Clin Pathol* 2004;121(2):254-63.

O'Donnell LR, Alder SL, Balis UJ, Perkins SL, Kjeldsberg CR. Immunohistochemical reference ranges for B lymphocytes in bone marrow biopsy paraffin sections. *Am J Clin Pathol* 1995;104(5):517-23.

Ocqueteau M, Orfao A, García-Sanz R, Almeida J, Gonzalez M, San Miguel JF. Expression of the CD117 antigen (c-Kit) on normal and myelomatous plasma cells. *Br J Haematol* 1996;95(3):489-93.

Oertel J, Oertel B, Schleicher J, Huhn D. Immunotyping of blasts in human bone marrow. *Ann Hematol* 1996;72(3):125-9.

Ogata K, Yoshida Y. Clinical implications of blast immunophenotypes in myelodysplastic syndromes [review]. *Leuk Lymphoma* 2005;46(9):1269-74.

Ogata K, Nakamura K, Yokose N, et al. Clinical significance of phenotypic features of blasts in patients with myelodysplastic syndrome. *Blood* 2002;100(12):3887-96.

Ohshima K, Suzumiya J, Sugihara M, et al. Clinical, immunohistochemical and phenotypic features of aggressive nodal cytotoxic lymphomas, including α/β, γ/δ T-cell and natural killer cell types. *Virchows Arch* 1999;435(2):92-100.

Orazi A, Chiu R, O'Malley DP. Chronic myelomonocytic leukemia: the role of bone marrow biopsy immunohistology [published online ahead of print October 13, 2006]. *Mod Pathol* 2006;19(12):1536-45.

Orazi A, O'Malley DP, Jiang J, et al. Acute panmyelosis with myelofibrosis: an entity distinct from acute megakaryoblastic leukemia. *Mod Pathol* 2005;18(5):603-14.

Osada S, Utsumi KR, Ueda R, et al. Assignment of a gene coding for a human T-cell antigen with a molecular weight of 40,000 daltons to chromosome 17. *Cytogene T-cell Genet* 1988;47(1-2):8-10.

Osuji N, Beiske K, Randen U, et al. Characteristic appearances of the bone marrow in T-cell large granular lymphocyte leukaemia. *Histopathology* 2007;50(5):547-54.

Pardanani A. Systemic mastocytosis: bone marrow pathology, classification, and current therapies [review]. *Acta Haematol* 2005;114(1):41-51.

Pellat-Deceunynck C, Barillé S, Jego G, et al. The absence of CD56 (NCAM) on malignant plasma cells is a hallmark of plasma cell leukemia and of a special subset of multiple myeloma. *Leukemia* 1998;12(12):1977-82.

Perea G, Domingo A, Villamor N, et al; CETLAM GroupSpain. Adverse prognostic impact of CD36 and CD2 expression in adult de novo acute myeloid leukemia patients. *Leuk Res* 2005;29(10):1109-16.

Peterson MR, Noskoviak KJ, Newbury R. CD5+ B-cell acute lymphoblastic leukemia. *Pediatr Dev Pathol* 2007;10(1):41-5.

Petrasch S, Perez-Alvarez C, Schmitz J, Kosco M, Brittinger G. Antigenic phenotyping of human follicular dendritic cells isolated from nonmalignant and malignant lymphatic tissue. *Eur J Immunol* 1990;20(5):1013-8.

Petrella T, Comeau MR, Maynadié M, et al. Agranular CD4+ CD56+ hematodermic neoplasm (blastic NK-cell lymphoma) originates from a population of CD56+ precursor cells related to plasmacytoid monocytes. *Am J Surg Pathol* 2002;26(7):852-62.

Petruch UR, Horny HP, Kaiserling E. Frequent expression of haemopoietic and non-haemopoietic antigens by neoplastic plasma cells: an immunohistochemical study using formalin-fixed, paraffin-embedded tissue. *Histopathology* 1992;20(1):35-40.

Pettersen RD, Bernard G, Olafsen MK, Pourtein M, Lie SO. CD99 signals caspase-independent T-cell death. *J Immunol* 2001;166(8):4931-42.

Pezzella F, Munson PJ, Miller KD, Goldstone AH, Gatter KC. The diagnosis of low-grade peripheral B-cell neoplasms in bone marrow trephines. *Br J Haematol* 2000;108(2):369-76.

Pileri SA, Ascani S, Milani M, et al. Acute leukaemia immunophenotyping in bone marrow routine sections. *Br J Haematol* 1999;105(2):394-401.

Pilichowska ME, Fleming MD, Pinkus JL, Pinkus GS. CD4+/CD56+ hematodermic neoplasm ('blastic natural killer cell lymphoma'): neoplastic cells express the immature dendritic cell marker BDCA-2 and produce interferon. *Am J Clin Pathol* 2007;128(3):445-53.

Pilozzi E, Pulford K, Jones M, et al. Co-expression of CD79a (JCB117) and CD3 by lymphoblastic lymphoma. *J Pathol* 1998;186(2):140-3.

Platzer B, Jörgl A, Taschner S, Höcher B, Strobl H. RelB regulates human dendritic cell subset development by promoting monocyte intermediates [published online ahead of print August 17, 2004]. *Blood* 2004;104(12):3655-63.

Polyak MJ, Ayer LM, Szczepek AJ, Deans JP. A cholesterol-dependent CD20 epitope detected by the FMC7 antibody. *Leukemia* 2003;17(7):1384-9.

Pruneri G, Bertolini F, Soligo D, et al. Angiogenesis in myelodysplastic syndromes. *Br J Cancer* 1999;81(8):1398-401.

Punnonen J, de Vries JE. Characterization of a novel CD2+ human thymic B-cell subset. *J Immunol* 1993;151(1):100-10.

Qi JC, Wang J, Mandadi S, et al. Human and mouse mast cells use the tetraspanin CD9 as an alternate interleukin-16 receptor [published online ahead of print September 6, 2005]. Blood. 2006;107(1):135-42.

Qiao X, Loudovaris M, Unverzagt K, et al. Immunocytochemistry and flow cytometry evaluation of human megakaryocytes in fresh samples and cultures of CD34+ cells. *Cytometry* 1996;23(3):250-9.

Rakozy CK, Mohamed AN, Vo TD, et al. CD56+/CD4+ lymphomas and leukemias are morphologically, immunophenotypically, cytogenetically, and clinically diverse. *Am J Clin Pathol* 2001;116(2):168-76.

Reddy VV. Topics in bone marrow biopsy pathology: role of marrow topography in myelodysplastic syndromes and evaluation of post-treatment and post-BM transplant biopsies [review]. *Ann Diagn Pathol* 2001;5(2):110-20.

Riccioni R, Rossini A, Calabrò L, et al. Immunophenotypic features of acute myeloid leukemias overexpressing the interleukin 3 receptor α chain. *Leuk Lymphoma* 2004;45(8):1511-7.

Richards ML, Katz DH. Biology and chemistry of low affinity IgE receptor (Fc ε RII/CD23) [review]. *Crit Rev Immunol* 1991;11(2):65-86.

Rimsza LM, Larson RS, Winter SS, et al. Benign hematogone-rich lymphoid proliferations can be distinguished from B-lineage acute lymphoblastic leukemia by integration of morphology, immunophenotype, adhesion molecule expression, and architectural features. *Am J Clin Pathol* 2000;114(1):66-75.

Robertson PB, Neiman RS, Worapongpaiboon S, John K, Orazi A. 013 (CD99) positivity in hematologic proliferations correlates with TdT positivity. *Mod Pathol* 1997;10(4):277-82.

Robillard N, Avet-Loiseau H, Garand R, et al. CD20 is associated with a small mature plasma cell morphology and t(11;14) in multiple myeloma. *Blood* 2003;102(3):1070-1.

Roozendaal R, Carroll MC. Complement receptors CD21 and CD35 in humoral immunity [review]. *Immunol Rev* 2007;219:157-66.

Rosenwasser LJ, Meng J. Anti-CD23 [review]. *Clin Rev Allergy Immunol* 2005 Aug;29(1):61-72.

Roullet MR, Paessler M, Choi JK. CD61 expression of rhabdomyosarcomas: a curious and cautionary tale. Abstract 1445. *Mod Pathol* 2007;20(suppl 2):314A.

Sadahira Y, Sugihara T, Yawata Y. Expression of p53 and Ki-67 antigen in bone marrow giant proerythroblasts associated with human parvovirus B19 infection. *Int J Hematol* 2001;74(2):147-52.

Sadahira Y, Kanzaki A, Wada H, Yawata Y. Immunohistochemical identification of erythroid precursors in paraffin embedded bone marrow sections: spectrin is a superior marker to glycophorin. *J Clin Pathol* 1999;52(12):919-21.

Sanderson RD, Lalor P, Bernfield M. B lymphocytes express and lose syndecan at specific stages of differentiation. *Cell Regul* 1989;1(1):27-35.

Sato N, Kishi K, Toba K, et al. Simultaneous expression of CD13, CD22 and CD25 is related to the expression of Fc ε R1 in nonlymphoid leukemia. *Leuk Res* 2004;28(7):691-8.

Sattentau QJ, Weiss RA. The CD4 antigen: physiological ligand and HIV receptor [review]. *Cell* 1988;52(5):631-3.

Schanberg LE, Fleenor DE, Kurtzberg J, Haynes BF, Kaufman RE. Isolation and characterization of the genomic human CD7 gene: structural similarity with the murine Thy-1 gene. *Proc Natl Acad Sci U S A* 1991;88(2):603-7.

Scheinecker C, Strobl H, Fritsch G, et al. Granulomonocyte-associated lysosomal protein expression during in vitro expansion and differentiation of CD34+ hematopoietic progenitor cells. *Blood* 1995;86(11):4115-23.

Schenkel AR, Liebman RM, Chen X, Muller WA: CD99 is used for transendothelial migration of monocytes. *FASEB J*. 2001;15:A1178.

References

Schlette E, Fu K, Medeiros LJ. CD23 expression in mantle cell lymphoma: clinicopathologic features of 18 cases. *Am J Clin Pathol* 2003;120(5):760-6.

Schlossman SF, Boumsell L, Gilks W, et al. CD antigens 1993. *J Immunol* 1994;152(1):1-2.

Schmidt-Wolf IG, Dejbakhsh-Jones S, Ginzton N, Greenberg P, Strober S. T-cell subsets and suppressor cells in human bone marrow. *Blood* 1992;80(12):3242-50.

Schwonzen M, Pohl C, Steinmetz T, Wickramanayake PD, Thiele J, Diehl V. Bone marrow involvement in non-Hodgkin's lymphoma: increased diagnostic sensitivity by combination of immunocytology, cytomorphology and trephine histology. *Br J Haematol* 1992;81(3):362-9.

Sebestyén A, Berczi L, Mihalik R, Paku S, Matolcsy A, Kopper L. Syndecan-1 (CD138) expression in human non-Hodgkin lymphomas. *Br J Haematol* 1999;104(2):412-9.

Seftalioglu A, Karakus S, Dundar S, et al. Syndecan-1 (CD138) expression in acute myeloblastic leukemia cells: an immuno electron microscopic study. *Acta Oncol* 2003a;42(1):71-4.

Seftalioglu A, Karakus S. Syndecan-1/CD138 expression in normal myeloid, acute lymphoblastic and myeloblastic leukemia cells. *Acta Histochem* 2003b;105(3):213-21.

Seliem RM, Freeman JK, Steingart RH, Hasserjian RP. Immunophenotypic changes and clinical outcome in B-cell lymphomas treated with Rituximab. *Appl Immunohistochem Mol Morphol* 2006;14(1):18-23.

Sezer O, Niemöller K, Eucker J, et al. Bone marrow microvessel density is a prognostic factor for survival in patients with multiple myeloma. *Ann Hematol* 2000;79(10):574-7.

Shin SS, Sheibani K, Kezirian J, et al. Immunoarchitecture of normal human bone marrow: a study of frozen and fixed tissue sections. *Hum Pathol* 1992;23(6):686-94.

Smith RG, Kitchens RL. Phenotypic heterogeneity of TDT+ cells in the blood and bone marrow: implications for surveillance of residual leukemia. *Blood* 1989;74(1):312-9.

Soligo D, Delia D, Oriani A, et al. Identification of CD34+ cells in normal and pathological BM biopsies by QBEND10 monoclonal antibody. *Leukemia* 1991;5(12):1026-30.

Sorg RV, Kögler G, Wernet P. Identification of cord blood dendritic cells as an immature CD11c− population. *Blood* 1999;93(7):2302-7.

Stamenkovic I, Seed B. The B-cell antigen CD22 mediates monocyte and erythrocyte adhesion. *Nature* 1990;345(6270):74-7.

Stevenson AJ, Chatten J, Bertoni F, Miettinen M. CD99 (p30/32 MIC2) neuroectodermal/Ewing's sarcoma antigen as an immunohistochemical marker: review of more than 600 tumors and the literature experience. *Appl Immunohistochem* 1994;2(4): 231-240.

Strobl H, Scheinecker C, Csmarits B, Majdic O, Knapp W. Flow cytometric analysis of intracellular CD68 molecule expression in normal and malignant haemopoiesis. *Br J Haematol* 1995;90(4):774-82.

Sundeen JT, Longo DL, Jaffe ES. CD5 expression in B-cell small lymphocytic malignancies: correlations with clinical presentation and sites of disease. *Am J Surg Pathol* 1992;16(2):130-7.

Sung CO, Ko YH, Park S, Kim K, Kim W. Immunoreactivity of CD99 in non-Hodgkin's lymphoma: unexpected frequent expression in ALK+ anaplastic large cell lymphoma. *J Korean Med Sci* 2005;20(6):952-6.

Takeuchi S, Furue M. Dendritic cells: ontogeny [review] [published online ahead of print August 1, 2007]. *Allergol Int* 2007;56(3):215-23.

Tan MAL, Chen W, Jones D, et al. Histological and immunophenotypical characterization of anti-immunoblastic T-cell lymphoma (AILT) involving the bone marrow. Abstract 1199. *Mod Pathol* 2007;20(suppl 2):261A-262A.

Tateyama H, Eimoto T, Tada T, Hattori H, Murase T, Takino H. Immunoreactivity of a new CD5 antibody with normal epithelium and malignant tumors including thymic carcinoma. *Am J Clin Pathol* 1999;111(2):235-40.

Terstappen LW, Safford M, Loken MR. Flow cytometric analysis of human bone marrow: III, neutrophil maturation. *Leukemia* 1990;4(9):657-63.

Thaler J, Denz H, Gattringer C, et al. Diagnostic and prognostic value of immunohistological bone marrow examination: results in 212 patients with lymphoproliferative disorders. *Blut* 1987;54(4):213-22.

Thiele JM, Kvasnicka HM. Diagnosis of polycythemia vera based on bone marrow pathology [review]. *Curr Hematol Rep* 2005;4(3):218-23.

Thiele JM, Hoffmann I, Bertsch HP, Fischer R. Myelodysplastic syndromes: immunohistochemical and morphometric evaluation of proliferative activity in erythropoiesis and endoreduplicative capacity of megakaryocytes. *Virchows Arch A Pathol Anat Histopathol* 1993;423(1):33-8.

Tiacci E, Pileri S, Orleth A, et al. PAX5 expression in acute leukemias: higher B-lineage specificity than CD79a and selective association with t(8;21)-acute myelogenous leukemia. *Cancer Res* 2004;64(20):7399-404.

Tonks NK, Charbonneau H, Diltz CD, Fischer EH, Walsh KA. Demonstration that the leukocyte common antigen CD45 is a protein tyrosine phosphatase. *Biochemistry* 1988;27(24):8695-701.

Torlakovic EE. MME (membrane metallo-endopeptidase). *Atlas Genet Cytogenet Oncol Haematol* 2007. Available at: http://AtlasGeneticsOncology.org/Genes/MMEID41386ch3q25.html. Accessed April 15, 2008.

Torlakovic E, Tenstad E, Funderud S, Rian E. CD10+ stromal cells form B-lymphocyte maturation niches in the human bone marrow. *J Pathol* 2005;205(3):311-7.

Torlakovic E, Torlakovic G, Brunning RD. Follicular pattern of bone marrow involvement by follicular lymphoma. *Am J Clin Pathol* 2002a;118(5):780-6.

Torlakovic E, Torlakovic G. Follicular colonization by follicular lymphoma. *Arch Pathol Lab Med* 2002b;126(9):1136-7.

Torlakovic E, Torlakovic G, Nguyen PL, Brunning RD, Delabie J. The value of anti-Pax-5 immunostaining in routinely fixed and paraffin-embedded sections: a novel pan pre-B and B-cell marker. *Am J Surg Pathol* 2002c;26(10):1343-50.

Torlakovic G, Langholm R, Torlakovic E. CD34/QBEND10 immunostaining in the bone marrow trephine biopsy: a study of CD34+ mononuclear cells and megakaryocytes. *Arch Pathol Lab Med* 2002d;126(7):823-8.

Toth B, Wehrmann M, Kaiserling E, Horny HP. Immunophenotyping of acute lymphoblastic leukaemia in routinely processed bone marrow biopsy specimens. *J Clin Pathol* 1999;52(9):688-92.

Trowbridge IS, Thomas ML. CD45: an emerging role as a protein tyrosine phosphatase required for lymphocyte activation and development [review]. *Annu Rev Immunol* 1994;12:85-116.

Tupitsyn NN, Mechetner EB, Baryschnikov AJ, et al. Two different anti-erythroid monoclonal antibodies in immunodiagnosis of human leukemias: a comparative study. *Int J Cancer* 1989;44(4):589-92.

Valent P, Schernthaner GH, Sperr WR, et al. Variable expression of activation-linked surface antigens on human mast cells in health and disease [review]. *Immunol Rev* 2001;179:74-81.

Valent P, Ashman LK, Hinterberger W, et al. Mast cell typing: demonstration of a distinct hematopoietic cell type and evidence for immunophenotypic relationship to mononuclear phagocytes. *Blood* 1989;73(7):1778-85.

van de Loosdrecht AA, Westers TM, Westra AH, Drager AM, van der Velden VH, Ossenkoppele GJ. Identification of distinct prognostic subgroups in low and intermediate-1 risk myelodysplastic syndromes by flow cytometry [published online ahead of print October 30, 2007]. *Blood* 2007;111(3):1067-77.

van der Valk P, Mullink H, Huijgens PC, Tadema TM, Vos W, Meijer CJ. Immunohistochemistry in bone marrow diagnosis. Value of a panel of monoclonal antibodies on routinely processed BM biopsies. *Am J Surg Pathol* 1989;13(2):97-106.

Vandersteenhoven AM, Williams JE, Borowitz MJ. Marrow B-cell precursors are increased in lymphomas or systemic diseases associated with B-cell dysfunction. *Am J Clin Pathol* 1993;100(1):60-6.

Vremec D, Pooley J, Hochrein H, Wu L, Shortman K. CD4 and CD8 expression by dendritic cell subtypes in mouse thymus and spleen. *J Immunol* 2000;164(6):2978-86.

Werner M, Kaloutsi V, Walter K, Buhr T, Bernhards J, Georgii A. Imunohistochemical examination of routinely processed BM biopsies. *Pathol Res Pract* 1992;188(6):707-13.

Wick MR. Immunohistology of neuroendocrine and neuroectodermal tumors [review]. *Semin Diagn Pathol* 2000;17(3):194-203.

Wilkins BS, Green A, Wild AE, Jones DB. Extramedullary haemopoiesis in fetal and adult human spleen: a quantitative immunohistological study. *Histopathology* 1994;24(3):241-7.

Wong KF, Chan JK, Matutes E, et al. Hepatosplenic γ/δ T-cell lymphoma. A distinctive aggressive lymphoma type [review]. *Am J Surg Pathol* 1995 Jun;19(6):718-26.

Wright MD, Tomlinson MG. The ins and outs of the transmembrane 4 superfamily [review]. *Immunol Today* 1994;15(12):588-94.

Wu L, D'Amico A, Winkel KD, Suter M, Lo D, Shortman K. RelB is essential for the development of myeloid-related CD8α− dendritic cells but not of lymphoid-related CD8α+ dendritic cells. *Immunity* 1998;9(6):839-47.

Wu L, Li CL, Shortman K. Thymic dendritic cell precursors: relationship to the T lymphocyte lineage and phenotype of the dendritic cell progeny. *J Exp Med* 1996;184(3):903-11.

Xu Y, McKenna RW, Kroft SH. Comparison of multiparameter flow cytometry with cluster analysis and immunohistochemistry for the detection of CD10 in diffuse large B-Cell lymphomas. *Mod Pathol* 2002;15(4):413-9.

Yaziji H, Battifora H, Barry TS, et al. Evaluation of 12 antibodies for distinguishing epithelioid mesothelioma from adenocarcinoma: identification of a three-antibody immunohistochemical panel with maximal sensitivity and specificity. *Mod Pathol* 2006;19(4):514-23.

Yefenof E, Klein G, Jondal M, Oldstone MB. Surface markers on human B and T-lymphocytes. IX: two-color immunofluorescence studies on the association between EBV receptors and complement receptors on the surface of lymphoid cell lines. *Int J Cancer* 1976;17(6):693-700.

Yoshida C, Takeuchi M. Histiocytic sarcoma: identification of its histiocytic origin using immunohistochemistry [published online February 1, 2008]. *Intern Med* 2008;47(3):165-9.

Yoshikawa K, Seto M, Ueda R, et al. Molecular cloning of the gene coding for the human T-cell differentiation antigen CD7. *Immunogenetics* 1991;33(5-6):352-60.

Yu IT, Rezania D, Messina JL, et al. Differentiating CD4+/CD56+ hematodermic neoplasm from acute monoblastic leukemia. Abstract 1292. *Mod Pathol* 2008;21(suppl 1);283A.

Zhang PJ, Barcos M, Stewart CC, Block AW, Sait S, Brooks JJ. Immunoreactivity of MIC2 (CD99) in acute myelogenous leukemia and related diseases. *Mod Pathol* 2000;13(4):452-8.

Chapter 4
OTHER COMMON MARKERS

4.1 Myeloperoxidase

Myeloperoxidase (MPO), lysozyme (LZ), and lactoferrin (LF) represent myeloid cell–associated lysosomal molecules with bactericidal activity and are widely regarded as specific myeloid lineage markers. Because LF is induced at later stages of the myeloid development, it is not used routinely like MPO and LZ in the detection of myeloid differentiation in acute leukemia or in general for immunohistochemical evaluation of BM biopsies. MPO is contained in primary, azurophilic neutrophil granules, but LF is stored in specific (secondary) granules of neutrophils. In contrast, LZ occurs in both granule types [Bainton 1971; Pryzwansky 1978]. Mature neutrophils express MPO, LZ, and LF, while CD14+ monocytes express MPO and LZ but lack LF [Knapp 1994]. However, MPO is only weakly expressed in the circulating monocytes. Despite low levels of MPO in monocytes, MPO can be demonstrated with IHC in tissue sections in monocytes. MPO also appears less expressed using immunological methods in more mature granulocytes. Some authors have attributed this low expression to the more compact content of secondary granules, with preserved histochemical activity, but less than optimal demonstration on immunohistochemistry [Dallegri 1978]. Myeloperoxidase may be deficient in both AML and CML [Bendix-Hansen 1983; Bendix-Hansen 1986]. In CML, this deficiency is difficult to appreciate with immunohistochemical methods. In myeloid hyperplasia, including myeloproliferative and myelodysplastic/myeloproliferative diseases, there is frequent finding of MPO+/hemoglobin A− cells in a paratrabecular position [Bartl 1982].

In the evaluation of acute leukemia, MPO is an essential marker that should not be substituted by, but appropriately complemented with, other myeloid markers (CD117, CD15, lysozyme, CD68, or other). Because of its high specificity, it remains the best marker of myeloid differentiation. However, it has been pointed out that MPO may not be so useful in evaluating cases in which the number of blasts is low, because MPO is expressed in all stages of myeloid differentiation [Orazi 2006]. Despite CD117, which is a myeloid marker regularly found in both benign and malignant mast cells, MPO is not expressed in mast cells [Dunphy 2007a; Jordan 2001]. However, few cases of cutaneous mast cell disease were found to express MPO [Li 1996].

F4.1.1 Myeloperoxidase in histologically normal bone marrow (BM)

This biopsy is from a 46-year-old man treated with imatinib for chronic myeloid leukemia that is now in histologic remission. The myeloid-erythroid ratio on the aspirate smear was 3.5:1 which is normal. Low magnification revealed a very large number of positive cells. Negative megakaryocytes and erythroid cells can be better appreciated using higher magnification. Early myeloid precursors (red arrow) show more intense staining than bands and segmented neutrophils (blue arrows).

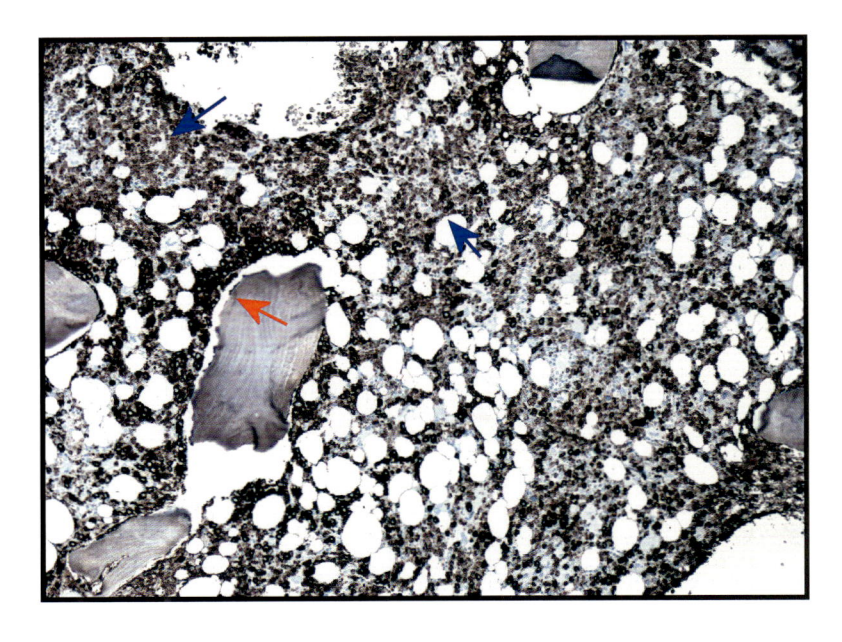

4: Other Common Markers

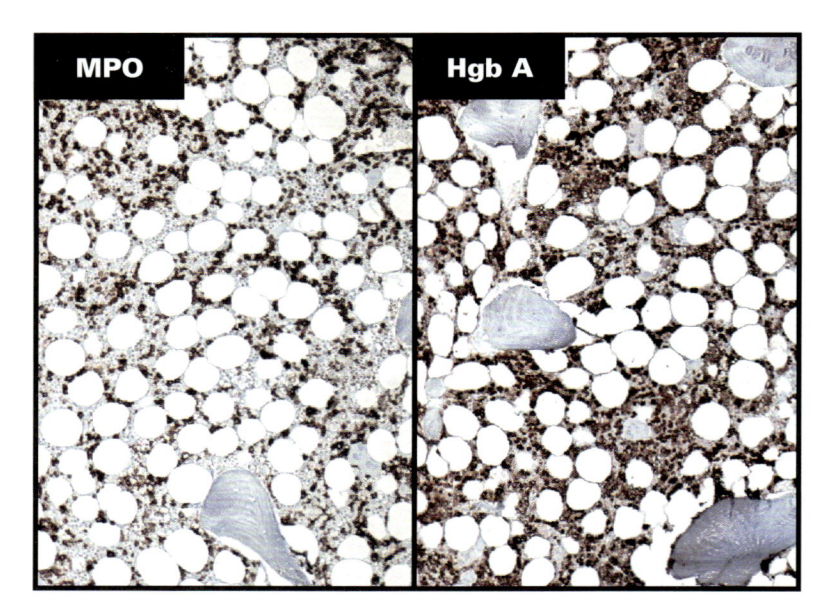

F4.1.2 The use of immunohistochemistry to determine myeloid-erythroid (M-E) ratio

This biopsy specimen is from a patient with neutropenia. The M-E ratio was 1:3 as estimated from myeloperoxidase-negative and hemoglobin A–stained sections. Cytogenetic analysis showed normal findings and there was no evidence of dyshematopoiesis, lymphoproliferative disease, or other malignancy, therefore, the cause was unknown. The correlation between low neutrophil count in the peripheral blood and myeloid hypoplasia is illustrated here, but such correlation is not always present.

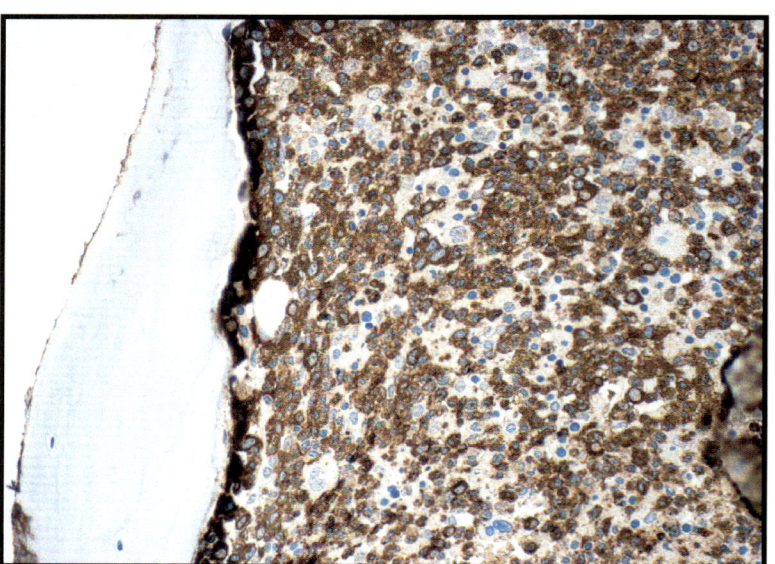

F4.1.3 Myeloperoxidase (MPO) shows the strongest expression in most immature neutrophils

This biopsy specimen is from a patient with chronic phase chronic myeloid leukemia (CML) and illustrates a higher expression of MPO in the myeloid precursors located in a paratrabecular location. This finding is frequently asymmetric and it is often not possible to show this differential expression of MPO in myeloid maturation. It may be easier to show this differential expression in CML, because some degree of MPO deficiency in neutrophils has been described in this disease.

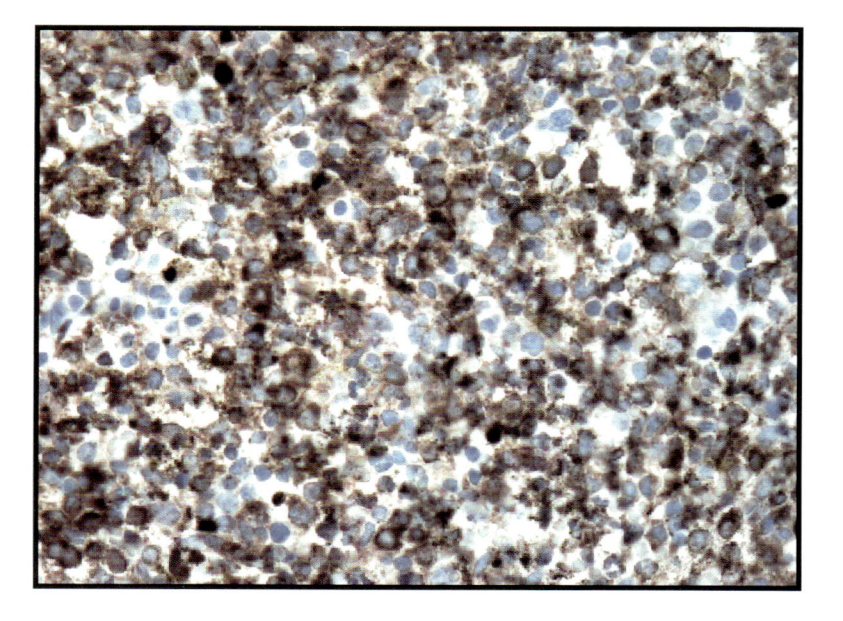

F4.1.4 Myeloperoxidase (MPO) in chronic myelomonocytic leukemia (CMML)

Some cases of CMML show weaker expression of MPO than that typically found in normal neutrophil precursors or in chronic myeloid leukemia (CML). This may be similar to difficulty in demonstrating monocytic markers (like CD68) in monocytic cells of CMML, which may be easier to demonstrate in CML than in CMML [Yang 2000].

4.1 Myeloperoxidase

F4.1.5 **Myeloperoxidase (MPO); suboptimal staining**

MPO is frequently expressed at high levels in most biopsies. Therefore, it may be difficult to optimally titrate the primary antibody dilution. It is tempting to go to higher dilutions to achieve more readable results and save money. The myeloid blasts in the biopsy specimen from a case of acute myeloid leukemia shown on the left are false negative. The staining is likely to have low sensitivity when more mature neutrophils are barely positive as illustrated here. Repeated staining showed that almost all blasts were positive. A true-negative case is illustrated on the right; even at low magnification, MPO is strongly positive in segmented neutrophils.

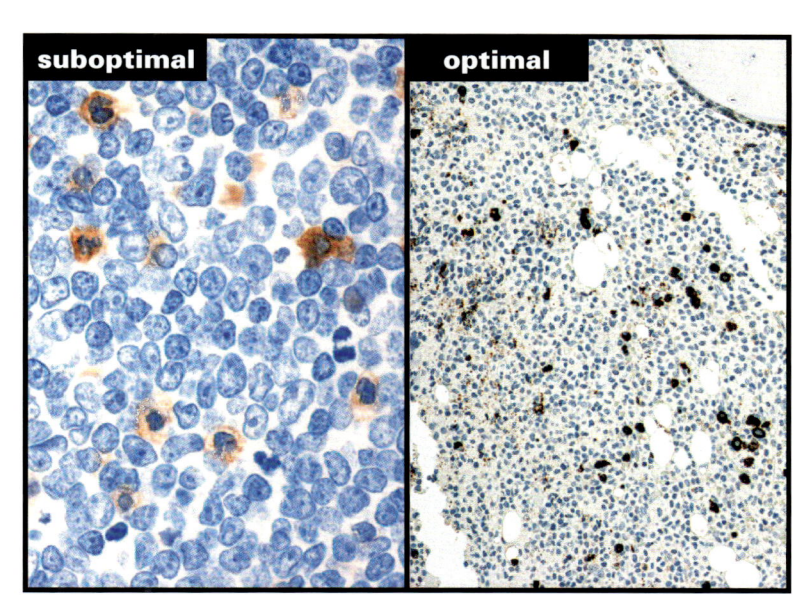

F4.1.6 **Myeloperoxidase in acute hypocellular leukemia**

While the cells have morphologic features consistent with blasts, the diagnosis may be difficult to establish with certainty without clear demonstration of markedly increased CD34+ cells, which accounted for 27% cells in a 500 cell count in this biopsy. Both aspirate smears and core biopsy imprints were inadequate because of marked dilution with peripheral blood. CD117 was also expressed in small interstitial blast clusters (arrow). Acute leukemias with hypocellular marrows are rare and almost always myeloid.

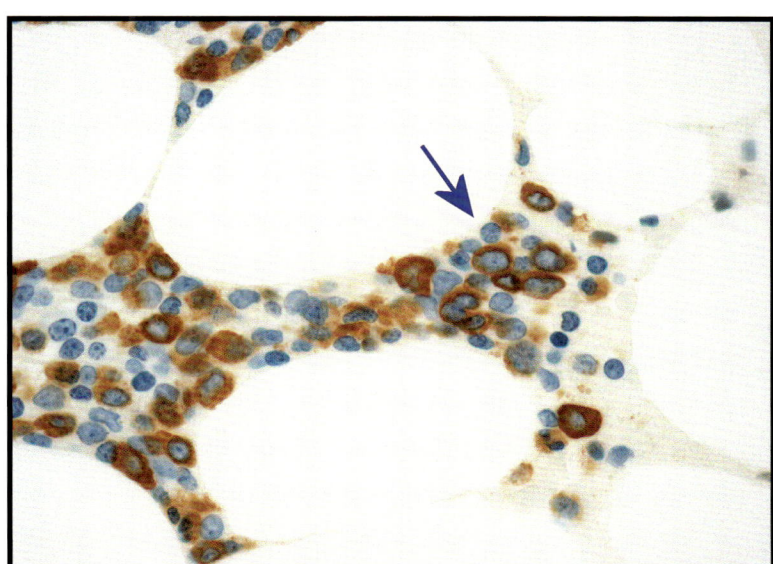

F4.1.7 **Comparison of CD15 and myeloperoxidase (MPO) expression in acute myeloid leukemia without maturation**

While MPO is consistently expressed in such leukemias, CD15 does not always give corresponding results. This illustrates the importance of using appropriate lineage markers for leukemia immunophenotyping with immunohistochemistry. MPO cannot simply be replaced by some other myeloid marker available in the laboratory.

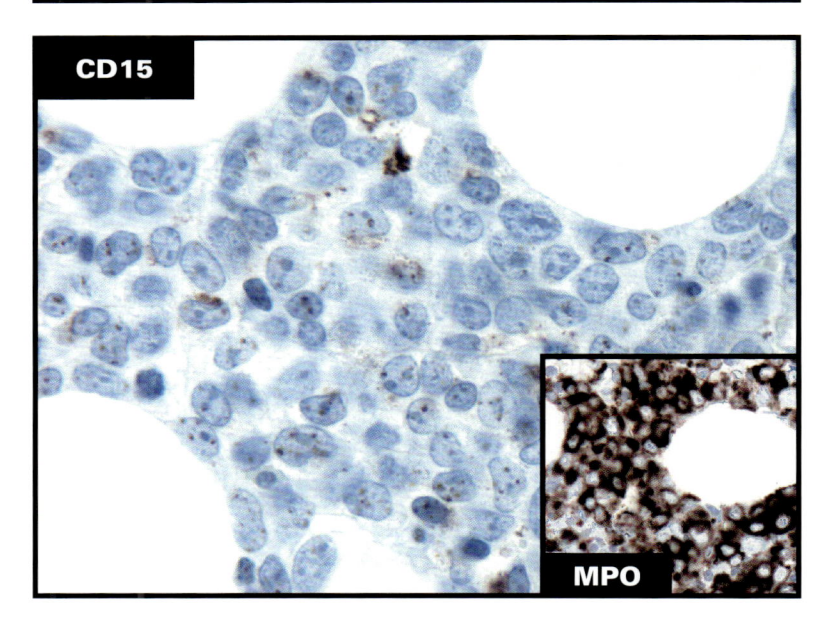

4: Other Common Markers

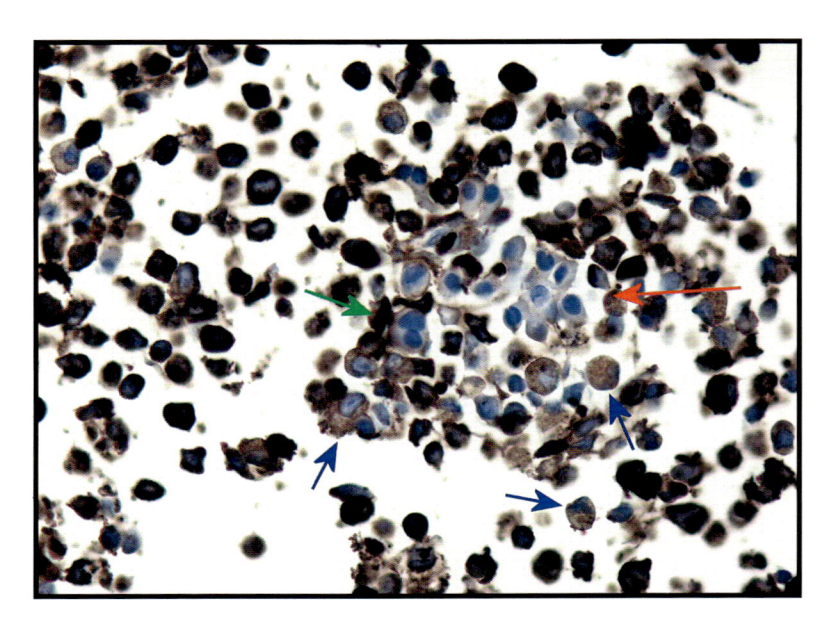

F4.1.8 Myeloperoxidase in acute myeloid leukemia with maturation

Only plasma cells (red arrow) that were focally increased and what appeared to be rare dysplastic megakaryocytes (green arrow) are negative for MPO. This unique case had increased, but morphologically normal eosinophils which expressed MPO (blue arrows). No inv16 or other abnormalities of chromosome 16 were demonstrated. Note that eosinophils here express relatively low levels of MPO.

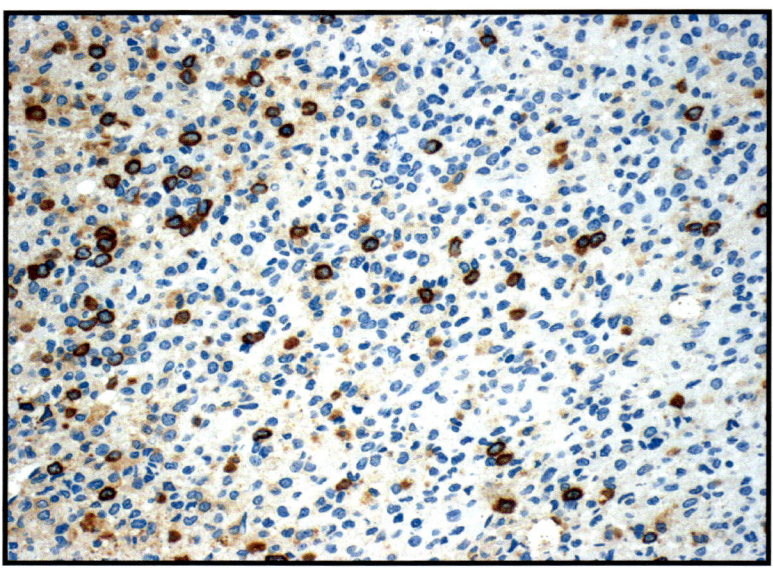

F4.1.9 Myeloperoxidase (MPO) in acute myelomonocytic leukemia

In myelomonocytic leukemia, immunohistochemistry often shows that neutrophil and monocytic areas are not fully intermixed, but areas with predominant neutrophil and predominant monocytic differentiation are present, as shown here. A predominantly monocytic area, negative for MPO, is illustrated. A transition area is also present (left). In the neutrophil areas, almost all cells are MPO-positive.

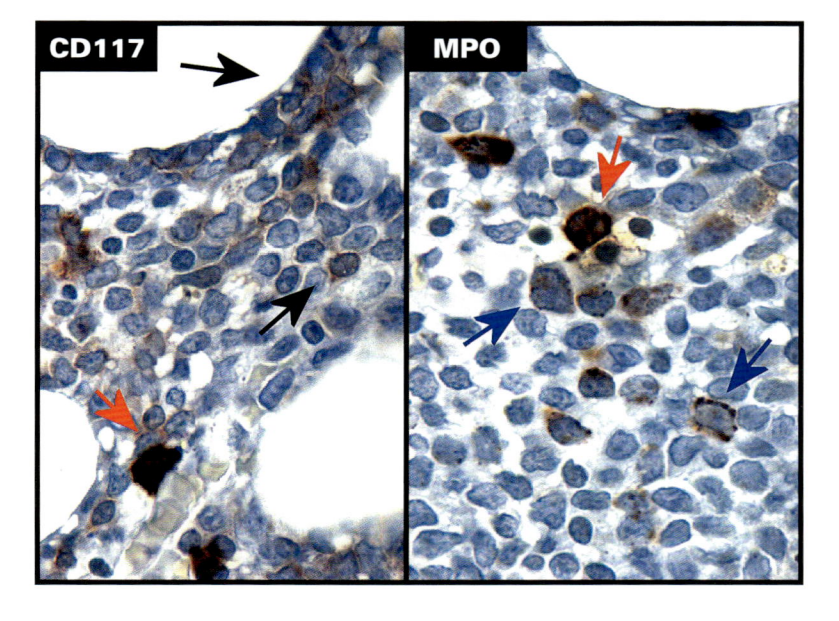

F4.1.10 Myeloperoxidase (MPO) compared with CD117 expression in biphenotypic acute leukemia (acute myeloid leukemia/precursor B-cell lymphoblastic leukemia)

On flow cytometry, both CD117 and MPO were positive, as well as several markers of precursor B-ALL. Such weak expression of CD117, as shown (black arrows), is not rare in immunohistochemistry in acute leukemia. MPO is found in fine cytoplasmic granules as expected (blue arrows). Red arrows point to mast cell in CD117 and neutrophil in MPO.

4.1 Myeloperoxidase

F4.1.11 Dotlike positivity for myeloperoxidase (MPO) in acute lymphoblastic leukemia (ALL)

In this CD13+ precursor B-cell lymhoblastic leukemia, rare cells show dotlike positivity for MPO, but the dots are clearly extracellular in other areas. This result should be interpreted as negative. If this case was truly positive for MPO, it would be classified as acute biphenotypic leukemia. If minimal or "dotlike cytoplasmic" positivity is used as evidence for disease classification, it has to be unequivocal and present in at least 10% of the leukemic blasts. The cytochemistry cutoff at 3% does not apply here.

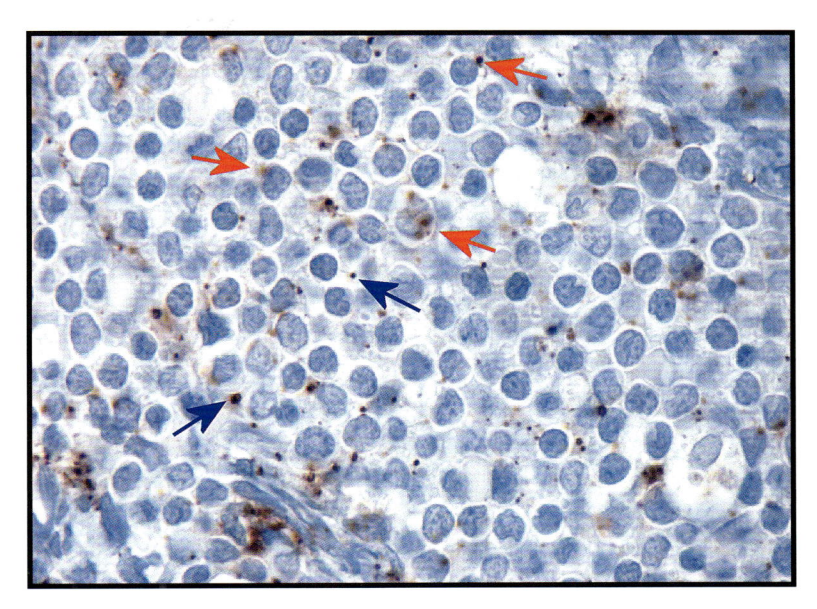

F4.1.12 Myeloperoxidase in precursor B-cell lymphoblastic leukemia day 7 after chemotherapy

There was no evidence of residual leukemic cells in this biopsy specimen. Early erythroid reconstitution is noted (blue arrows) and rare early myeloid precursors are found. In this particular case at this stage of myeloid reconstitution, the positive cells were not adjacent to bony trabeculae, but rather in close association with dilated sinuses (red arrows). Very strong staining is typical of very early myeloid precursors.

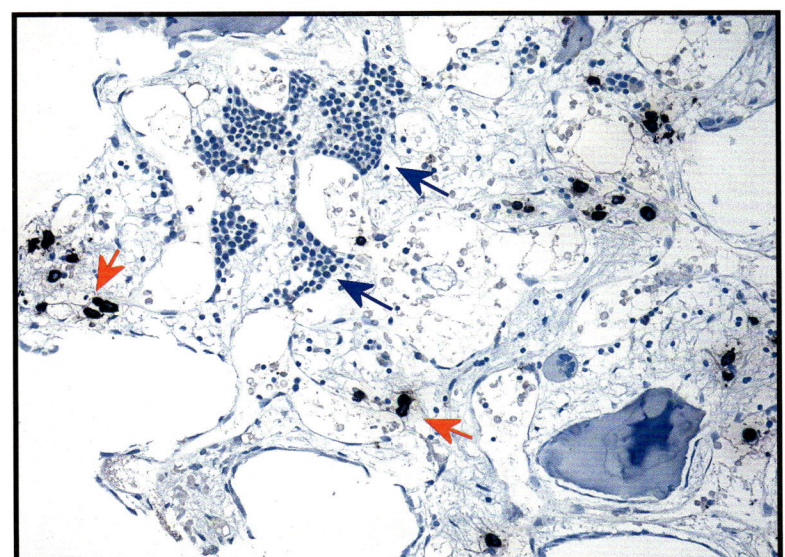

4.2 Hemoglobin A (HgbA)

Detection of HgbA with IHC has been in use for many years [Pinkus 1981; Forni 1983]. The optimization of the protocols has been difficult and some laboratories report high background and therefore do not find it to be a very useful and informative marker [Dunphy 2007a]. In optimized protocols, HgbA is a very useful marker in the evaluation of the M-E ratio together with MPO, and also in immunophenotyping of acute leukemias. HgbA concentration increases as red blood cells mature and is highest in the non-nucleated red blood cells [Dover 1980]. However, nucleated red blood cell precursors in BM sections stain stronger than non-nucleated circulating red blood cells. The earliest erythroid precursors show weak expression, which dramatically changes in intermediate and late nucleated erythroid cells. Suddenly, for reasons that are not clear, the staining of non-nucleated red blood cells becomes weak again despite their high HgbA content. This is likely to be related to tissue processing and possible leakage of the HgbA out of the cells. In any case, this phenomenon works well because mature red blood cell interference is minimized and much less prominent than in sections stained by glycophorin A.

When erythroid hyperplasia or predominance is detected, BM recovery should be considered along with other pathologic cases of inverted M-E ratio. In particular, after chemotherapy, erythroid precursors proliferate more rapidly than myeloid cells, which has been reported after treatment with virtually all chemotherapeutic agents [Khalil 2007; Adelstein 1985].

Hemoglobin F may also find use in evaluation of the bone marrow biopsies since it is reported to be expressed in most hypoplastic myelodysplastic syndromes, but only rarely so in anaplastic anemia [Choi 2002; Iwasaki 2008].

4: Other Common Markers

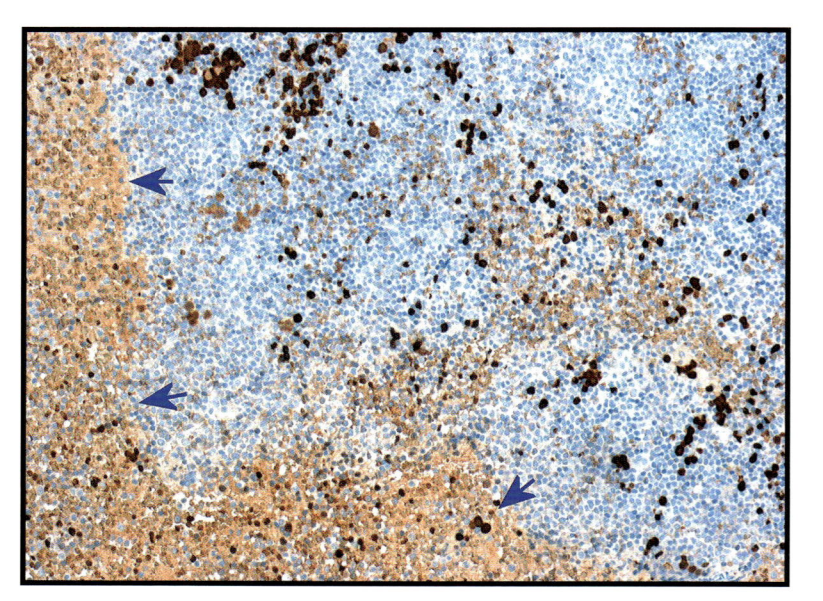

F4.2.1 Hemoglobin A (HgbA) in hypercellular bone marrow with neutrophil hyperplasia

In contrast to glycophorin (see F4.2.2), HgbA staining is stronger in nucleated red blood cells in the bone marrow than in circulating red blood cells. This image shows a clot specimen and the blue arrow indicates the border between the BM particle and clotted blood. However, optimization of anti-HgbA antibodies can be difficult. Demonstration of HgbA rather than glycophorin A is recommended for determination of the myeloid-to-erythroid ratio.

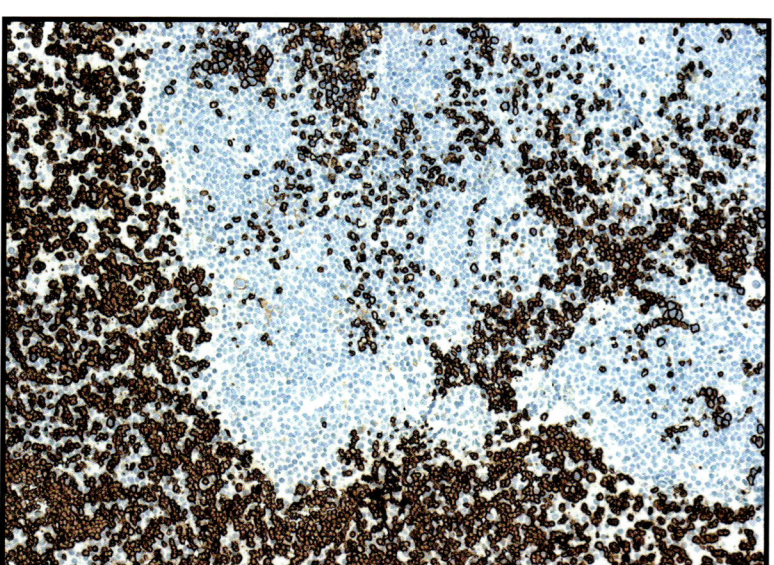

F4.2.2 Glycophorin A in hypercellular bone marrow with myeloid hyperplasia

Glycophorin A antibodies are generally technically non-problematic. The drawback is that all nucleated and non-nucleated red blood cells show strong expression and therefore the myeloid-erythroid ratio may be difficult to estimate (for comparison see F4.2.1). However, this is an excellent choice for demonstration of erythroleukemia, when blasts are present in sheets and the contaminating mature red blood cells are very few.

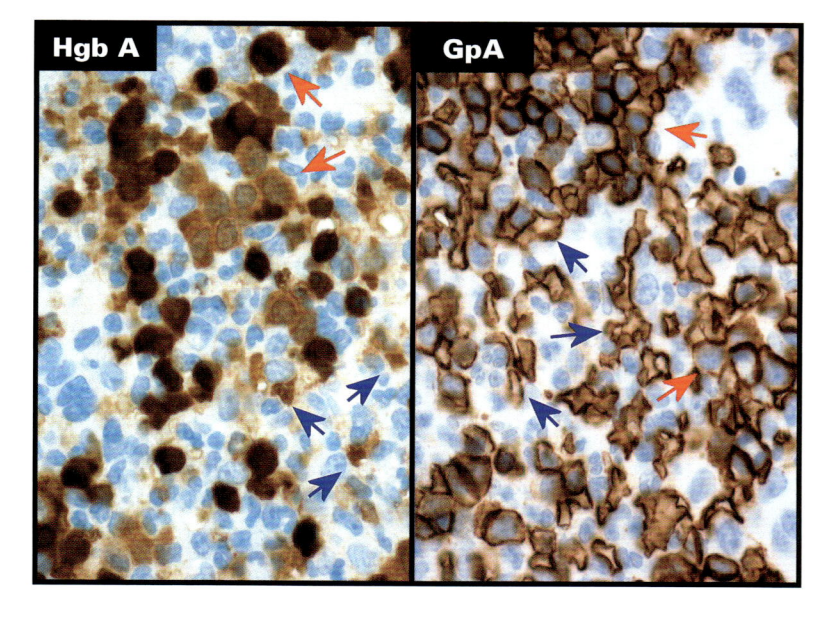

F4.2.3 Hemoglobin A vs glycophorin A

Hemoglobin A clearly highlights nucleated red blood cells (red arrows) more than non-nucleated red blood cells (blue arrows), which is not the situation with glycophorin A staining, where high magnification examination is necessary to distinguish the two.

4.2 Hemoglobin A

F4.2.4 Hemoglobin A in thin tissue sections

In widely distributed antigens with a high level of expression, it is difficult to optimize protocols. Thin tissue sections are very helpful in such optimization because they enable interpretation of the results even in heavily stained cells side by side with negative and weakly positive cells. Sections of 2 to 4 μm appear to be the best; sections in routine work often have a thickness of 8 to 15 μm.

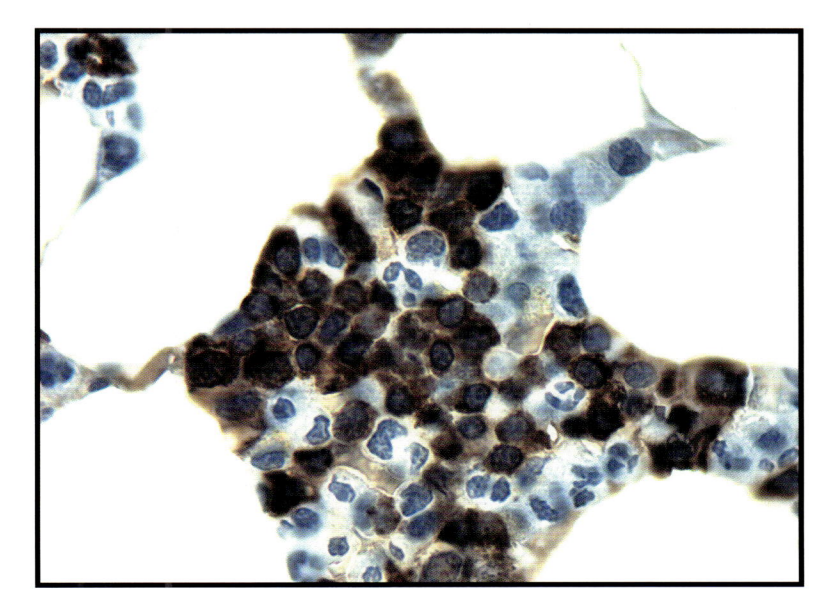

F4.2.5 Differential expression of hemoglobin A (HgbA) in erythroid maturation

Six groups of red blood cells (erythrons) are demonstrated. In erythroid maturation, as cells acquire more hemoglobin, the nucleus becomes more pyknotic, and the cell decreases in size. Non-nucleated red blood cells should have the highest HgbA concentration. However, they are weakly stained similar to very early precursors (blue arrow). Moderate (green arrow) and intense staining (red arrows) are generally found in intermediate stages.

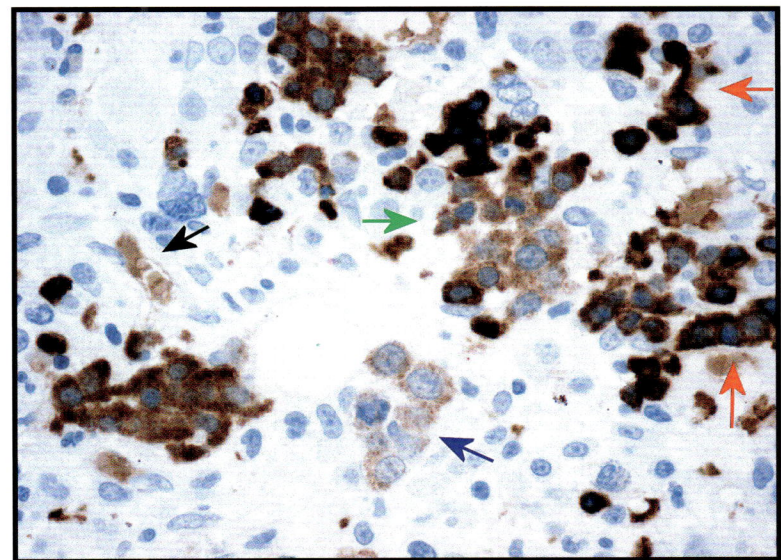

F4.2.6 Hemoglobin A (HgbA) in suboptimally fixed clot sections

Clot sections have a high content of peripheral blood, which can be more or less successfully removed before the tissue is fixed. A high content of blood impedes prompt fixation, which may result in poor antigen preservation. The image on the left shows a suboptimally fixed clot specimen with quite strong HgbA staining, but poor localization of the antigen. The image on the right shows the same biopsy section that was optimally fixed. The signal-to-noise ratio and the antigen localization are better.

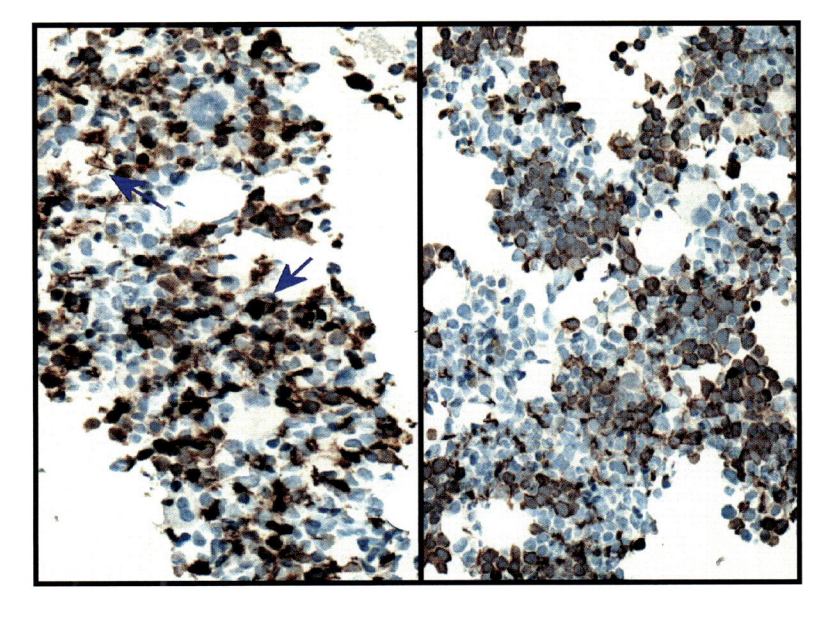

4: Other Common Markers

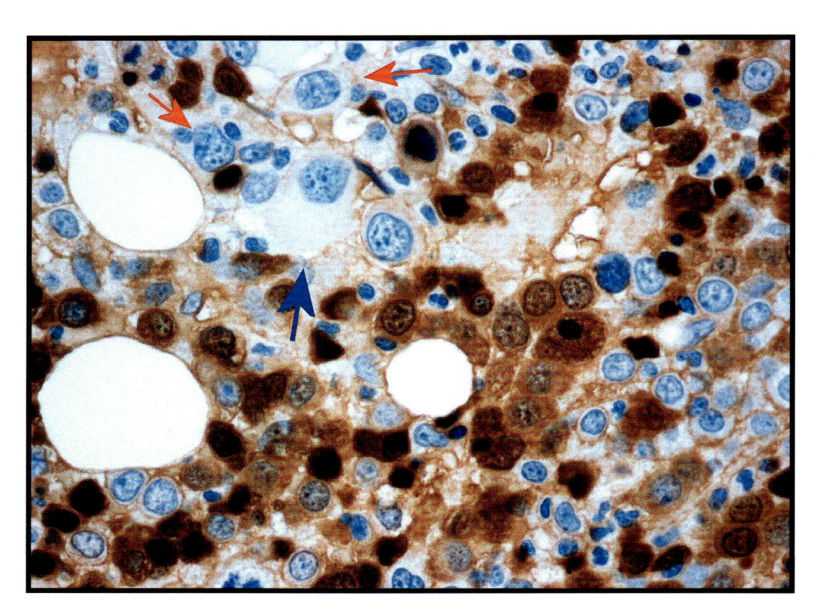

F4.2.7 Hemoglobin A (HgbA) in myeloid/erythroid leukemia

This case of acute myeloid/erythroid leukemia shows variable expression of HgbA. Erythroid markers are more expressed in pure erythroid leukemia than in the myeloid/erythroid variant. In this field, a few possible erythroid precursors appear negative for HgbA (red arrow). Compare this with the variable glycophorin A expression in myeloid/erythroid leukemia in F3.34.5. Blue arrow points to a possible small megakaryocyte.

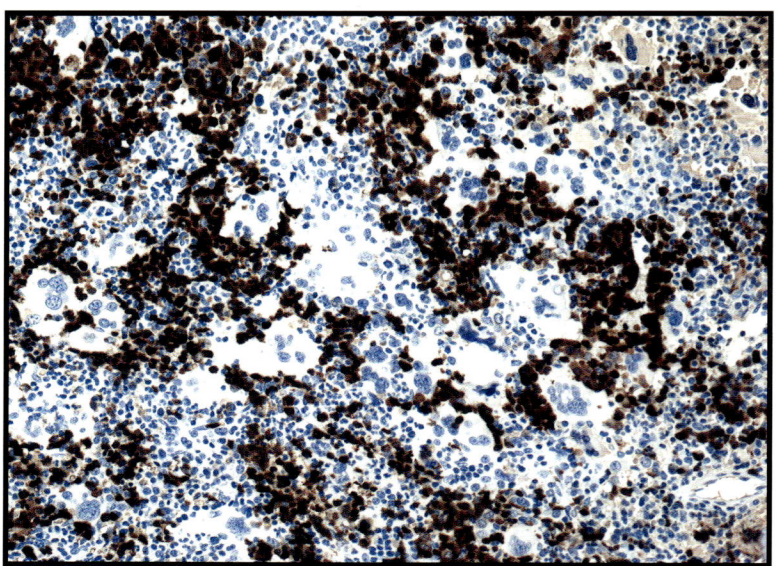

F4.2.8 Hemoglobin A (HgbA) in erythroid hyperplasia in myeloproliferative disease

This biopsy specimen is from a 72-year-old woman with prefibrotic stage chronic idiopathic myelofibrosis. As erythroid areas increase in size, they start to arborize, as shown here. Megakaryocyte localization shows no predilection for either myeloid or erythroid zones and they appear to be present equally in both.

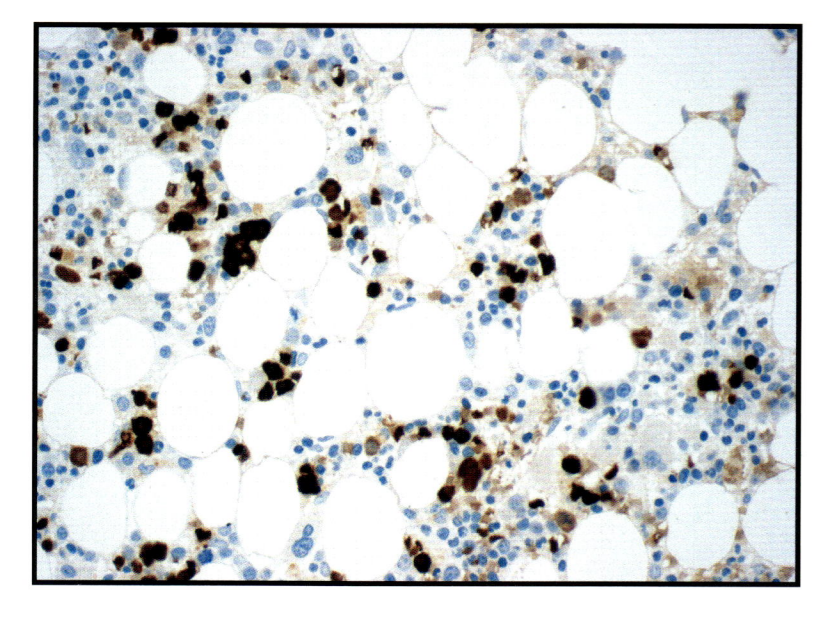

F4.2.9 Hemoglobin A (HgbA) in hypoplastic bone marrow with aplastic anemia

This specimen is from a 57-year-old woman with pancytopenia. The overall BM cellularity was estimated at 20%. A follow-up biopsy revealed further decrease in the BM cellularity and overall findings were most compatible with aplastic anemia.

4.3 Mast Cell Tryptase

Two types of human mast cells have been identified based on their composition of neutral proteases. MC_{TC} cells contain tryptase in their secretory granules and are the predominant type in alveolar walls of the lung and small intestinal mucosa. MC_{TC} cells contain tryptase in addition to chymase and human mast cell carboxypeptidase. MC_{TC} cells are the predominant type of mast cell present in the skin and in the submucosa of the small intestine [Irani 1991; Horny 2007]. Therefore, mast cell tryptase (MCT) IHC will detect all mast cells and has been established as a sensitive and specific marker of both benign and malignant mast cells [Horny 1998]. However, it has also been demonstrated in basophilic granulocytes as well as in myeloid blasts [Samorapoompichit 2001; Sperr 2001]. Even though mast cell disorders are diagnosed by morphologic examination, the task is simplified by using IHC for MCT. Mast cells can be detected with IHC using a murine monoclonal antitryptase antibody, which is a more sensitive method than detection of metachromasia with toluidine blue [Irani 1989]. Finding of round cell infiltrates that are MCT+ does not designate such cells as mast cells [Horny 2006]. This finding, termed TROCI-BM by Horny et al [2006], refers to tryptase-positive round cell infiltrates in the BM, which were found in 6 different rare myeloid neoplasms. 2D7 is an Ag that is specific for basophilic granulocytes and may be helpful, but it is not widely available.

The WHO classification of mastocytosis includes 7 categories: cutaneous mastocytosis (CM), indolent systemic mastocytosis (ISM), SM with an associated clonal hematological non–mast cell lineage disease (SM-AHNMD), aggressive SM (ASM), mast cell leukemia (MCL), mast cell sarcoma, and extracutaneous mastocytoma [Valent 2001]. If neoplastic mast cells are detected in the BM, the patient has systemic mastocytosis (SM) with or without skin or other organ involvement. Mast cell disease can be associated with various other hematologic neoplasms designated SM with an associated non–mast cell clonal hematologic disease (SM-AHNMD). If mastocytosis is detected/confirmed with MCT (+/− other markers), the BM needs to be further evaluated to exclude other hematologic malignancies [Horny 2007]. Compared with MDS, MPD more often shows increased mast cells without evidence of SM and often spindled/dyspoietic mast cells [Dunphy 2005].

F4.3.1 Mast cell tryptase (MCT) in histologically normal bone marrow

This biopsy specimen is from a 48-year-old man with recently diagnosed follicular lymphoma. This BM specimen was obtained for staging. There was mild myeloid hyperplasia. This image illustrates a small number of unremarkable mast cells, which is a normal finding. One possible slightly spindled mast cell was noted histologically (arrow).

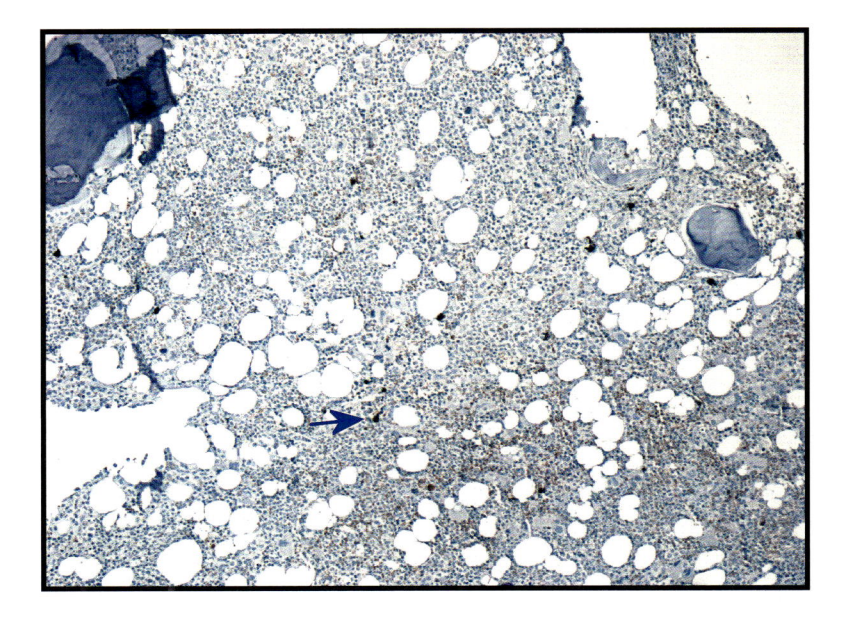

4: Other Common Markers

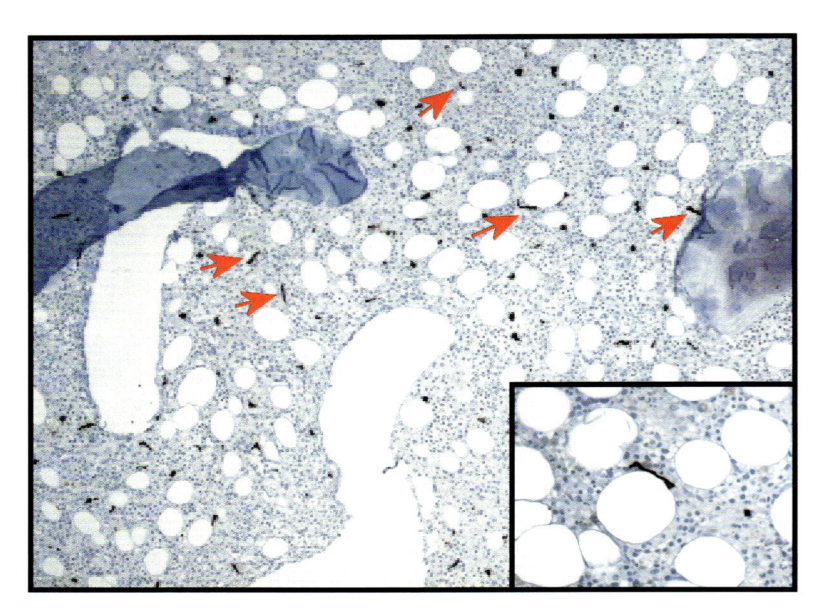

F4.3.2 **Mast cell tryptase in reactive bone marrow in 37-year-old patient with rheumatoid arthritis**

This patient had no clinical evidence of mast cell disease. However, a small population of spindled mast cells was present throughout the BM core biopsy specimen. Rare spindled mast cells were also found in the aspirate smears. Two years later, there was no evidence of mast cell disease, suggesting that the spindle cell morphology of rare/occasional mast cells is not in itself sufficient for the diagnosis of mast cells disease.

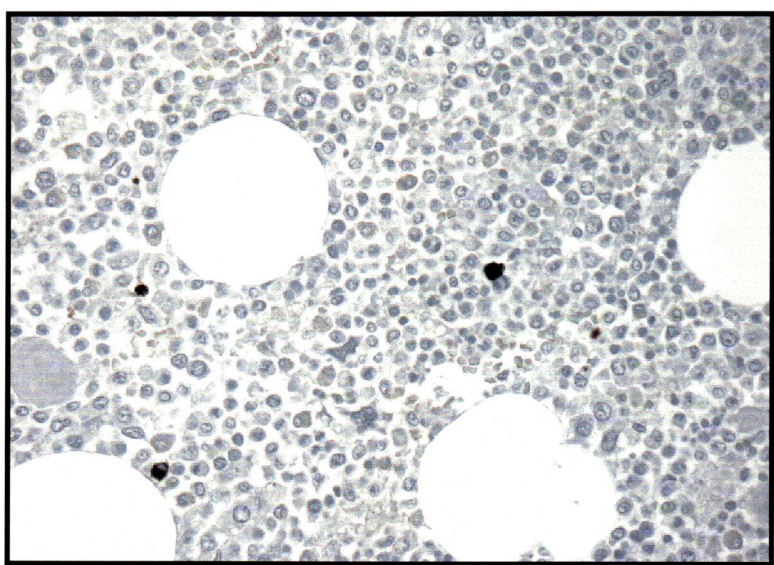

F4.3.3 **Mast cell tryptase (MCT) in a postmortem bone marrow specimen**

Despite autolytic changes, the MCT antigen appears well preserved and can be easily detected with immunohistochemistry in autopsy samples. Mast cells are rare, small, and round, which is a normal finding.

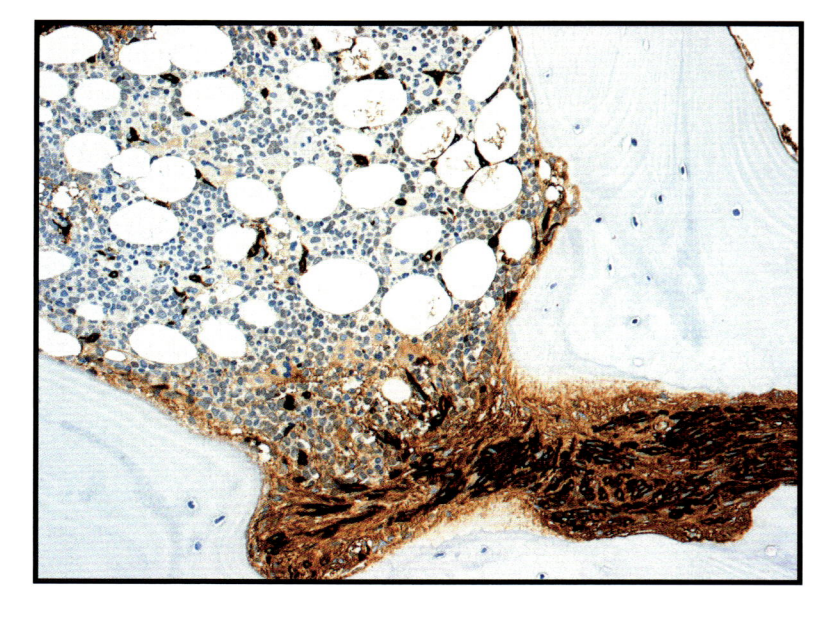

F4.3.4 **Mast cell tryptase (MCT) in systemic mastocytosis (SM)**

Atypical spindled cells strongly positive for MCT are present in a paratrabecular location and somewhat smaller forms interstitially. This is very typical of systemic mastocytosis. This image illustrates one major and one minor criterion for the diagnosis of SM: a solid tight aggregate of more than 15 mast cells (major criterion) and prominent spindle cell morphology (minor criterion), which is sufficient for diagnosis.

F4.3.5 Mast cell tryptase in systemic mastocytosis

Even though the number of atypical mast cells is very low and in the range of reactive changes, the extensive margination along the bony trabecula by mast cells and their spindle cell morphology satisfy the diagnostic criteria without the use of other specific markers of atypical mast cells such as CD25. CD2 is of limited value because of difficulties in interpretation, while there are no definite guidelines for CD35 immunohistochemistry.

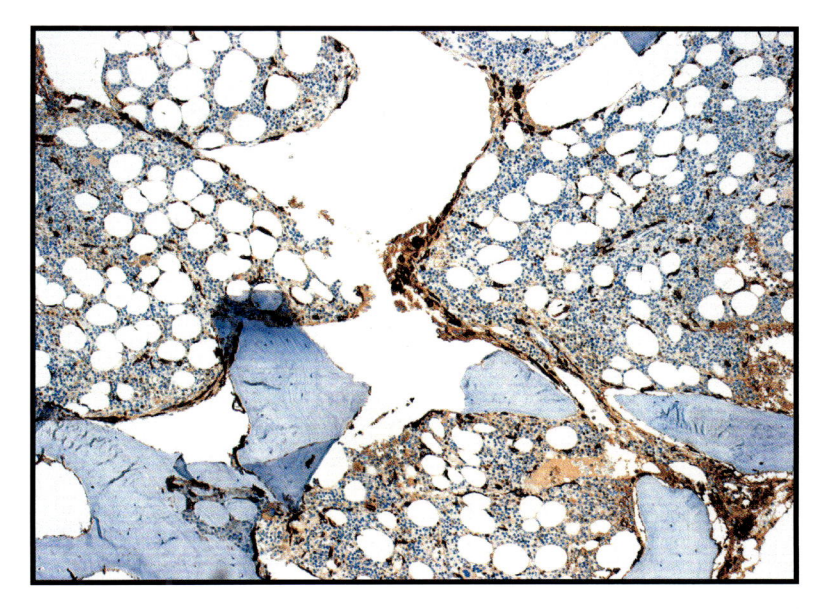

F4.3.6 Mast cell tryptase in systemic mastocytosis

These patchy infiltrates were CD117+; serum tryptase was increased, and many spindled mast cells were identified in the aspirate smears. When patchy infiltrates that are not associated with bone are found in the bone marrow, an important mimicker of mastocytosis should be considered (tentatively termed "fibromastocytic lesion" by Prof P Horny). In this condition, there is focal fibrosis and mast cells are not so numerous (not illustrated here).

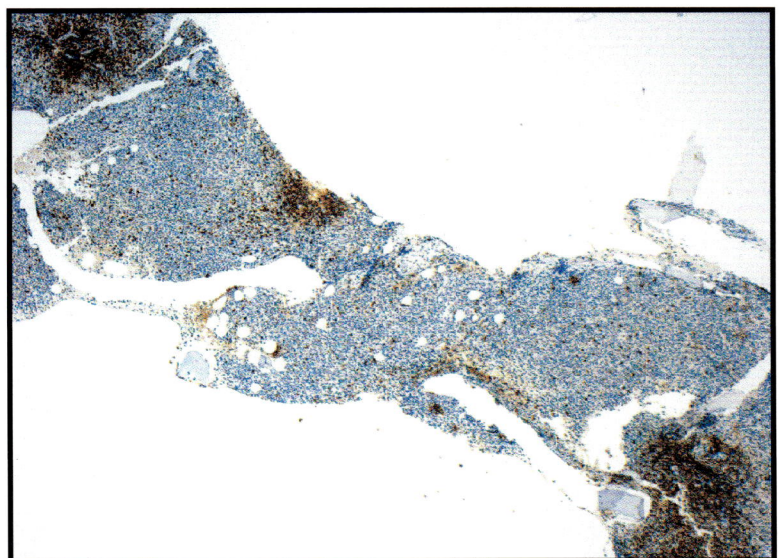

F4.3.7 Mast cell tryptase (MCT) in systemic mastocytosis

These 2 different cases illustrate malignant mast cells with round cell morphology and variability of MCT expression. The intensity of staining may also significantly vary from cell to cell in each case. Blasts in acute myeloid leukemia and basophils can also be positive for MCT; therefore, when only round cell infiltrates are present, further investigation as recommended for TROCI-bone marrow is required.

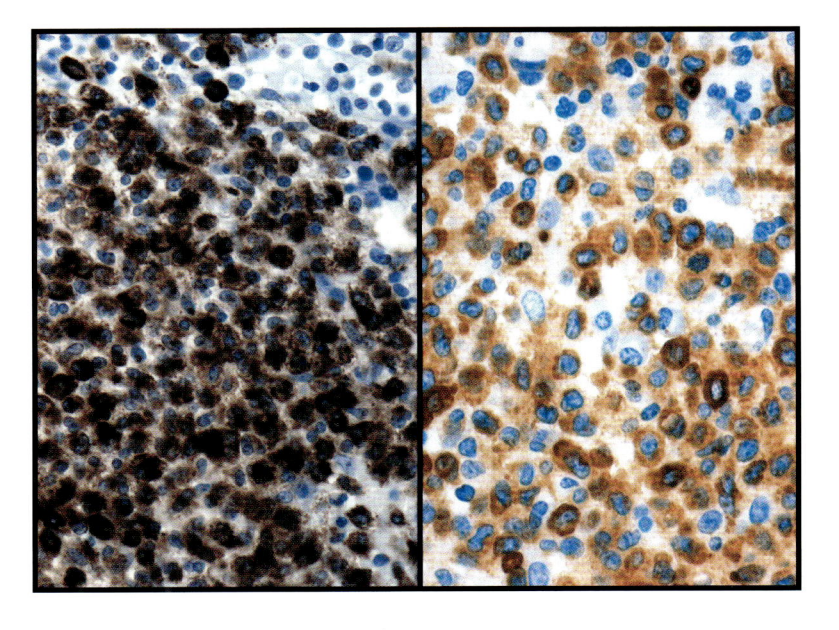

4: Other Common Markers

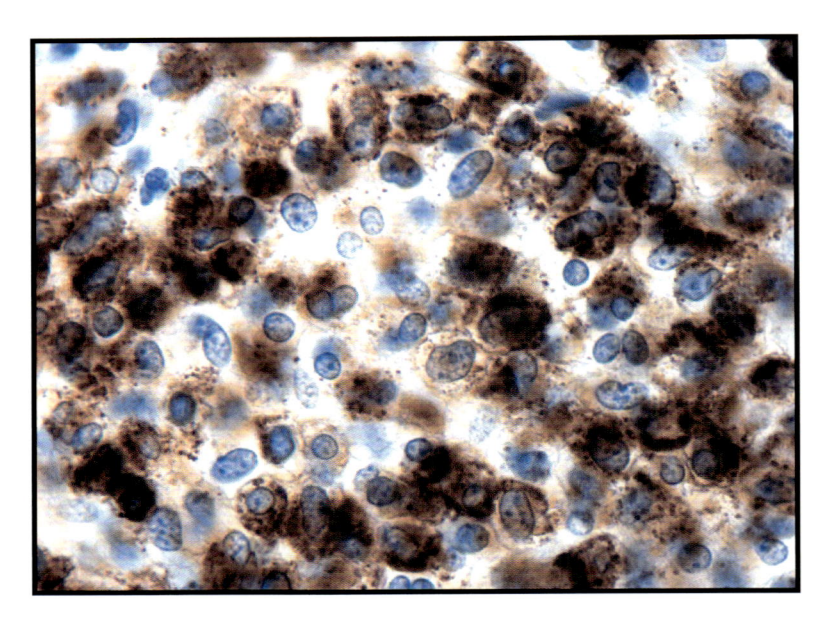

F4.3.8 Mast cell tryptase (MCT) in systemic mastocytosis–associated in non–mast cell clonal hematologic disease (slide courtesy of P Horny, MD, Institute of Pathology, Ansbach, Germany)

There is weak and very irregular distribution of MCT positivity. In such cases it is obvious that MCT is confined to mast cell (secretory) granules. As a result, cases with hypogranular mast cells usually show weaker staining. Even if the cells show no metachromasia on toluidine blue staining, they may turn significantly positive with MCT immunohistochemistry.

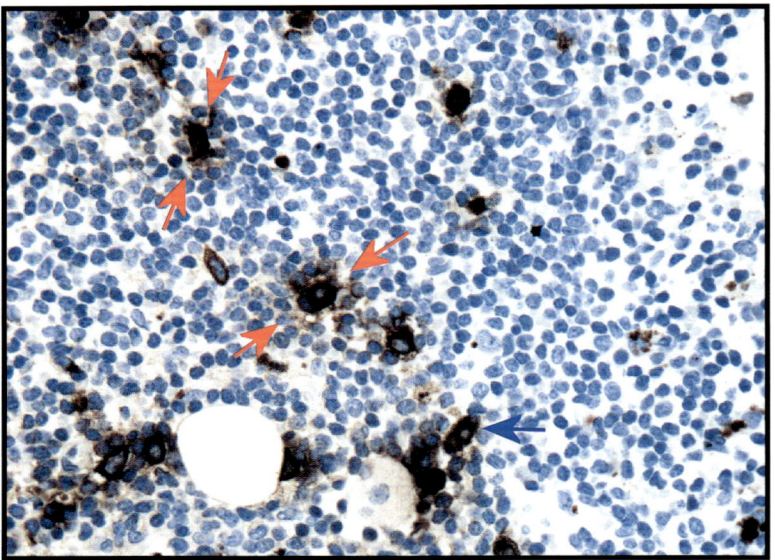

F4.3.9 Chymase in mast cells (slide courtesy of P Horny, MD, Institute of Pathology, Ansbach, Germany)

While mast cell tryptase is present in all cells, chymase is found only in a subset. The staining results are identical, including the overshoot of weak positivity because of leakage of the antigen around the cells in all strongly positive mast cells (red arrows), which show borders of weak positivity extending beyond cell borders. Some positive cells do not show this phenomenon (blue arrow).

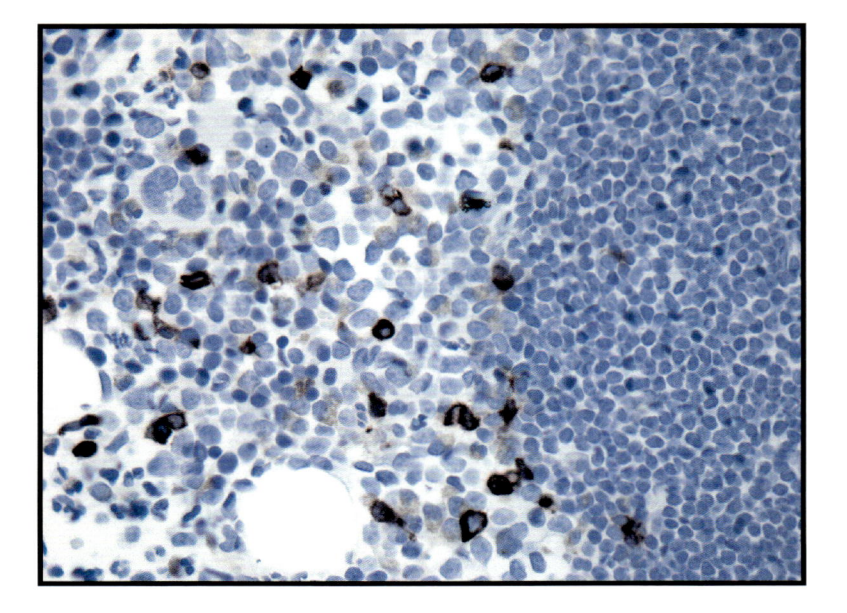

F4.3.10 Mast cell tryptase around lymphoid aggregates

Both benign and malignant lymphoid aggregates can be surrounded by increased mast cells that are usually benign but may also be malignant. Therefore, when lymphoid aggregates and mast cells are seen together, both components should be given separate consideration. This chronic lymphocytic leukemia aggregate is associated with a local increase in mast cells.

F4.3.11 Mast cell tryptase (MCT) in rare cells in chronic myeloid leukemia (CML)

Mast cells are not increased in Ph+ CML and many other myeloid or lymphoproliferative disorders. Basophils also stain with MCT, but this case had far more eosinophils than basophils. Only one case of Ph+ CML associated with systemic mastocytosis has been reported [Agis 2005].

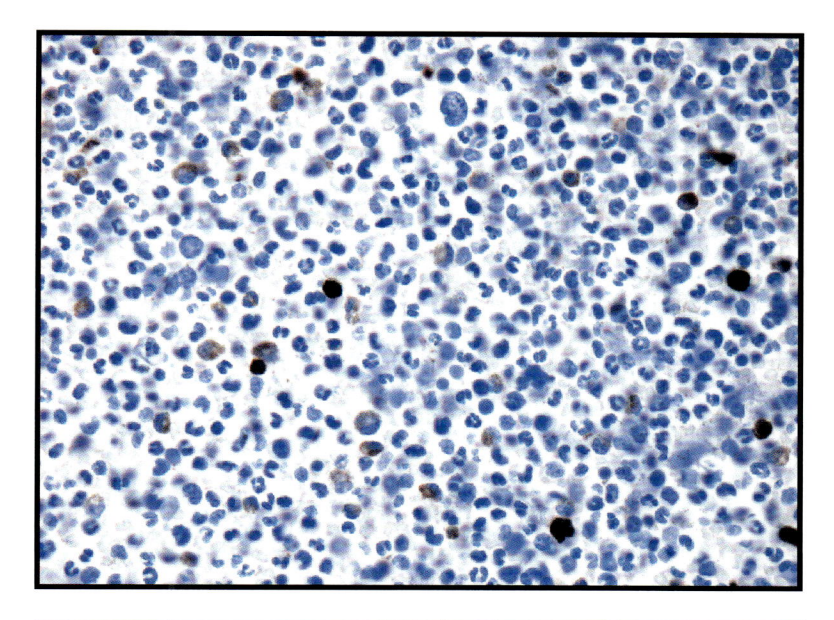

F4.3.12 Mast cell tryptase (MCT) in chronic myeloid leukemia (CML) in histologic remission after imatinib therapy

This is an example of TROCI-bone marrow in CML, but probably the smallest focus that can still be designated as such. TROCI-BM consists of a compact aggregate of round cells that are positive for MCT. The cells were negative for CD34 and CD117. However, 2D7 antibody was not available to confirm the basophilic nature of the cells. At the time of this writing, 3 years later, there is no progression of disease.

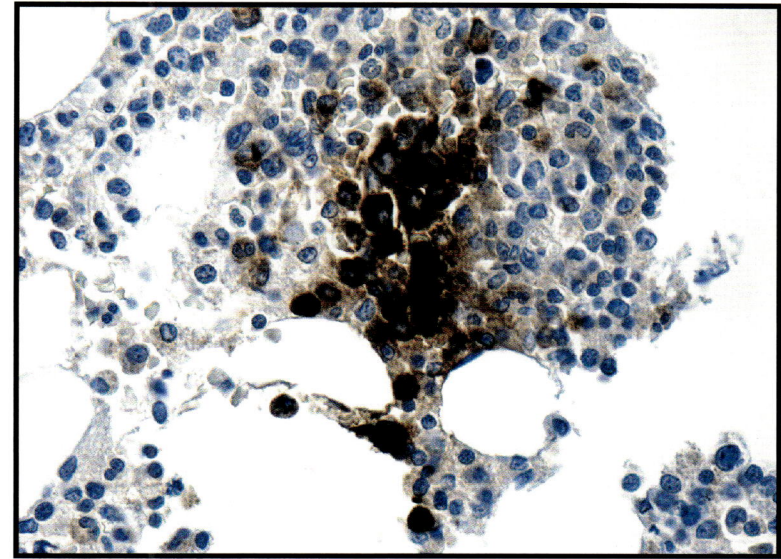

F4.3.13 Mast cell tryptase (MCT) in chronic myeloid leukemia (CML; slide courtesy of P Horny, MD, Institute of Pathology, Ansbach, Germany)

It is not possible to determine with certainty the cell type of very strongly MCT+ cells, but they are probably mast cells (blue arrows). Weaker positive cells (red arrows) are likely to represent basophils, which are increased in CML. Widely available staining for CD117 may help distinguish the two (see F4.3.14).

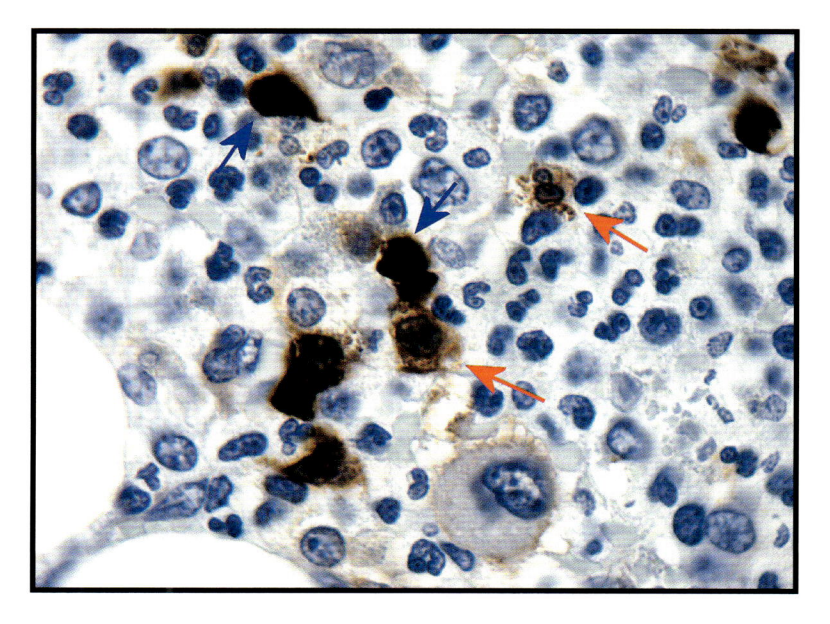

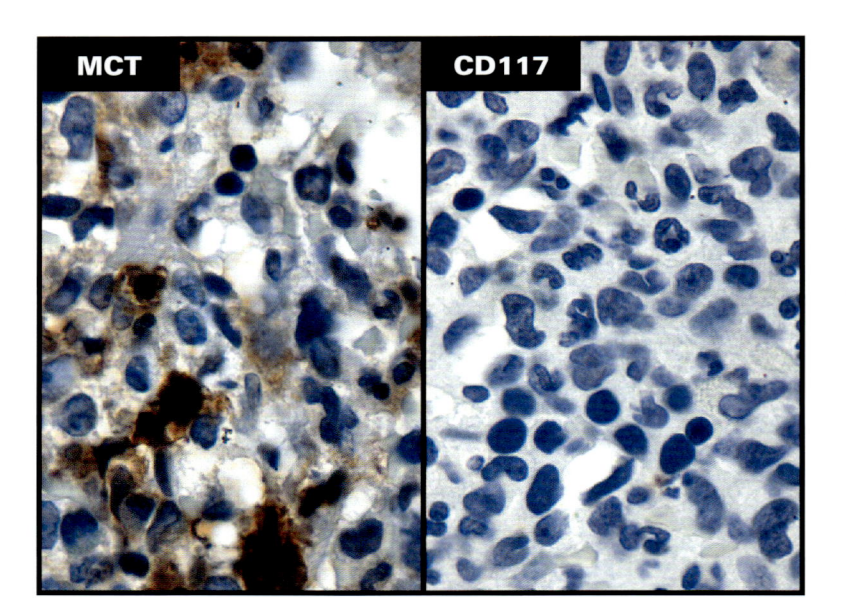

F4.3.14 Mast cell tryptase (MCT) and CD117 in chronic myeloid leukemia (slide courtesy of P Horny, MD, Institute of Pathology, Ansbach, Germany)

MCT shows large number of positive cells. Serial staining with CD117 revealed that none of the cells in the exact same area is positive for CD117. This excludes mast cells and confirms that the staining is because of reactivity of basophilic granulocytes with anti-MCT antibody. While myeloid blasts can also be positive for MCT, they would most likely be positive for CD117 and/or CD34.

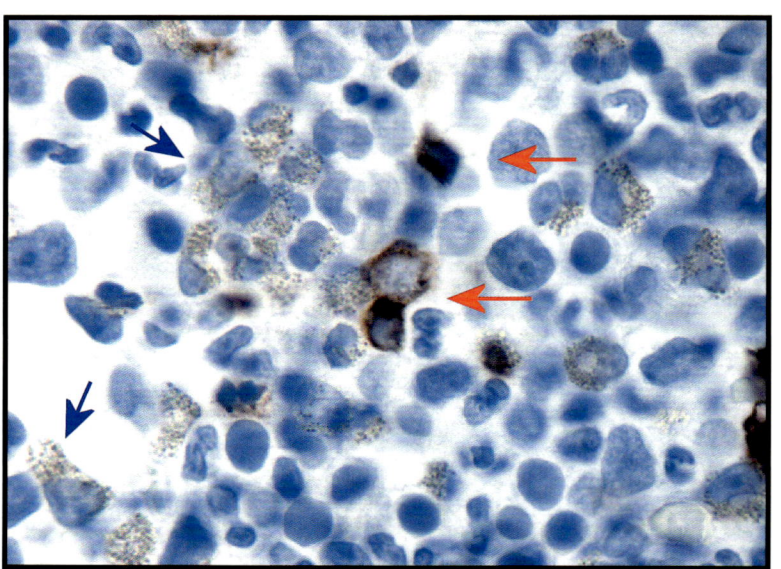

F4.3.15 Mast cell tryptase in immature cells in chronic myelomonocytic leukemia (CMML)

This biopsy specimen is from a 57-year-old man who presented with persistent monocytosis. CMML type 2 was diagnosed. Few immature appearing cells (red arrows), some of which may be myeloid blasts that were increased at 12% showed weak cytoplasmic staining. The number of positive blasts was about 3% in a 500-cell count. Eosinophils were focally increased (blue arrows). Peripheral eosinophil count was less than $1.5 \times 10^9/L$ and therefore, the criterion for "CMML with eosinophilia" was not fulfilled.

4.4 Terminal Deoxynucleotidyltransferase (TdT)

Terminal deoxynucleotidyltransferase (TdT) is also known as DNA nucleotidylexotransferase and nucleosidetriphosphate:DNA deoxynucleotidylexotransferase (OMIM). TdT is a DNA polymerase that catalyzes the addition of deoxyribonucleotides onto the 3'-hydroxyl end of DNA primers without template direction [Landau 1984]. It is expressed in immature thymocytes, lymphoid precursors in the BM, in very small numbers in peripheral lymphoid tissues, lymphoblastic leukemias and lymphomas, and also aberrantly in a subpopulation of many Merkel cell carcinomas [Sening 2004; Strauchen 2003; Strauchen 2001; Hsu 1985; Orazi 1994; Sur 2007]. In precursor B cells, it is expressed in pro-B cells but its expression declines at the pre-B-cell stage, when heavy-chain gene rearrangement is complete and light-chain gene rearrangement has commenced. TdT is a marker of lymphoblastic leukemia. With that said, it must be emphasized that some myeloid leukemias express TdT. Because acute promyelocytic leukemia (APL) is the most differentiated AML, TdT is typically not expressed in this subtype of AML, but it has been reported in rare variant APLs [Chapiro 2006]. TdT expression as a singular event does not designate cells as lymphoblastic. However, in the great majority of lymphoblastic leukemias/lymphomas, its expression is typically very high in every cell. Variable and weakly expressed TdT or TdT expression in a small number of cells should be interpreted with caution. However, the detection of a small number of positive cells may be significant because groups of 5 or more clearly TdT+ cells have been reported in patients at risk for impending relapse in childhood ALL [Rimsza 1998]. In optimized protocols, only rare cases of precursor B or precursor T-ALL can be found to express lower levels of TdT. Overall, normal TdT+ cells are about 1000-fold more frequent in the marrow than in the blood. More than 75% of TdT+ cells in both the blood and marrow are precursor B cells. TdT+ cells in the BM express T-cell antigens in less than 0.2% cells, while in the blood, there are about 4% TdT+ precursor T cells. This suggests that lineage-uncommitted and/or thymus-destined TdT+ cells are selectively released from the marrow into the circulation [Smith 1989]. TdT+ cells in the BM can be significantly increased in reactive bone marrow in children in different clinical settings. These may include infections, metastatic tumors like neuroblastoma, and other conditions associated with reactive bone marrow changes. They are also reported in large numbers in some healthy infants and young children. They may be significantly increased in adults including those with autoimmune diseases, regenerative bone marrow state, acquired immunodeficiency syndrome (AIDS), and other conditions [Davis 1994]. Not all hematogones are TdT+, but when hematogones are very increased and account for about 50% of the bone marrow cellularity, the number of TdT+ hematogones will also be very high. Flow cytometry is very helpful in distinguishing hematogones from precursor B lymphoblastic leukemia [Davis 1994; McKenna 2001]. On IHC, TdT+ hematogones tend to form rows, rather than rounded aggregates, which occasionally may also favor hematogones over leukemic cells [Torlakovic 2005a].

F4.4.1 TdT in histologically normal bone marrow

This biopsy specimen is from a 54-year-old woman with classical Hodgkin lymphoma. The BM is not involved. A small number of TdT+ cells can be observed throughout the life span including old age.

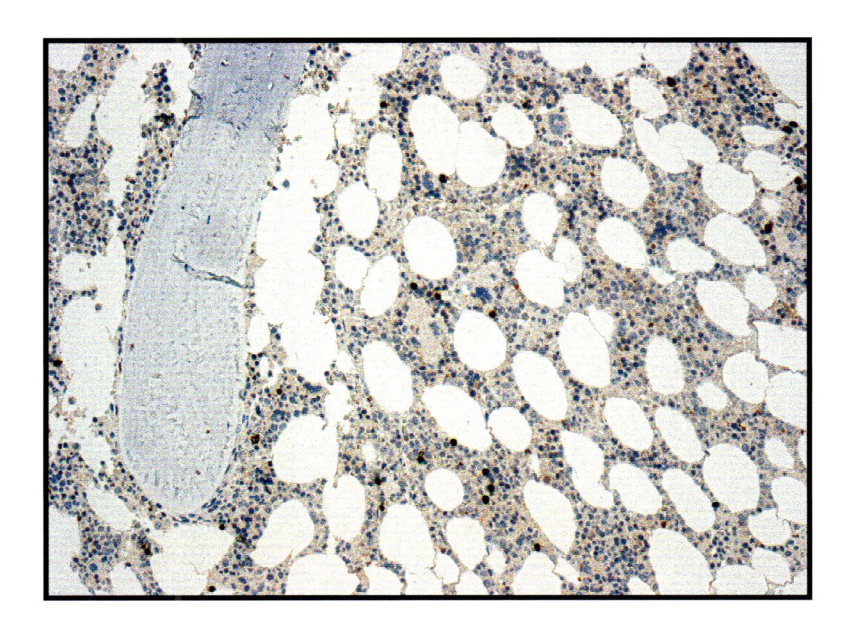

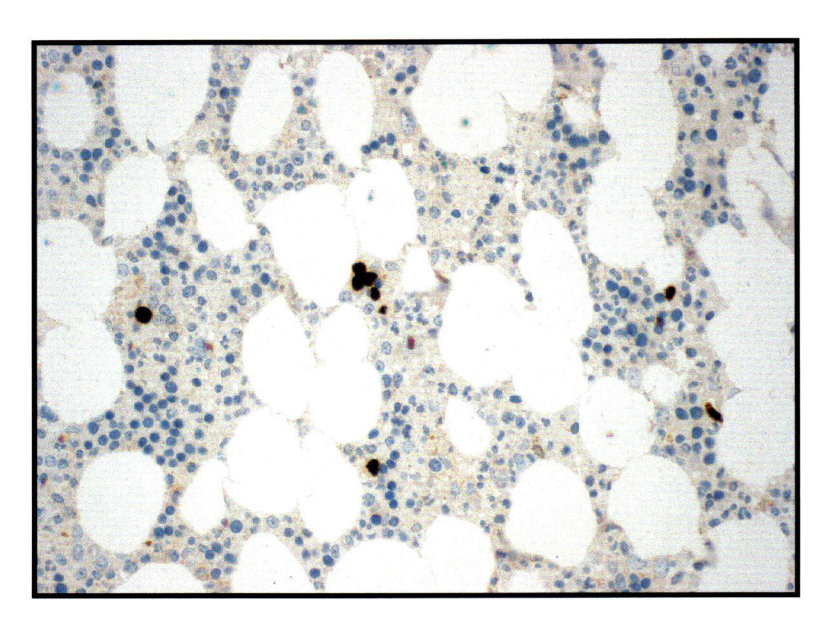

F4.4.2 TdT in histologically normal bone marrow

Similar to CD34+ cells, the TdT+ cells do not form round clusters if they are benign cells. This cluster contains 3 or 4 cells. Finding clusters of 5 or more positive cells has been described as a pathological finding and predictive of an early relapse in acute lymphoblastic leukemia [Rimsza 1998].

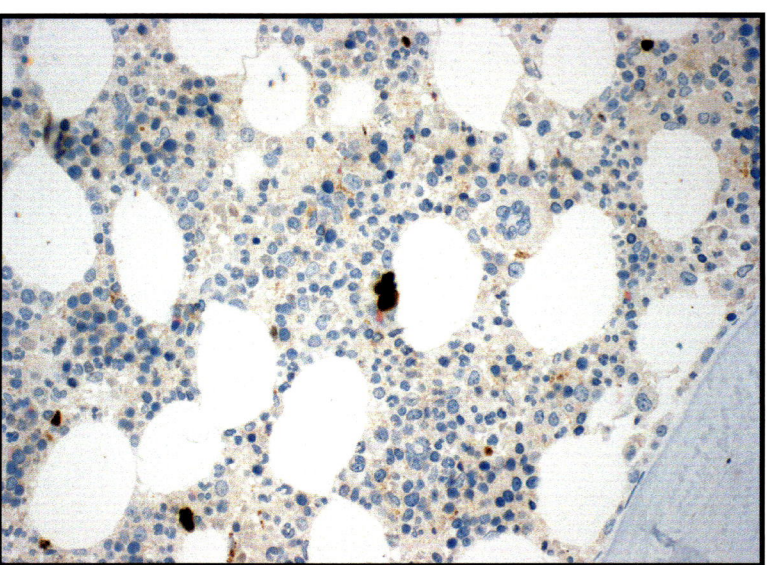

F4.4.3 TdT in histologically normal bone marrow

A cluster of 3 TdT+ cells is demonstrated here. It appears that this is the beginning of a maturational row of hematogones [Torlakovic 2005a]. Hematogones form maturational rows (see section 4.6 [Pax-5]). The rest of the maturational row cannot be demonstrated with TdT, but is easily highlighted with Pax-5 or CD79a.

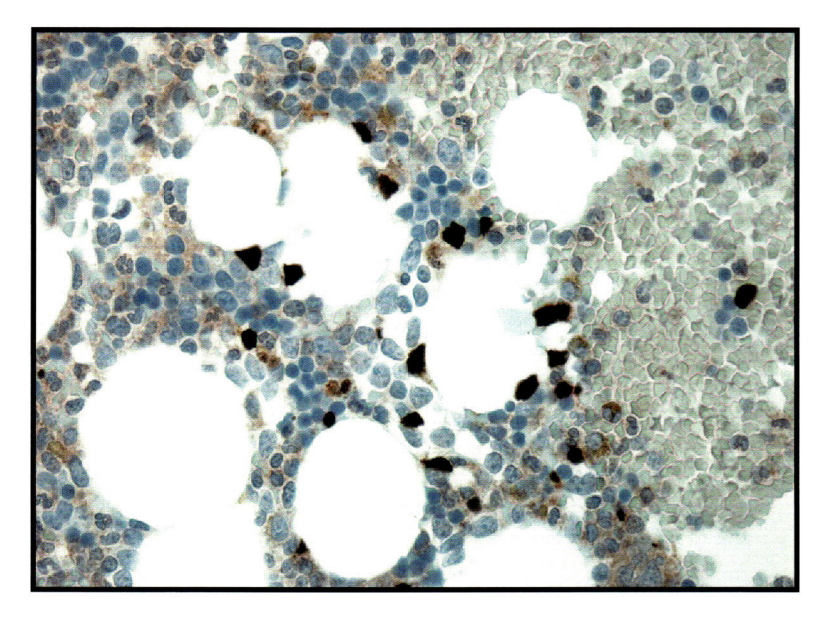

F4.4.4 TdT in histologically normal bone marrow

In many, if not most BM biopsy specimens with a normal population of TdT+ cells, there is a pronounced tendency for association with adipocytes. The biological background of this phenomenon is not clear. This is termed here as "nipple sign" and it is not unique to TdT+ cells (see also **F3.10.2** and **F3.33.1**).

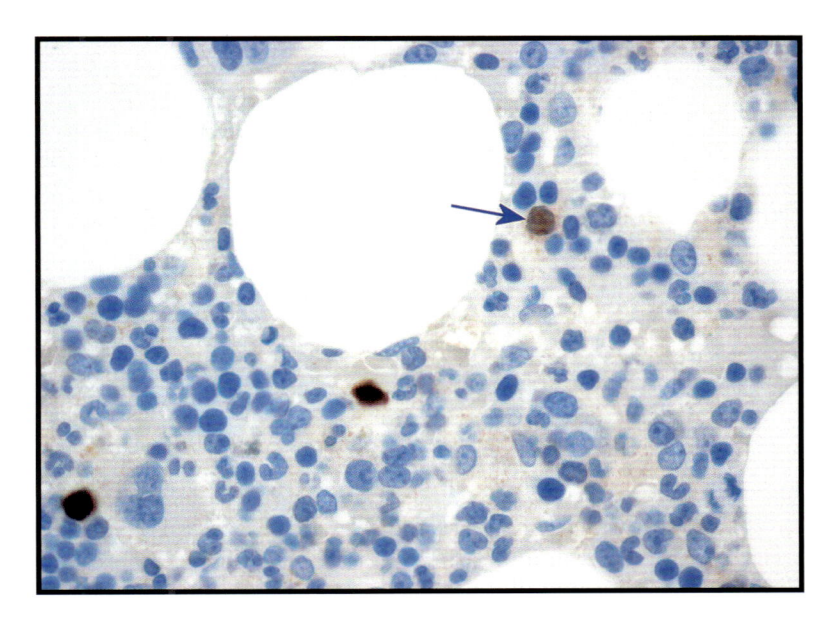

F4.4.5 TdT in histologically normal bone marrow

As lymphoid precursors mature, the content of TdT rapidly decreases. Occasionally, this normal downregulation of TdT may be observed with immunohistochemistry as weak staining in rare cells (arrow). These are regularly B-cell precursors. T-cell precursors express TdT in thymus and are unlikely to be found with downregulated TdT in the BM biopsy.

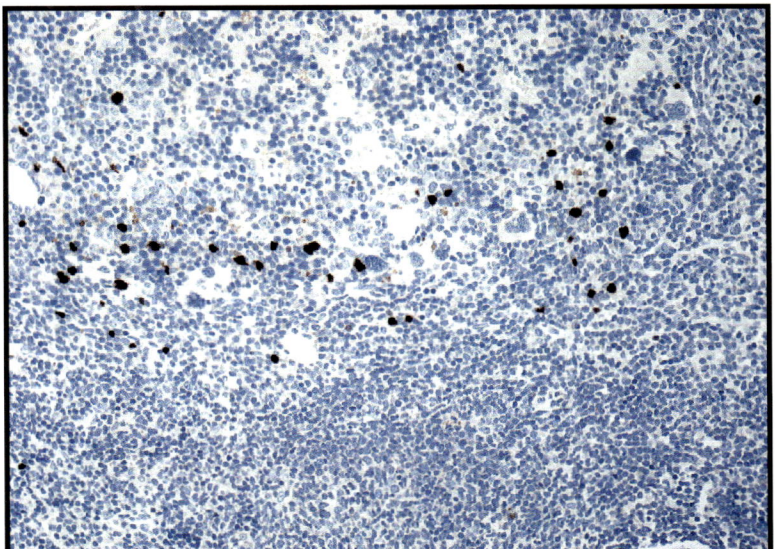

F4.4.6 TdT induction around lymphoid aggregates

This biopsy specimen is from a 49-year-old woman with follicular lymphoma involving the bone marrow. An ill-defined band of TdT+ cells developed around the large lymphoid aggregates between the malignant cells and histologically normal BM. Biological basis of this phenomenon is not clear.

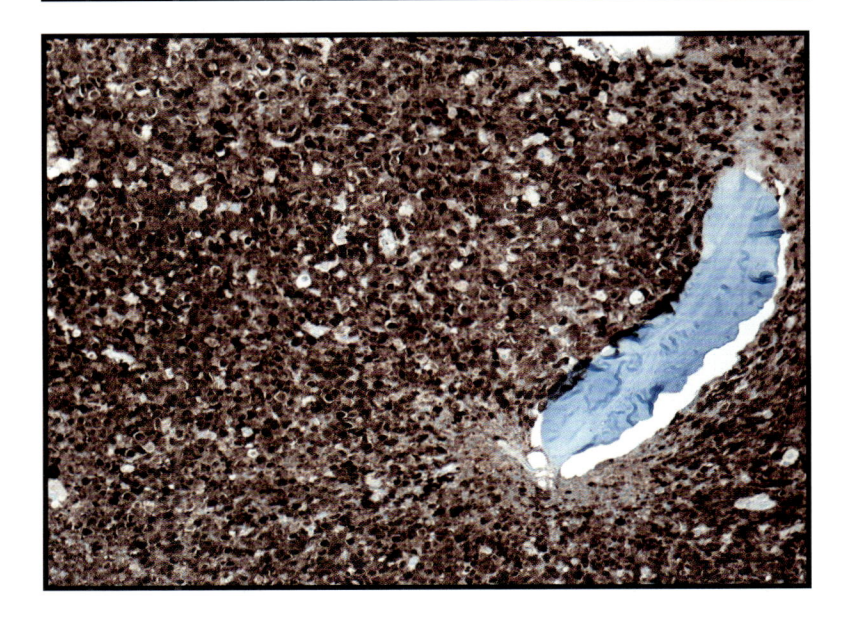

F4.4.7 TdT in precursor B acute lymphoblastic leukemia (precursor B-ALL).

In classic cases, demonstration of TdT positivity is used to support the diagnosis of lymphoblastic leukemia, whether it is of precursor T or precursor B type. It has to be emphasised that the interpretation of weak and variable expression of TdT may be difficult. TdT is not specific enough to differentiate between acute lymphoblastic and myeloid leukemia and TdT has also been found in some cases of Merkel cell carcinoma, which can be also Pax-5+.

4: Other Common Markers

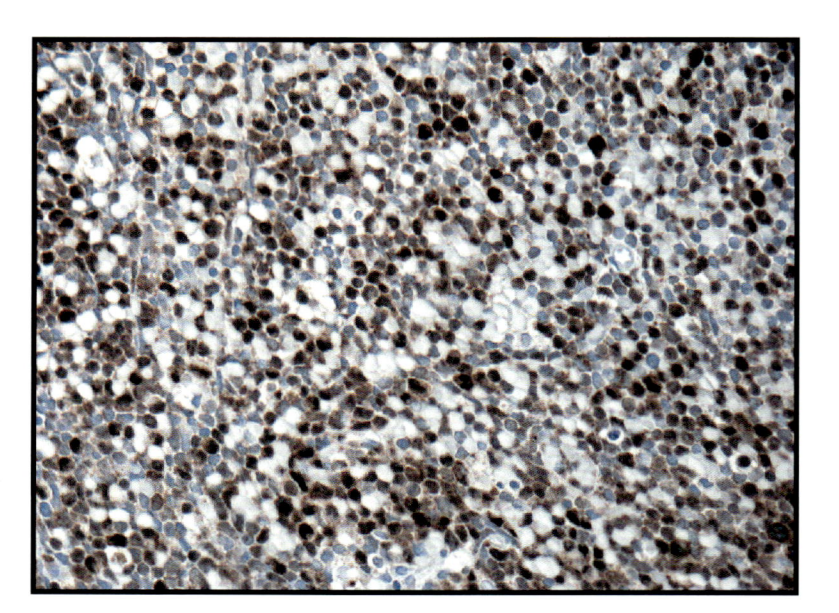

F4.4.8 TdT in precursor B-cell acute lymphoblastic leukemia (weak to moderate expression).

Compared with the intensity of TdT staining seen in **F4.4.7**, this specimen shows weak to moderate positivity in about half of the leukemic cells. If the percentage of positive cells is very low, one should first consider that these cells may not represent the neoplastic population. On the other hand, if very weak staining is present diffusely, it is most likely representative of the neoplastic population, but it still has to be interpreted with caution.

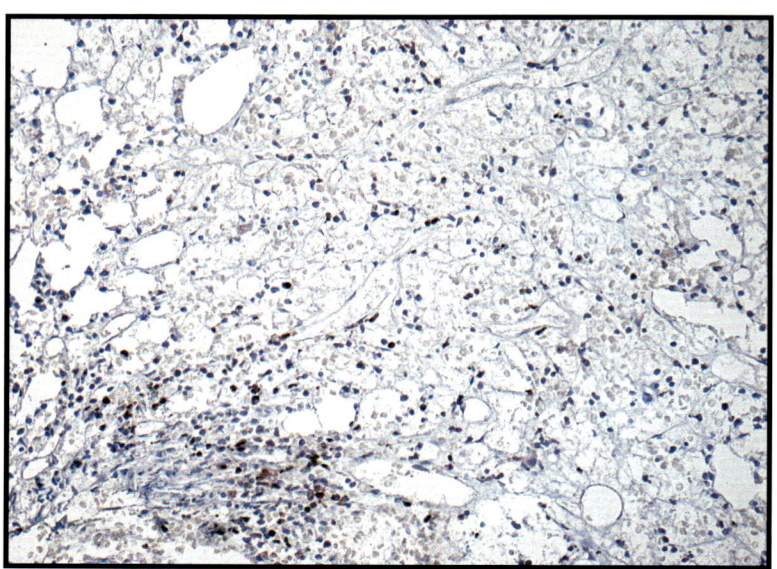

F4.4.9 TdT in precursor B-cell acute lymphoblastic leukemia 7 days after induction chemotherapy

This bone marrow specimen is basically acellular; a few TdT+ cells are present (left lower corner). Their significance at this phase of therapy is not clear. In some patients, the increased TdT+ cells regress with marrow regeneration and declare themselves as hematogones, but in others these cells may represent a residual lymphoblastic population.

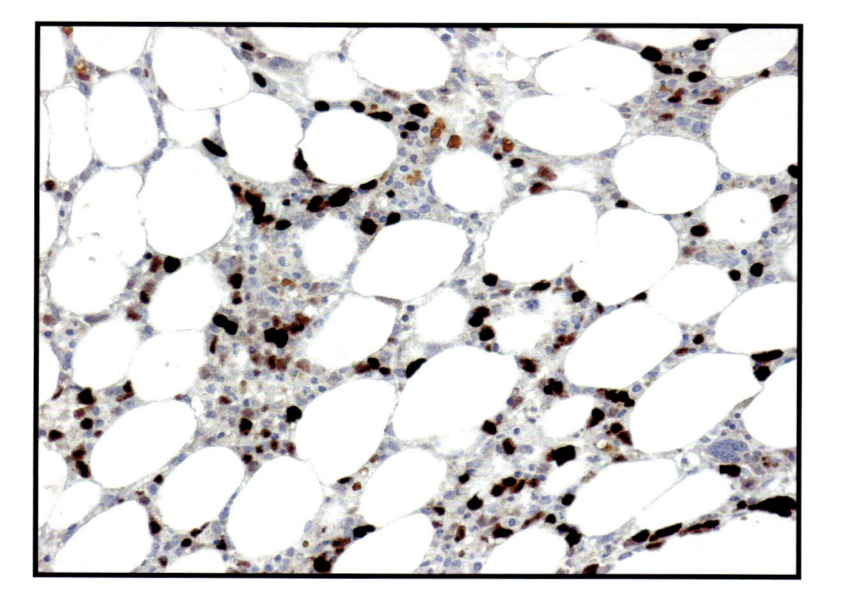

F4.4.10 TdT in precursor B-cell acute lymphoblastic leukemia (B-ALL) relapse

This specimen is from an adult patient with Ph+ precursor B-ALL. These TdT+ cells were detected approximately 7 months after chemotherapy was completed and were interpreted as evidence of relapse.

F4.4.11 TdT in precursor B-cell acute lymphoblastic leukemia 14 days after induction chemotherapy

In this specimen 14 days after chemotherapy, the bone marrow was completely replaced by leukemic blasts. There was no evidence of TdT or CD34+ expression at this time.

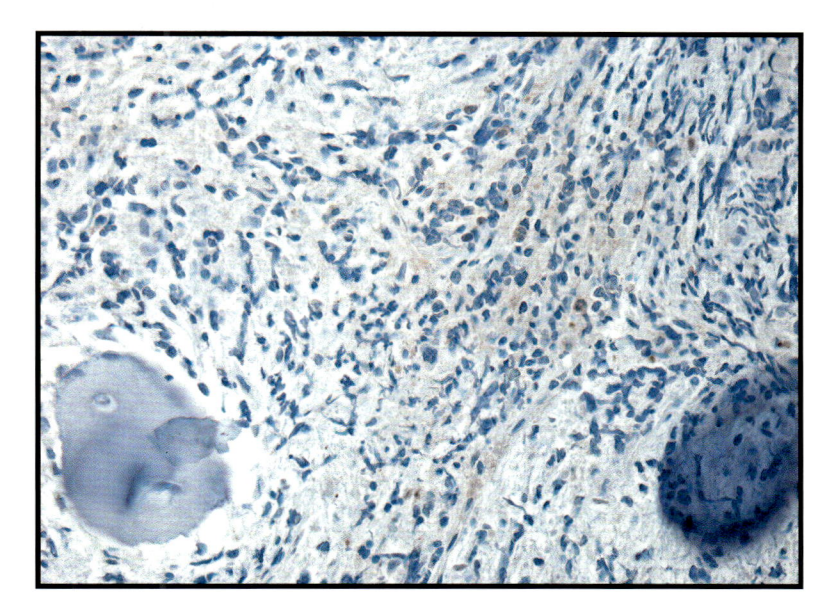

F4.4.12 TdT in acute biphenotypic leukemia (acute myeloid leukemia/precursor T-cell acute lymphoblastic leukemia)

This biopsy specimen is from a 67-year-old man with pancytopenia. On flow cytometry, CD5, cytoplasmic CD3 and TdT were expressed by the blasts as well as several myeloid markers. Note variable expression of TdT in leukemic cells.

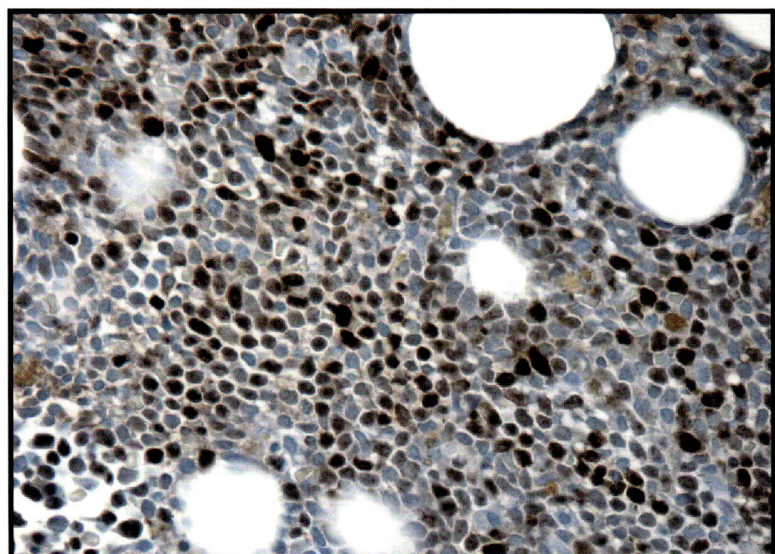

F4.4.13 TdT expression in acute biphenotypic leukemia (acute myeloid leukemia/precursor B-cell acute lymphoblastic leukemia)

In contrast to relatively weak expression of TdT illustrated in F4.4.12, this case of acute biphenotypic leukemia displays very high TdT expression.

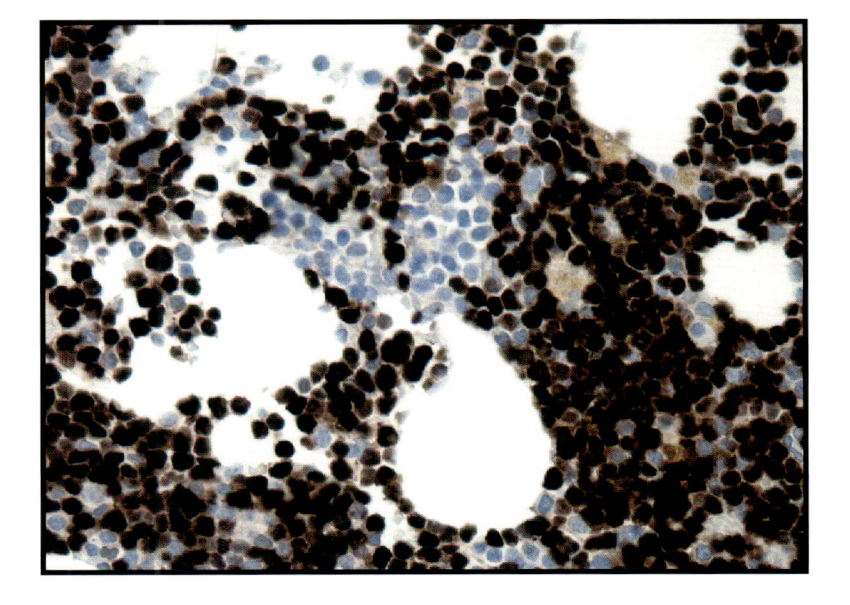

4: Other Common Markers

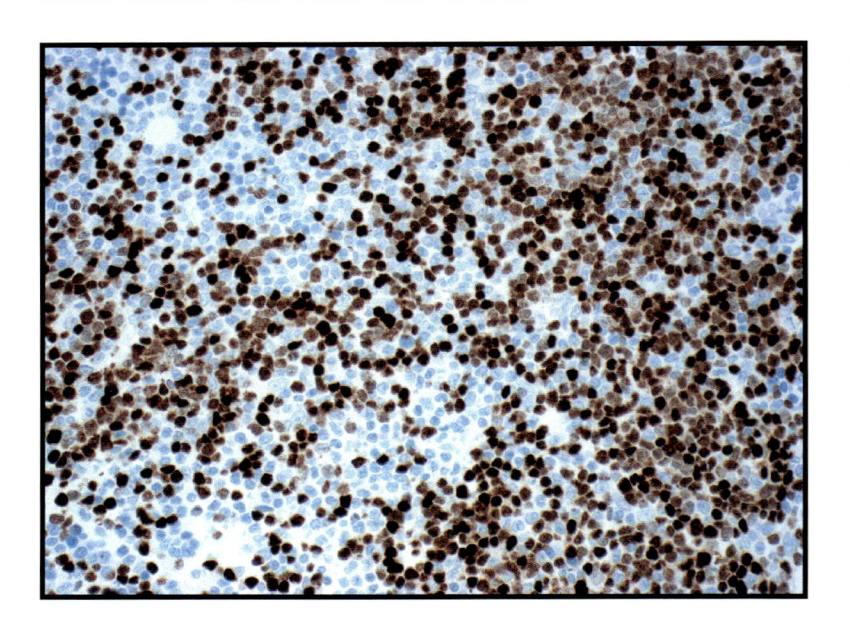

F4.4.14 TdT expression in acute bilineal leukemia

Tissue sections reveal 2 blast populations: TdT+ and TdT−. Flow cytometric analysis revealed that the TdT+ population of blasts also expressed markers of B-cell differentiation (cCD22, CD19) and the TdT− population markers of myeloid differentiation (CD13+, CD33+, CD11b+, and CD64+). Both blast populations were CD34+. In tissue sections, these 2 separate populations are clearly demonstrated.

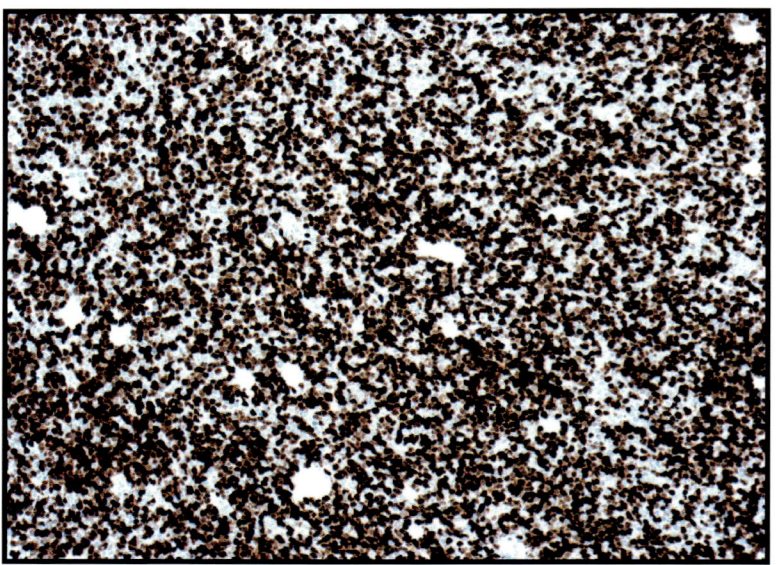

F4.4.15 Strong TdT expression in acute myeloid leukemia (AML) without maturation

This illustrates a case of AML with flow cytometric and immunohistochemical immunophenotyping. The only "lymphoid marker" that was unequivocally demonstrated was TdT. Occasionally, AML blasts can express levels of TdT as high as those found in lymphoblastic leukemia.

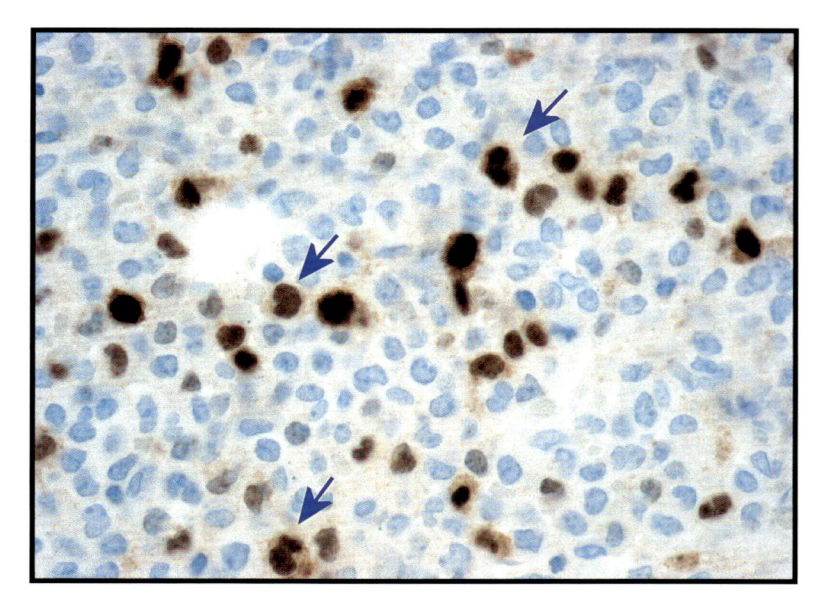

F4.4.16 TdT in acute promyelocytic leukemia

This type of leukemia does not express TdT and this is not the type of acute myeloid leukemia that is seen as a component of either biphenotypic or bilineal leukemia. The t(15;17)(q22;q21) was demonstrated by cytogenetic analysis. Occasional positive cells shown here appear to be promyelocytes with TdT expression (blue arrows). The number of cells is too low to classify the case as "TdT+".

4.4 Terminal Deoxynucleotidyltransferase

F4.4.17 TdT expression in acute myelomonocytic leukemia

This specimen from an 84-year-old woman showed morphological and immunophenotypical evidence of myelomonocytic leukemia. There is strong expression of TdT as illustrated. No other lymphoid markers were detected with flow cytometry or immunohistochemistry (IHC). Flow cytometry showed no evidence of TdT+ cells. This discrepancy is rarely encountered, and both flow cytometry and IHC should be repeated.

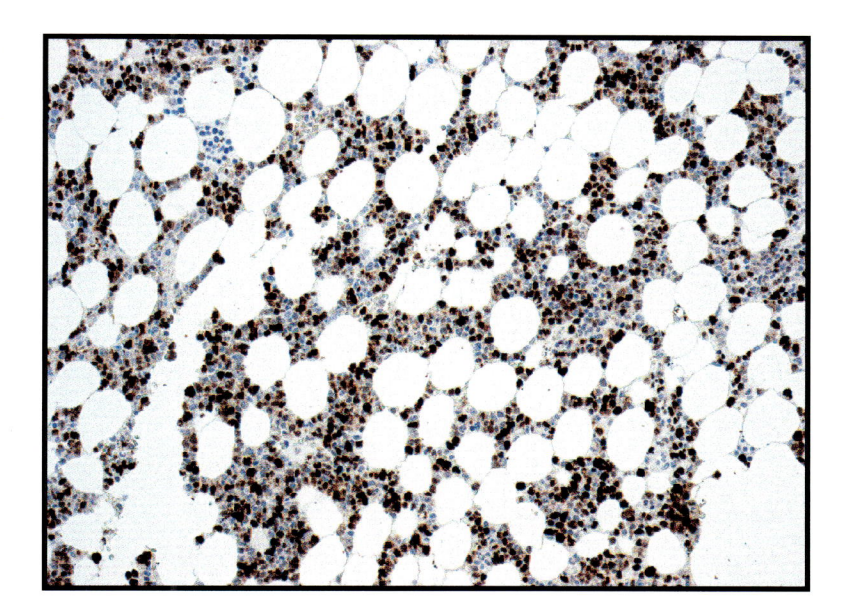

F4.4.18 TdT in otherwise undifferentiated acute leukemia

This specimen is from a 55-year-old man with acute leukemia. The bone marrow was completely replaced by blasts. Flow cytometry and immunohistochemistry were uninformative. TdT as shown here was interpreted as equivocal with scattered borderline positive cells. This type of positivity is not sufficient for designation of lineage.

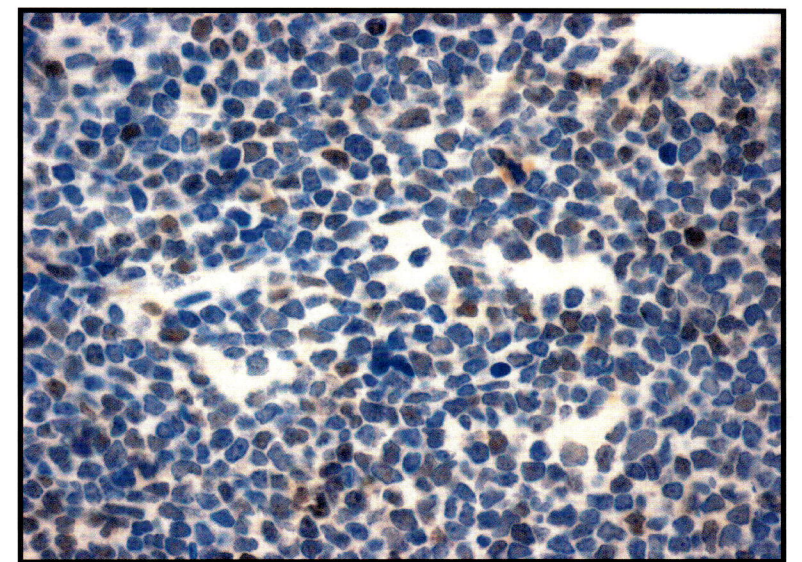

4.5 Factor 8-Related Antigen (von Willebrand Factor)

F8-ra is a marker of endothelial cells, megakaryocytes, and platelets [Sadler 1998]. F8-ra, or more correctly, vWF is a large, multimeric glycoprotein that is found in platelet α-granules and endothelial cell cytoplasm and is secreted toward plasma and subendothelial connective tissue. vWF performs essential functions in hemostasis: it mediates platelet aggregation and the adhesion of platelets to subendothelial connective tissue, and it binds factor VIII [Sadler 1998]. vWF is made by endothelial cells throughout the body and by megakaryocytes [Jaffe 1974; Nachman 1977;]. Up to 95% of vWF is secreted, whereas the remainder is stored in cytoplasmic granules called Weibel-Palade bodies [Wagner 1982]. In endothelial cells, the vWF within granules contains very large multimers made almost exclusively of mature vWF subunits, whereas the vWF that is secreted constitutively contains mostly small multimers and a high proportion of unprocessed pro-vWF subunits [Sporn 1986]. Chuang et al [Chuang 2000] showed that for routine practice, vWF is the most reliable marker for identifying atypical megakaryocytes, especially in the cases of 5q– syndrome and agnogenic myeloid metaplasia. We have observed that CD61, CD42b, and also vWF can all be downregulated in myelodysplastic syndromes. vWF is an important marker of endothelial and megakaryoblastic differentiation and it is recommended for use in an acute leukemia panel. CD9 and CD31, which are both expressed by megakaryocytes and endothelial cells, in addition to the surface expression, also colocalize in platelet α granules with wWF [Cramer 1994].

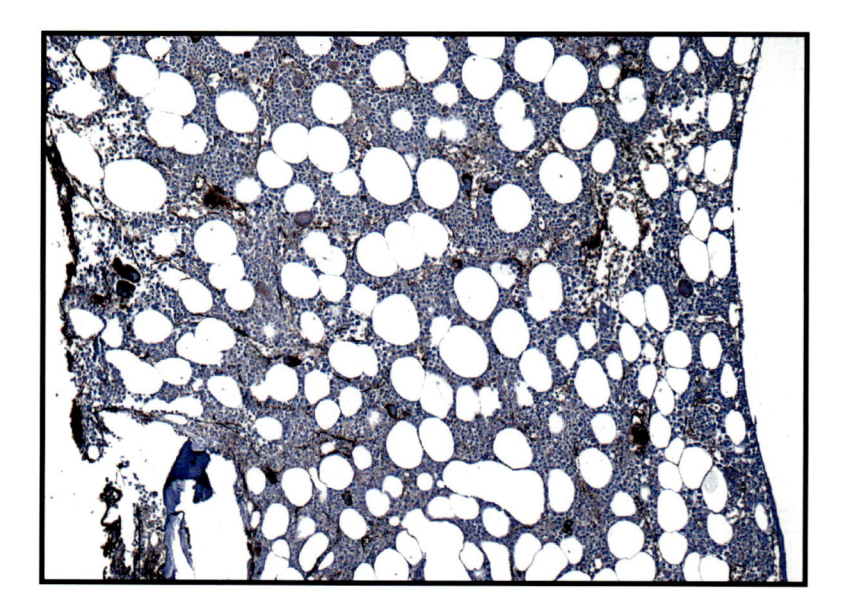

F4.5.1 von Willebrand factor (vWF) in histologically normal bone marrow

Only the megakaryocytes at the edge of the biopsy are stained suggesting a technical problem. Endothelial cells are also poorly stained. Immunohistochemistry demonstration of vWF may be technically difficult and protocols should be carefully optimized to achieve the best possible signal-to-noise ratio.

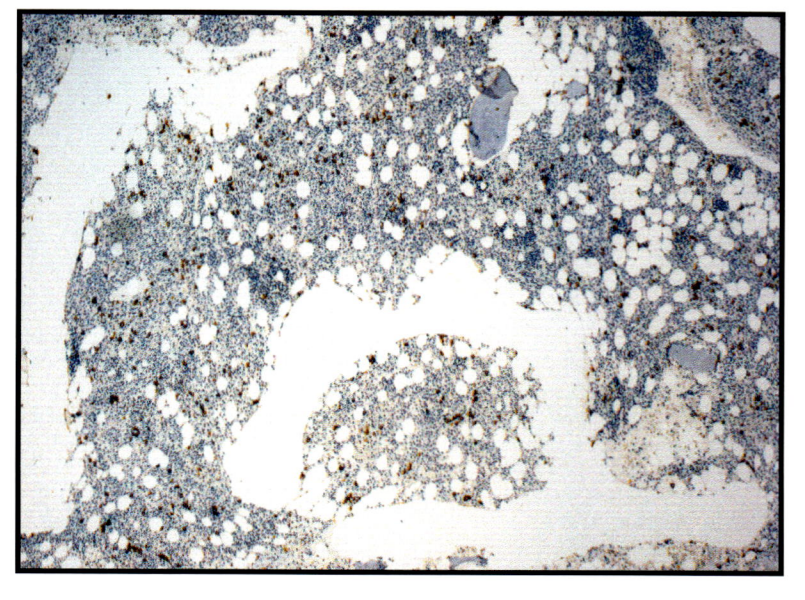

F4.5.2 Optimal staining for von Willebrand factor (vWF)

The staining intensity of megakaryocytes should be uniform throughout the bone marrow specimen. In most biopsy specimens megakaryocytes show strong expression of vWF and this positivity is easily visualized even on low power examination.

4.5 Factor 8-Related Antigen (von Willebrand Factor)

F4.5.3 Weak expression of von Willebrand factor in megakaryocytes

In optimal protocols (left) it is still possible to identify weakly stained megakaryocytes, especially in myelodysplasia. This may be a uniform phenomenon throughout the biopsy specimen or only in a subpopulation of megakaryocytes. In optimal protocols, endothelial cells are strongly stained (blue arrows). If megakaryocyte staining is weak because of technical problems, endothelial cells will also be weakly stained or negative (red arrows).

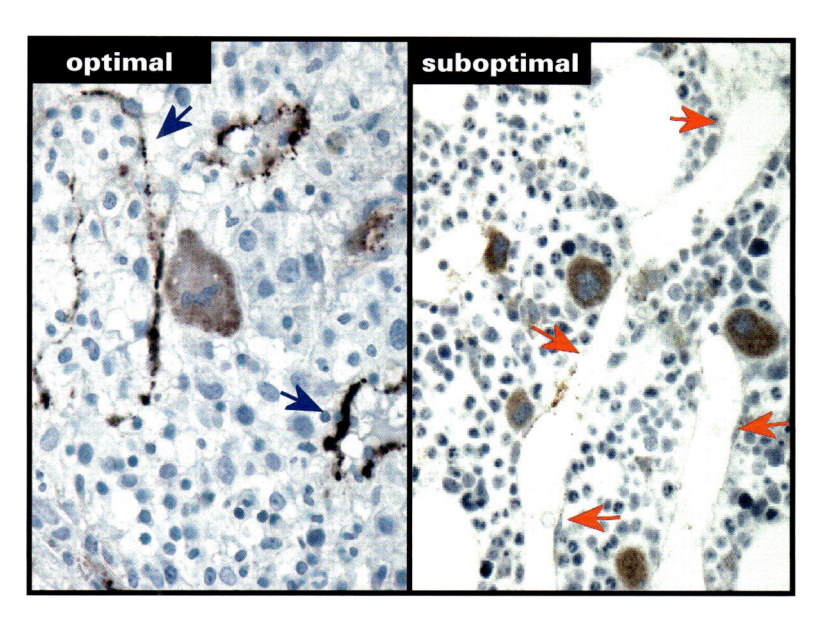

F4.5.4 von Willebrand factor (vWF) in endothelial cells (optimized protocol)

vWF is synthesized by endothelial cells and megakaryocytes. In endothelial cells, most of the vWF is secreted and only 10% is stored in Weibel-Palade bodies. Secreted vWF is detected in the lumen.

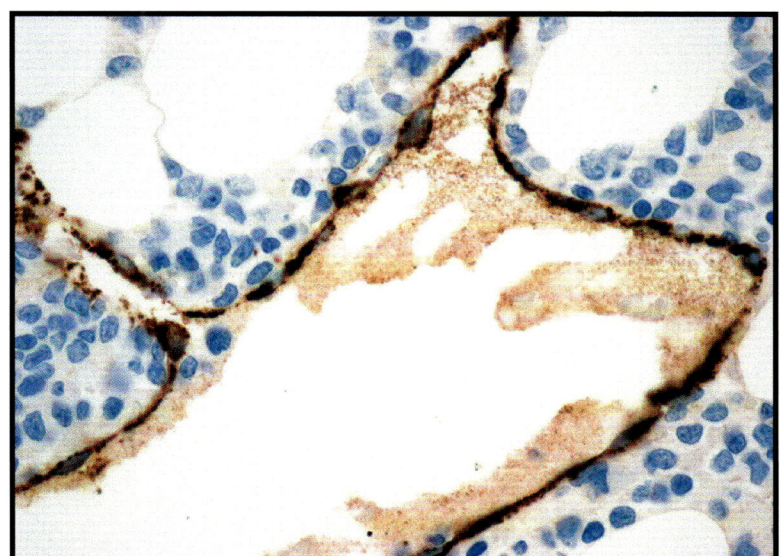

F4.5.5 von Willebrand factor in small megakaryocytes

This biopsy specimen is from a 58-year-old man with anemia. The number of megakaryocytes is normal, but some were small, and some had hypolobated nuclei. They are present in small groups. The intensity of staining is similar to that of normal megakaryocytes (in optimized protocols). Most of the megakaryocytes appear clearly associated with endothelial cells, which contain strong granular positivity (arrows).

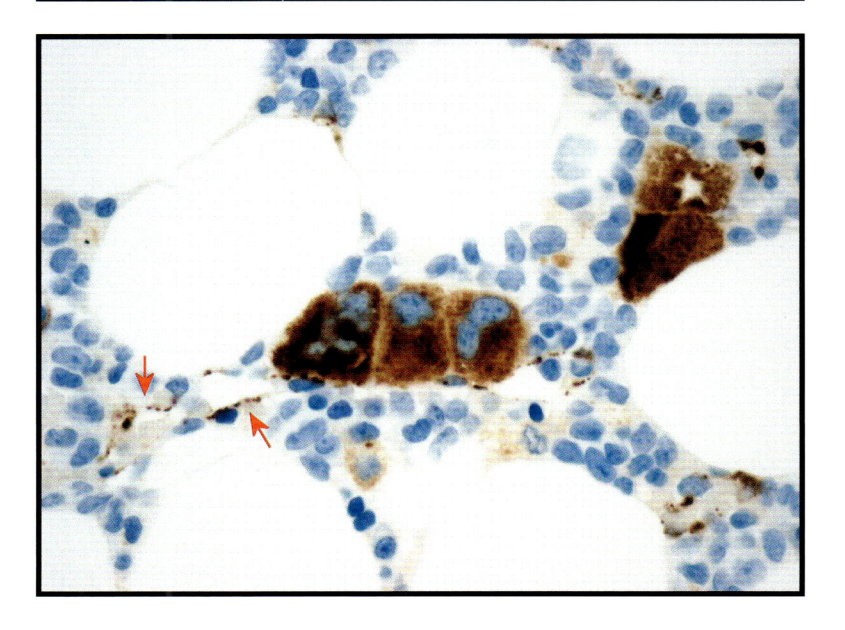

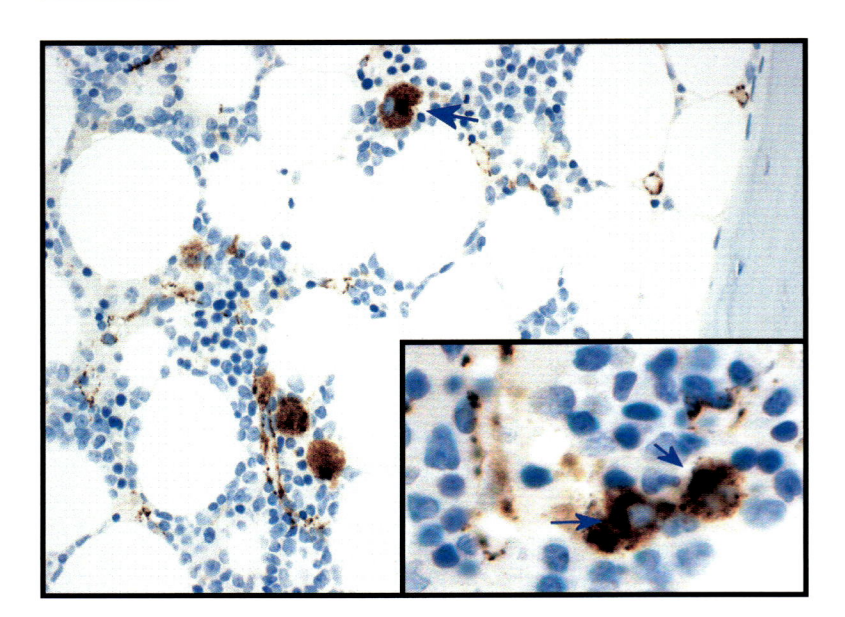

F4.5.6 von Willebrand factor (vWF) in Golgi area

Golgi concentration of vWF may be detected in dysplastic megakaryocytes. Golgi-type reactivity cannot be clearly demonstrated in the endothelial cells.

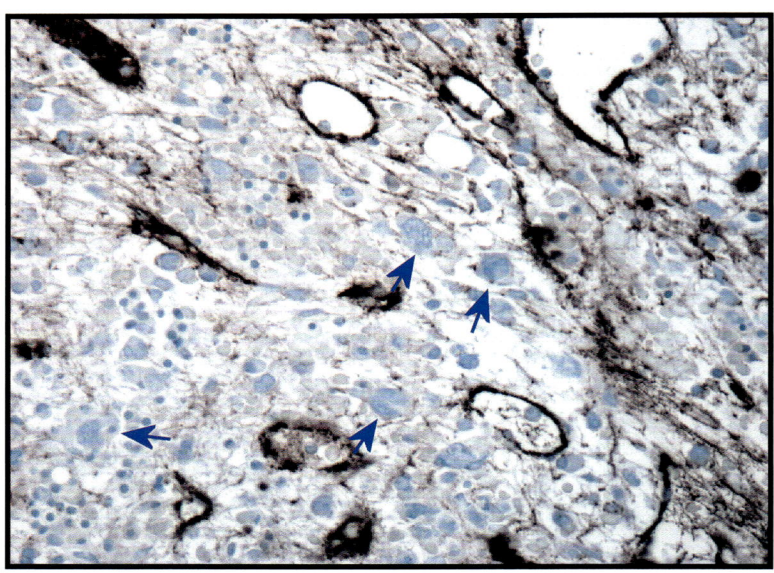

F4.5.7 von Willebrand factor (vWF) may be decreased in megakaryocytes after induction chemotherapy for precursor B-cell lymphoblastic leukemia (B-ALL)

This biopsy specimen is from a 2-year-old boy with precursor B-ALL with no residual blasts 14 days after chemotherapy. Megakaryocytes are increased (arrows) and do not express vWF. This is not a false negative result because vWF is clearly demonstrated in endothelial cells.

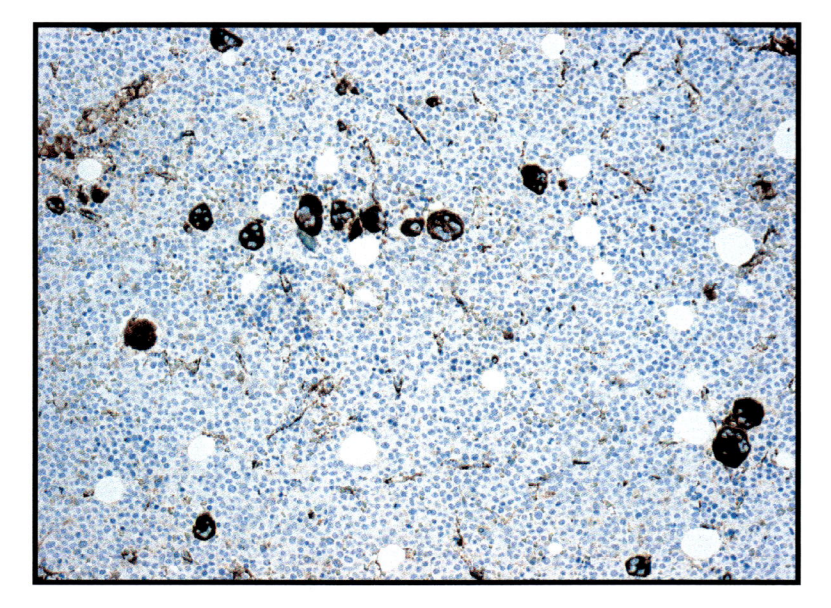

F4.5.8 von Willebrand factor highlights a linear distribution of megakaryocytes

This biopsy specimen is from an 83-year-old patient with acute promyelocytic leukemia. The megakaryocytes are overall decreased, resulting in thrombocytopenia. Many remaining megakaryocytes showed a linear pattern of distribution. Some of the megakaryocytes are clearly linked to endothelial cells, which are decreased.

F4.5.9 Megakaryocytes are associated with endothelial cells of the bone marrow sinusoids

This image shows that all neoplastic megakaryocytes in transforming essential thrombocythemia are associated with endothelial cells of the BM sinusoids. Many hypolobated, small megakaryocytes, and microkaryocytes are present. This and a few previous images demonstrate how neoplastic conditions occasionally help clarify the basic biology of the BM. Retrospectively, in many histologically normal BM biopsy specimens, megakaryocytes are also found associated with endothelial cells.

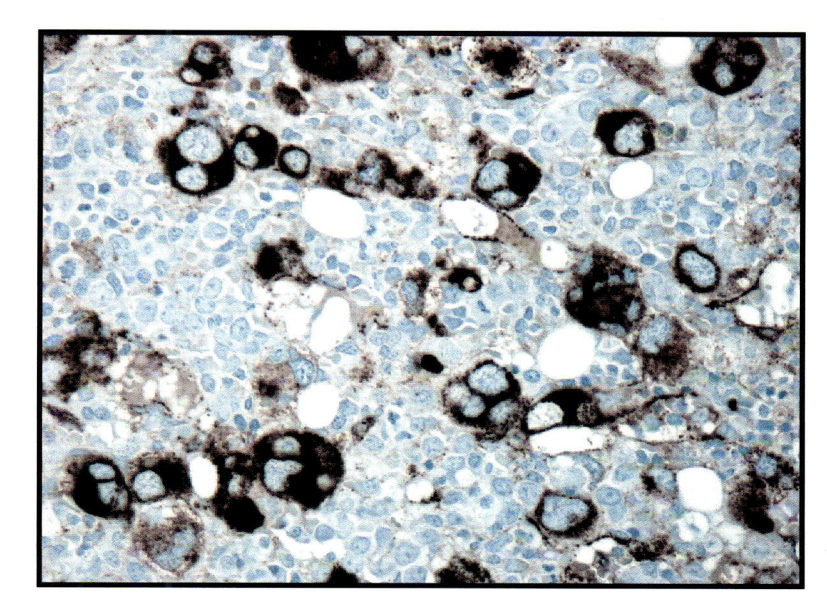

F4.5.10 von Willebrand factor in myelodysplastic syndrome associated with systemic mastocytosis

This bone marrow biopsy specimen was involved by systemic mastocytosis and also displayed trilinear dyshematopoiesis. Many of the megakaryocytes have dysplastic features and show the presence of micromegakaryocytes (arrows). Megakaryocyte markers facilitate the detection of micromegakaryocytes in the tissue sections.

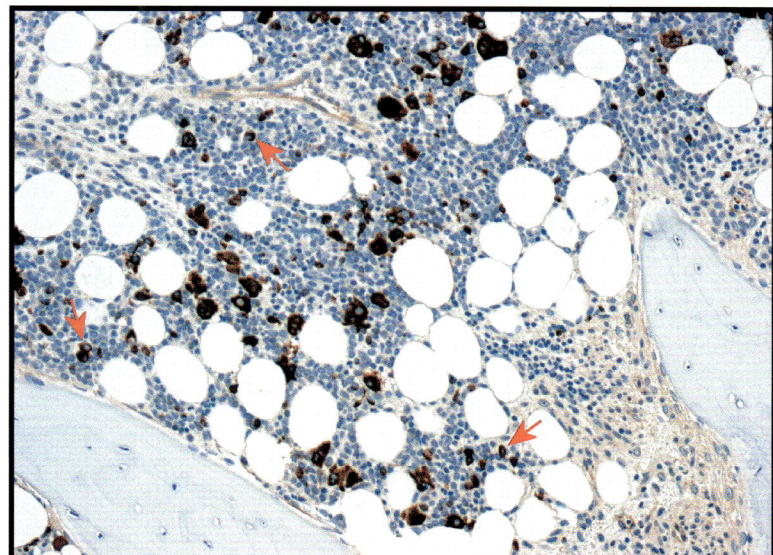

F4.5.11 von Willebrand factor (vWF) in acute megakaryoblastic leukemia

This biopsy specimen is from a 4-year-old boy with thrombocytosis. All blasts show weak to moderate cytoplasmic expression of vWF. Flow cytometric analysis revealed expression of CD117, CD13, CD41, and CD36. All other markers were negative. CD61 was also detected in the cytoplasm with immunohistochemistry.

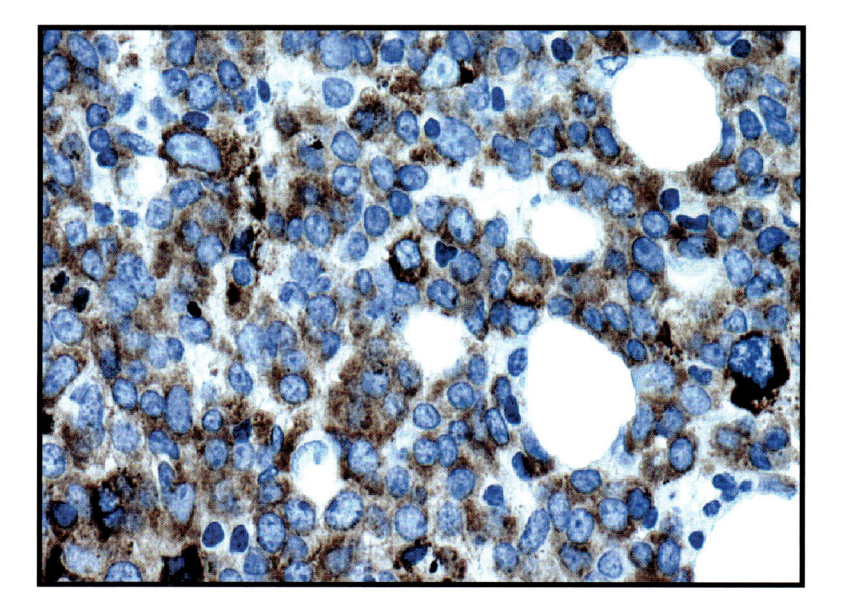

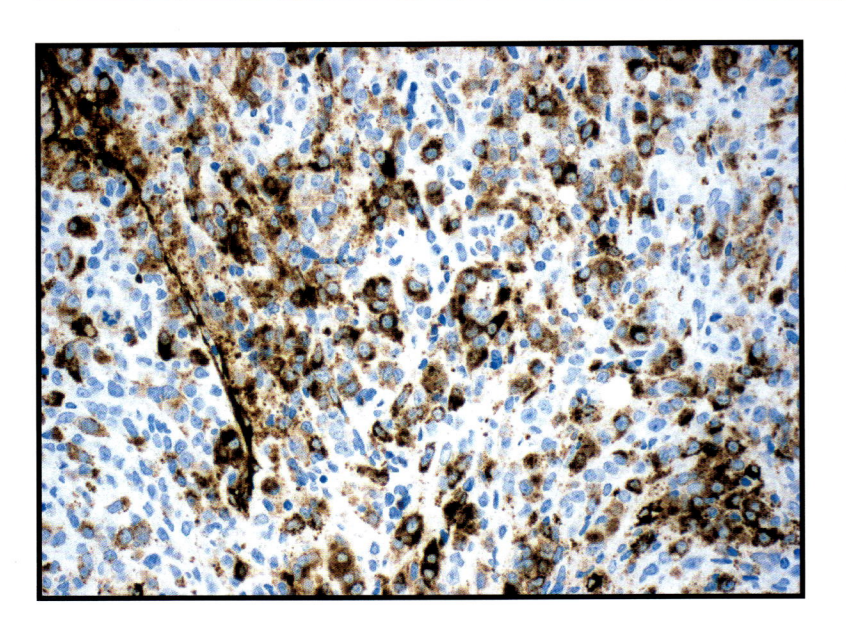

F4.5.12 von Willebrand factor (vWF) in acute megakaryoblastic leukemia

This bone marrow specimen is from a 2-year-old boy. Because of fibrosis of the BM, no specimen could be aspirated for flow cytometry. Immunohistochemistry revealed expression of vWF and CD61 with only a subpopulation of blasts positive for CD34. CD117 was also positive in a subpopulation of blasts.

4.6 Pax-5

Pax-5 is also known as a B-cell-specific activator protein (BSAP) [Adams 1992]. In normal hematopoiesis, Pax-5 is expressed only by B cells and is downregulated in plasma cells. Similary, Pax-5 is expressed in precursor B-ALL and mature B-cell neoplasms, but is not present in the great majority of cases of plasma cell malignancies [Torlakovic 2002]. Pax-5 binds to regulatory regions of CD19, CD79a, and also is a regulator of IgH isotype switching at later stages of differentiation [Kozmik 1992; Fitzsimmons 1996; Hagman 2000]. Pax-5 is required for the differentiation of the earliest B-lineage–committed precursor cells in the fetal liver. In contrast, B-cell development in the adult bone marrow progresses up to an early pro–B-cell stage in the absence of Pax-5 function. The PAX5 gene is commonly altered by deletion or by point mutation in precursor B-ALL [Mullighan 2007]. This results in reduced transcriptional activity, demonstrating that the mutations of PAX5 lead to loss of function. The PAX5 gene is also involved in several chromosomal translocations that occur in cases of B-progenitor lymphoblastic leukemia including PAX5-ETV6, PAX5-EVI3, and PAX5-ELN [Cobaleda 2007]. It has been shown that the PAX5-ENL protein inhibits the function of the wild-type PAX5 protein [Bousquet 2007]. However, practically all the clinical cases of precursor B-ALL evaluated thus far show Pax-5 expression [Torlakovic 2002; Kröber 2003; Anderson 2007; Harashima 2005; Tiacci 2004]. Pax-5 may also be detected in AML, in particular in t(8;21)-AML [Tiacci 2004; Gibson 2006; Valbuena 2006]. Pax-5 is also expressed in the great majority of Hodgkin lymphomas and in the BM, it can be used to differentiate between Hodgkin cells and megakaryocytes [Torlakovic 2002]. Pax-5 should not be used instead of CD20 or CD79a. Despite great overlap between these markers, they all provide somewhat different information and selection of pan-B-cell markers is determined by the (patho)biology of the process being evaluated.

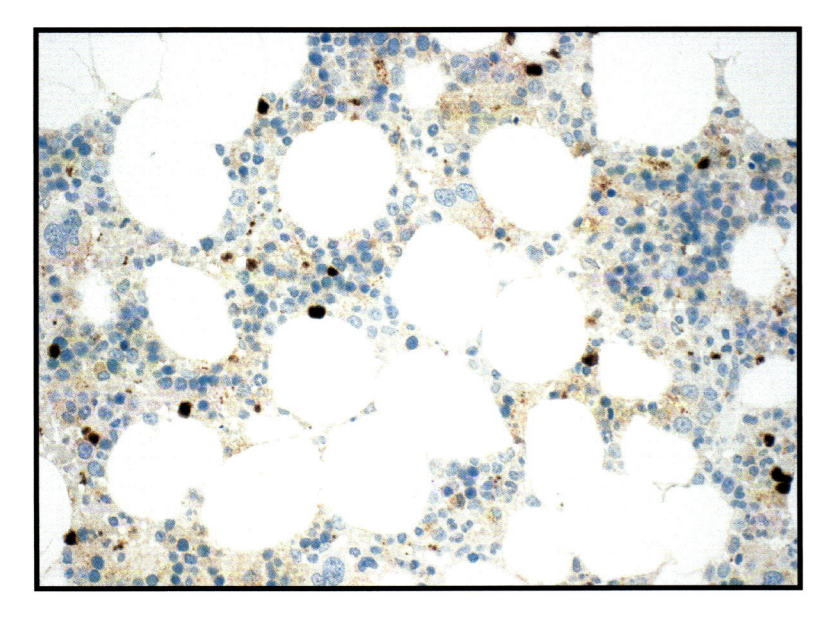

F4.6.1 Pax-5 in histologically normal bone marrow

This biopsy specimen is from a 42-year-old woman with recently diagnosed marginal zone lymphoma of the skin. The BM showed a small number of Pax-5+ cells, which is interpreted as a normal finding.

4.6 Pax-5

F4.6.2 Comparison of Pax-5 and TdT

In non-neoplastic hematopoiesis, including normal hematopoiesis and hematopoiesis in reactive conditions, the Pax-5+ cells are usually more numerous than TdT+ cells, and both are more numerous than CD34+ cells. There is about 80% more Pax-5+ than TdT+ cells in this image, which was representative of the entire specimen.

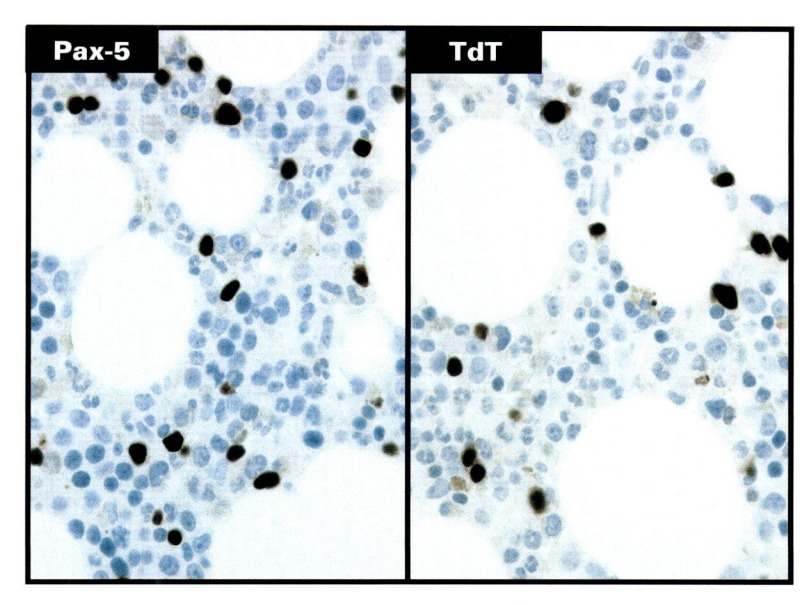

F4.6.3 Pax-5 in chronic myelomonocytic leukemia (CMML) type I

Every normal bone marrow should have evidence of B-cell hematopoiesis as shown in **F4.6.1**. However, in a rare specimen, it is not possible to find any Pax-5+ cells, as in this case of CMML. To our knowledge, there are no studies that address an absence of Pax-5+ cells in the BM in different conditions and what, if any, clinical significance this finding may have.

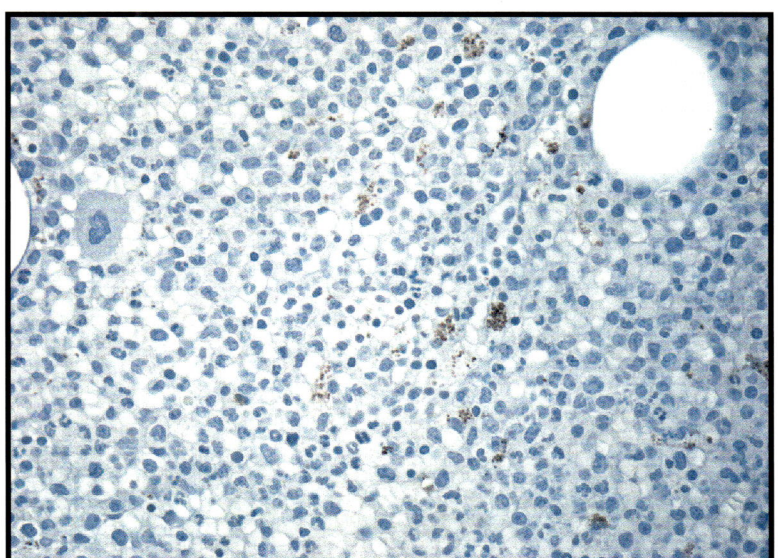

F4.6.4 Pax-5 in linear arrangements

This specimen is from a patient with follicular lymphoma (FL) that was recently treated with rituximab. CD20 was completely negative (see **F4.6.5)**. Pax-5+ cells were increased, but they should not be interpreted as evidence of FL. No paratrabecular infiltrates and no round aggregates of Pax-5+ cells were found. Many Pax-5+ cells in linear arrangements were detected. This distribution strongly suggests increased hematogones, which was confirmed with flow cytometry.

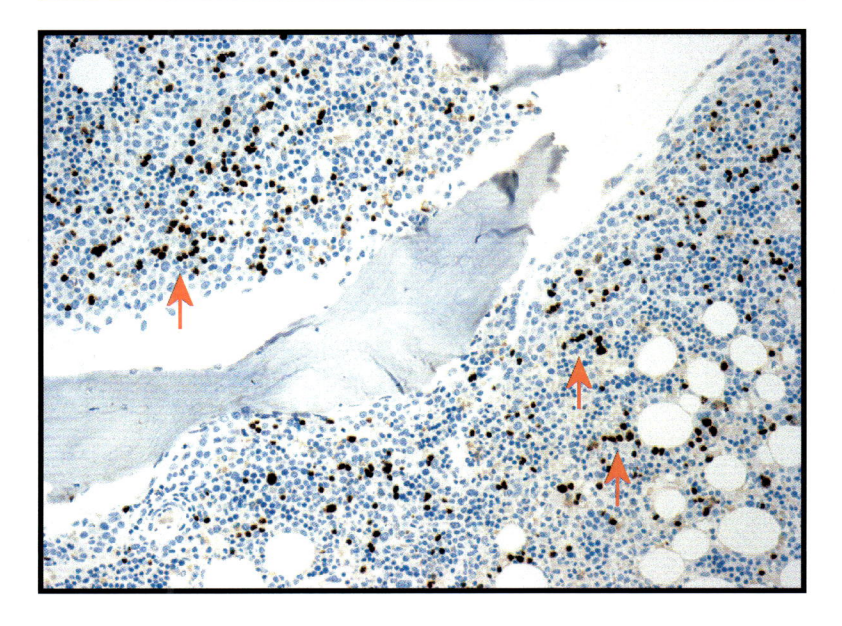

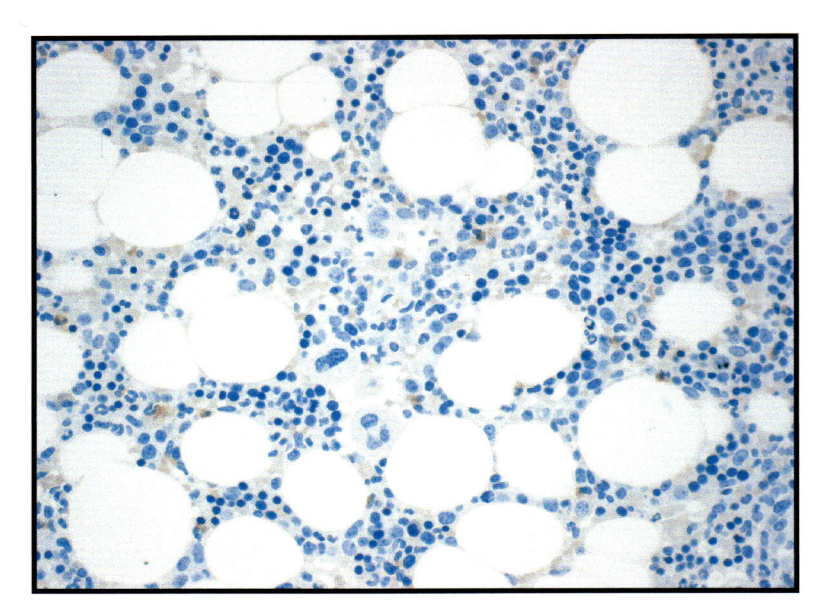

F4.6.5 CD20 in bone marrow with Pax-5+ cells in linear arrangements

In BM biopsy specimens that have increased hematogones, they regularly have variable numbers of CD20+ cells, but in much smaller numbers than Pax-5+ cells. However, in this biopsy specimen from a patient who recently received treatment with rituximab, no CD20+ cells were found. Pax-5 and CD79a may be useful markers after rituximab therapy, but their results should be interpreted with caution.

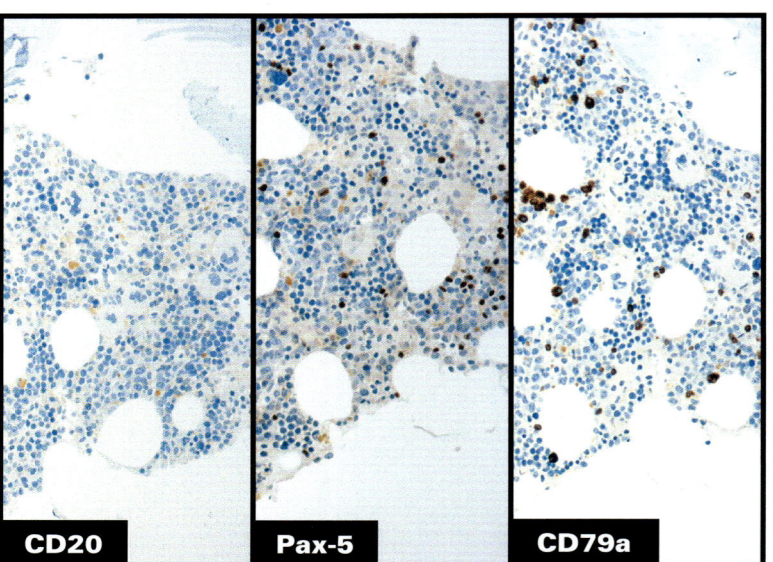

F4.6.6 B-cell markers compared in rituximab-treated patient with mild plasmacytosis

This specimen is from a different patient than that shown in **F4.6.5**. While CD20 was completely negative after rituximab therapy, Pax-5 detects B-cell precursors and mature B cells. CD79a had the highest positivity because CD79a is also expressed by terminally differentiated B cells (plasma cells), while Pax-5 is not. CD79a has the broadest range of positivity in B-cell lineage, which includes very early precursors, mature B cells, and plasma cells. A panel of antibodies is required for the appropriate evaluation of rituximab-treated B-cell lymphomas [Aumeller 2008].

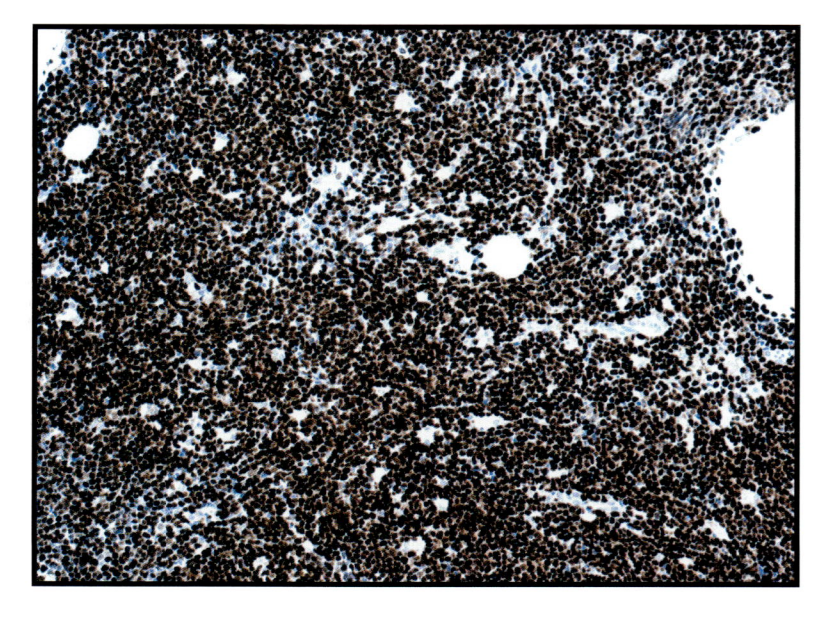

F4.6.7 Pax-5 in precursor B-cell lymphoblastic leukemia

This specimen is from a 3-year-old girl with precursor B-cell lymphoblastic leukemia. Most precursor B-lymphoblastic leukemia cases, both in children and adults (including lymphoblastic blast crisis of CML), show high expression of Pax-5. Such a high level of Pax-5 expression is also seen in occasional B-cell precursors in normal hematopoiesis.

4.6 Pax-5

F4.6.8 Weakly expressed Pax-5 in precursor B-ALL

In this biopsy specimen, the Pax-5 immunostaining is very weak. No aberrant markers were found with flow cytometry. PU.1, CD19, CD20, and CD79a were all weakly expressed. This finding could represent an indication of genetic alterations of Pax-5, which are common in precursor B-ALL [Mullighan 2007].

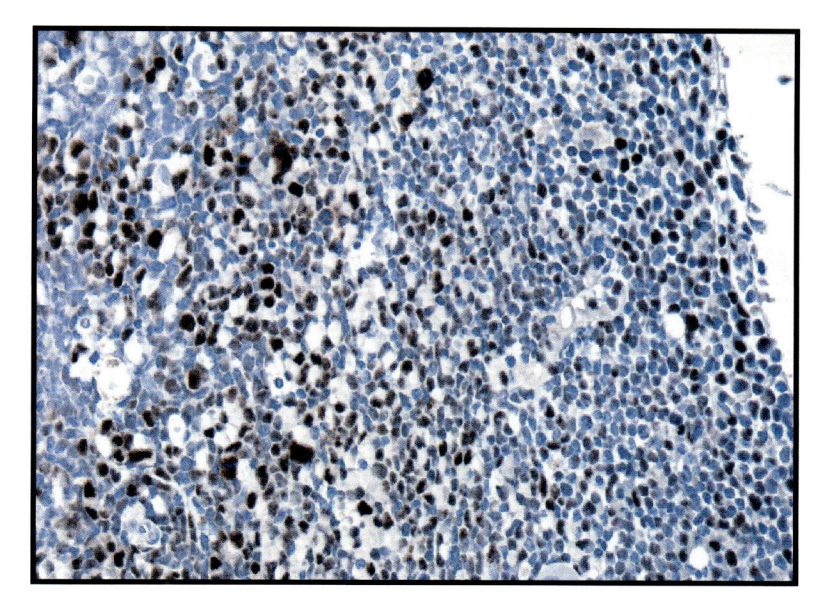

F4.6.9 Pax-5 in precursor B-cell acute lymphoblastic leukemia (ALL) after induction chemotherapy

This biopsy specimen is from a patient with residual leukemia 14 days after induction chemotherapy for precursor B-cell ALL. About 45% blasts were seen in the aspirate smears. However, these cells expressed only CD20 and CD10 and no Pax-5 or TdT were detected. This indicates that ALL can change immunophenotype after chemotherapy. Correlation with morphologic findings is essential for the interpretation of immunohistochemistry results.

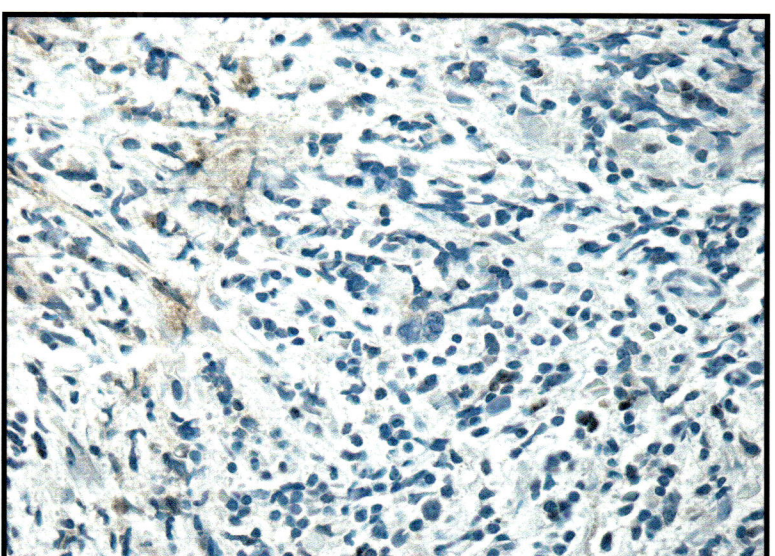

F4.6.10 Pax-5 in acute erythroid leukemia

The blast population shows no expression of Pax-5. Small lymphoid cells are strongly positive and represent normal B-cell maturation. The great majority of acute myeloid leukemia (AML) cases do not express Pax-5. Even though erythroid and megakaryocytic leukemias are rare and were not systematically studied for evidence of Pax-5 expression, we have never observed these types of AML to express Pax-5.

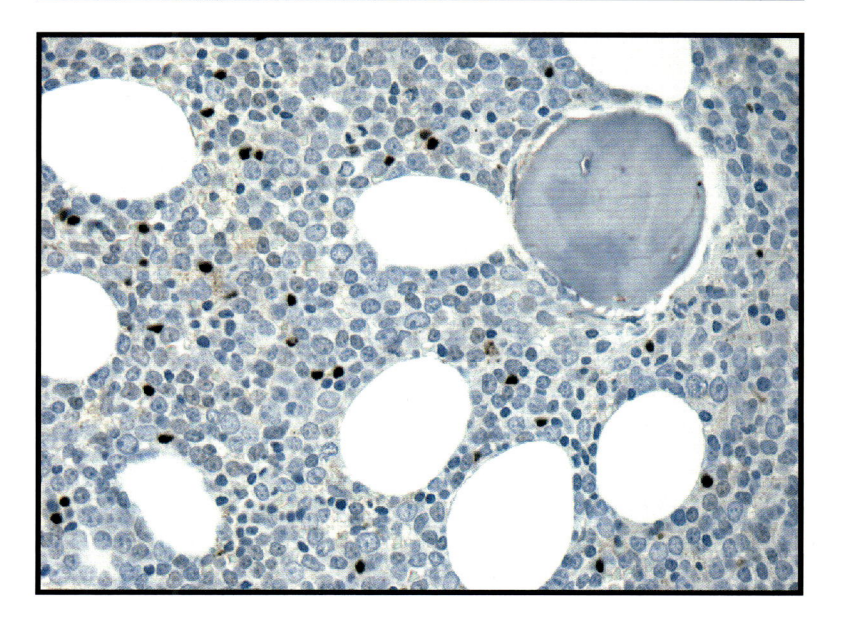

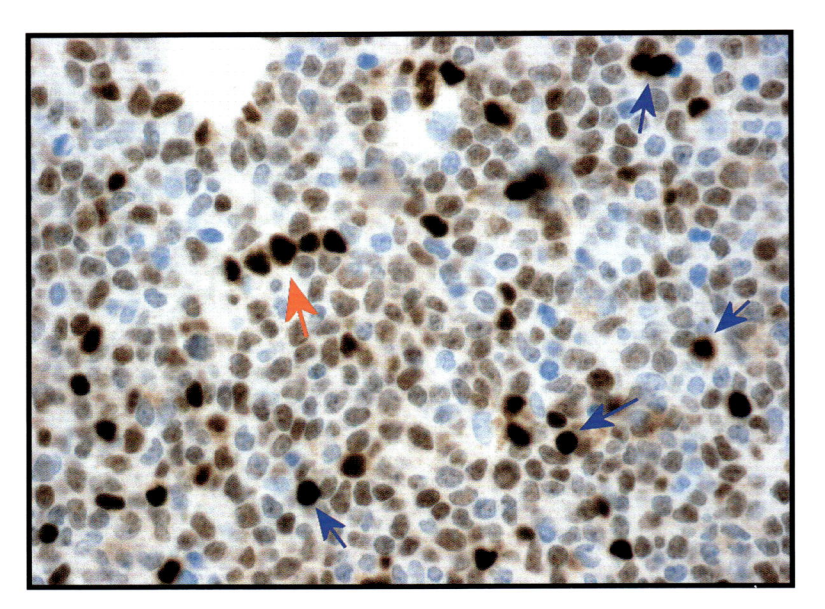

F4.6.11 Pax-5 expression in minimally differentiated acute myeloid leukemia (AML) without t(8;21)/AML1-ETO rearrangement

Weak expression of Pax-5 was found in this case of minimally differentiated AML. There was no evidence of aberrant expression of other B-cell markers with flow cytometry. Most of the cells show weak positivity. A small number of strongly positive cells are present (blue arrows) and occasionally form linear arrangements (red arrow). These cells may represent normal B-cell precursors.

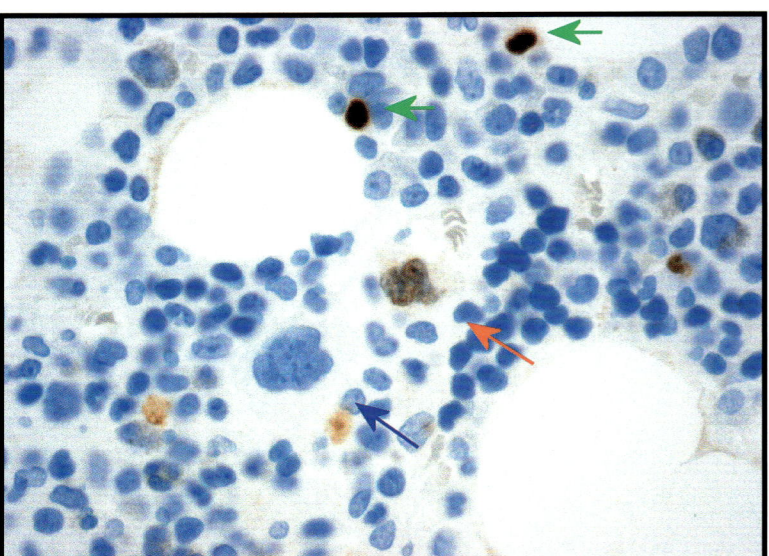

F4.6.12 Pax-5 in classical Hodgkin lymphoma

When bone marrow involvement is obvious and accompanied by fibrosis, it is good practice to confirm CD30+/Pax-5+/CD15+ positivity in the large cells. When there is no fibrosis and BM involvement is minimal, it may be difficult to differentiate Hodgkin cells from megakaryocytes. Pax-5 clearly distinguishes between the two (red arrow) with megakaryocytes always being negative (blue arrow). Non-neoplastic B cells are also detected (green arrows).

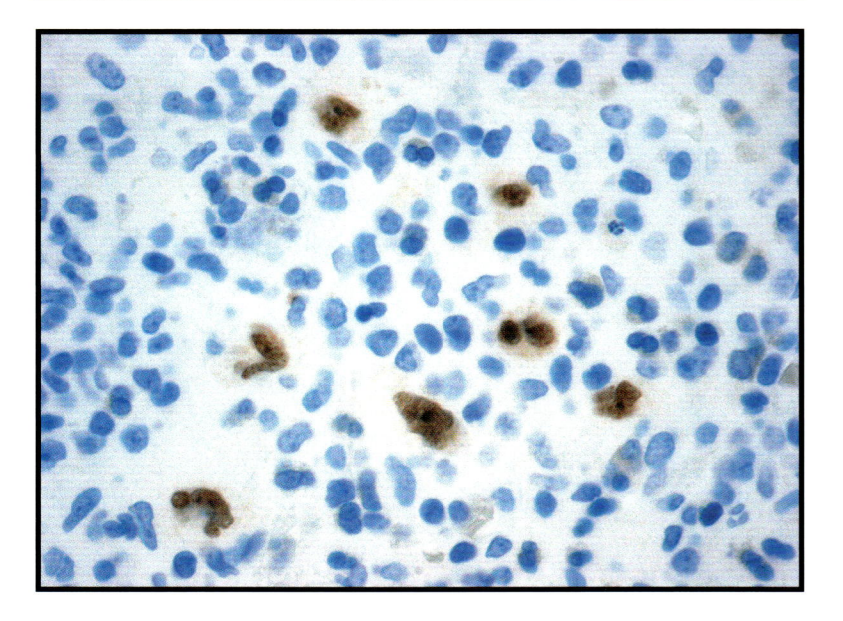

F4.6.13 Pax-5 in classical Hodgkin lymphoma (cHL)

Some of the Hodgkin cells can be easily confused for megakaryocytes in this field. Interestingly, CD30 was variably expressed in this cHL and several of the Hodgkin cells in this field are CD30-negative. This may more often present as a problem in bone marrow biopsy specimens fixed in B5 because CD30 antigen is better preserved in formalin-fixed than in B5-fixed tissue.

4.6 Pax-5

F4.6.14 Pax-5 in mature B-cell lymphoma

This is a case of follicular lymphoma (FL) with minimal paratrabecular involvement of the bone marrow. Both CD20 and Pax-5 will demonstrate FL cells in the BM. Pax-5 appears significantly more positive only because more lymphoma cells are present at this deeper level. The selection of pan B-cell antibody may depend on the specific purpose to be achieved by immunostaining or personal preference. In general, CD20 is adequate for evaluating most mature B-cell lymphoproliferative disorders.

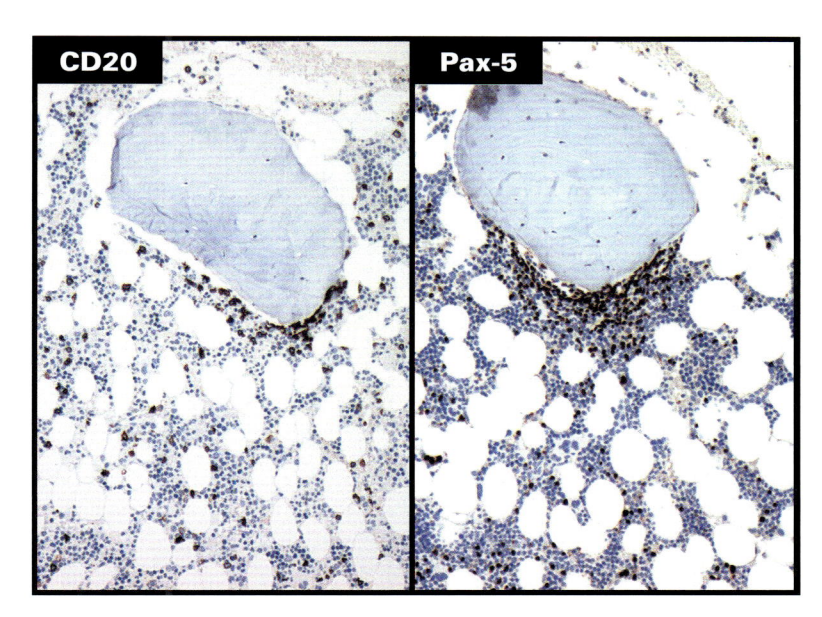

F4.6.15 Pax-5 in mature B-cell lymphoma

It may be useful to evaluate Pax-5 staining in lymphomas in which it may be difficult to determine the cell size or when CD20 is negative. Only a single large cell was found in this follicular lymphoma involving the bone marrow (arrow), which aids in grading. This may be useful in crushed tissue. An insert shows Pax-5 staining in diffuse large B-cell lymphoma which was CD20−. In such cases, the use of either Pax-5 or CD79a may be critical for identification of tumor cells.

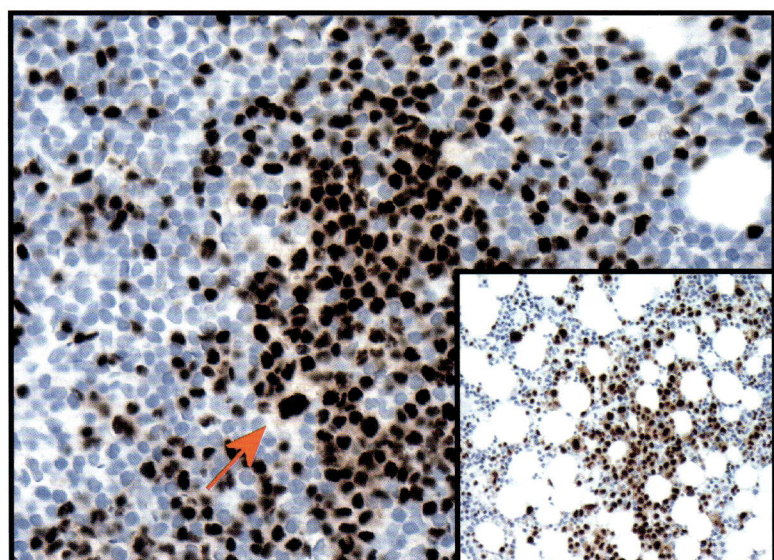

F4.6.16 Pax-5 in follicular lymphoma (FL)

As noted in F4.6.15, Pax-5 helps determine cell size, and although it may be clearly visualized even on low magnification, CD20 is much better for determining the total tumor volume, which tends to be downgraded by nuclear markers such as Pax-5. Therefore, CD20 is the marker of first choice in identifying mature B-cell lymphomas. Other pan-B-cell markers could be used as needed in addition to CD20.

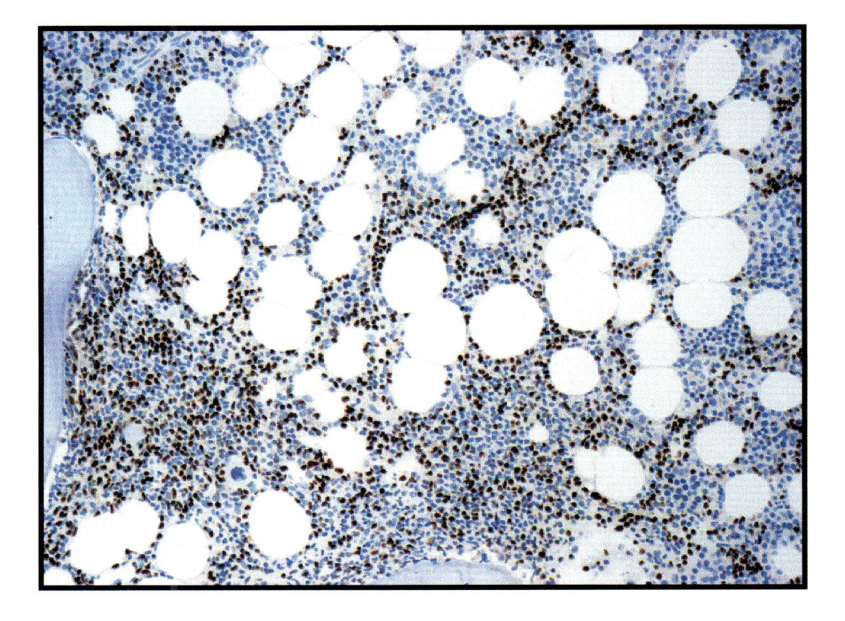

4: Other Common Markers

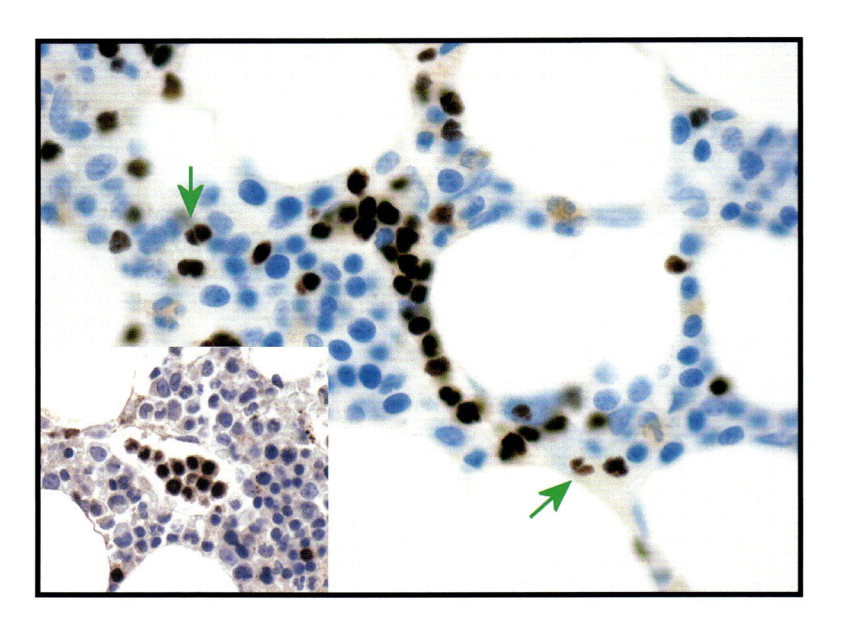

F4.6.17 **Pax-5 highlights intrasinusoidal distribution of B-cell lymphoma**

This figure illustrates Pax-5 in follicular lymphoma (FL) with focal intrasinusoidal distribution. Because Pax-5 is a nuclear marker, there will always be a space between the B-cell nucleus and another cell including endothelial cells. Nuclear features of small cleaved cells of FL are also demonstrated (arrows). Inset: Intravascular marginal zone lymphoma detected with Pax-5.

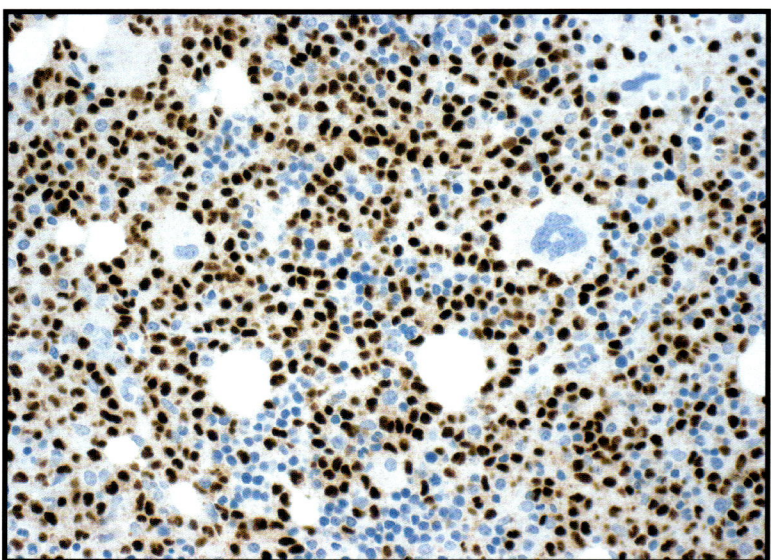

F4.6.18 **Pax-5 in hairy cell leukemia (HCL)**

Pax-5 is moderately expressed in most leukemic cells in this case of HCL. Pax-5 expression is often somewhat less intense in mature B-cell lesions than in precursor B-cell lymphoblastic leukemia.

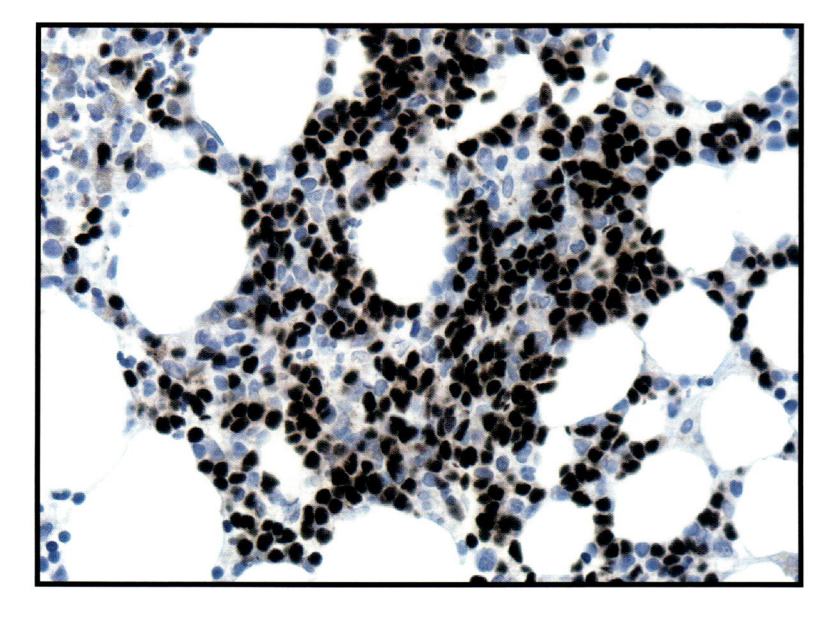

F4.6.19 **Pax-5 in mantle cell lymphoma (MCL)**

Both CD20 and Pax-5 are generally strongly expressed in MCL. Pax-5 in MCL appears to be expressed at higher levels than in most cases of CLL. However, Pax-5 detection is not indicated in routine evaluation of either MCL or chronic lymphocytic leukemia.

F4.6.20 Pax-5 in mantle cell lymphoma

In this bone marrow biopsy specimen, this rare small cluster of Pax-5+ cells is the only B-cell aggregate found. This finding is insufficient to establish a diagnosis of B-cell lymphoma. However, the same aggregate was cyclin D1+ and CD5+, thereby confirming MCL despite minimal involvement (<10% malignant cells). Such small aggregates may be difficult to detect in the BM, especially if there is erythroid hyperplasia. Either CD20 or Pax-5 would clearly identify these cells.

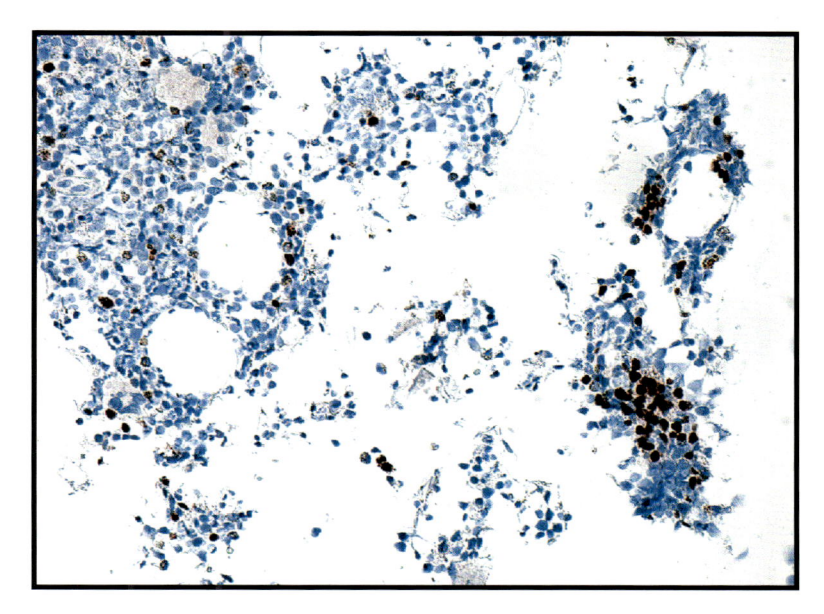

F4.6.21 Pax-5 in marginal zone lymphoma (MZL)

This biopsy specimen shows small interstitial clusters of Pax-5+ cells. Such clusters are suspicious for malignant lymphoma. Clot section from the same biopsy specimen showed large B-cell aggregates of MZL. In some cases of MZL, CD20 and Pax-5 may not detect cells with plasmacytoid differentiation. As a result, CD79 would be a better choice in such cases, which is also the best choice for demonstration of all lymphoma cells in lymphoplasmacytic lymphoma.

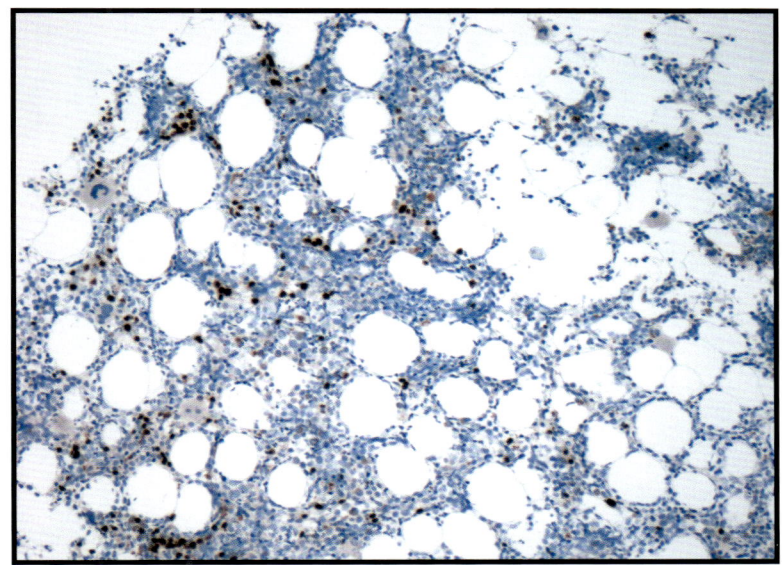

4.7 PU.1

PU.1 is also known as SPI1 in humans and it is an Ets transcription factor essential for development of multiple hematopoietic lineages [Scott 1994]. It is expressed in hematopoietic stem cells (HSCs) and common myeloid and lymphoid precursors. In contrast to Pax-5, whose expression designates a commitment to B-cell lineage, PU.1 transcription factor is likely to be more important for differentiation rather than for commitment of different cell lineages [Dakic 2007]. PU.1 loss or downregulation in the HSCs and early lymphomyeloid progenitors below a critical threshold required for efficient differentiation and tumor suppression is associated with leukemogenesis [Dakic 2007]. For instance, all-trans retinoic acid (ATRA) treatment resolves the differentiation block in acute promyelocytic leukemia by restoring PU.1 expression in otherwise PU.1-deficient leukemic promyelocytes [Mueller 2006]. Megakaryocytes, erythroid precursors, and mature NK and T cells show no expression of PU.1. Very early NK and T-cell precursors also normally express PU.1 and, as expected, some precursor T-ALL cases express PU.1. PU.1 is also required for plasmacytoid dendritic cell development [Marafioti 2008; Schotte 2004]. In the normal BM, PU.1 is found strongly expressed in granulocytes and their precursors, monocyte/macrophages, mast cells, and osteoclasts, but not in erythroid precursors, megakaryocytes, mature T and NK cells, or plasma cells [Walsh 2002]. It is also weakly expressed in precursor and mature B cells. While PU.1 plays an important role in B-cell development, PU.1 is not essential for the development of functional B lymphocytes beyond the pre-B stage [Polli 2005]. PU.1 is expressed in various B-cell neoplasms including precursor B-ALL, the vast majority of mature B-cell lymphomas and leukemias with the exception of rare PU.1-negative DLBCLs, and nodular lymphocyte predominant Hodgkin lymphoma, but not in cHL [Feldman 2008; Torlakovic 2006a; Marafioti 2004; Pileri 2003a; Loddenkemper 2004; Pileri 2003b; Torlakovic 2001]. PU.1 is also regularly expressed at high levels in histiocytic and dendritic cell lesions [Lehtonen 2005; Iwama 2002].

4: Other Common Markers

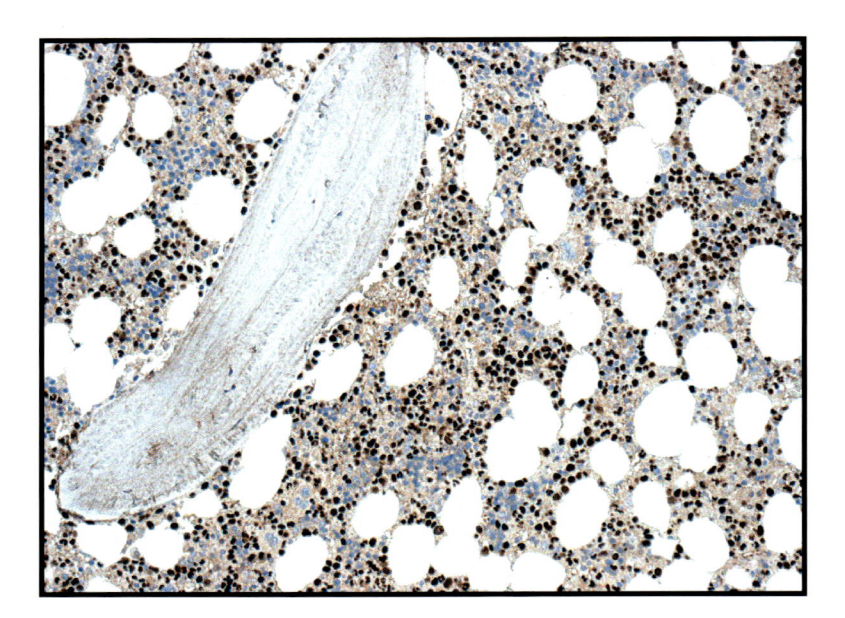

F4.7.1 PU.1 in histologically normal bone marrow (ADVANCE)

PU.1 transcription factor is expressed in myeloid cells including neutrophils, monocytes, macrophages, myeloid dendritic cells, and B cells. The appearance at low magnification is similar to that of myeloperoxidase because the great majority of positive cells in the normal BM are neutrophils and precursors.

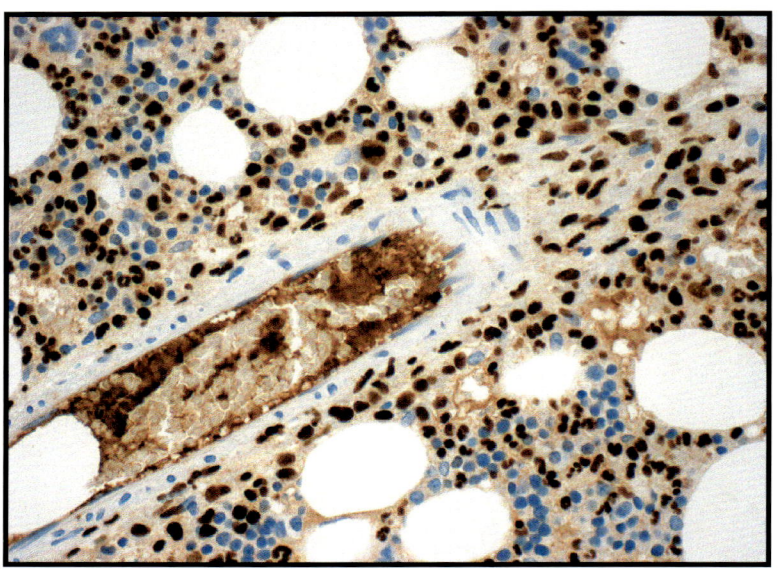

F4.7.2 PU.1 in histologically normal bone marrow

Perivascular population of PU.1+ mononuclear cells is demonstrated and probably corresponds to CD14+ perivascular monocytic cells. (See also **F3.10.9**.)

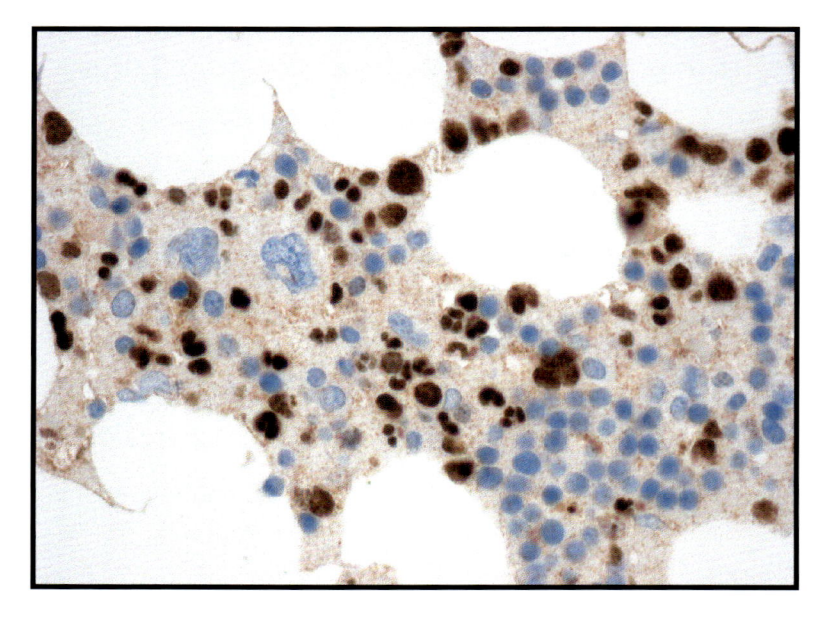

F4.7.3 PU.1 in histologically normal bone marrow

This biopsy specimen shows focal erythroid predominance. In such areas, very few neutrophils are noted and most appear to be mature cells. It appears that the largest round cells with very strong PU.1 expression and a few smaller round cells with intermediate expression of PU.1 represent normal B-cell precursors. While cytoplasmic positivity for PU.1 can be occasionally found in some cells, this is not usually found in megakaryocytes or red blood cells.

4.7 PU.1

F4.7.4 PU.1 staining in extracellular spaces

This biopsy specimen shows acute myeloid leukemia with very weak PU.1 expression. Intense multifocal staining can be noted in the extracellular spaces. It is not clear why PU.1 immunohistochemistry staining is frequently found in extracellular spaces in most tissues resembling similar and expected results for Ig light chains.

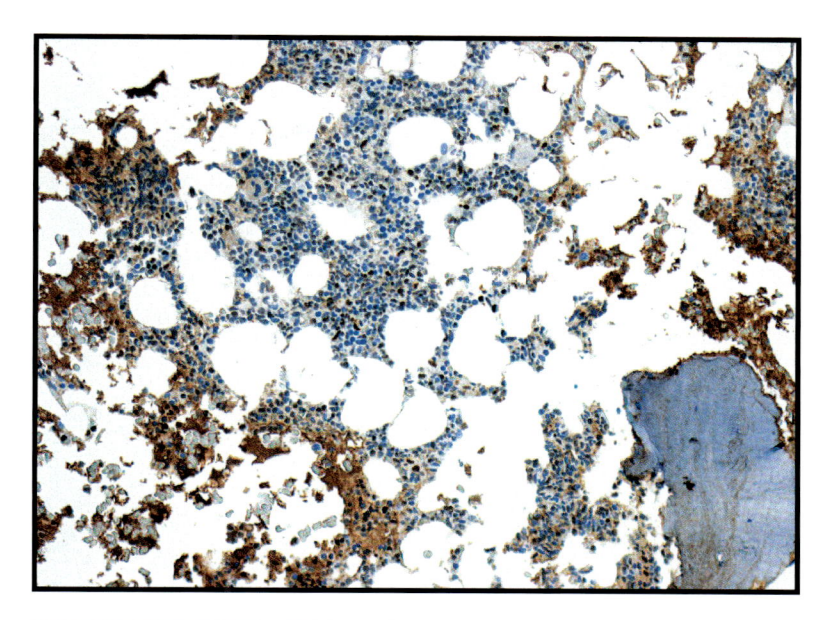

F4.7.5 PU.1 in undifferentiated acute leukemia

This biopsy specimen is from a 57-year-old woman. Expression of PU.1 is weak. PU.1 is not a lineage marker and its expression, weak or strong, is insufficient for lineage determination even though its levels of expression are critical for appropriate myeloid (high levels) and B lymphoid (low levels) development.

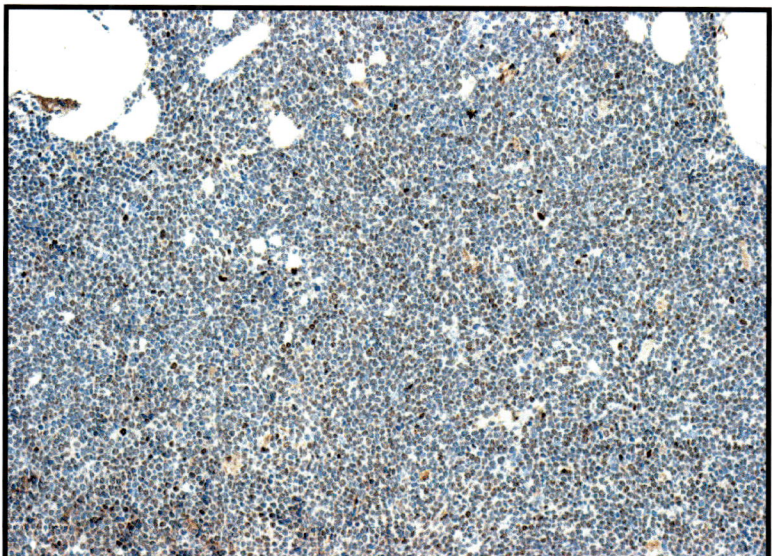

F4.7.6 PU.1 in acute myeloid leukemia (AML) without maturation

PU.1 is regularly expressed in many AMLs (M0 to M5 by FAB classification). We have also observed some cases of weakly positive erythroid and megakaryoblastic acute leukemias.

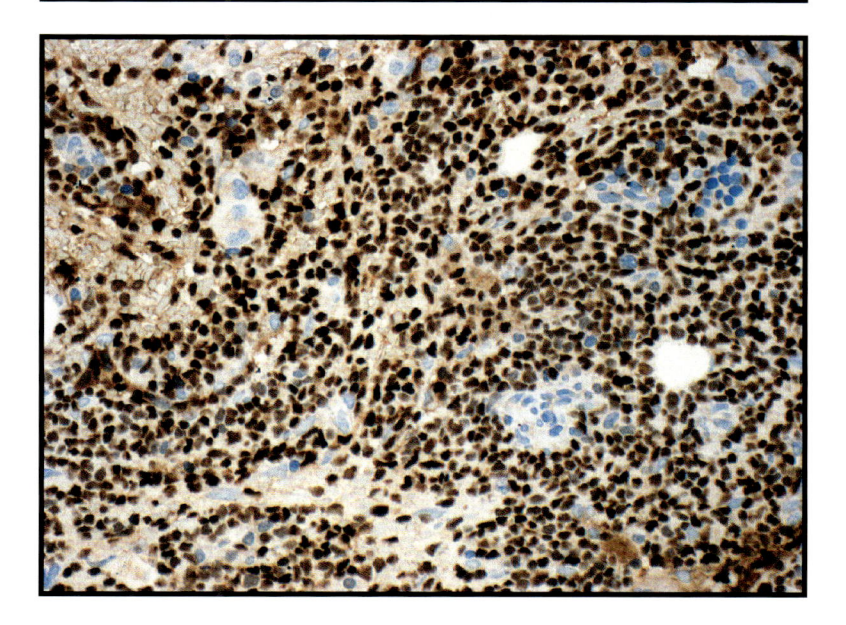

4: Other Common Markers

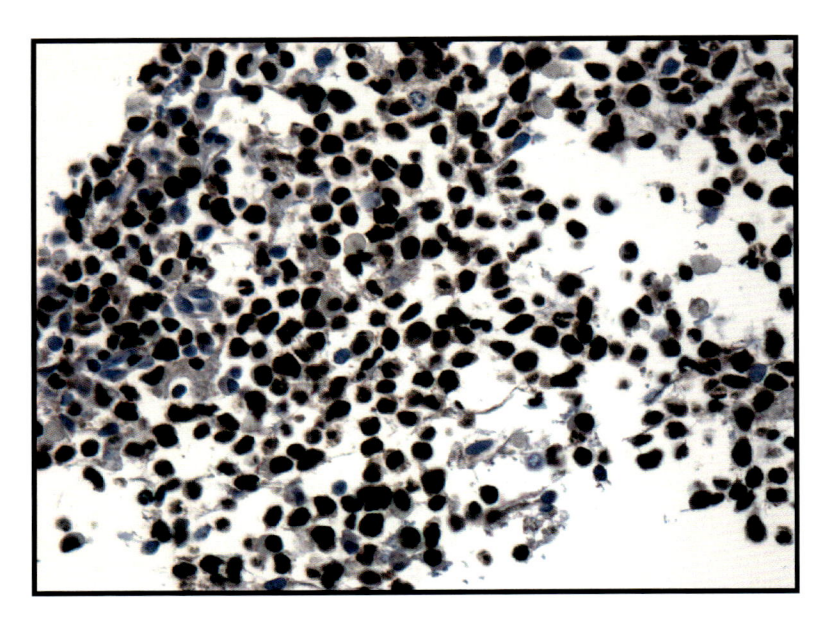

F4.7.7 PU.1 in acute myeloid leukemia (AML) with maturation

This 6-year-old boy was diagnosed with AML with maturation. No aberrant markers were identified with flow cytometry, and cytogenetic analysis revealed normal karyotype. PU.1 is strongly expressed in all leukemic blasts as well as in more mature myeloid cells.

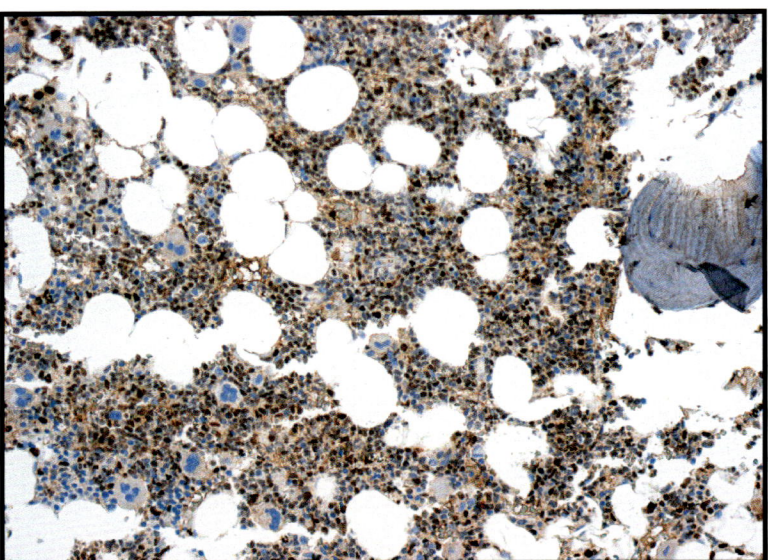

F4.7.8 PU.1 in CD4+/CD56+ hematodermic neoplasm involving bone marrow

This specimen is from a 56-year-old man with a leukocyte count of 22.0×10^9/L, anemia, and thrombocytopenia. The leukemic cells resembled monoblasts. PU.1 is weakly to moderately expressed in this case of CD4+/CD56+ hematodermic neoplasm. PU.1 is expressed in normal plasmacytoid dendritic cells and accordingly could be found in CD4+/CD56+ hematodermic neoplasm, which is a tumor of plasmacytoid dendritic cells.

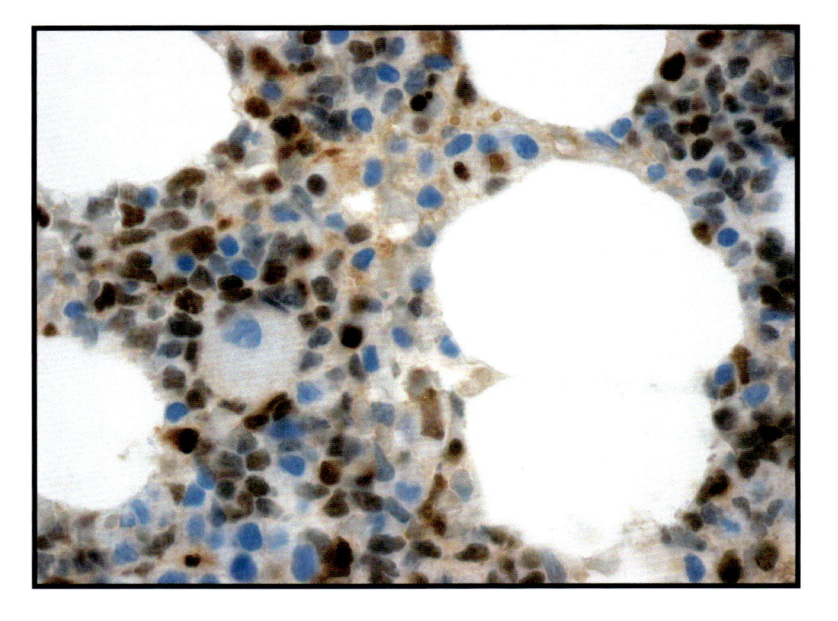

F4.7.9 PU.1 in CD4+/CD56+ hematodermic neoplasm

This is a high magnification image of the case shown in F4.7.8. A spectrum of positivity for PU.1 is detected. While a few megakaryocytes and erythroid cells can be recognized and do not stain with PU.1, most of the negative cells are probably mature infiltrating T cells, which normally do not express PU.1.

F4.7.10 PU.1 in precursor B-cell lymphoblastic leukemia

The strongest positive cells are probably monocytes or other benign myeloid or lymphoid precursors. The leukemic blasts appear to express weak uniform positivity in this case of precursor B-cell lymphoblastic leukemia. The level of expression is comparable to that expected in B cells in general.

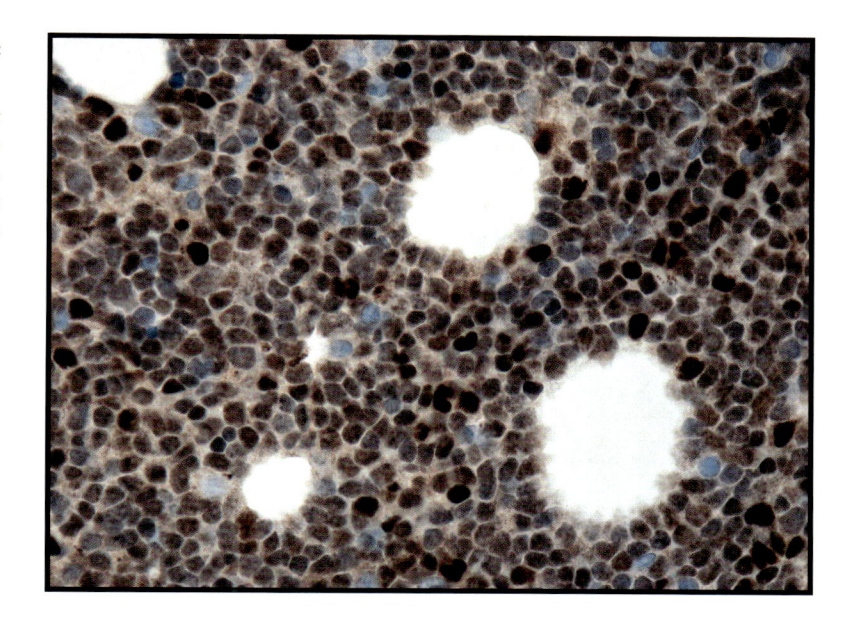

F4.7.11 PU.1 in chronic myelomonocytic leukemia type 2

More mature granulocytes are recognizable. Large cells with intermediate positivity correspond to myeloid precursors and some of which are possibly blasts. The cells of intermediate size and having the highest expression of PU.1 would be expected to be monocytic cells.

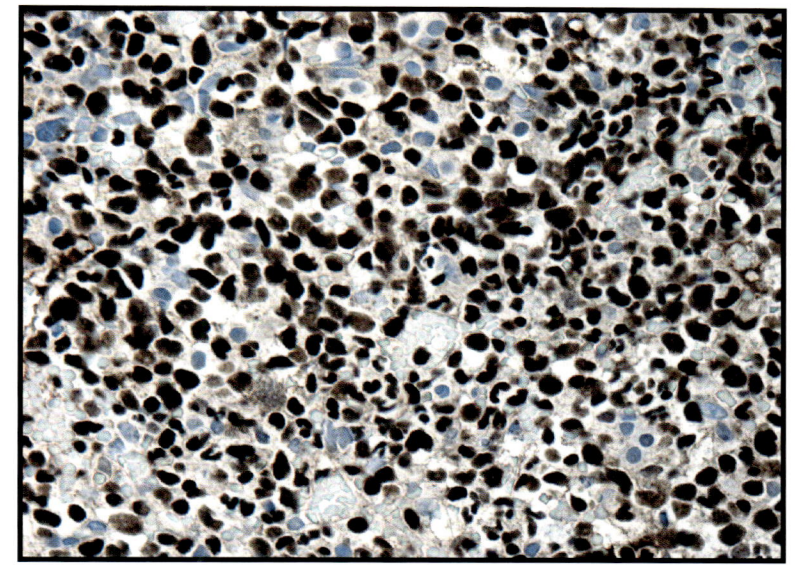

F4.7.12 PU.1 in chronic myelomonocytic leukemia (CMML) type 1

Compared with the specimen shown in F4.7.11, this CMML shows very weak expression of PU.1 in all cells. This finding should not be interpreted as a biological variation or differential expression between CMML type 1 and type 2, before a technically suboptimal result is ruled out. Prolonged decalcification was shown to be the cause of suboptimal staining in this case.

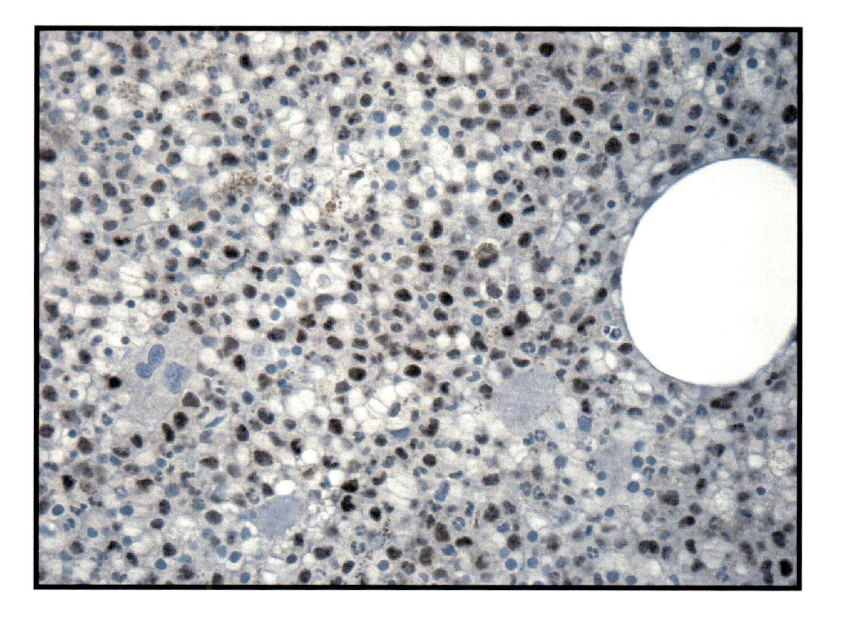

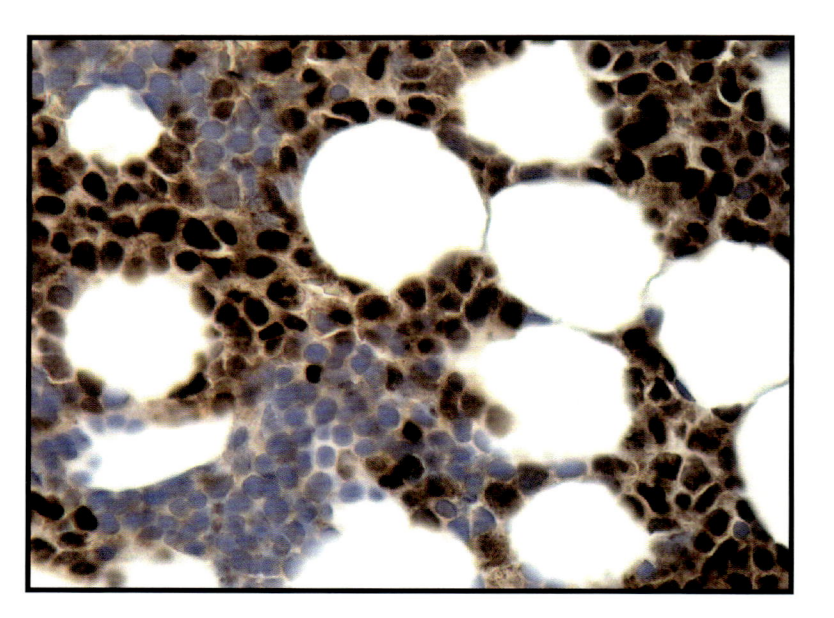

F4.7.13 PU.1 in myeloid/erythroid leukemia

In this type of erythroid leukemia, the blasts express some myeloid markers and, as illustrated in this case, PU.1 was also present. Erythroid precursors comprised about 60% of all cells in the aspirate smears and large erythroid islands were found in tissue sections. The large groups of negative cells are erythroid cells. The strongest positive cells are myeloid cells. Blasts show weak to moderate expression of PU.1.

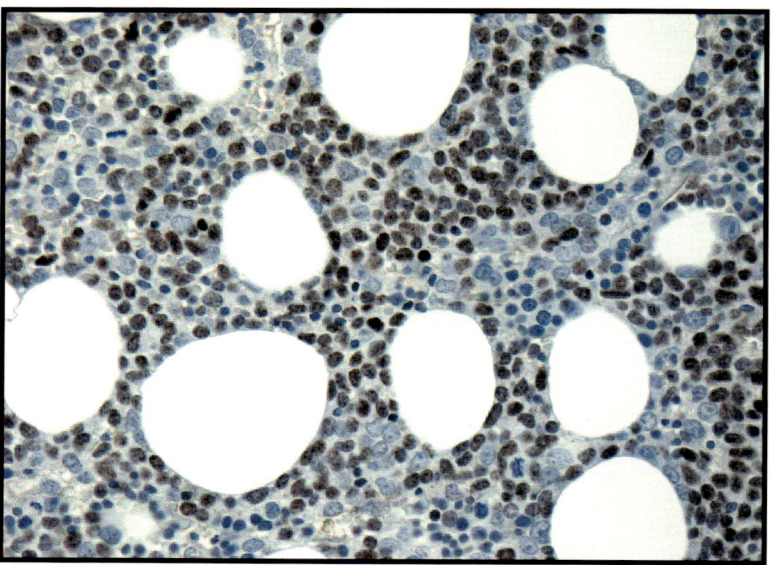

F4.7.14 PU.1 in acute pure erythroid leukemia

Most erythroblasts show very weak expression of PU.1. While PU.1 expression was linked to Friend murine erythroleukemia, there is no such evidence in humans. Expression of PU.1 in erythroblasts is an abnormal finding because erythroid cells do not express PU.1 in normal hematopoiesis. Erythroid differentiation does not proceed before PU.1 is downregulated by GATA-1. Hypothetically, a block of erythroid differentiation by PU.1 may represent an oncogenic property of PU.1 in this case.

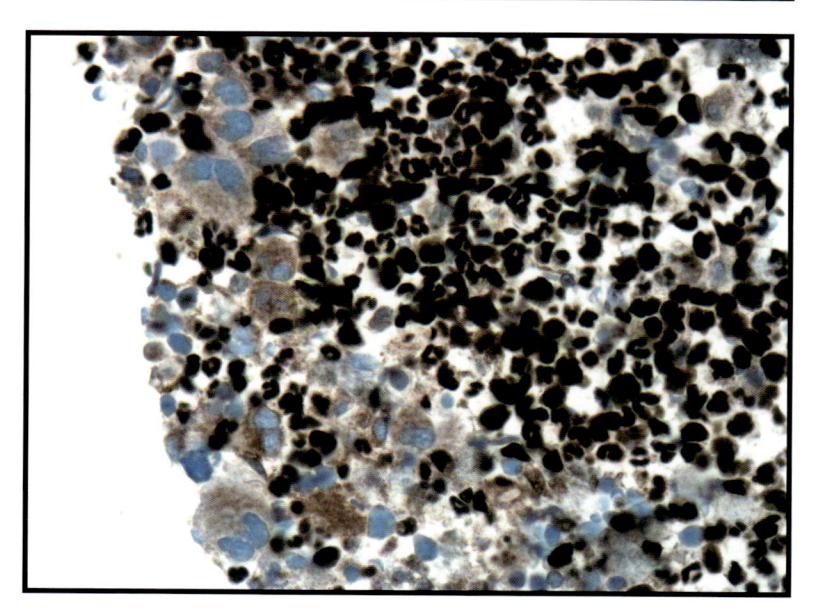

F4.7.15 PU.1 in chronic myeloid leukemia (CML)

Most of the cells in CML are neutrophils and precursors. Megakaryocytes normally do not express PU.1, not even in the cytoplasm. It is not clear if cytoplasmic PU.1 in megakaryocytes in this case has biological significance. Nonspecific staining related to technical problems is the proposed interpretation.

4.8 Fli-1

Fli-1 is an Ets transcription factor involved in cell proliferation and oncogenesis and in humans its role is best recognized in Ewing sarcoma because the *FLI1* gene is implicated in t(11;22)(q24:q12). *EWS-FLI-1* fusion protein is believed to behave as an aberrant transcriptional activator [Prasad 1992; Riggi 2007]. Fli-1 is expressed by lymphoid cells including even very early precursors of NK cells and T cells, but also B cells. It is also expressed by neutrophils, megakaryocytes, and endothelial cells [Anderson 1999]. Its expression in the BM appears significant and it is present at high levels in positive hematopoietic cells. It is strongly expressed in all stages of megakaryocyte development and in humans, it is hemizygously deleted in patients with thrombocytopenia [Hart 2000]. Overexpression of Fli-1 in myeloproliferative disease has been described only in megakaryocytes, but not in other myeloid cells [Bock 2006]. Overexpression of Fli-1 has also been identified in progression of mycosis fungoides as well as in some cases of melanoma [Quick 2006; Torlakovic 2006b]. In our experience, Fli-1 is also regularly detected in B-cell and T-cell lymphomas including both non-Hodgkin and Hodgkin lymphoma; 1 study reported its expression in only a small number of malignant lymphomas [Mhawech-Fauceglia 2007]. Because so many hematopoietic cells express Fli-1 in the BM, it probably would not be helpful to use Fli-1 IHC to screen for rare Ewing sarcoma metastatic cells in the BM even though the great majority of cases of this sarcoma express high levels of Fli-1 [Llombart-Bosch 2001]. In benign BM, the difference between megakaryocytes and red blood cells is distinct because normal red blood cells are never positive and megakaryocytes express very high levels of Fli-1. The difference in megakaryoblastic and erythroid leukemia is possibly less clear because we have observed that it may also be expressed to some degree in rare erythroid leukemia, while in megakaryoblastic leukemia its level of expression may be less than in normal megakaryocytes. Interestingly, it was shown that constitutive expression of Fli-1 in HB60 cells (erythroblastic cells) blocks Epo-induced differentiation while promoting Epo-induced proliferation, which is similar to what happens in retroviral insertional activation of Fli-1 observed in Friend murine leukemia virus (F-MuLV)-induced erythroleukemia [Pereira 1999]. Its oncogenic properties should be further investigated in human erythroid and megakaryoblastic leukemia [Truong 2000]. Expression in endothelial cells can also be observed in the BM, but just like in the rest of the body, the benign endothelial cells show weak expression of Fli-1, while higher levels are readily observed in angiosarcomas [Folpe 2001; Folpe 2000]. Fli-1 is equally expressed in lymphatics and blood vessels [Pusztaszeri 2006].

F4.8.1 Fli-1 in histologically normal bone marrow

This biopsy specimen is from a 43-year-old man with mixed cellularity classical Hodgkin lymphoma. There was no BM involvement. Fli-1 staining reveals numerous positive cells; this Ets transcription factor is expressed by neutrophils and their precursors and lymphoid cells, but in contrast to PU.1, it is also expressed by megakaryocytes and endothelial cells.

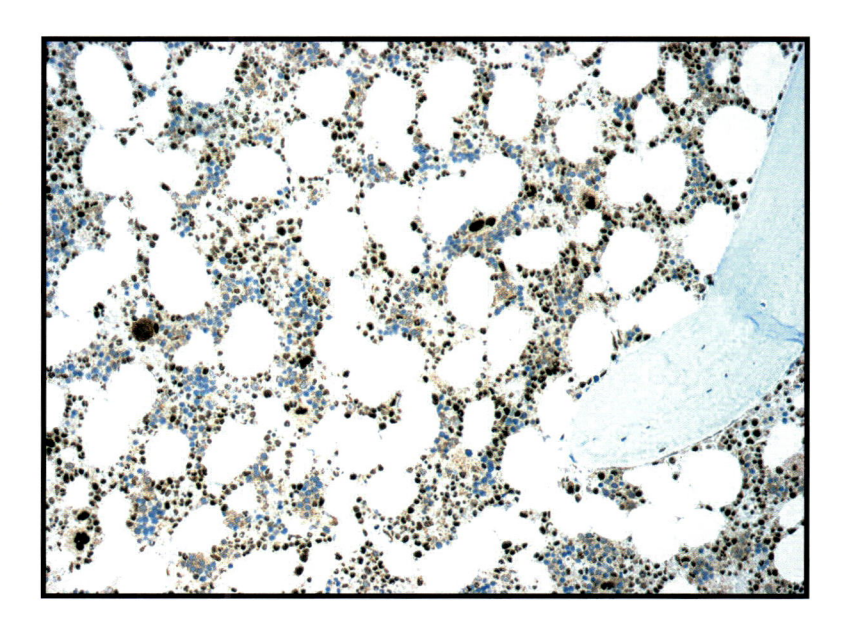

4: Other Common Markers

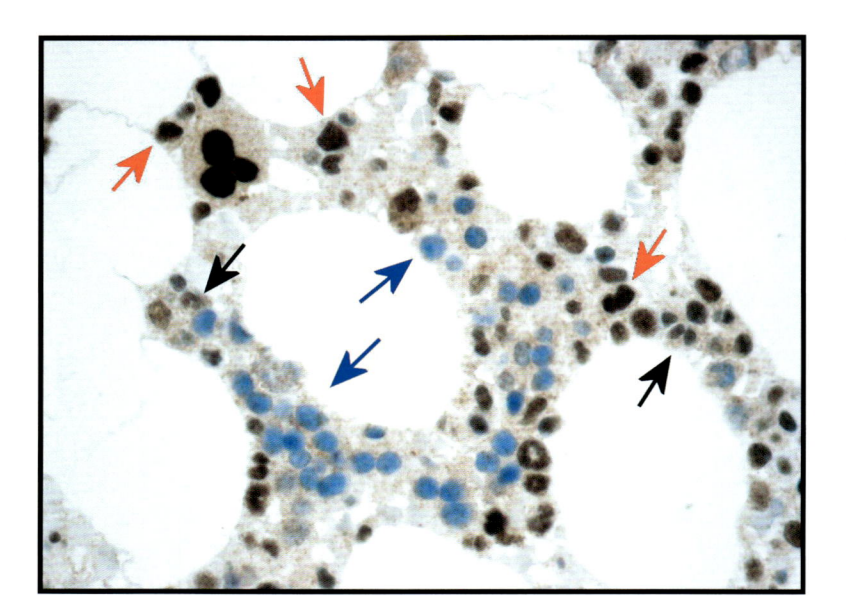

F4.8.2 Fli-1 in histologically normal bone marrow

Erythroid precursors are clearly negative. A single illustrated megakaryocytes (left upper corner) is strongly positive. Neutrophils vary in expression from strong in early precursors (red arrows) to moderate or weak in more mature cells (black arrows). This image and other images here demonstrate that Fli-1 should not be used to search for rare Ewing sarcoma cells in the BM; it is perfectly legitimate to use Fli-1 to confirm the diagnosis when there is diffuse involvement by the tumor.

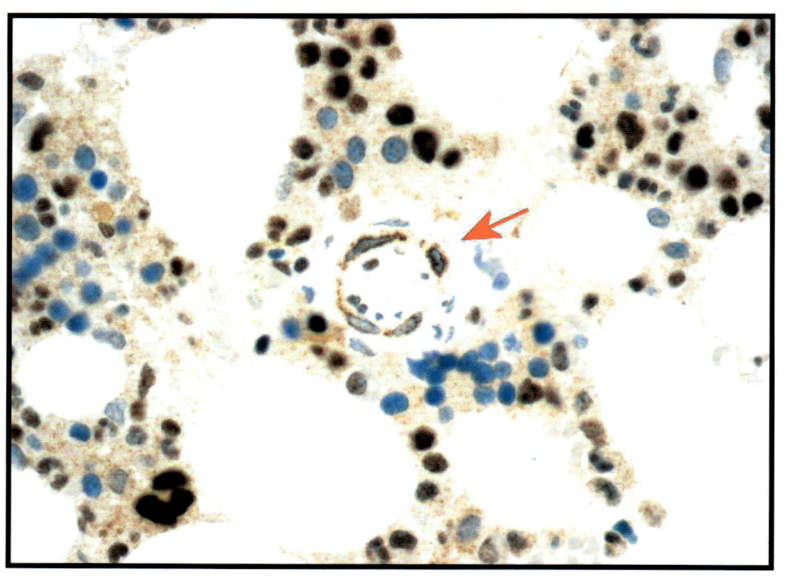

F4.8.3 Fli-1 in endothelial cells

The arrow points to a cross-section of a vessel. The endothelial cells are, as expected, weakly positive, but also show some cytoplasmic expression. This is not a constant finding. In contrast to a normal weak Fli-1 expression in benign endothelial cells, angiosarcomas express high levels of Fli-1.

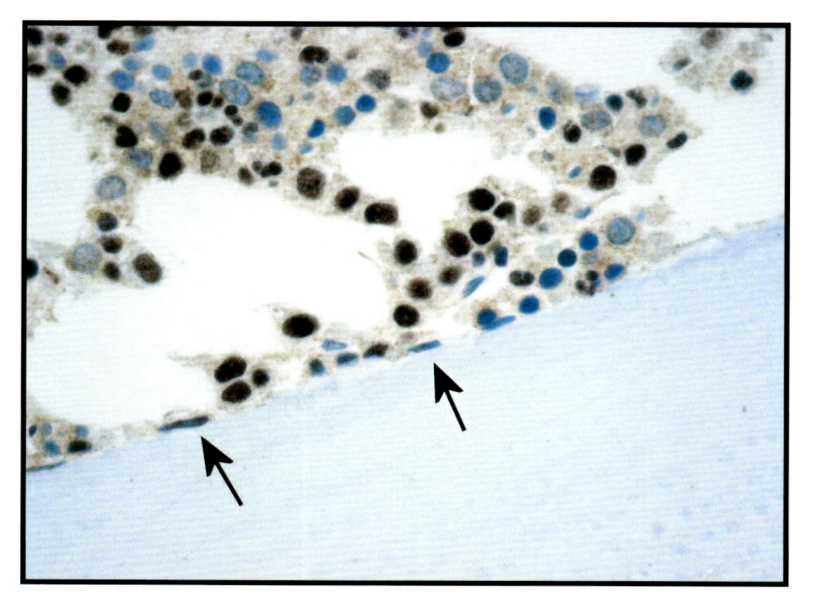

F4.8.4 Fli-1 in endosteal lining cells

Fli-1 is not expressed in flat endosteal cells that line subcortical and trabecular surfaces (black arrows) or osteoblasts.

F4.8.5 Fli-1 in acute myeloid/erythroid leukemia

Fli-1 is highly expressed by abnormal megakaryocytes. More mature erythroid forms show no expression of Fli-1; this field also shows a population of larger round cells interpreted as blasts, which are weakly positive.

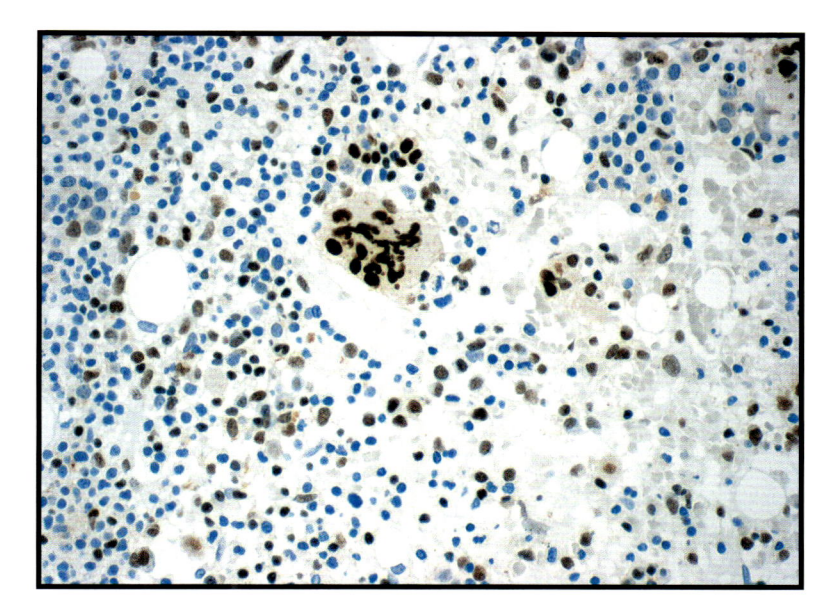

F4.8.6 Fli-1 in essential thrombocythemia (ET) in transformation to acute leukemia

Fli-1 is markedly overexpressed in atypical megakaryocytes and it is also expressed in many relatively large blasts that were also positive for CD61 and von Willebrand factor. However, note that many blasts actually appear to stain less intensely than the abnormal megakaryocytes. Overexpression of Fli-1 in megakaryocytes in myeloproliferative disease has been previously described [Bock 2006].

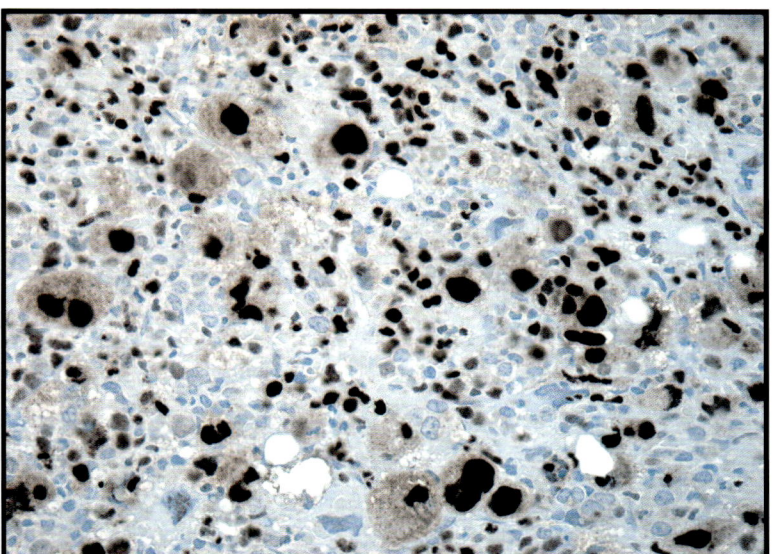

4.9 Cyclin D1

Cyclin D1 is also known as BCL1; PRAD1; U21B31; D11S287E (Entrez Gene). Cyclin D1 forms a complex with CDK4 or CDK6 kineses, whose activity is required for cell cycle G1/S transition. It interacts with tumor suppressor protein Rb. Mutations, amplification, and overexpression of this gene, which alters cell cycle progression, are observed frequently in various tumors (Entrez Gene). In hematologic disorders, cyclin D1 has an important role in the biology of some B-cell malignancies where its overexpression has been associated principally with t(11;14)(q13;q32) [Liu 2004]. Cyclin D1 can be detected with IHC in a wide variety of benign and malignant human tissues, but its role in diagnostic hematopathology is limited to the diagnosis of MCL and its variants [Yatabe 2001; Torlakovic 2005b]. It has to be emphasized that cyclin D1 is often expressed in multiple myeloma and also in hairy cell leukemia, but these 2 entities have very characteristic clinical and pathological features and practically never are in the differential diagnosis of MCL [Troussard 2000; Bosch 1995; Bosch 1994]. Cyclin D1 expression in MCL does not need to be very high and the staining may be weak, but its presence in the nuclei has to be unequivocal and it has to be present diffusely in at least some areas where sheets of cells show definite positivity. With this nuclear marker, randomly distributed occasional positive cells do not support the diagnosis of MCL. While many epithelial and stromal cells can express cyclin D1, its expression in the benign BM is limited to stromal cells. It appears that cyclin D1 expression in the benign cells of the BM can be induced by various benign or malignant lesions that involve BM. This induction of high expression of cyclin D1 in stromal cells has been described in follicular dendritic cells of follicular lymphoma and nodular sclerosis cHL [Torlakovic 2005b]. Cyclin D1 gene expression in vascular endothelial cells is regulated by a dual system: one is inducible in the G(1) phase, and the other is constitutively active; the later regulatory mechanism is probably reponsible for common detection of weak expression of cyclin D1 in endothelial cells throughout the body including the BM [Nagata 2001]. It is known that parathyroid hormone upregulates cyclin D1 in osteoblasts [Datta 2007]. Differentiated adipocytes would be expected to have reduced proliferative potential and no expression of cyclin D1. However, elevated levels of cyclin D1 expression were described in mature adipocytes in the subcutaneous tissue and are dependent on insulin [Kim 2001]. Cyclin D1 detection is frequently used in the evaluation of non-Hodgkin lymphoma. It is particularly helpful in diagnosing variant forms of MCL [Dunphy 2007b; Athanasiou 2001; Miranda 2000; Viswanatha 2000; Vasef 1997].

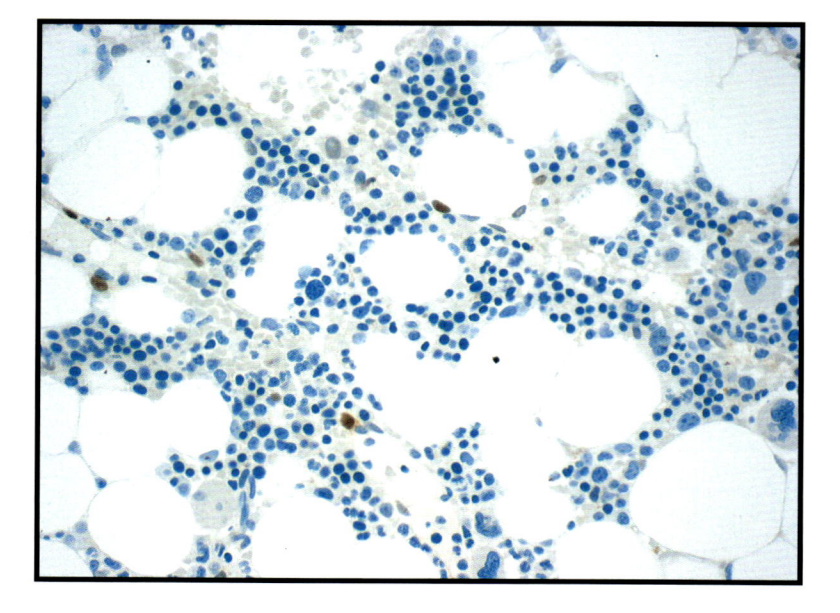

F4.9.1 Cyclin D1 in histologically normal bone marrow

In normal BM, occasional stromal cells can always be found to express cyclin D1. Hematopoietic cells do not show detectable expression of cyclin D1 on immunohistochemistry even with highly sensitive methods.

4.9   Cyclin D1

F4.9.2 Cyclin D1 in histologically normal bone marrow

Endothelial cells (arrows) frequently express cyclin D1. However, the staining is very variable and the number of positive cells varies greatly from area to area as well as from one biopsy to another.

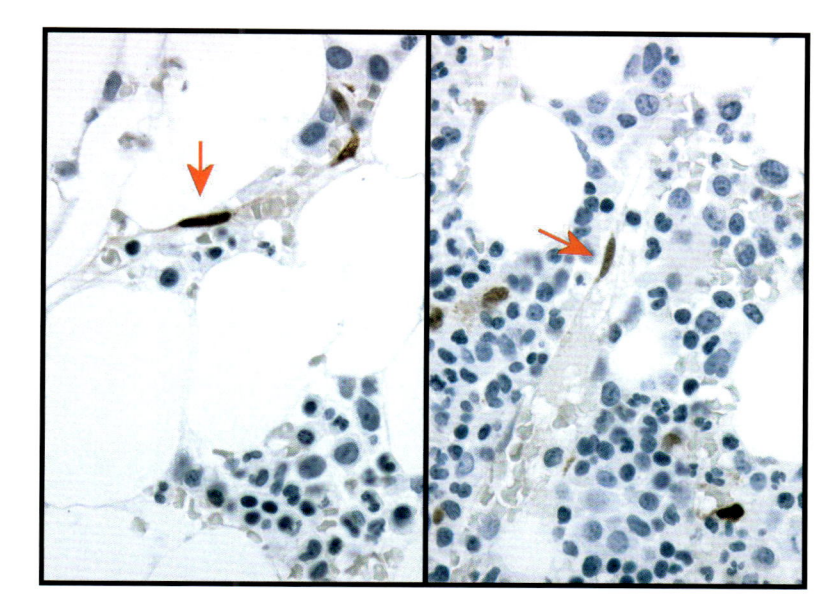

F4.9.3 Cyclin D1 in osteoblasts

Cyclin D1 can be strongly expressed by normal osteoblasts. Its expression is often limited to small groups of cells and many osteoblasts in the same biopsy specimen do not express cyclin D1.

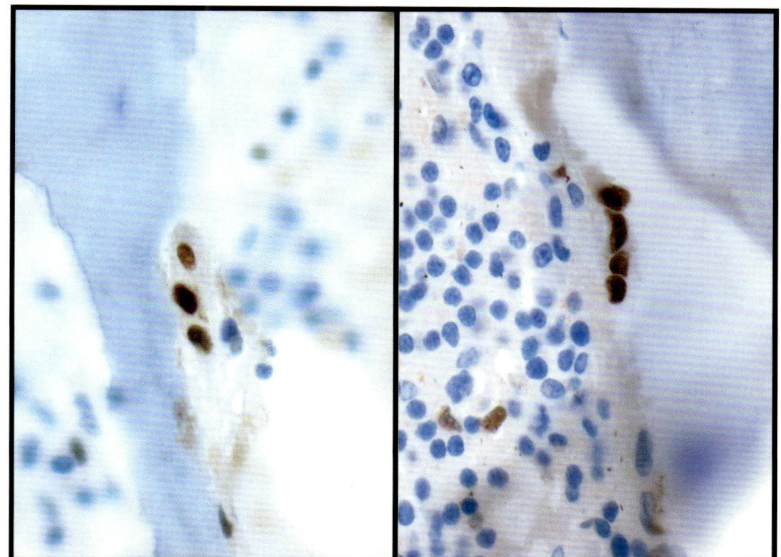

F4.9.4 Cyclin D1 in adipocytes

Mature adipocytes in the bone marrow may show cyclin D1 expression in various conditions (arrows). Differentiated adipocytes would be expected to have reduced proliferative potential and no expression of cyclin D1. However, elevated levels of cyclin D1 expression were described in mature adipocytes in the subcutaneous tissue and are dependent on insulin.

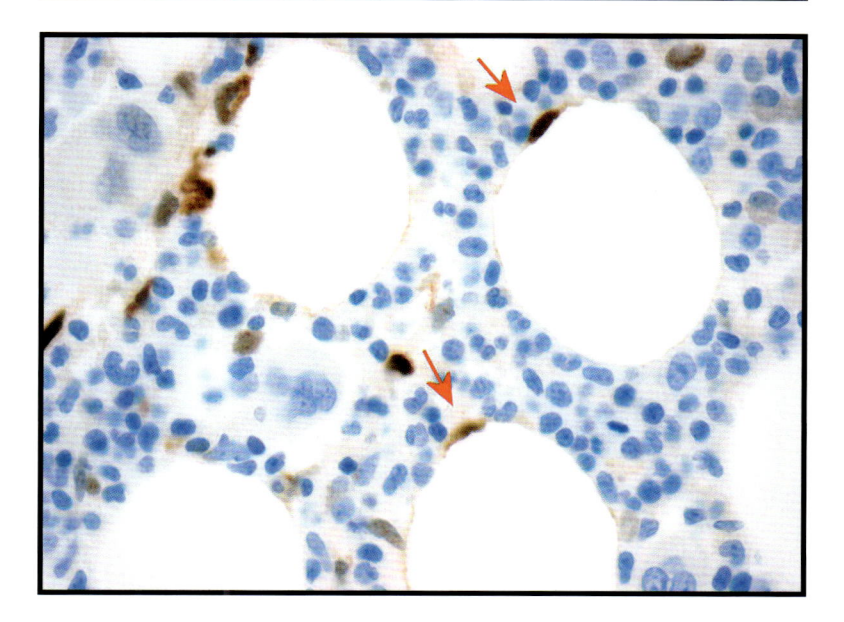

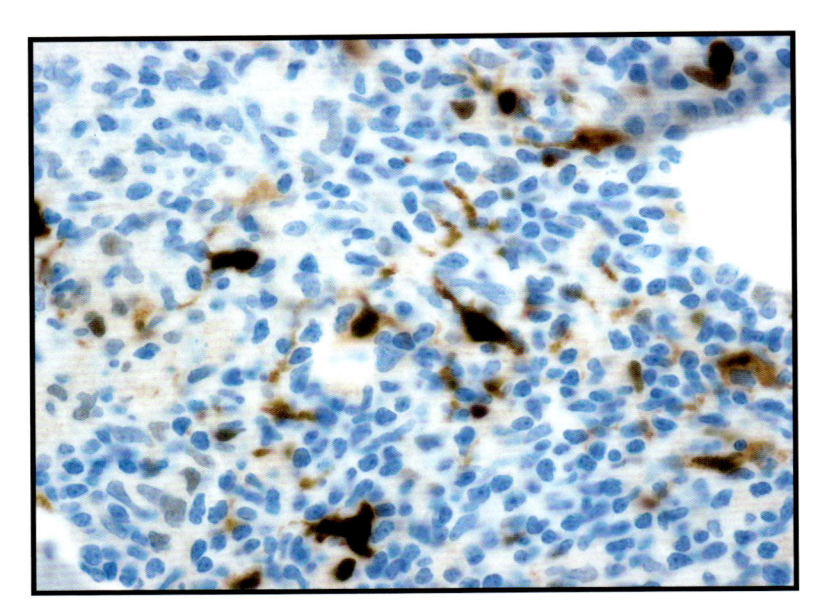

F4.9.5 Cyclin D1 in dendritic cells

This biopsy specimen is involved by a peripheral T-cell lymphoma. In the areas of involvement by lymphoma, a population of dendritic cells with both cytoplasmic and nuclear positivity for cyclin D1 is shown. Their biological significance is not clear. Similar cyclin D1+ dendritic cells have been described in the lymph node biopsy specimens with classical Hodgkin lymphoma and follicular lymphoma.

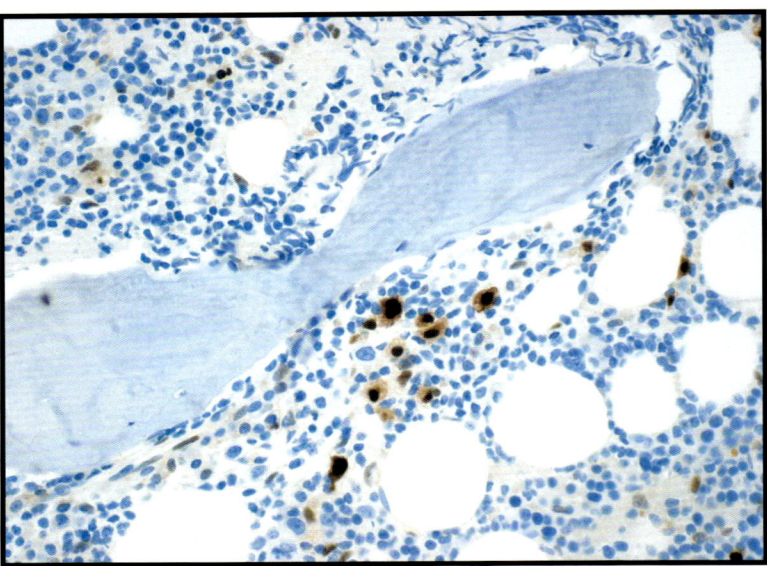

F4.9.6 Cyclin D1 in dendritic cells associated with follicular lymphoma (FL)

This image illustrates several strongly cyclin D1+ cells associated with a paratrabecular infiltrate of FL. Their nature is not clear, but they may be compatible with stromal dendritic cells or macrophages (note relatively low nuclear-cytoplasmic ratio). FL cells are negative as expected.

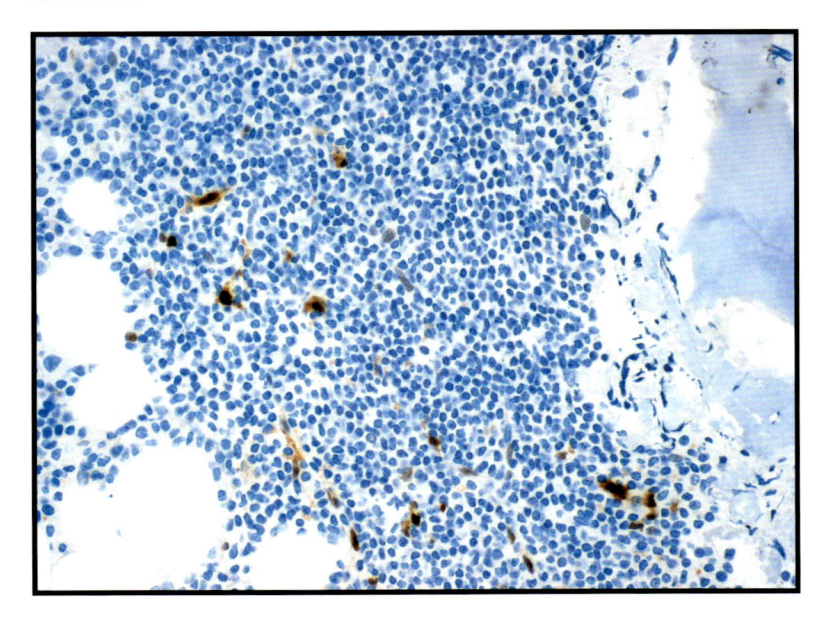

F4.9.7 Cyclin D1 in atypical lymphoid aggregate of uncertain biological potential

This biopsy specimen is from an adult HIV-negative patient with a fever of unknown origin. A single large atypical lymphoid aggregate was identified, but the immunophenotype of mixed T and B cells was not abnormal and IgH and T-cell receptor–γ gene rearrangement tests by PCR were negative. Cyclin D1 highlights occasional dendritic cells with nuclear and cytoplasmic positivity. These cells were not present outside the lymphoid aggregate.

F4.9.8 Cyclin D1 in chronic lymphocytic leukemia (CLL)

Cyclin D1+ dendritic cells are also identified in the bone marrow involved by CLL. It appears that cyclin D1+ dendritic cells are regularly found in the areas infiltrated by lymphocytes and do not represent follicular dendritic cells.

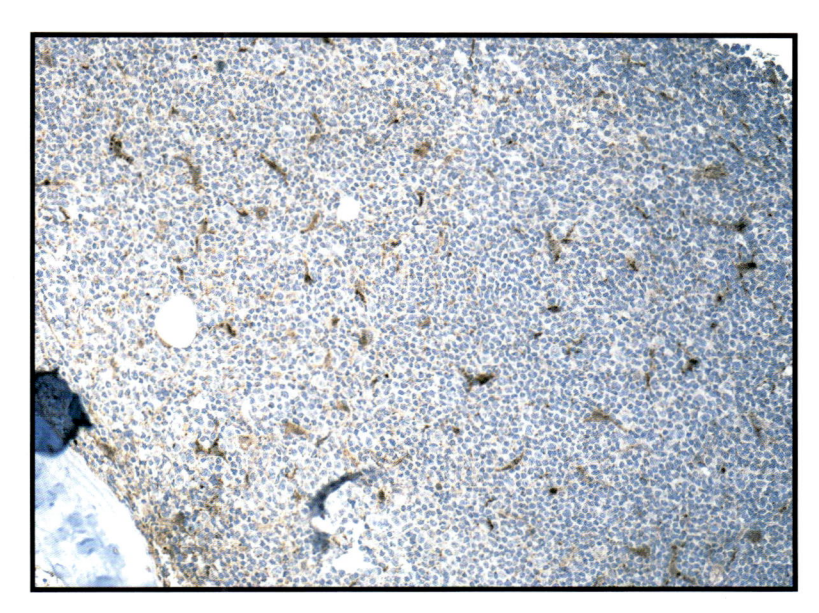

F4.9.9 Cyclin D1 in hairy cell leukemia (HCL)

This figure illustrates cyclin D1 expression in HCL. HCL frequently shows cyclin D1 expression, which is typically variable as shown here. Dendritic cells positive for cyclin D1 are not present in this case of HCL.

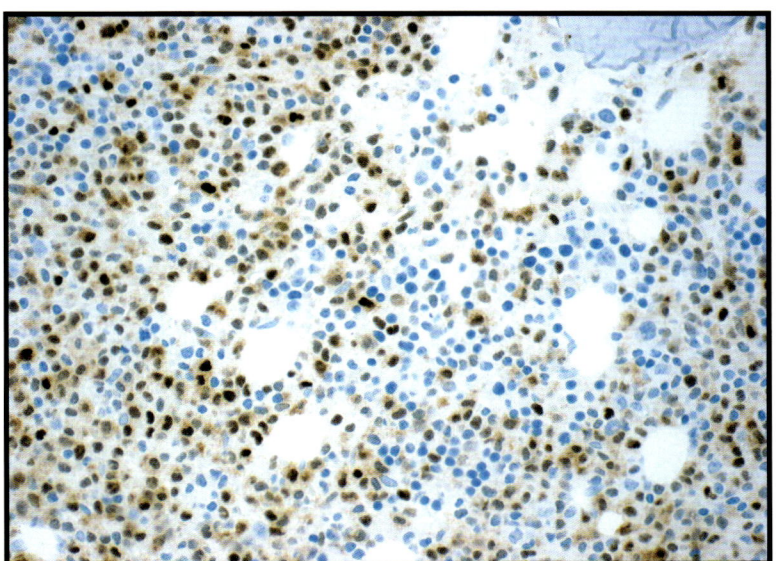

F4.9.10 Cyclin D1 in mantle cell lymphoma (MCL)

This biopsy specimen is from a 45-year-old man with primary nodal MCL. Multiple malignant lymphoid aggregates are identified. Cyclin D1 is expressed in the majority of malignant cells, but the degree of its expression varies considerably in MCL using immunohistochemistry methods.

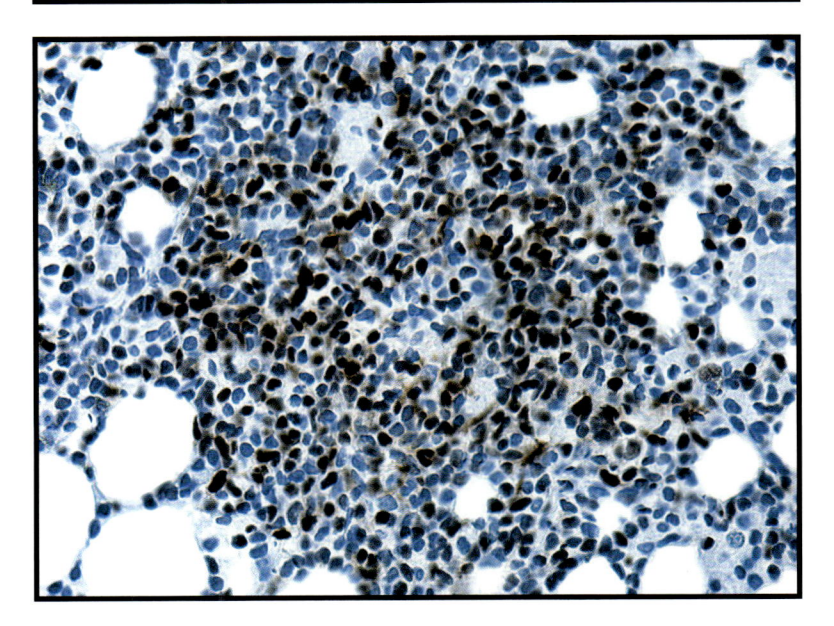

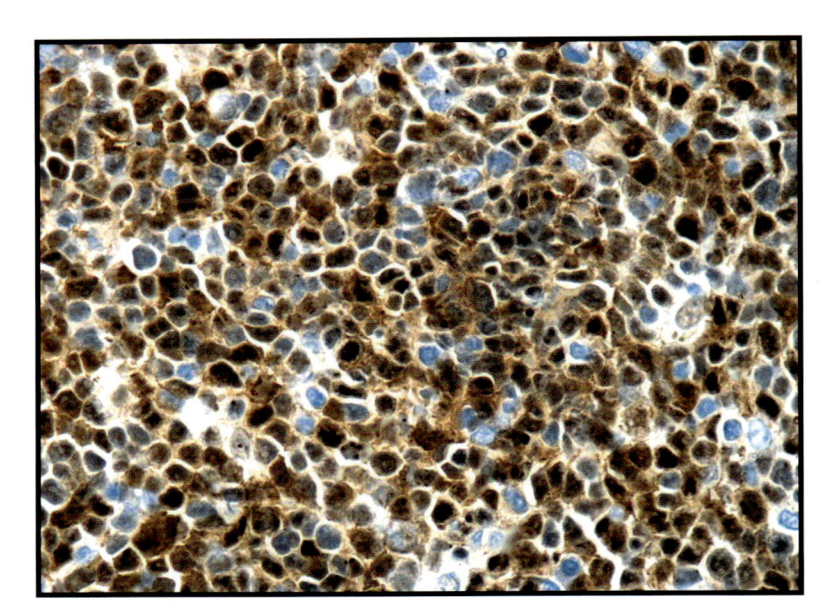

F4.9.11 Cyclin D1 in blastic variant of mantle cell lymphoma (MCL)

This bone marrow specimen is diffusely infiltrated by malignant large lymphocytes with blastic nuclear features. Demonstration of cyclin D1 and CD5 expression in this variant of MCL is critical for the correct classification of this disease.

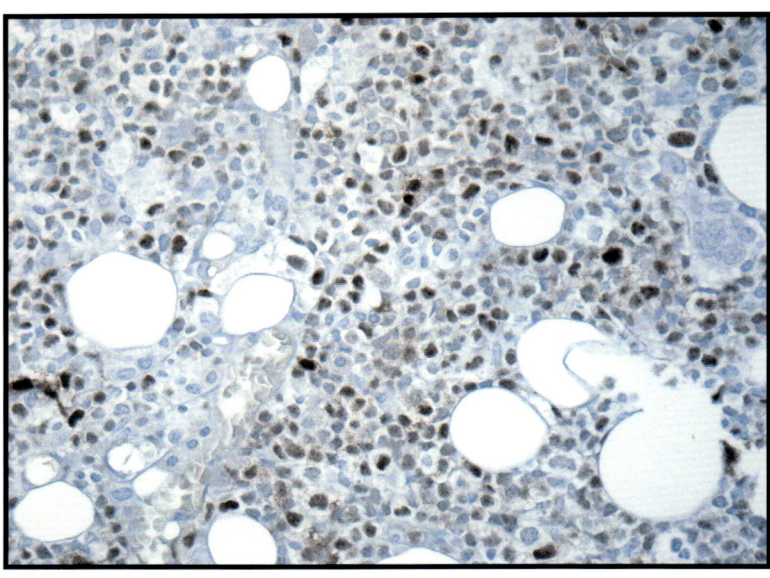

F4.9.12 Cyclin D1 in pleomorphic variant of mantle cell lymphoma (MCL)

This bone marrow biopsy specimen is involved by MCL. Cyclin D1 is positive, but only weakly. This type of positivity was common before the SP4 clone was available because most other primary anti–cyclin D1 antibodies have lower sensitivity. Suboptimal tissue processing caused weak results in this case stained by SP4 because no usual stromal cyclin D1+ cells are found. However, occasional MCL can truly express this low level of cyclin D1.

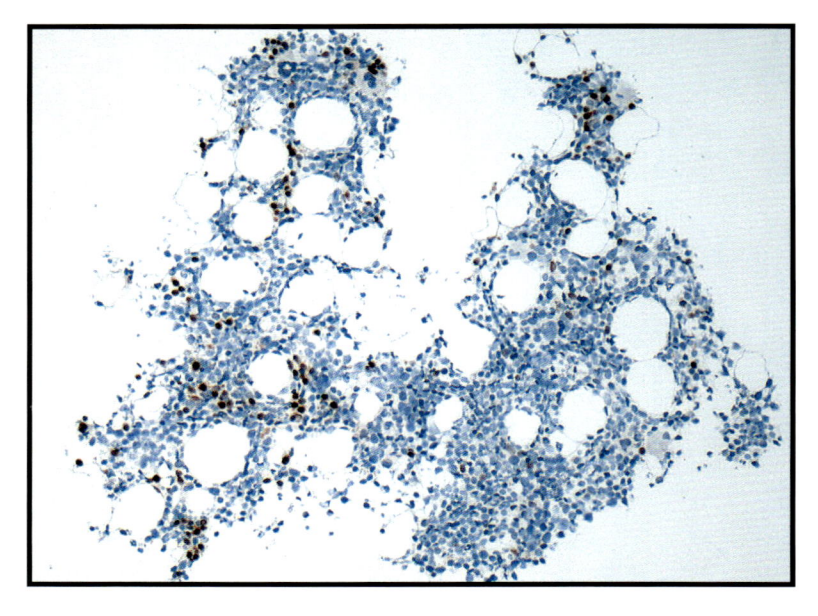

F4.9.13 Cyclin D1 in mantle cell lymphoma (MCL)

Cyclin D1 detection is very useful for confirmation of the bone marrow involvement when only small groups of interstitial B cells are present. CD5 expression by small B cells was also identified in this case.

4.9　Cyclin D1

F4.9.14 Cyclin D1 in IgA-κ multiple myeloma with t(11;14)

Malignant plasma cells show variable expression of cyclin D1. Some degree of variable cytoplasmic positivity is common in cyclin D1+ myeloma. Rare elongated positive cells are endothelial cells. While t(11;14) is found in up to 20% of cases, cyclin D1 can be identified with immunohistochemistry in up to 50% of myelomas. However, uniform and strong expression is highly predictive of t(11;14) cases.

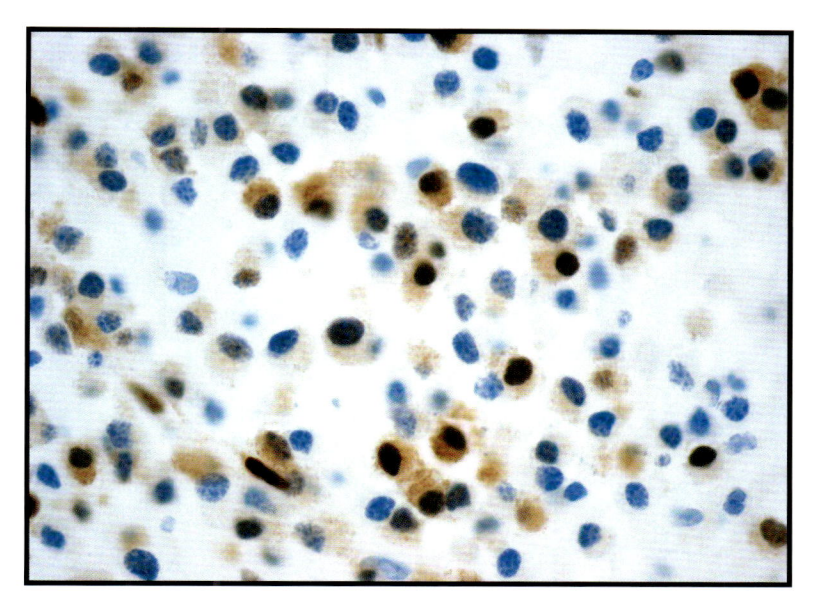

F4.9.15 Cyclin D1 in myeloma after autologous stem cell transplantation

Several malignant plasma cells are identified in this field. Cyclin D1 is a nuclear marker that highlights Dutcher bodies (arrows).

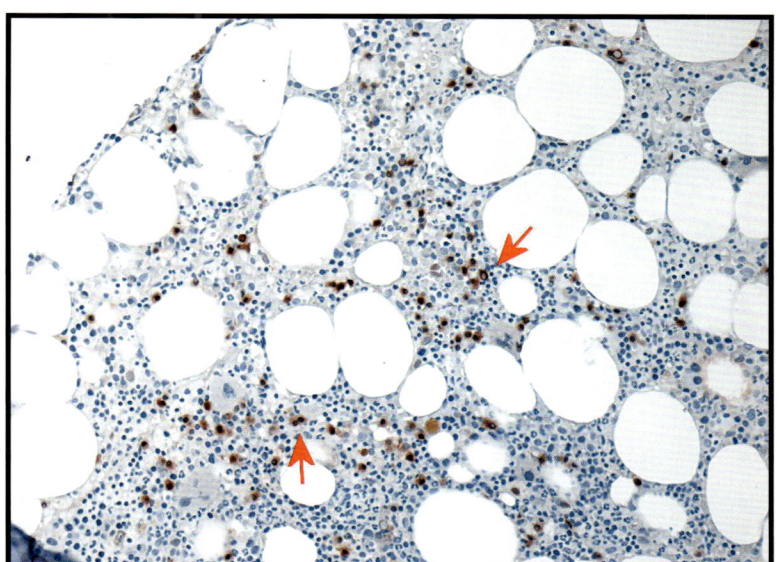

4.10 Lysozyme

Even though lysozyme (LZ) and myeloperoxidase (MPO) are both myeloid cell–associated lysosomal molecules with bactericidal activity, are expressed very early in myeloid differentiation, and are widely regarded as specific lineage markers, these 2 molecules cannot be used interchangably in myeloid differentiation. MPO is contained in primary, azurophilic neutrophil granules, but LZ occurs in both granule types [Bainton 1971; Pryzwansky 1978]. Mature neutrophils and mature monocytes both express MPO and LZ [Knapp 1994]. MPO and LZ are frequently coexpressed in many BM diseases. However, this is not always the case and it is not recommended to use LZ as a replacement for MPO and neither should be used as a replacement for CD117 in IHC studies.

4: Other Common Markers

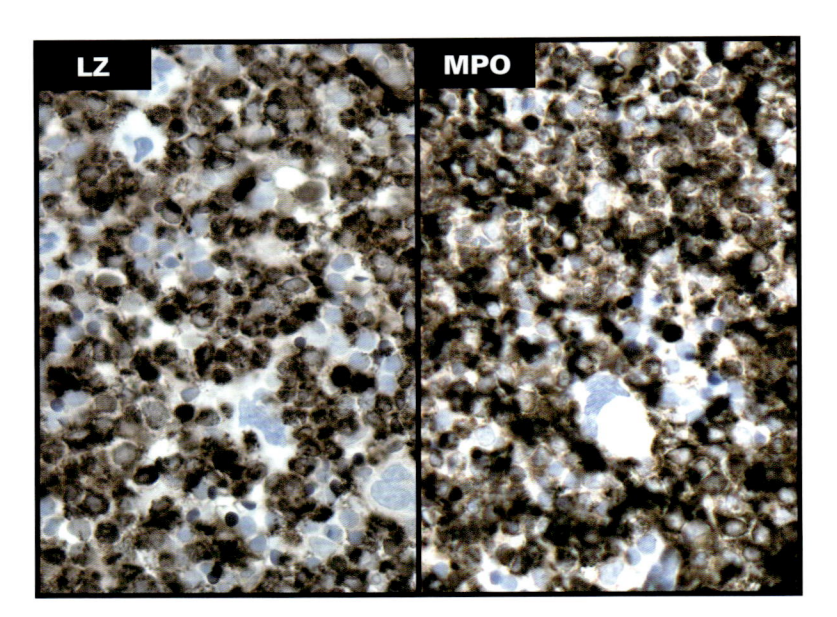

F4.10.1 Lysozyme (LZ) and myeloperoxidase (MPO) in chronic myelomonocytic leukemia (CMML) type 1

There is no significant difference in the staining between LZ and MPO in normal bone marrow and many different conditions including myeloproliferative and myeloproliferative/myelodysplastic diseases. In CMML, the staining with LZ and MPO correlate well and typically show great variation from cell to cell with both markers. It is not certain, however, that LZ and MPO correlate in each individual cell.

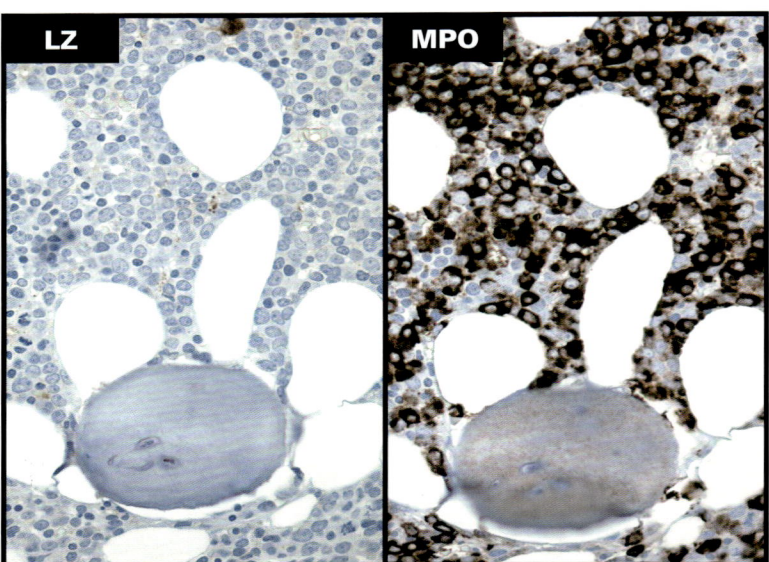

F4.10.2 Lysozyme (LZ) and myeloperoxidase (MPO) in acute myeloid/erythroid leukemia

MPO is expressed in the blasts, but LZ is entirely negative. LZ and MPO are not interchangeable in the evaluation of the bone marrow. This is particularly true for the evaluation of acute leukemia.

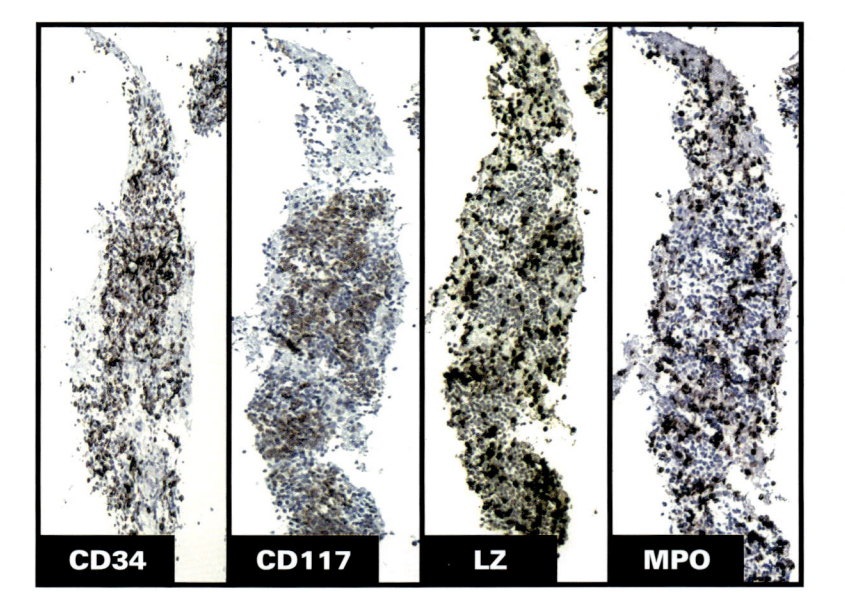

F4.10.3 Lysozyme (LZ) compared with myeloperoxidase (MPO) and CD117 in acute myeloid leukemia without maturation

The extent of leukemic cells is shown with CD34 staining. CD117 is positive; LZ and MPO are substantially less positive. When evaluating acute leukemia with immunohistochemistry, it may be necessary to use several myeloid markers. LZ should not be used alone as a myeloid marker in acute leukemia.

4.11 Bcl-6

Bcl-6 stands for B-cell lymphoma 6 and is also known as zinc finger protein 51 (ZNF51) and lymphoma-associated zinc finger gene on chromosome 3 (LAZ3) (OMIM). Bcl-6 is a zinc finger transcription factor and contains an N-terminal POZ domain. This protein acts as a sequence-specific repressor of transcription and can interact with various POZ-containing proteins that function as transcription corepressors (Entrez Gene). Structural alterations of the Bcl-6 are found in about 40% of DLBCLs and up to 10% FLs [Cattoretti 1995]. BCL-6 protein is predominantly expressed in the B-cell lineage where it is present in mature B cells topographically restricted to germinal centers including all centroblasts and centrocytes. The BCL-6 protein is also detectable in inter- and intra-follicular CD4+ T cells. Human myeloid and monocytic cells express Bcl-6, but in a much lower degree than B cells [Yu 2005; Yamochi 1997; Toney 2000]. In T cells, Bcl-6 is expressed in precursor T-cell lymphoblastic lymphoma and in its normal counterpart in the thymus [Hyjek 2001]. Various B-cell lymphomas express Bcl-6. Most commonly, Bcl-6 is detected in FLs and DLBCLs [Dogan 2000; Skinnider 1999; Capello 2000; West 2002]. FLs can express detectable levels of Bcl-6 in the BM biopsy specimen, but the levels of expression usually parallel those of CD10 and are low when malignant cells of FL reside in tissues unsupported by follicular dendritic cells [Eshoa 2001]. Follicular type of peripheral T-cell lymphoma with Bcl-6 expression has also been described [de Leval 2001].

F4.11.1 Bcl-6 in normal bone marrow (ADVANCE)

This biopsy specimen shows monocytes and more mature neutrophils with weakly positive nuclei (arrow). Using the same clone of the primary antibody, no cells were positive by EnVision+. Accordingly, the expression of Bcl-6 is very weak and is usually not detected with the usual methods. The mRNA expression in benign and malignant monocytes/macrophages has previously been described.

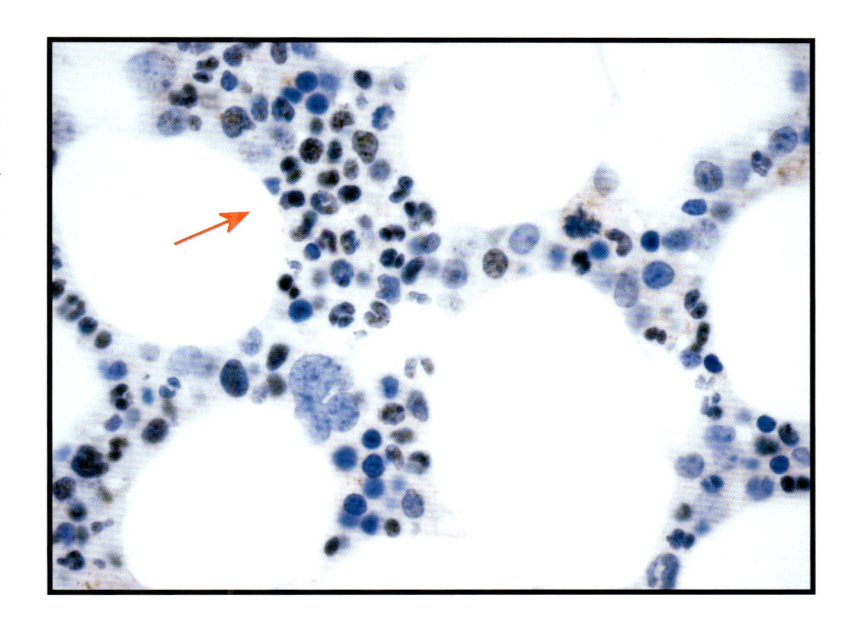

F4.11.2 Bcl-6 in monocytic cells and endothelial cells in marginal zone lymphoma (ADVANCE)

Bcl-6 is not expressed in the malignant lymphocytes. Monocytic/histiocytic (red arrows) cells show variable expression. In addition, weak/borderline nuclear expression is detected in the cells with elongated nuclei, which are presumably endothelial cells (blue arrows).

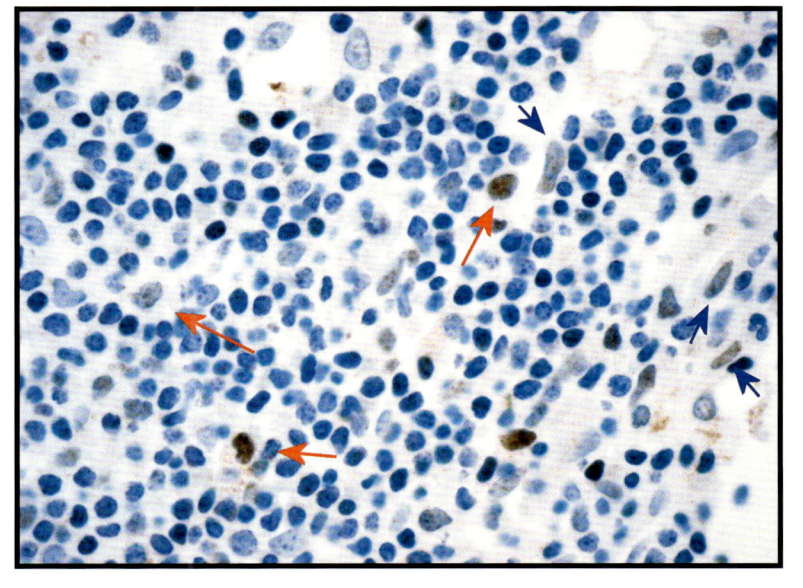

4: Other Common Markers

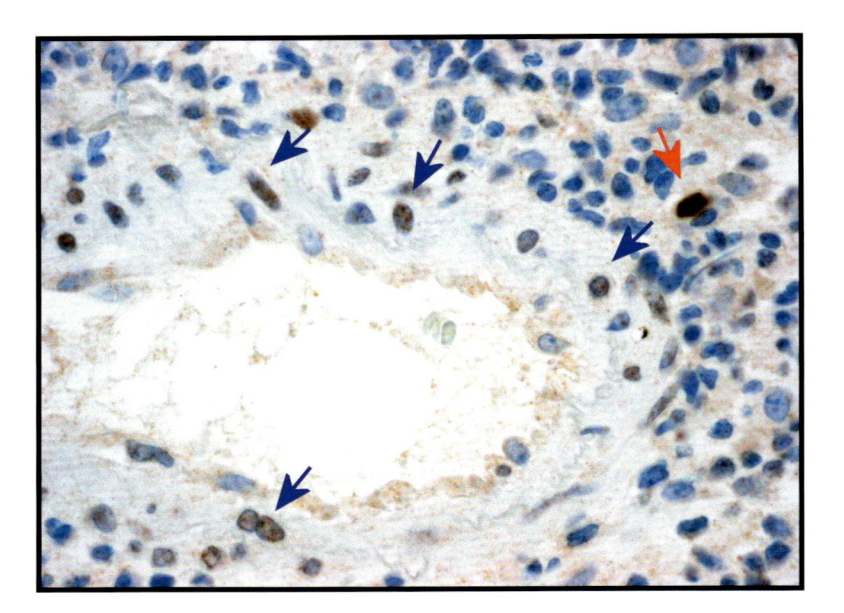

F4.11.3 Bcl-6 expression in perivascular monocytes (ADVANCE)

The CD14+ monocytic cells are identified with immunohistochemistry in many organs including bone marrow. These cells show weak expression of Bcl-6 like other monocytic cells (blue arrows). Bcl-6 expression in these perivascular cells is very weak compared with rare monocytic cells not related to vascular structures (red arrow). (See also **F3.10.9**. and **F4.7.2**.)

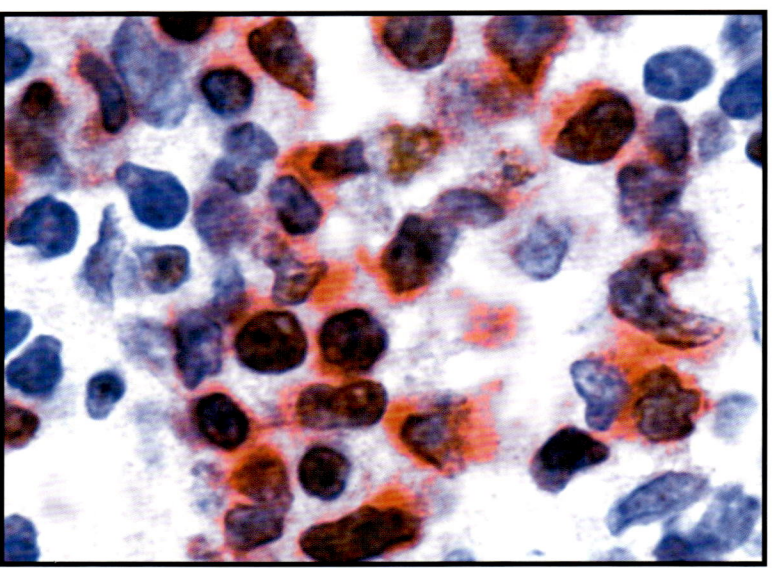

F4.11.4 Bcl-6 in peripheral T-cell lymphoma

Some peripheral T-cell lymphomas may express Bcl-6 as in this angioimmunoblastic T-cell lymphoma involving bone marrow. To demonstrate that Bcl-6 is indeed expressed by T cells and there is no concurrent B-cell process, double immunostaining was used. The CD3 is demonstrated in red and the Bcl-6 with brown chromogen.

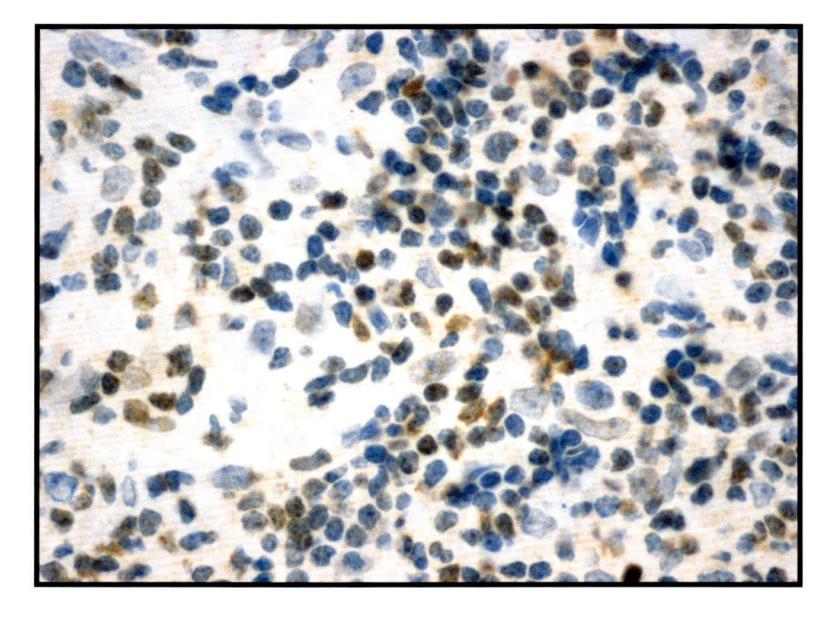

F4.11.5 Bcl-6 in follicular lymphoma (FL) with transformation to diffuse large B-cell lymphoma (DLBCL)

This biopsy specimen is from a 57-year-old man with a long history of FL. Only a subpopulation of small cleaved cells of FL shows weak and variable expression of Bcl-6. The largest cells in this field are generally negative. In other areas of this biopsy specimen with large lymphoid aggregates of DLBCL, no Bcl-6 expression was detected. In this case, the transformation to DLBCL was associated with loss of Bcl-6 expression.

F4.11.6 Bcl-6 in diffuse large B-cell lymphoma (DLBCL) involving bone marrow
This biopsy specimen is from a 54-year-old woman with a history of follicular lymphoma (FL). The transformation to DLBCL was documented only in the BM. Bcl-6 expression was higher in the DLBCL component than in the FL component and it was easily demonstrated in this BM biopsy specimen.

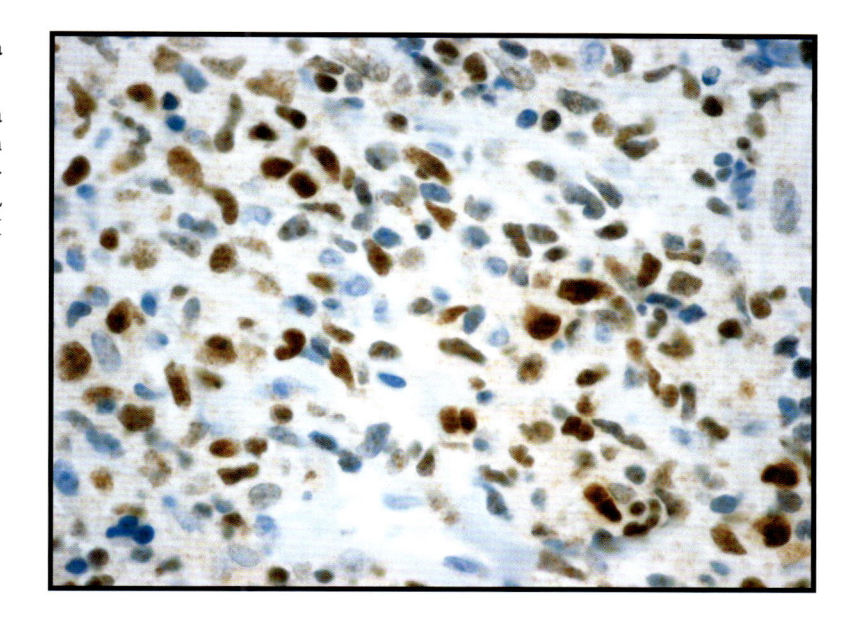

4.12 Immunoglobulins

Immunoglobulins (Ig) are antibody (Ab) proteins synthesized by B cells. Essentially, human Ab is composed of one or more basic units consisting of 2 identical heavy chains and 2 identical light chains. Heavy chains are μ, δ, γ, α, or ε; light chains are κ and λ. B-cell Ig genes undergo a strictly programmed series of gene rearrangements in the BM during B-cell development. Ig heavy-chain gene rearrangement begins in early pro-B cells, and when successfully completed, the cell progresses to become a pre-B-cell. A successful rearrangement means that intact μ chains are produced. These cells are large (large TdT+ cells in normal BM). After the transient expression of the rearranged heavy chain as part of a pre-B-cell receptor complex (μ chains + surrogate light chain + CD79a + CD79b), these cells start to divide. After a burst of proliferation, the cells then undergo the transition to small resting pre-B cells, in which the light-chain locus can be rearranged [Janeway 2008]. Often, the κ light chain gene rearranges, and if unsuccessful, the λ light chain gene undergoes rearrangement. Most κ rearrangements are successful and therefore, in humans, a typical κ:λ ratio is 65:35. For diagnostic purposes in IHC, the κ:λ ratio must be quite high to confirm the monotypic nature of the plasma cells. A ratio of 16:1 was recommended previously [Peterson 1986]. We use a ratio of 10:1 for predominant κ and a ratio of 1:6 for predominant λ populations. It may be prudent to use a higher ratio for smaller plasma cell populations. Once light chain is successfully rearranged, IgM is formed and expressed on the surface together with CD79a and CD79b to form a functional B-cell receptor, and the pre-B-cell becomes immature B-cell. If the cell at this point is not self-reactive, it continues to mature. Mature B cells produce a δ heavy chain as well as a μ heavy chain by a mechanism of alternative mRNA splicing and are marked by the additional appearance of IgD on the cell surface [Janeway 2008]. Mature B cells express surface Ig until they reach terminal B-cell differentiation, when surface Ig is replaced by cytoplasmic Ig, which is secreted by the plasma cell. The activation of B cells and their terminal differentiation into Ab-secreting plasma cells is triggered by antigen.

The morphologically and immunophenotypically transitional stage(s) between the mature B cell and plasma cell are known as "plasmacytoid" and "plasmacytic" lymphocytes. Plasmacytoid cells are lymphocytes with a minor resemblance to plasma cells, but begin to express cytoplasmic Ig (cIg) before other mature B-cell antigens are fully downregulated. Plasmacytic cells are those that have almost complete plasma cell morphology, a higher level of cIg, but still express some B-cell antigens including CD20 and Pax-5 to a variable degree.

Most commonly, only light chains are evaluated by IHC, but occasionally IgG, IgA, IgM, IgD, and rarely IgE may provide diagnostically useful information. IgM myeloma is a very rare entity and it appears to frequently be CD56−/CD117−/cyclin D1+ [Feyler 2008]. All other possibilities must be excluded before the diagnosis of IgM myeloma is established; in particular, lymphoplasmacytic lymphoma with plasmacytic morphology and plasmablastic lymphoma need to be ruled out. Neoplastic plasma cells occasionally do not express heavy chains (light chain disease) or produce Ig and are nonsecretory; in these cases, results of serum electrophoresis are negative, but the BM biopsy shows Ig+ plasma cells [Preud'Homme 1976; Stavem 1976].

It is difficult to demonstrate cytoplasmic μ chain in hematogones with IHC. It is also difficult to demonstrate surface Ig in mature B cells and their malignant counterparts. Ig can be most successfully detected in plasma cells as well as plasmacytoid and plasmacytic lymphocytes, all of which have a component of cIg. Lymphoplasmacytic lymphomas and marginal zone lymphomas with plasmacytoid differentiation usually express sufficient cIg to be detected with IHC [Wong 2002; Feiner 1990; Berger 2005; Pangalis 2005;]. Plasmacytoid differentiation has also been described in CLL, FL, and very rare MCL [Vago 1985; Sen 2002]. In addition, plasmablastic lymphoma, posttransplant and age-related EBV-associated lymphoproliferative diseases, and some DLBCLs also may show detectable cIg as evidence of some degree of terminal B-cell differentiation [d'Amore 1991; Knowles 1999; Diebold 2002; Simonitsch-Klupp 2004; Chetty 2003; Teruya-Feldstein 2005].

4: Other Common Markers

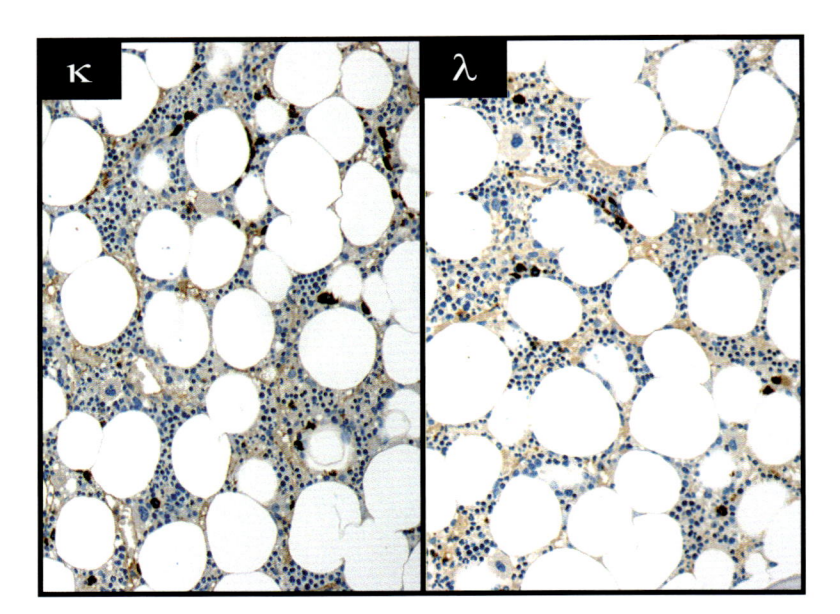

F4.12.1 Ig light chains in slightly hypocellular bone marrow

This biopsy specimen is from a 65-year-old man with a history of non-Hodgkin lymphoma. No evidence of lymphoma was detected. The plasma cells were few and were polytypic, as seen here. The κ Ig light chain was detected in a larger number of plasma cells than λ Ig light chain. When the κ:λ ratio is inverted or more than or equal to 10, a monotypic population of plasma cells is probable.

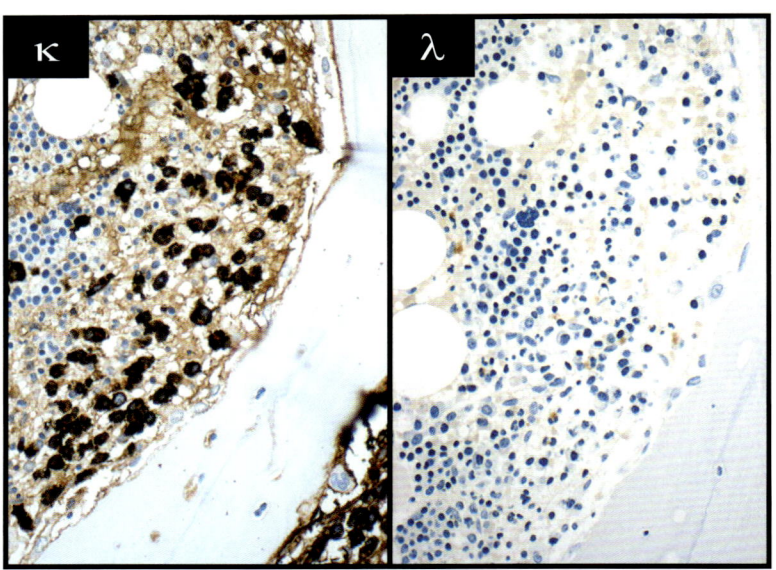

F4.12.2 Demonstration of an Ig light chain restricted lesion

A κ monotypic plasma cell population is illustrated. In bone marrow biopsies, immunohistochemistry is frequently used to demonstrate a monoclonal plasma cell population. Ig antigenicity is well preserved for cytoplasmic Ig and less so for surface Ig. The κ:λ ratio should be quite high or quite low to be certain that the population in question is monotypic.

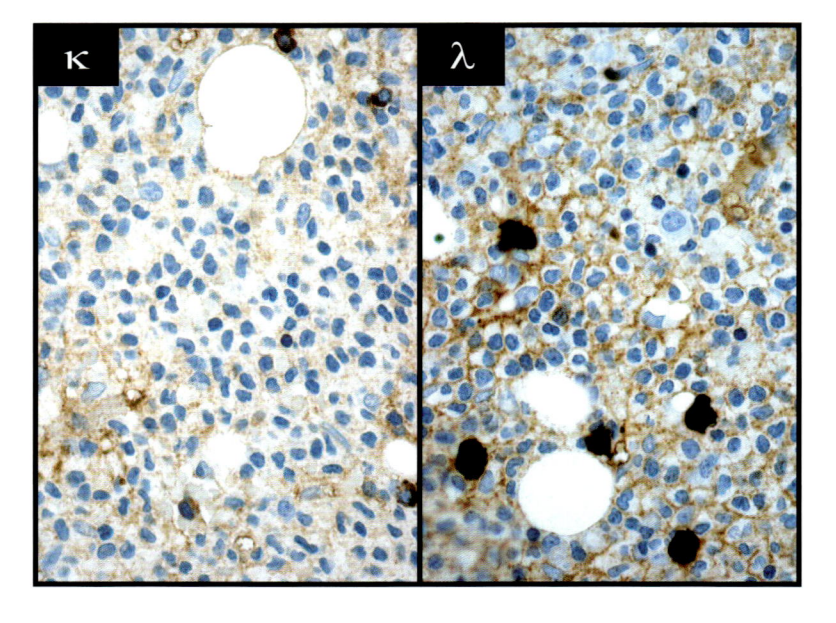

F4.12.3 Surface Ig light chain λ restriction in hairy cell leukemia (HCL)

In formalin-fixed–paraffin embedded sections it is much easier to demonstrate cytoplasmic Ig (cIg) than surface (membranous) Ig (sIg). However, in optimized protocols, it may be possible to demonstrate sIg. This HCL expressed λ light chain. In both κ and λ slides, extracellular positivity is obvious, but only the λ antibody shows a membranous pattern. Considerable caution should be used not to overinterpret artefacts as surface positivity.

4.12   Immunoglobulins

F4.12.4 Reactive plasmacytosis with predominant IgA heavy chain

In most cases of reactive plasmacytosis, IgG plasma cells are the most numerous in the bone marrow. However, as illustrated here, in some cases other Ig may be predominantly expressed and this should not in itself be interpreted as a sign of malignancy.

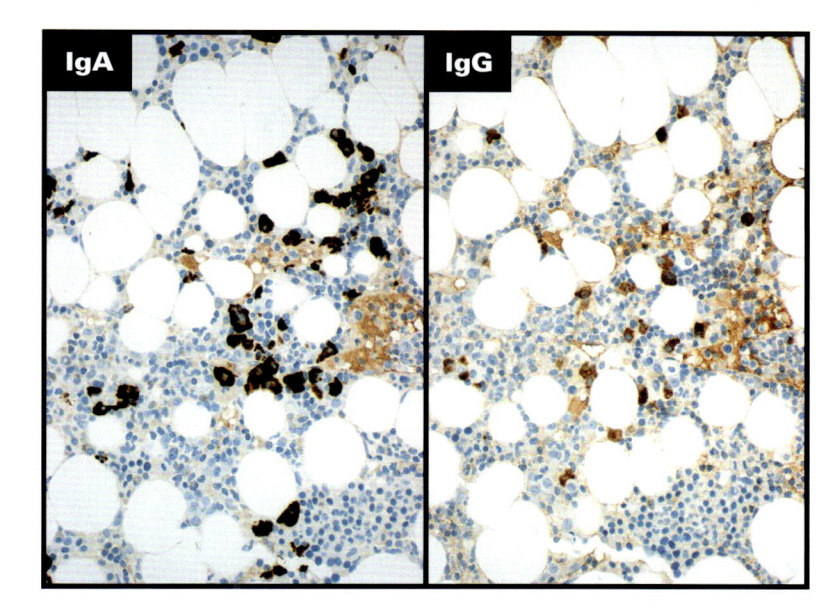

F4.12.5 IgG+ multiple myeloma

While myeloma cells are often easily detected with Ig immunohistochemistry, the expression of cytoplasmic Ig is often less than that in normal plasma cells. This figure illustrates a small population of plasma cells with very high expression of IgG, which probably represents a residual population of benign plasma cells (blue arrows); morphologically malignant plasma cells with prominent nucleoli show weak to moderate IgG expression (red arrow).

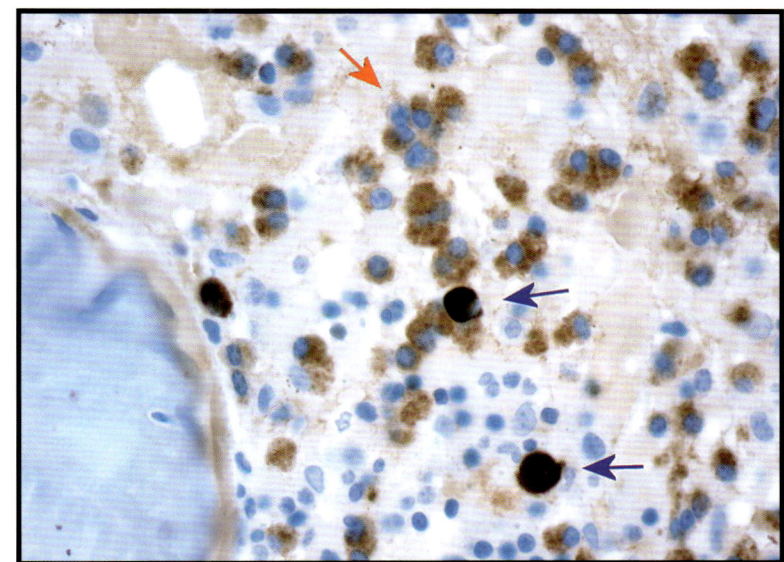

F4.12.6 IgA-κ+ multiple myeloma

This figure illustrates a case of IgA-κ myeloma after chemotherapy. The cytoplasmic reactivity was dotlike; the appearance is not consistent with Golgi-type positivity but is rather targetoid with clear halos around the dense core. Optimization of the Ig immunohistochemistry is critical for interpretation. A good signal-to-noise ratio facilitates detection of a precise localization of the signals.

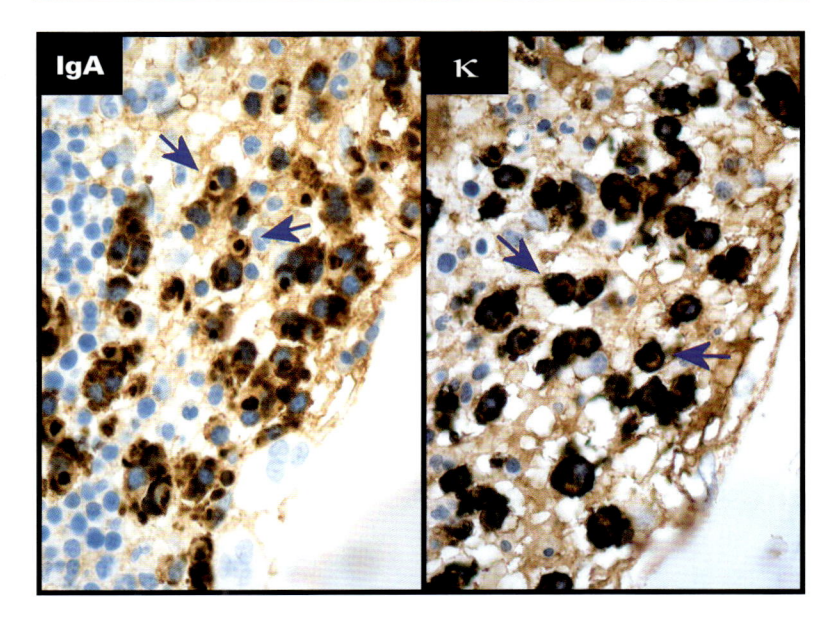

4: Other Common Markers

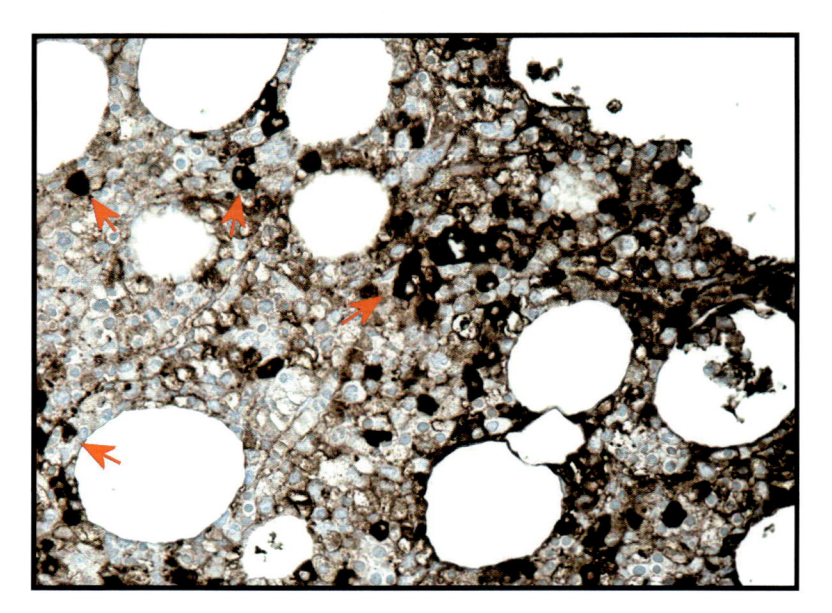

F4.12.7 IgA in diffuse large B-cell lymphoma (DLBCL)

Some DLBCLs express significant cytoplasmic Ig (cIg), which can be readily detected with immunohistochemistry as shown here. Benign and malignant plasma cells with complete terminal B-cell differentiation are not the only hematopoietic cells that express cIg. Marginal zone lymphoma, lymphoplasmacytic lymphoma, some Epstein-Barr virus–associated lymphoproliferative diseases, and rare cases of other lymphomas including chronic lymphocytic leukemia, may show detectable cIg.

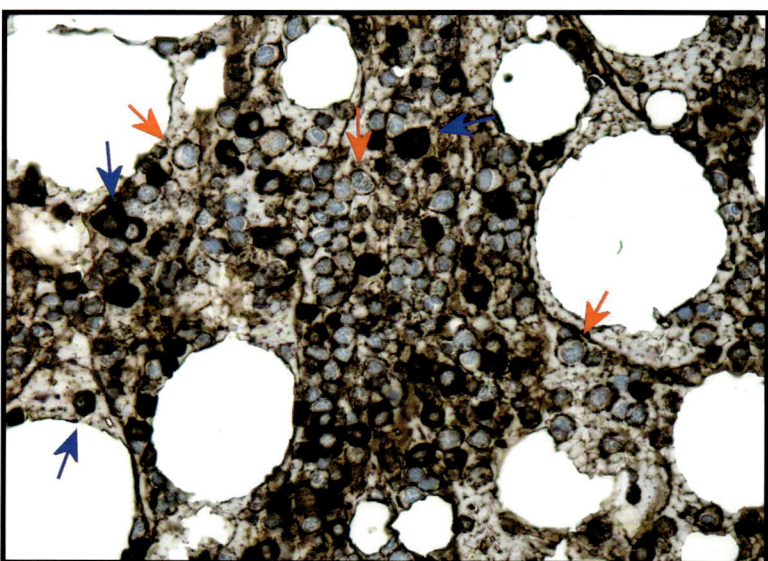

F4.12.8 IgM in lymphoplasmacytic lymphoma (LPL)

IgM is typically found in LPL, but other heavy chains may rarely be expressed by LPL. The blue arrows point to plasmacytoid cells with cytoplasmic IgM. The red arrows point to cells that appear to have membranous IgM, but most are myeloid cells and the staining comes from a large amount of secreted extracellular Ig. Higher dilutions of the primary antibody would probably be helpful, but this cannot be determined a priori.

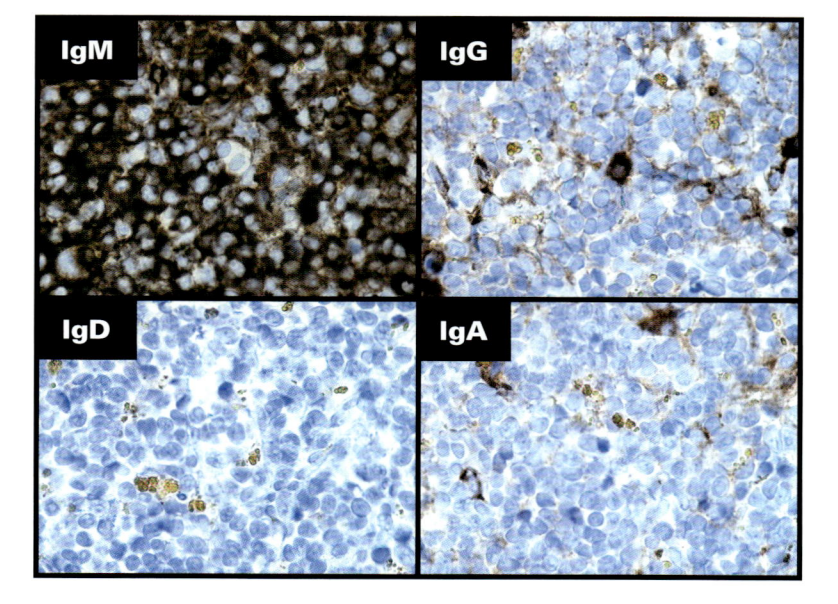

F4.12.9 IgM in lymphoplasmacytic lymphoma (LPL)

This specimen from a case of LPL shows high expression of IgM. Other heavy chains are absent. The cells of LPL may show a spectrum of lymphoplasmacytic differentiation, which varies from cell to cell and from case to case. In this case, most cells appear to show a uniform stage of differentiation, most being true lymphoplasmacytic cells with very few plasma cells or mature B cells without cytoplasmic Ig.

4.12   Immunoglobulins

F4.12.10 IgM in lymphoplasmacytic lymphoma

Morphologic and immunophenotypic variation is illustrated in this case. The malignant cells are forming large interstitial lymphoid aggregates that were CD20+ with occasional cells with weak or dotlike cytoplasmic IgM-κ. There is also an IgM-κ monotypic plasma cell population surrounding lymphoid aggregates and interstitially through the bone marrow. Often neoplastic mature B cells tend to form lymphoid aggregates, while more terminally differentiated cells are dispersed interstitially.

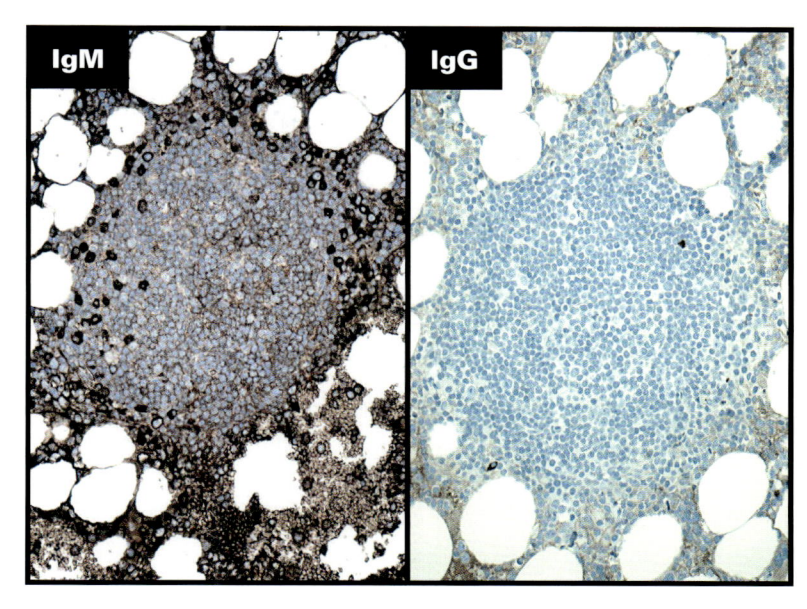

F4.12.11 IgM in marginal zone lymphoma (MZL)

The small lymphoid cells show cytoplasmic and focally membranous expression of IgM and IgD. MZL often shows some degree of plasmacytoid differentiation and patients may have increased IgM paraprotein in the serum; it is usually found in significantly lower levels than in lymphoplasmacytic lymphoma (LPL). Many times the distinction between MZL and LPL is challenging, and in some cases it may be impossible to differentiate between the two. Clinicopathological correlation is essential for correct interpretation in such cases.

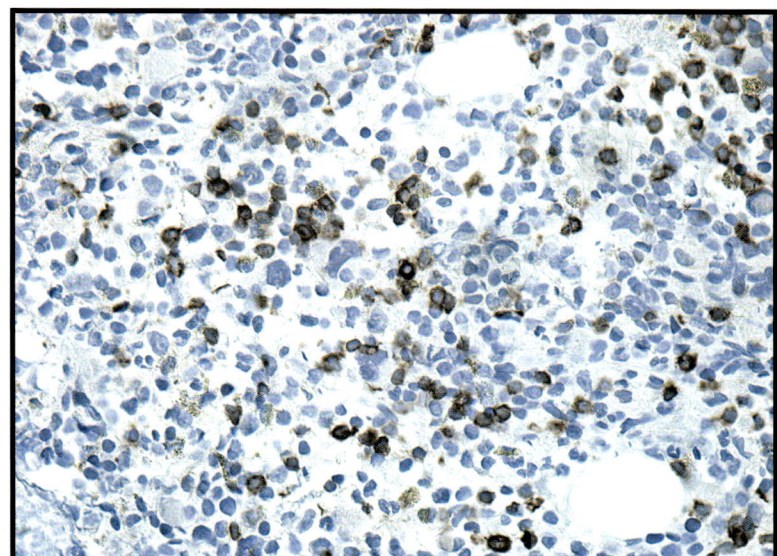

F4.12.12 IgD in mantle cell lymphoma (MCL)

This biopsy specimen is from a patient with MCL. Bone marrow involvement was marked. The MCL expresses surface IgD. Surface IgD is usually easier to demonstrate than other Ig heavy chains. Possibly, the recognized epitope is better preserved than those of other Ig heavy chains after fixation, decalcification, and embedding in paraffin.

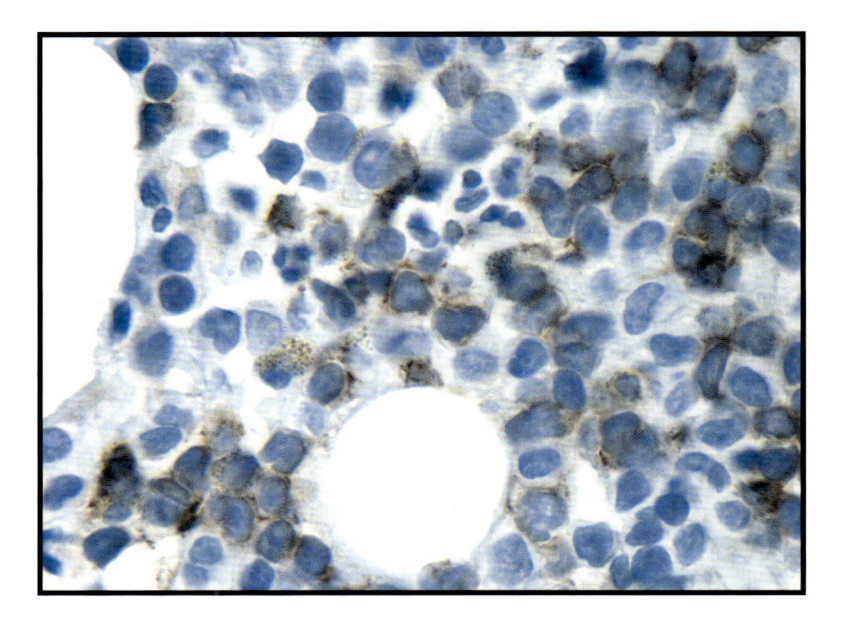

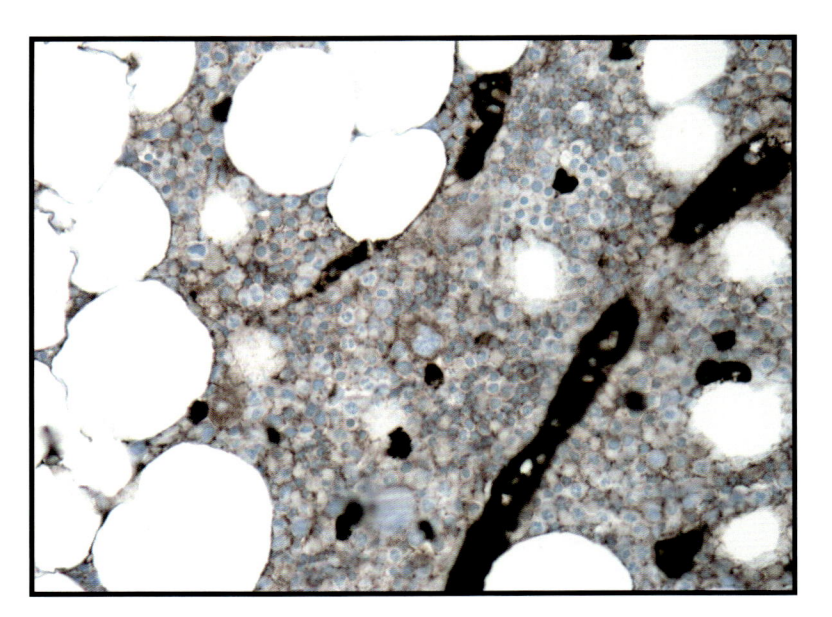

F4.12.13 Ig light chain λ in chronic myelomonocytic leukemia type 1

Rare benign plasma cells have very strong cytoplasmic expression. Vascular spaces contain blood with Ig and hence the staining is specific. There is also a weak staining between the cells, resulting in a false impression of a weak surface Ig expression. However, the cells illustrated are clearly myeloid or erythroid precursors. If lymphoid aggregates were present, interpretation could be difficult.

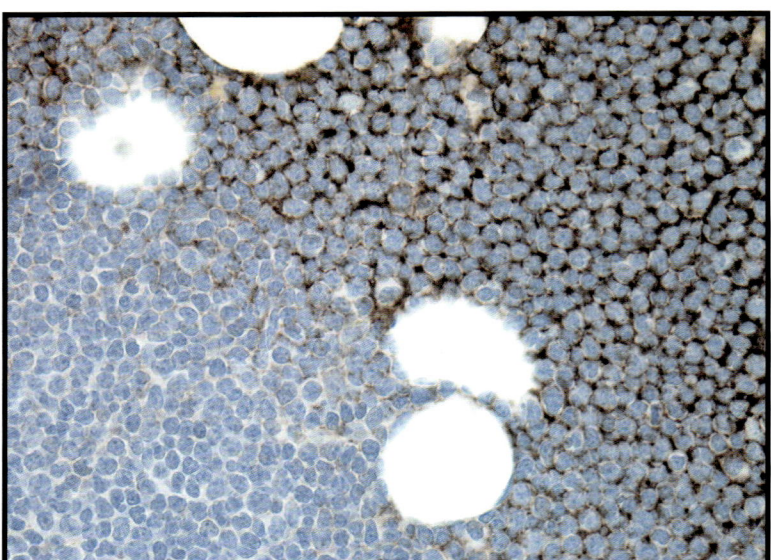

F4.12.14 IgM in acute myeloid leukemia

The compactness of the biopsy specimen often determines results obtained with Ig immunohistochemistry staining. Areas with closely spaced cells show no evidence of staining, while Ig staining can be detected in those areas with more widely spaced cells where plasma or whole blood are allowed to penetrate. Caution should be exercised not to interpret this as evidence of membranous positivity.

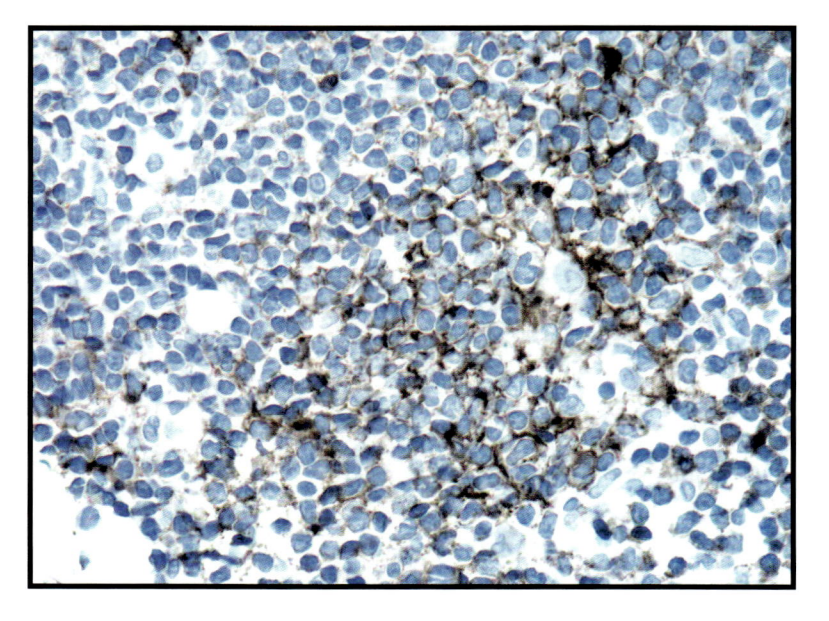

F4.12.15 IgM in mantle cell lymphoma (MCL)

Impression of possible focal membranous IgM expression is present. Examination revealed positivity in the extracellular fluid. The true membranous positivity is present only when the entire circumference of the plasma membrane is positive and only if this is consistently identified between the closely apposed lymphoid cells. (See also **F4.12.3** and **F4.12.12**.)

4.13 Ki-67

Ki-67 is also known as MKI67 or KIA (Entrez Gene). This nuclear antigen is expressed in proliferating cells but not in quiescent cells. Ki-67 is expressed preferentially during the G1, S, G2, and M phases of the cell cycle and it cannot be detected during the G0 phase (OMIM) [Schlüter 1993]. While there are some other commercially available antibodies, MIB-1 clone is most commonly used in diagnostic practice in paraffin-embedded tissues [Gerdes 1983]. It is not often necessary to detect Ki-67 in diagnostic practice in BM pathology. One reason is that normal BM has a very high proliferation fraction that varies from 60% to 90% or more depending on the functional state of the BM and the cell lineage, the highest being recorded in the normal erythroid maturation with over 90% positivity [Thiele 1993; Pellegrini 1995; Cattoretti 1993; Apte 1990]. As a result, the interpretation of the proliferation index will be hampered by the "background" signals. Areas involved by various tumors usually show much lower expression of Ki-67, and if testing is done to confirm a low proliferation rate, detection of Ki-67 may offer some diagnostic information. For instance, in CLL the proliferation rate is very low [Thaler 1987]. This is similar for most small B-cell lymphoproliferative disorders and also the great majority of metastatic tumors to the BM [Schlimok 1990; Falini 1988; Thaler 1987]. Even acute luekemias have comparatively lower rates than the normal BM [Ito 1995; Ito 1992; Hirt 1992]. The levels of Ki-67 are lower in children than adults with ALL [Xu 2006]. In both age groups, the expression in precursor T-ALL and My(+) ALL are higher than that in precursor B-ALL and null-ALL and complete remission rate was higher in cases with lower Ki-67 values [Xu 2006; Nowicki 2002]. Childhood precursor B-cell ALL was reported to have a mean Ki-67 labeling index of only about 18% to 25% [Ito 1992; White 1994]. More importantly, the proliferation fraction was highest (mean 57%) in cases with unfavorable predictive factors and those with complex karyotype abnormalities. Good prognosis, high hyperdiploidy cases showed significantly lower proliferation rates [Ball 1999]. Ki-67 positivity is typically higher than 90% in Burkitt and Burkitt-like lymphomas [Nomura 2008; Chuang 2007].

F4.13.1 Ki-67 in normal adult bone marrow

In the adult BM, a higher proliferation rate is usually seen in the erythroid lineage; the neutrophil lineage also has a high proliferation rate; the rate in megakaryocytes is very variable. The number of positive cells is not significantly higher in myeloproliferative disease (MPD). In MPD, the largest increase in proliferation is usually seen in the megakaryocytic lineage. Some weak positivity may be observed even in segmented neutrophils (arrows), which is unexpected in these postmitotic cells.

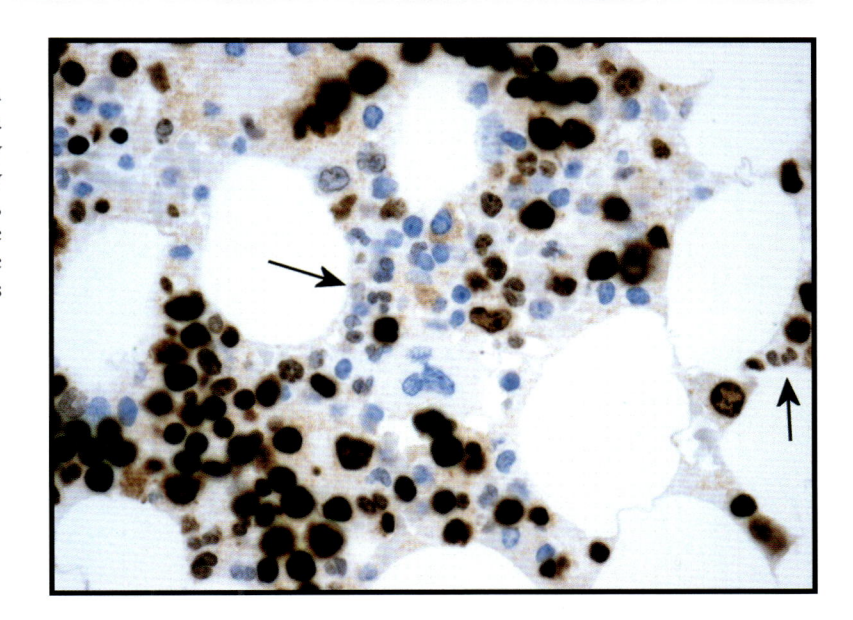

F4.13.2 Ki-67 in non-neoplastic adult bone marrow from a 38-year-old man (staging for non-Hodgkin lymphoma)

Although the Ki-67 proliferation rate in normal BM is high in this age group, it can be somewhat variable from field to field. Note that endosteal lining cells are flattened and show no definite expression of Ki-67 antigen (arrows).

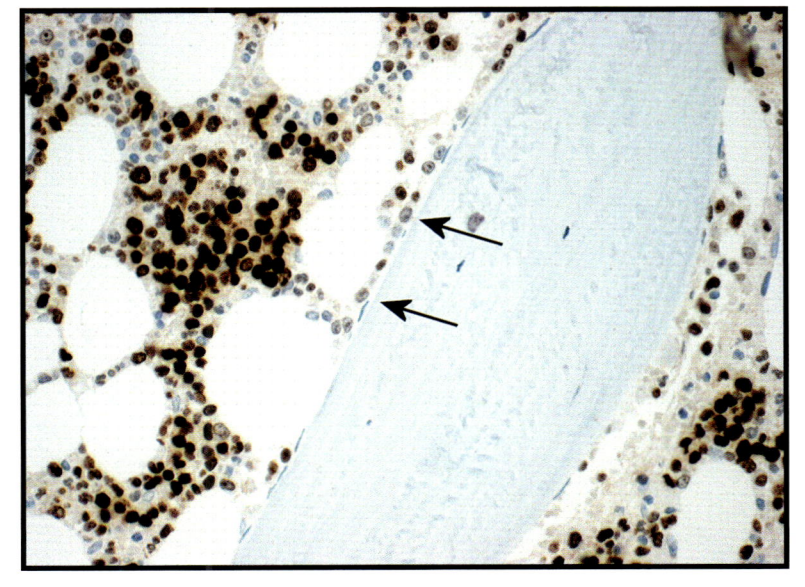

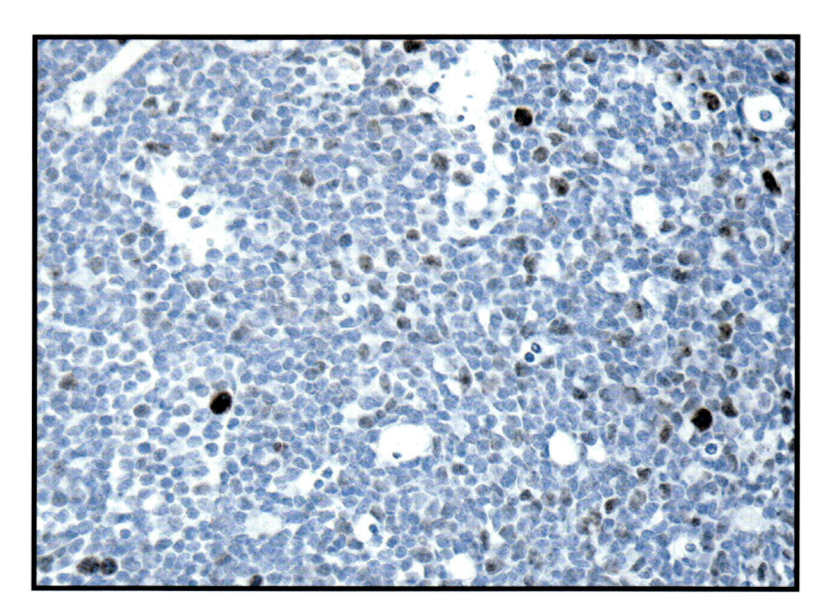

F4.13.3 Ki-67 in precursor B-cell acute lymphoblastic leukemia (B-ALL)

The proliferation rate as measured with Ki-67 immunohistochemistry is higher in ALL than in acute myeloid leukemia (AML); it is generally higher in precursor T-ALL than in precursor B-ALL. Values in precursor B-ALL are higher in adults than in children [Schlüter 1993]]. Overall, the rate in precursor B-ALL is low, with an average of about 25% [Thiele 1993; Pellegrini 1995]. the low proliferation rate is illustrated in this case of common precursor B-ALL in a 9-year-old girl.

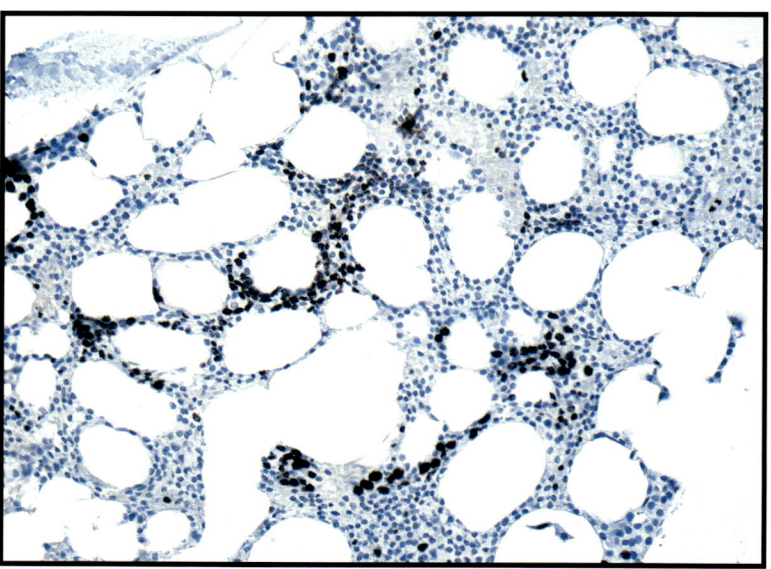

F4.13.4 Ki-67 in a 65-year-old man with newly diagnosed hairy cell leukemia (HCL)

HCL is a low-grade B-cell lymphoproliferative disease, in which the proliferation rate is very low. The Ki-67 usually highlights residual hematopoiesis rather than the cells of HCL, as in this illustration.

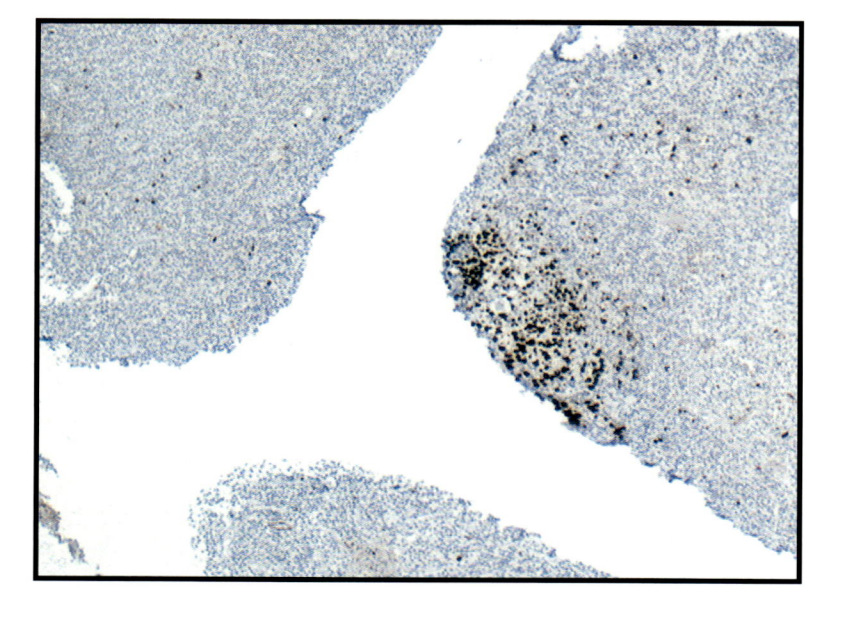

F4.13.5 Ki-67 in multiple myeloma

This biopsy specimen is from a 77-year-old man with massive involvement by myeloma resistant to chemotherapy. The tumor cells show a very low proliferation fraction; in contrast to the myeloma, a small focus of residual hematopoiesis shows brisk proliferation. Myelomas with Ki-67 proliferation rate higher than 8% may have more aggressive disease.

4.14 Cytotoxic Molecules

T-cell intracellular antigen-1 (TIA-1), granzymes, and perforin are cytotoxic molecules stored in cytoplasmic granules. Cytotoxic molecules induce apoptosis of targeted cells [Froelich 1998; Liu 1995; Smyth 1995]. TIA-1 is also known as granule membrane protein of 17 kDa (GMP-17). Expression of TIA-1 can be detected in all cytotoxic cells regardless of their activation status, whereas granzyme B and perforin expression can be detected in high levels only in activated cytotoxic cells [Liu 1995; Smyth 1995]. However, low levels of perforin and granzymes are present in γ-δ T cells, and NK cells constitutively [Froelich 1998]. TIA-1 is expressed in all monocytes and granulocytes, in activated CD4+ T-cell clones and activated NK cell clones, and in Con A–activated thymocytes. TIA-1 is not expressed by B lymphocytes or B-cell lines. In the normal BM, many cells show reactivity for TIA-1, while only a few cells are positive for granzyme B or perforin. Determination of cytotoxic molecules may be very helpful in the evaluation of T-cell and NK-cell neoplasms [Kinney 2007]. Aggressive NK-cell leukemia, subcutaneous panniculitislike T-cell lymphoma, enteropathy-type T-cell lymphoma, and extranodal NK/T-cell lymphoma, nasal type express both TIA-1 and granzyme B/perforin. T-cell large granular lymphocytic leukemia, hepatosplenic T-cell lymphoma, and T-cell prolymphocytic leukemia are usually positive for TIA-1 only [Morice 2002; Kumar 1998]. HTLV-1 associated adult T-cell leukemia/lymphoma is typically negative for all cytotoxic molecules. Cytotoxic molecules may be expressed in more advanced stages and in CD8+ mycoses fungoides [Berti 1999; Vermeer 1999]. CD4+/CD56+ hematodermic tumor does not express cytotoxic molecules [Herling 2007].

F4.14.1 TIA-1 in refractory anemia with excess blasts and T lymphocytosis

The level of expression in this biopsy specimen is comparable to that found in histologically normal bone marrow in which almost every cell appears positive. TIA-1 is expressed in all cells possessing cytolytic potential including all monocytes and granulocytes, cytotoxic CD8+ T cells, activated CD4+ T-cell clones, and activated NK cell clones. However, if the population of interest is present in solid sheets, the expression of TIA-1 still may be accurately determined.

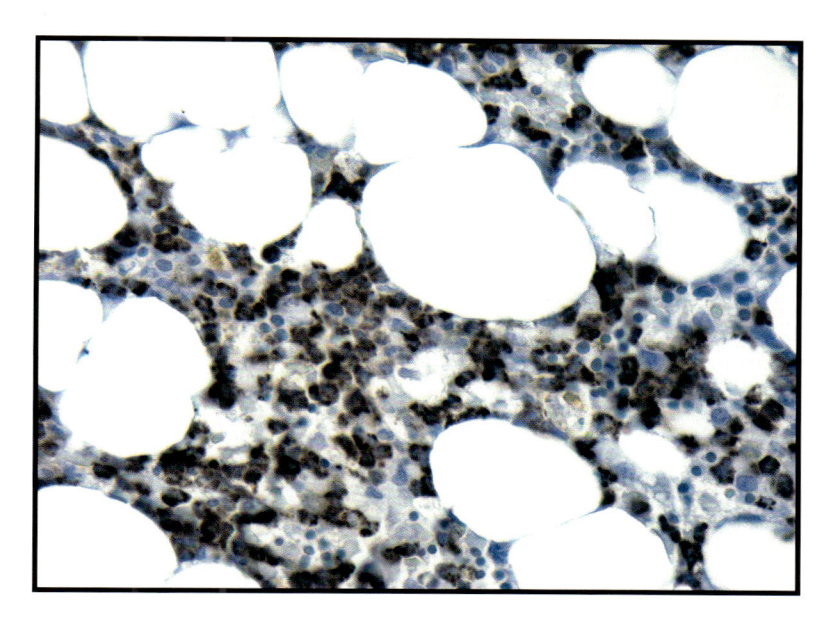

F4.14.2 TIA-1 in refractory anemia with excess blasts

Myeloid cells (black arrow) show variable, but generally weak expression of TIA-1. Morphologically, cells compatible with blasts and early myeloid precursors, as well as erythroid precursors are negative. Occasional cytotoxic lymphocytes (red arrow) are very strongly stained.

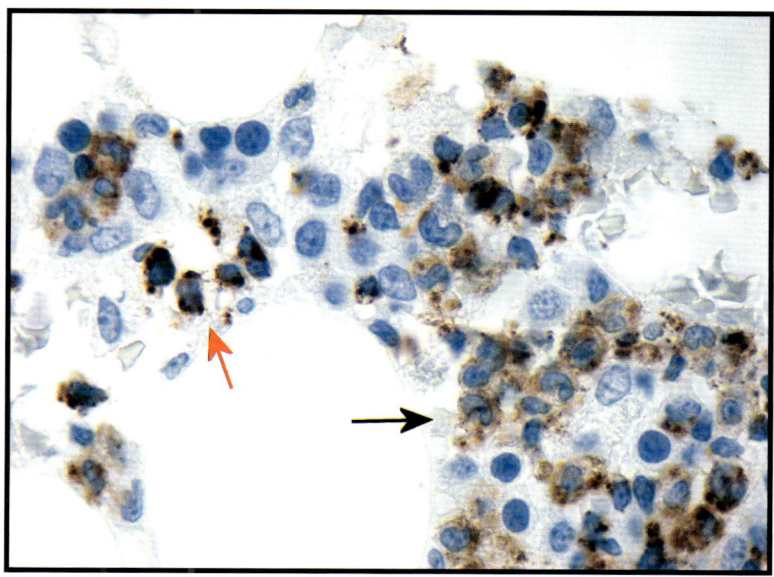

4: Other Common Markers

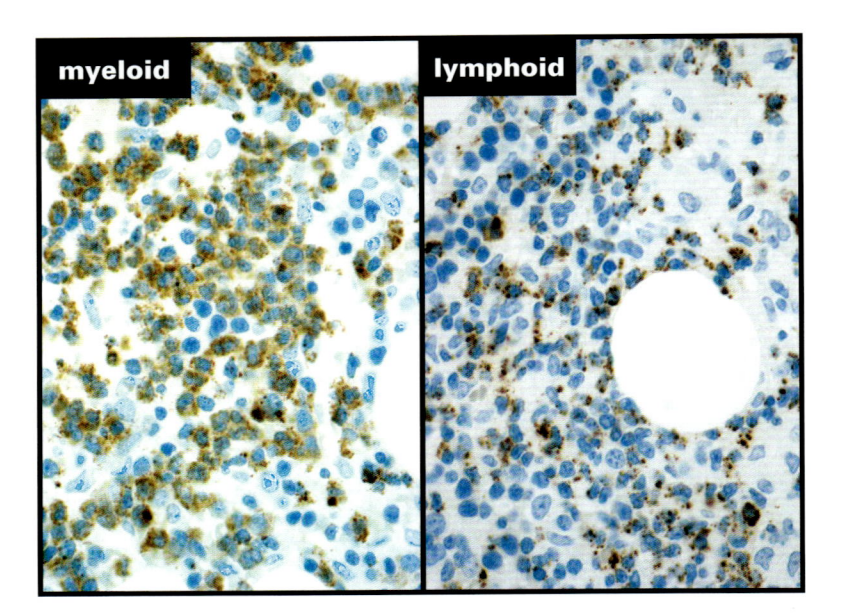

F4.14.3 TIA-1 in peripheral T-cell lymphoma (PTCL)

As expected in TIA-1+ PTCL with partial involvement of the bone marrow, the positivity is found in both noninvolved areas where myeloid cells are positive and in large lymphoid aggregates where neoplastic T cells are positive. In this case, myeloid cells are more consistently positive, but neoplastic T cells show more distinct granular cytoplasmic positivity.

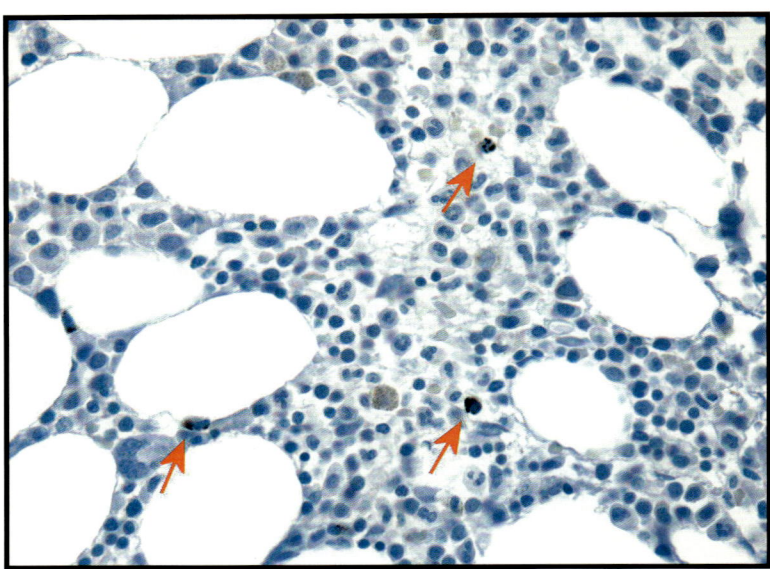

F4.14.4 Granzyme B in histologically normal bone marrow

In contrast to TIA-1, granzyme B expression is restricted to NK cells or activated cytotoxic lymphocytes that are very few in the normal BM. This field shows 3 positive cells (arrows), while other areas have even fewer. Granzyme B, like TIA-1, is found only in the cytoplasm and typically in a granular distribution if antigen localization is good.

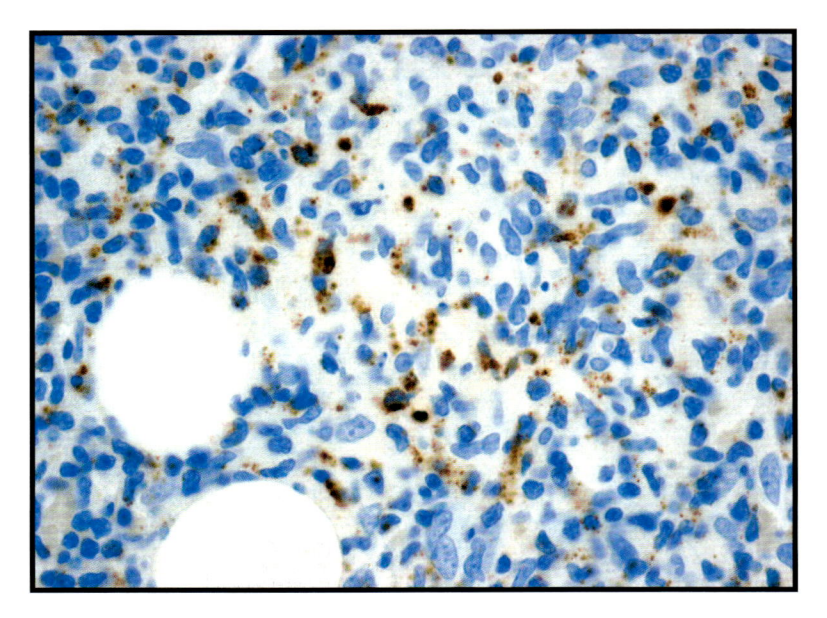

F4.14.5 Granzyme B in peripheral T-cell lymphoma (PTCL)

This biopsy specimen is from a 55-year-old man with cutaneous cytotoxic PTCL. The disease progressed rapidly and the bone marrow was involved about 1 year after the presentation. Positive granzyme B is much easier to interpret than positive TIA-1 because there is no interference by myeloid cells. The distribution of perforin generally parallels granzyme B.

F4.14.6 Cytotoxic molecules in T-cell large granular lymphocyte leukemia (T-LGL)
This biopsy specimen is from a 73-year-old man with T-LGL. The bone marrow contains only slightly increased CD8+ T cells. T-LGL is negative for granzyme B in about 30% cases, as seen in this case. In contrast, TIA-1 is negative in only 10% of cases. When a small number of neoplastic cells is present, it may be impossible to determine whether the neoplastic T cells are positive for TIA-1.

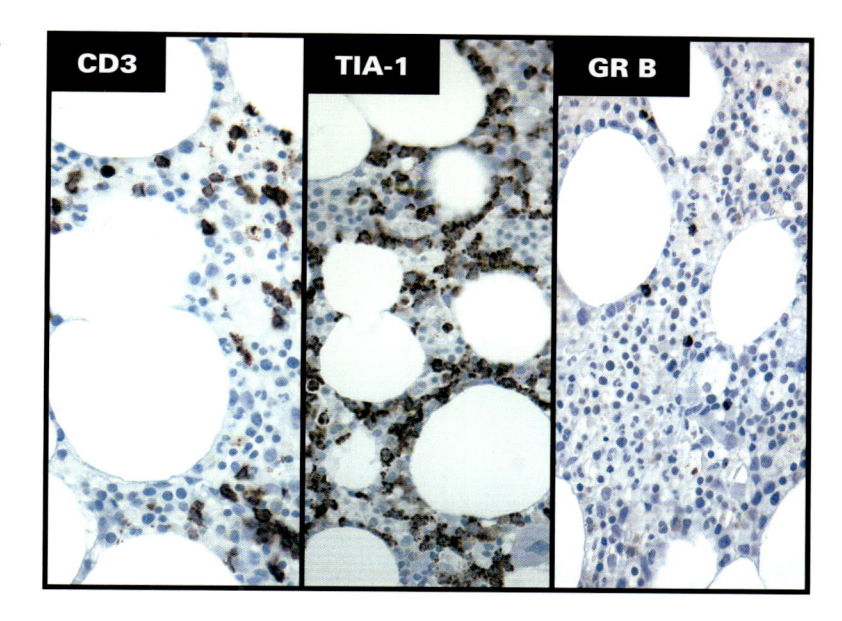

4.15 Stromal Markers

BM stroma is complex and is a dynamic anatomic compartment where changes can rapidly develop in reactive and neoplastic conditions [Anjos-Afonso 2007; Benayahu 2007; Direkze 2006; Bianco 2001]. It is derived from mesenchyme and contains mesenchymal stem/progenitor cells that gives rise to skeletal tissue components such as cartilage and bone, adipocytes, and hematopoiesis supporting stromal cells [Dennis 1999]. The Mesenchymal and Tissue Stem Cell Committee of the International Society for Cellular Therapy proposed 3 minimal criteria to define human mesenchymal stem cell (MSC) as follows:

1. MSC must be plastic-adherent when maintained in standard culture conditions;
2. MSC must express CD105, CD73, and CD90, and lack expression of CD45, CD34, CD14 or CD11b, CD79α or CD19, and HLA-DR surface molecules; and
3. MSC must differentiate to osteoblasts, adipocytes, and chondroblasts in vitro [Dominici 2006].

While we are used to visualizing CD34+ hematopoietic progenitors in bone marrow tissues, CD105, CD73, and CD90 have not been widely evaluated in pathologic conditions in the BM and are currently not used in diagnostic hematopathology. Therefore, this chapter will address only some markers of terminally differentiated stromal cells, including vimentin, desmin, smooth muscle actin, laminin, and VCAM. Several other markers that are not exclusively stromal, but also detect stromal cells, are described in the respective chapters (see CD10, CD31, CD34, CD68, cyclin D1, and other). Because immunoreactivity of tumor cells in bone marrow biopsy specimens for nonhemopoietic antigens, including stromal markers, does not exclude a diagnosis of acute leukemia, it is important to consider expression of stromal epitopes in normal and diseased BM [Ruck 1995].

Vimentin is the most abundantly present mesenchymal intermediate filament protein. Vimentin is found in stellate stromal cells present in a small number among the hematopoietic cells and in granulopoietic cells [Dennis 1999]. Intense staining of endothelial cells of sinusoids and capillaries and of monohistiocytic cells can be demostrated. However, vimentin expression in normal BM is not limited to stromal cells only. Very early progenitors from each lineage express vimentin, which differs strikingly as the cells mature. T lymphocytes, monocytes, and granulocytes retain vimentin expression at all stages of maturation. B lymphocytes also express vimentin, but tend to lose its expression later when they mature into plasma cells. In contrast, megakaryoblasts lose vimentin expression at a very early stage of differentiation and erythroblasts at variable stages between the committed erythroid cell and the mature red blood cell [Dellagi 1983]. If the BM is involved with a process with differential diagnosis that includes Hodgkin lymphoma and T-cell/histiocyte-rich B-cell lymphoma, it may be useful to know that vimentin is regularly expressed in cHL, but not in T-cell/histiocyte-rich B-cell lymphoma or nodular lymphocyte predominant Hodgkin lymphoma [Rüdiger 1998].

Desmin immunoreactivity was identified in stromal cells, endothelial cells, and smooth muscle cells of larger blood vessels and weak cytoplasmic staining was seen in all cells of the various hematopoietic lineages [Loyson 1997]. Evaluation of in vitro cultures of bone marrow stromal cells by IHC both in resting state and after activation with interferon γ and tumor necrosis factor α could not confirm wide expression of desmin in BM stroma [Lisignoli 1996].

The presence of α smooth muscle–positive cells (myoid cells, myofibroblastic cells) in human bone marrow has been observed during hematopoiesis in embryonic life. During adult life, it is strictly related to pathologic conditions such as metastatic carcinoma, Hodgkin lymphoma, hairy cell leukemia, and to some degree, chronic myeloproliferative diseases [Papadopoulos 2001]. A smooth muscle actin is regularly observed in smooth muscle cells of larger blood vessels [Loyson 1997]. Actin is increased in bone marrow stroma as myofibroblasts are generated in response to metastatic tumors, but it is not increased in other fibrotic conditions in the BM including HIV/AIDS-related BM fibrosis or chronic idiopathic myelofibrosis [Fang 2003; O'Malley 2005]. Expression of smooth muscle actin was also described expressed in osteoblasts and bone-lining cells [Kinner 2002].

Laminin and collagen type IV are extracellular matrix proteins that colocalize in the BM extracellular matrix with the bone marrow vessels, including arterioles, veins, and sinuses; they are also present in the periosteum [Nilsson 1998; Balduino 2005]. Laminin and collagen can be strikingly increased in MPD, in particular chronic idiopathic myelofibrosis [Lisse 1991; Apaja-Sarkkinen 1986; Thiele 2006].

Vascular cell adhesion molecule-1 (VCAM-1 or CD106) is expressed on a subpopulation of BM stromal cells that have a hematopoietic supportive role and are also termed as "reticular stromal" cells [Dittel 1995; Funk 1995 Dittel 1995; Funk 1995]. If VCAM-1 is experimentally ablated in the BM stromal cell population, the BM cellularity is increased as is the progenitor content, which supports the role of VCAM-1 in progenitor BM retention during homeostasis [Ulyanova 2007]. VCAM-1 has also been identified on a subpopulation of blasts in AML and ALL, but not on normal CD34+ BM precursor cells [Reuss-Borst 1995].

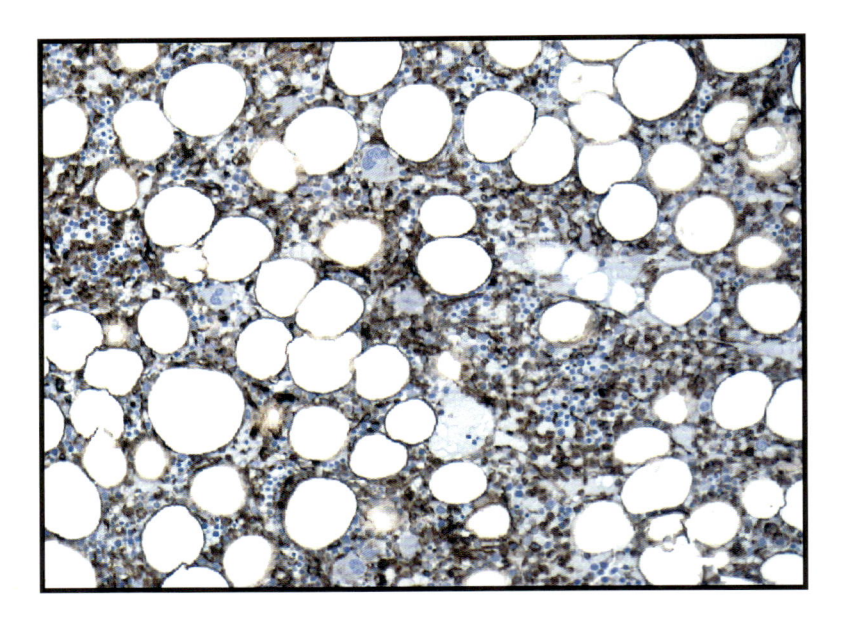

F4.15.1 Vimentin in histologically normal bone marrow

This normal BM biopsy specimen is from a 15-year-old child with a soft tissue mass of the left lower extremity. Vimentin staining reveals that many of the hematopoietic cells are negative, while stromal cells are positive. The soft tissue mass was benign.

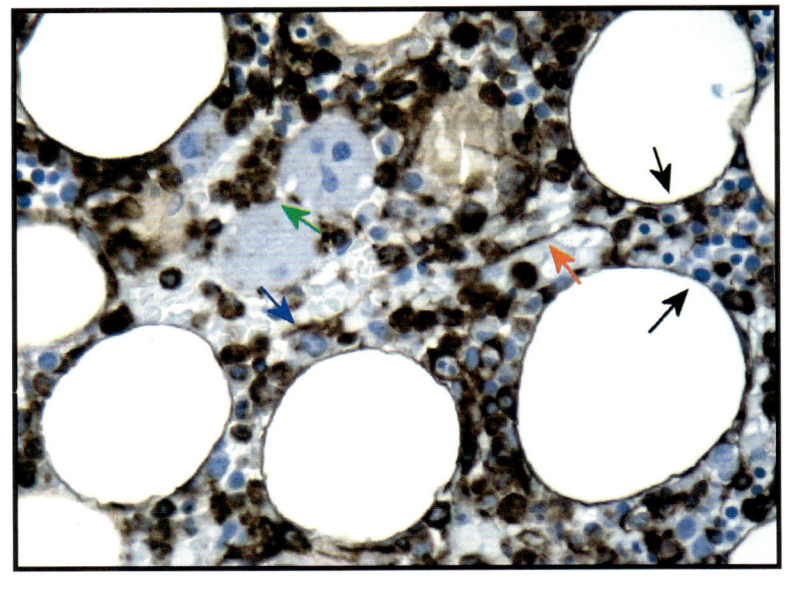

F4.15.2 Vimentin in histologically normal bone marrow

Same specimen as illustrated in F4.15.1. Megakaryocytes are negative. Black arrows point to negative red blood cell precursors. Neutrophils and neutrophil precursors are positive with intermediate forms being most strongly stained. Groups of mature neutrophils are moderately stained (green arrow). A possible promyelocyte with Golgi-type positivity is identified (blue arrow). Endothelial cells (red arrow) and other stromal cells are strongly positive.

4.15 Stromal Markers

F4.15.3 Vimentin in B cells (lymph node)

Early B cells express more vimentin than mature B cells. Variable, but weak expression is demonstrated in mantle zones (between red arrows), but it is not present in the centroblasts and centrocytes of the germinal center (GC). Only follicular dendritic cells show strong vimentin expression. Similarly, vimentin expression varies in various B-cell neoplasms. Monocytes and histiocytes express a very high level of vimentin (yellow arrow pointing to a cluster of epitheliod histiocytes).

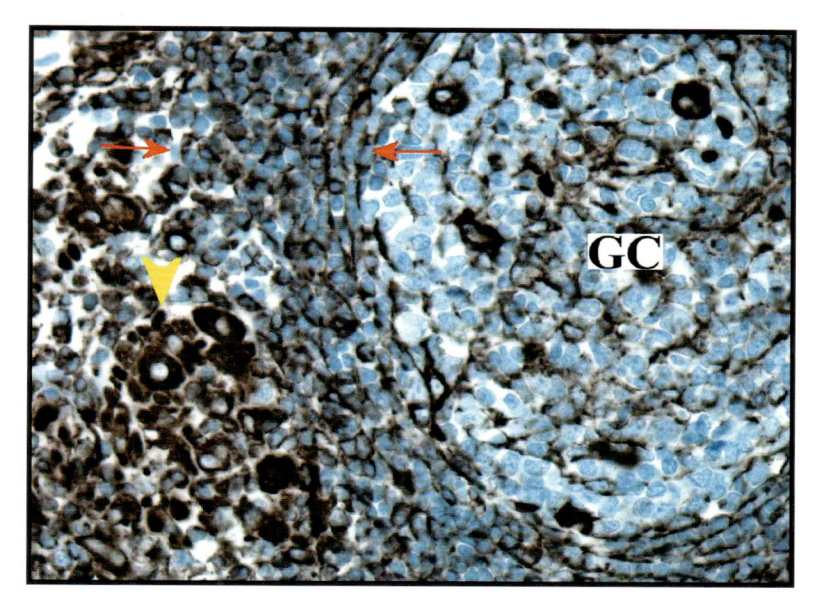

F4.15.4 Vimentin in myeloid hypoplasia

This specimen is from a 72-year-old man. It illustrates significantly reduced vimentin in a bone marrow specimen with a predominant erythroid population. Stromal cells are accentuated, but are not increased.

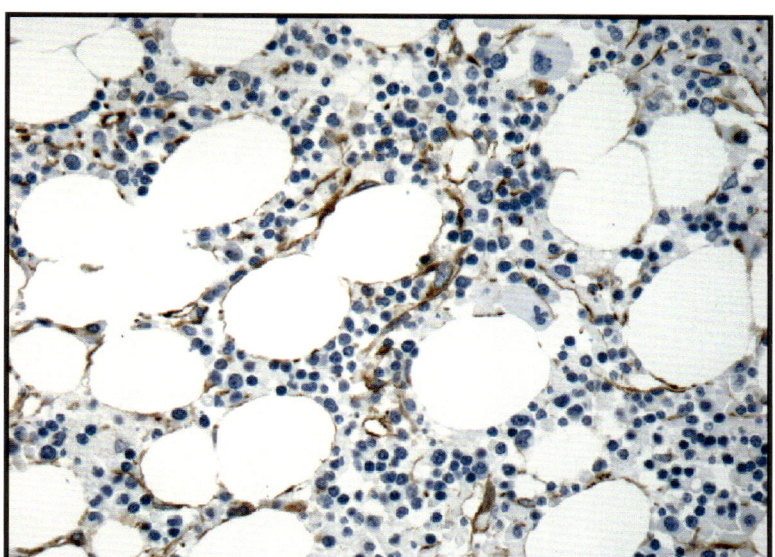

F4.15.5 Vimentin in acute myeloid/erythroid leukemia

Dysplastic megakaryocytes are strongly positive in this biopsy specimen, which is an abnormal finding because vimentin is downregulated very early in megakaryopoiesis. Vimentin expression cannot be detected in neutrophil precursors, which is also an abnormal finding. Compare with the specimen shown in F4.15.2.

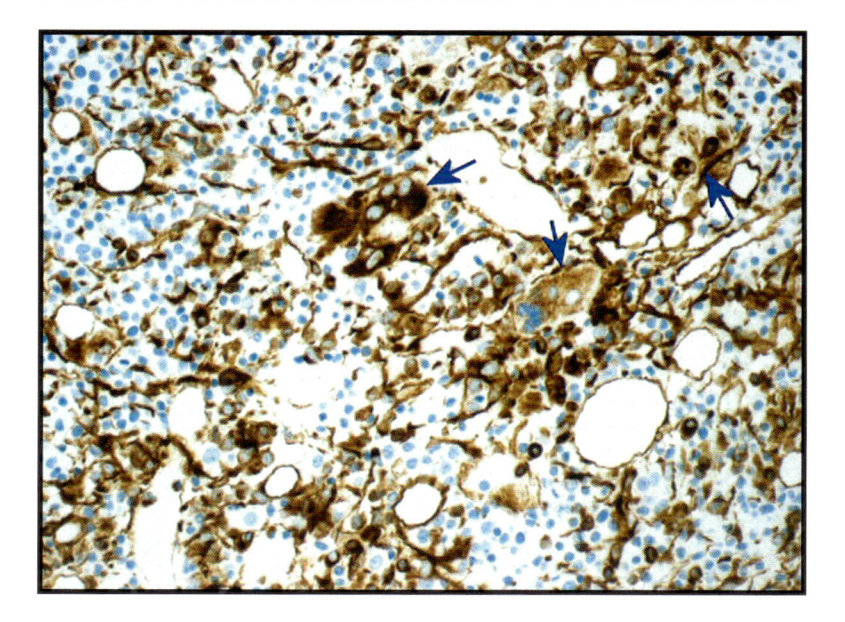

215

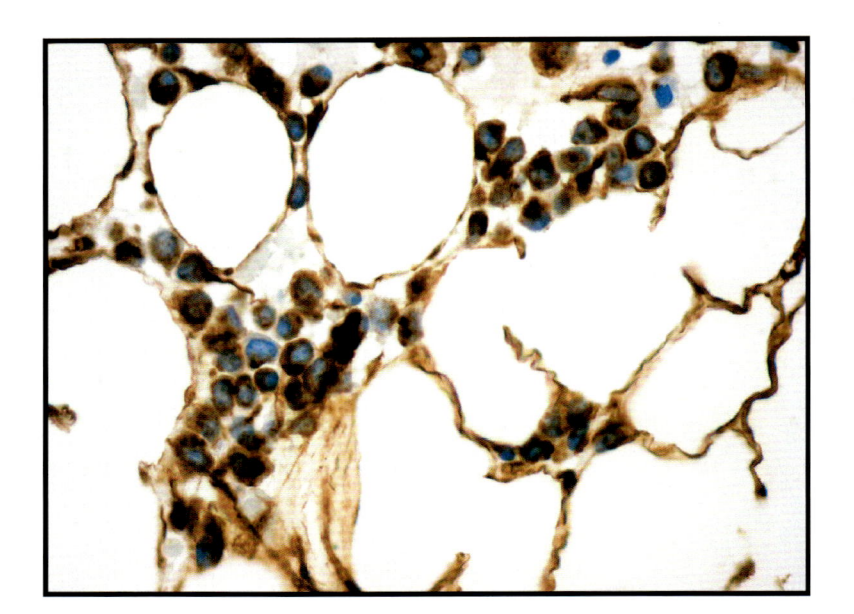

F4.15.6 Vimentin in acute myeloid leukemia (AML)

A case of hypocellular AML is illustrated. The blasts are positive for vimentin in most cases of AML. Vimentin expression in AML blasts and its biological significance, if any, has not been evaluated.

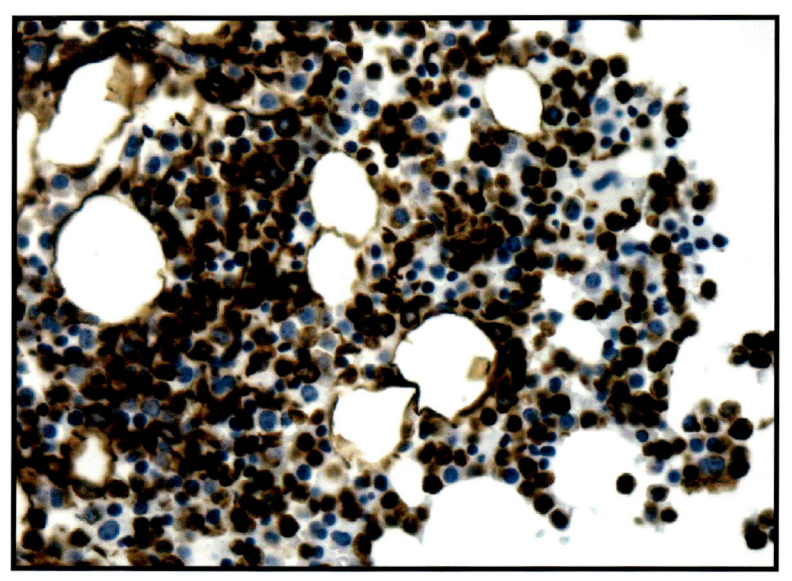

F4.15.7 Vimentin in refractory anemia with myeloid hyperplasia

Vimentin staining highlights myeloid hyperplasia. Intermediate forms of neutrophil precursors appear to show the strongest staining for vimentin and this population is particularly increased in most cases of myeloid hyperplasia, neoplastic or otherwise.

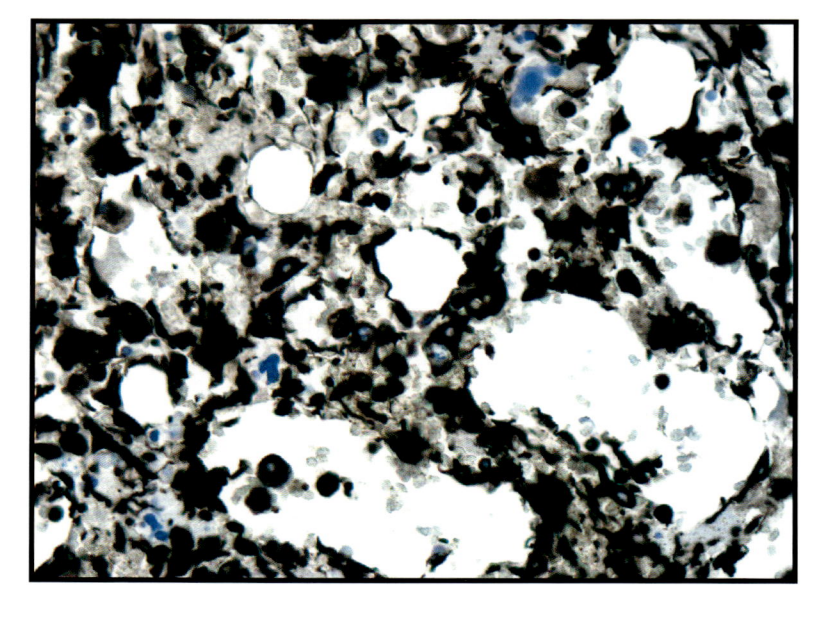

F4.15.8 Vimentin in hemophagocytic syndrome

This biopsy specimen is from a 10-year-old child who died secondary to virally induced phagocytic syndrome. In the bone marrow, vimentin is highly expressed in normal monocytes and megakaryocytes. Even though this is a postmortem sample, the staining is very strong (same protocol as in F4.15.7). Upregulation of vimentin in stromal cells and monocyte/macrophage cells cannot be ruled out.

4.15 Stromal Markers

F4.15.9 Desmin in bone marrow (ADVANCE)

This biopsy specimen is from a 37-year-old man with classical Hodgkin lymphoma stage 1. Only smooth muscle cells lining blood vessels express desmin in normal BM. Occasionally peculiar images occur because of tangentional cutting as shown here. Weak background staining is often present when using ADVANCE even in optimized systems.

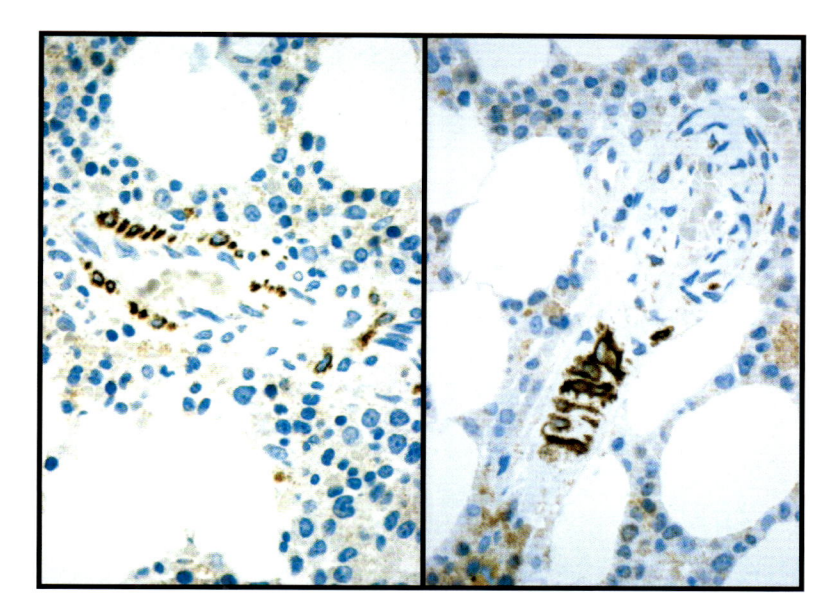

F4.15.10 Smooth muscle actin (ADVANCE)

Smooth muscle actin is found in smooth muscle cells of vessels. It is not expressed by endothelial cells (arrow), but it is expressed by pericytes. There is a difference in the appearance between the smooth muscle actin and desmin staining in the vessel wall (for comparison see **F4.15.9**).

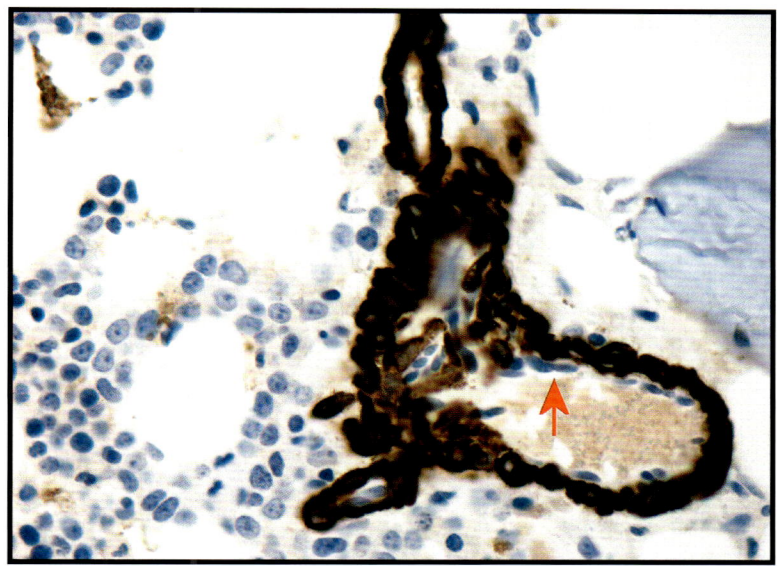

F4.15.11 Smooth muscle actin (ADVANCE)

Smooth muscle actin is occasionally identified in bone marrow stromal cells with dendritic morphology, which are associated with adipocytes. Careful inspection rules out segmental expression of small muscle actin by adipocytes.

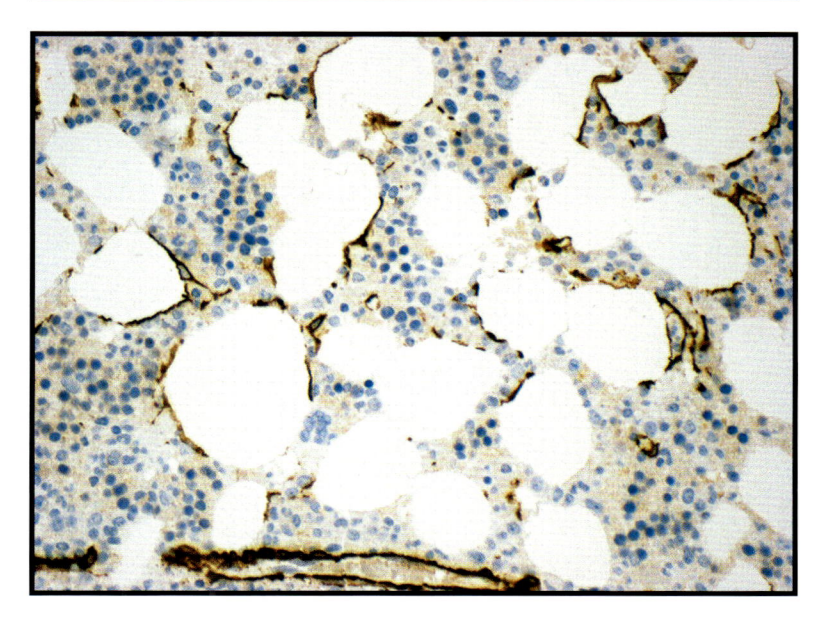

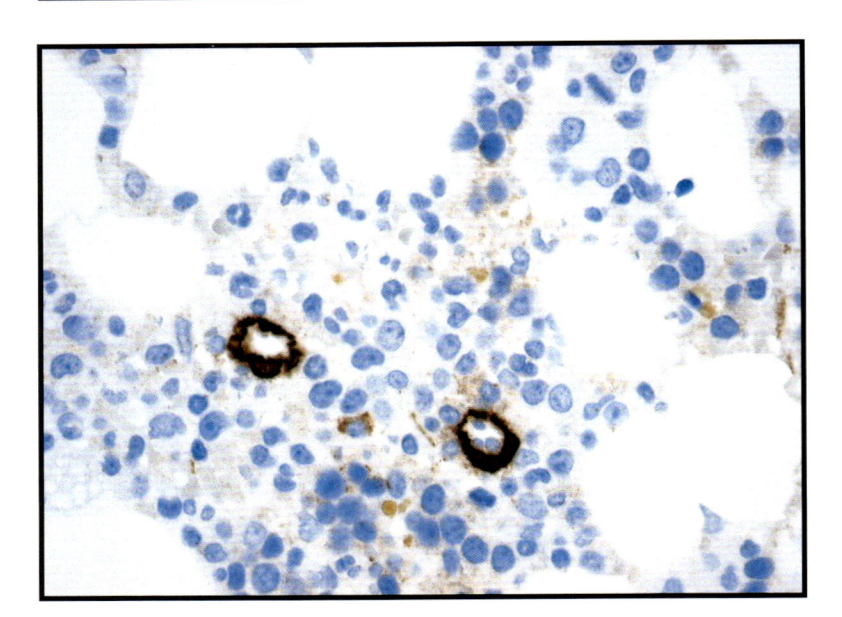

F4.15.12 Smooth muscle actin (ADVANCE)

This bone marrow biopsy specimen was obtained for non-Hodgkin lymphoma staging in a 38-year-old woman; there is no evidence of disease. Two small vascular spaces are highlighted by smooth muscle actin staining. In this calibre vessel, only pericytes are present and these would be negative for desmin, which in normal conditions is restricted to smooth muscle cells.

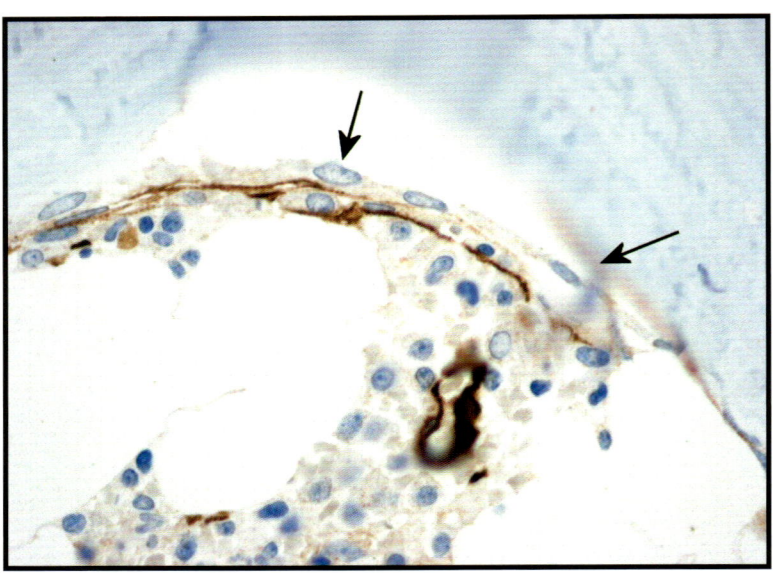

F4.15.13 Smooth muscle actin (ADVANCE)

Smooth muscle actin is expressed by endosteal lining cells, but not osteoblasts. This, however, is not a constant finding and its biological significance is not clear.

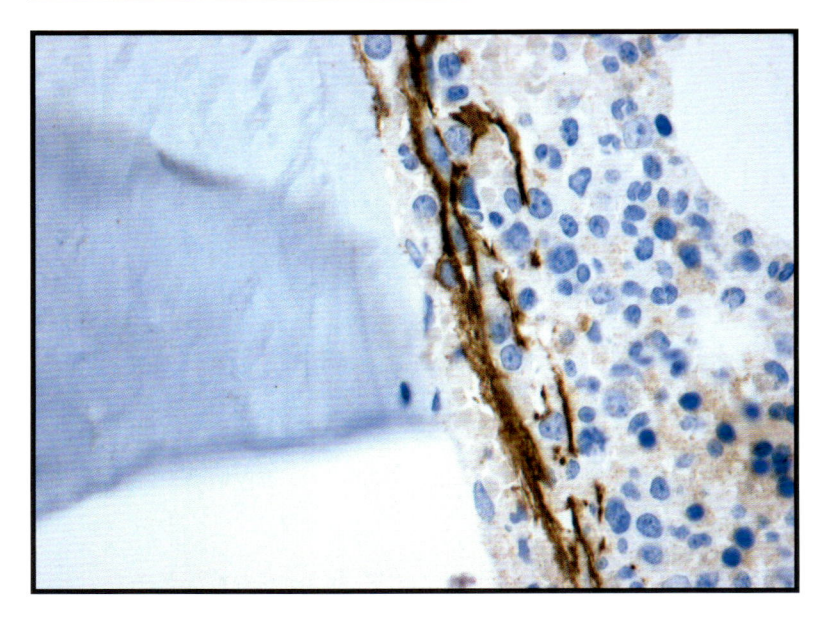

F4.15.14 Smooth muscle actin (SMA) in paratrabecular lining cells (ADVANCE)

This biopsy specimen is from a 27-year-old woman with stage I classical Hodgkin lymphoma. The paratrabecular SMA+ cells appear more numerous in this area. These cells do not line vascular lumens and are hyperplastic endosteal lining cells.

4.15 Stromal Markers

F4.15.15 S-100 in histologically normal bone marrow

In the normal BM, adipocytes are positive. In addition, very few other cells, all presumably stromal cells, express S-100 protein. Megakaryocytes, erythroid cells, and neutrophils are all negative.

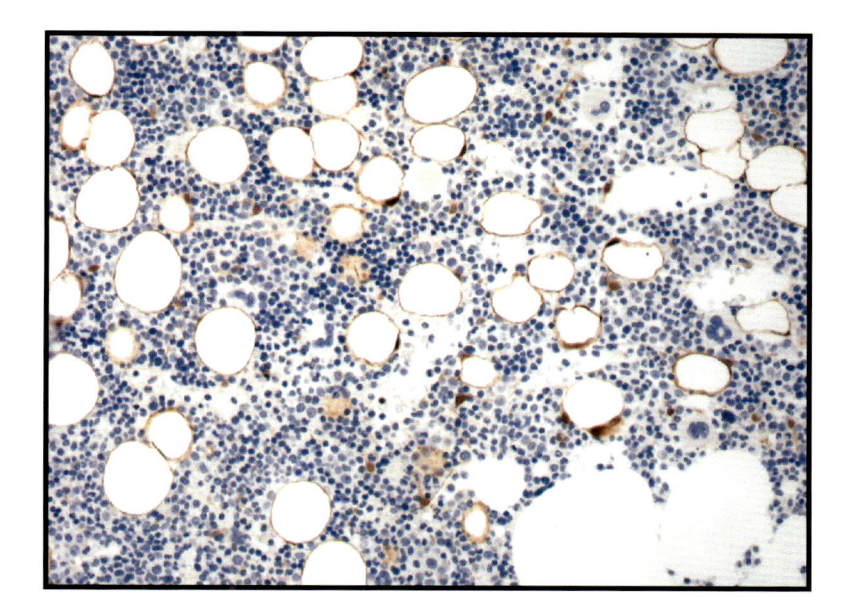

F4.15.16 S-100 in adipocytes

Adipocytes show both nuclear and cytoplasmic expression of S-100 protein. S-100 is a calcium-binding protein and belongs to the EF hand family, to which calretinin (not shown here) also belongs. When expressed in various cell types, calretinin also shows identical cellular distribution with nuclear and cytoplasmic localization.

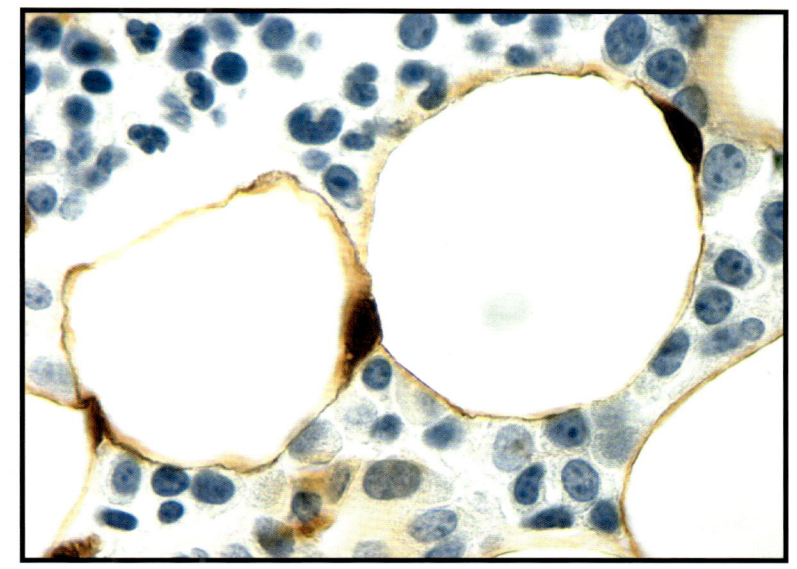

F4.15.17 S-100 in small stromal cells in lymphoid aggregates

A benign small juxtatrabecular lymphoid aggregate is shown. Strong nuclear-cytoplasmic staining for S-100 is demonstrated in a population of cells that show cellular extensions and are compatible with dendritic cells, which may suggest bone marrow stromal response to lymphoid infiltration. However, these are not follicular dendritic cells because no germinal center is present and no cells are positive for either CD21 or CD23.

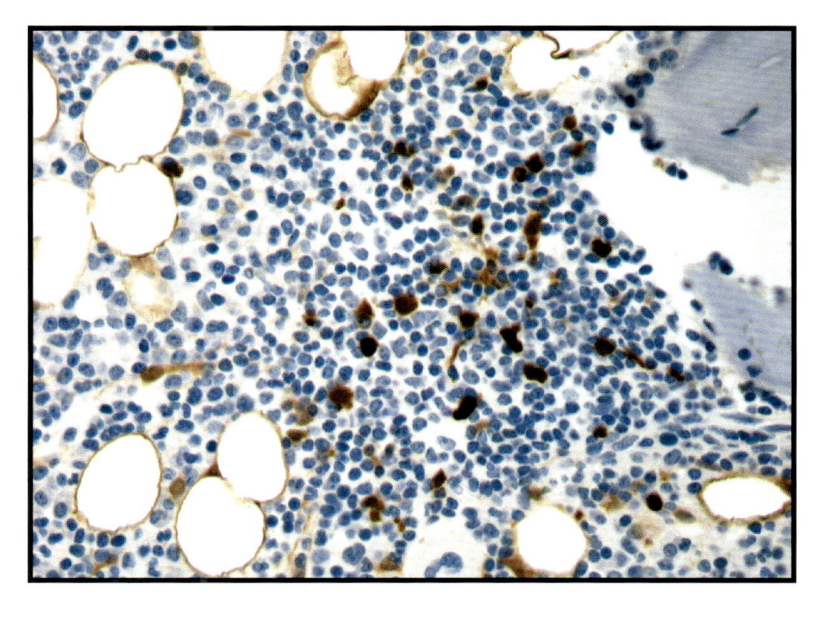

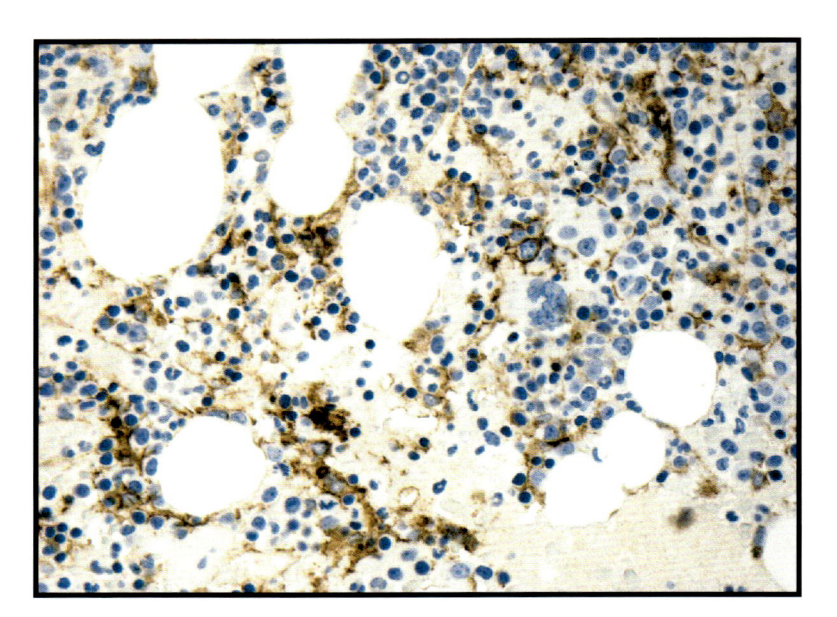

F4.15.18 Vascular cell adhesion molecule (VCAM-1) in histologically normal bone marrow

Stromal cells of the BM are heterogeneous. VCAM-1 staining highlights prototypic BM stromal cells with complex dendritic extensions found in contact with cells belonging to all 3 lineages.

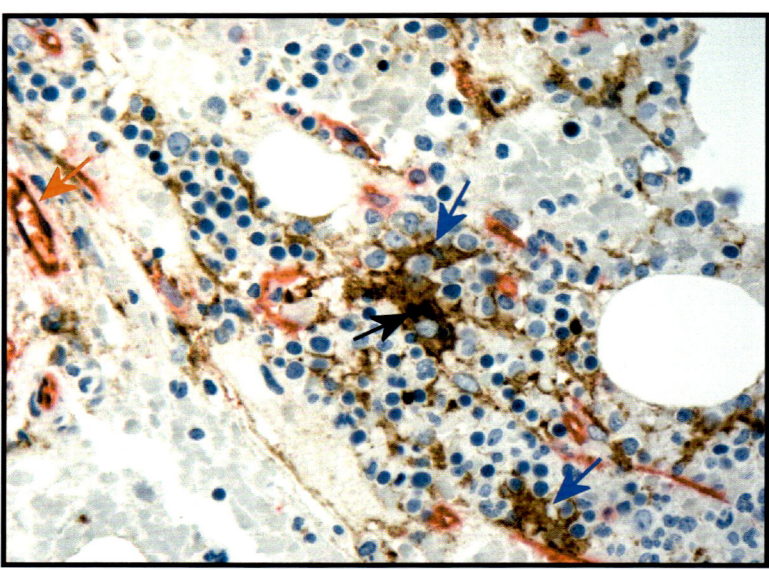

F4.15.19 VCAM-1 (brown) + CD34 (red)

VCAM-1 is expressed by large stromal cells with low nuclear-cytoplasmic ratio and large cell bodies with numerous irregular and complex dendritic extensions (blue arrows). The Golgi area is usually stained stronger than the rest of the cell body (black arrow) and dendritic extensions vary in intensity of staining. The red arrow points to endothelial cells that demonstrate expression of both VCAM-1 and CD34. Most likely all endothelial cells express both markers, but with variable intensity.

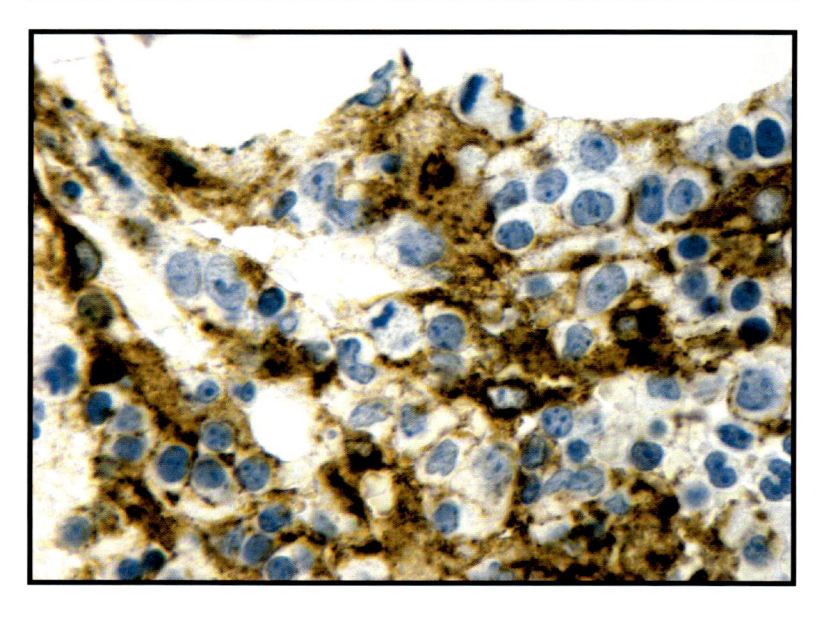

F4.15.20 VCAM-1 in histologically normal bone marrow

Occasionally, normal BM shows a larger number of VCAM-1+ dendritic cells, present in clusters (as shown here). Their dendritic extensions appear to delicately envelope all maturing hematopoietic cells. Most cells in this field appear to be neutrophils.

4.15 Stromal Markers

F4.15.21 Laminin in histologically normal bone marrow

Left, laminin can be found in the internal (red arrow) and external (blue arrow) lamina in the vascular walls and adipocytes (green arrow). Right, laminin is found weakly expressed in the lining of the BM sinusoids (blue arrow) and also in rare stromal cells in close contact with BM sinusoids (red arrow).

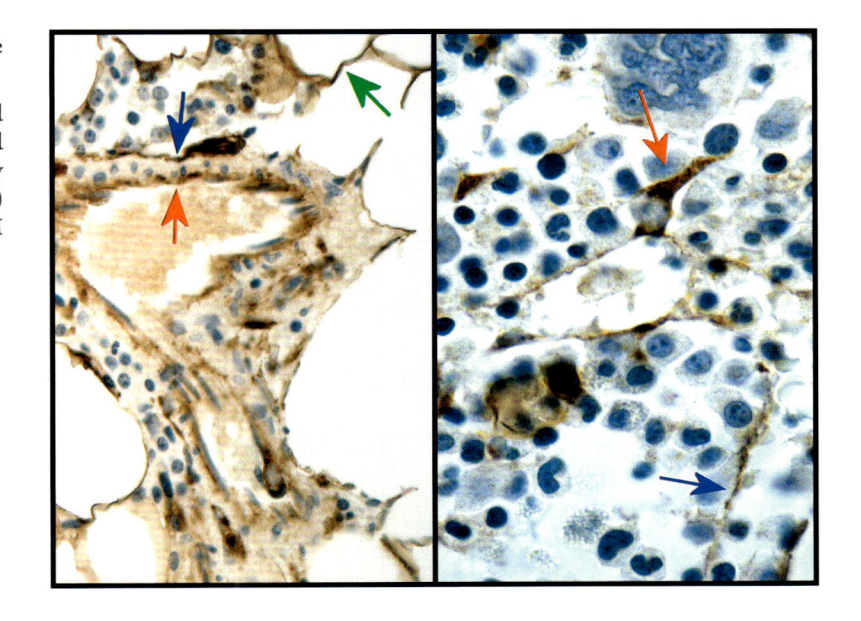

4.16 MUM1

MUM1 (multiple myeloma oncogene 1)/*IRF4* (interferon regulatory factor 4) gene is an oncogene transcriptionally activated by a t(6;14)(p25;q32) chromosomal translocation in multiple myeloma (MM) and it is localized in the nucleus [Iida 1997]. However, MUM1 is widely expressed by benign plasma cells and MM [Heintel 2008; Claudio 2002]. It is a useful marker of cHL [Carbone 2002]. It is also considered to be a marker of activated B-cell subtype of DLBCL, but it is also detected in activated T cells as well as in some T-cell lymphomas [Falini 2000; Yamada 2001]. CD138, which is most frequently used for identification and quantitation of benign and malignant plasma cells, is also expressed by epithelial cells. If morphologic or other evidence of terminal B-cell differentiation is lacking and Ig light chains are difficult to interpret, an additional plasma cell marker may be needed. In this situation MUM1 could be useful. Although it is a nonspecific marker expressed in various lymphoproliferative disorders, it is never expressed by epithelial neoplasms [Tsuboi 2000]. MUM1 is also used for subtyping of DLBCL, where its expression in CD10-negative tumors indicates activated B-cell type of lymphoma [Hans 2004]. Its expression was also described relatively frequently in CLL, in particular in proliferation centers, and occasionally in grade 3 FL [Naresh 2007; Chang 2002; Craig 2008]. Plasmablastic lymphomas, plasmablastic myeloma, and post-transplant lymphoproliferative disorders also express MUM1 [Colomo 2004; Vega 2005; Capello 2005].

F4.16.1 MUM1 in hypocellular bone marrow

This biopsy specimen is from a 44-year-old woman with a slightly hypocellular BM and reactive plasmacytosis. The plasma cells were polytypic. In non-neoplastic BM, only plasma cells show expression of MUM1.

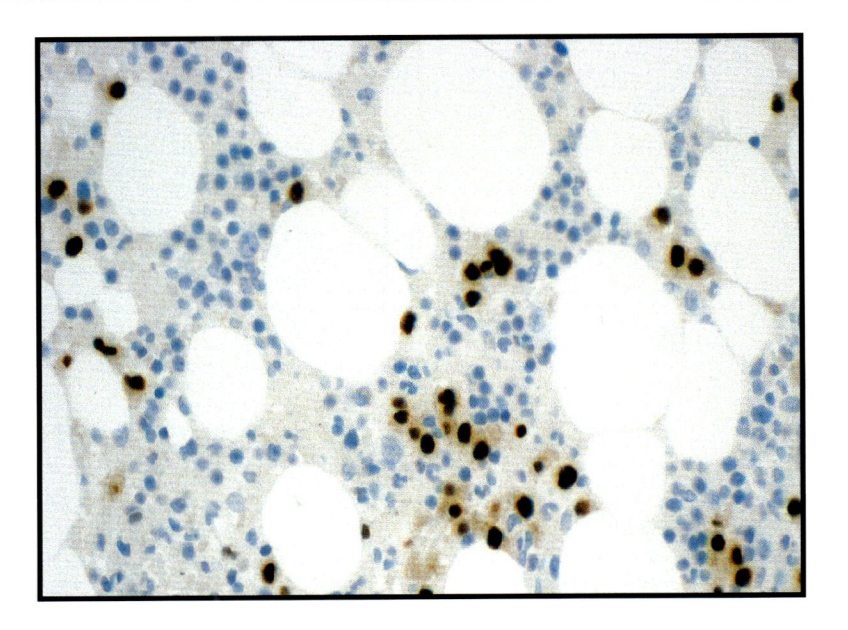

4: Other Common Markers

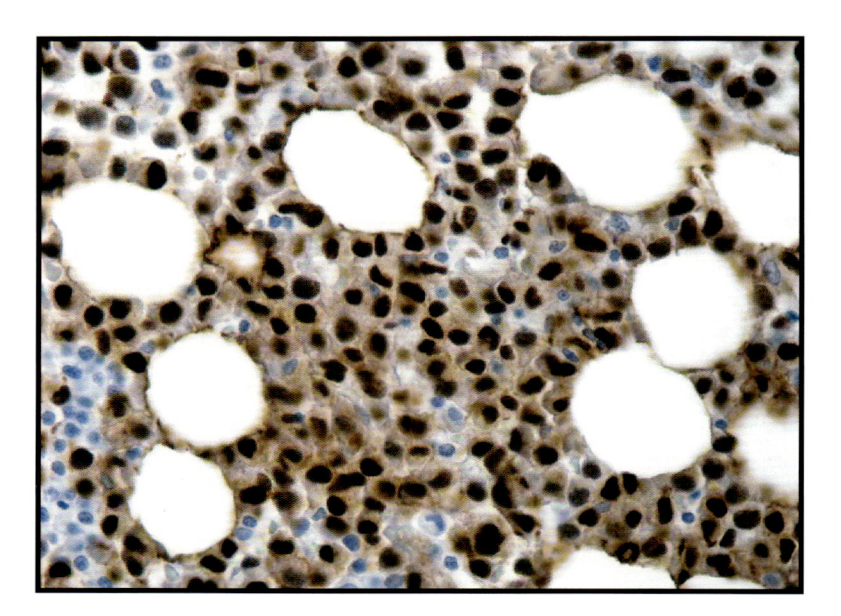

F4.16.2 MUM1 in IgG-κ multiple myeloma (MM)

This biopsy specimen is from a 54-year-old woman with MM. The plasma cells comprised 75% of the bone marrow cellularity and expressed CD138+ and IgG-κ. MUM1 is a transcription factor important for terminal B-cell differentiation and should be localized to the nucleus as illustrated. Some associated cytoplasmic staining is very common.

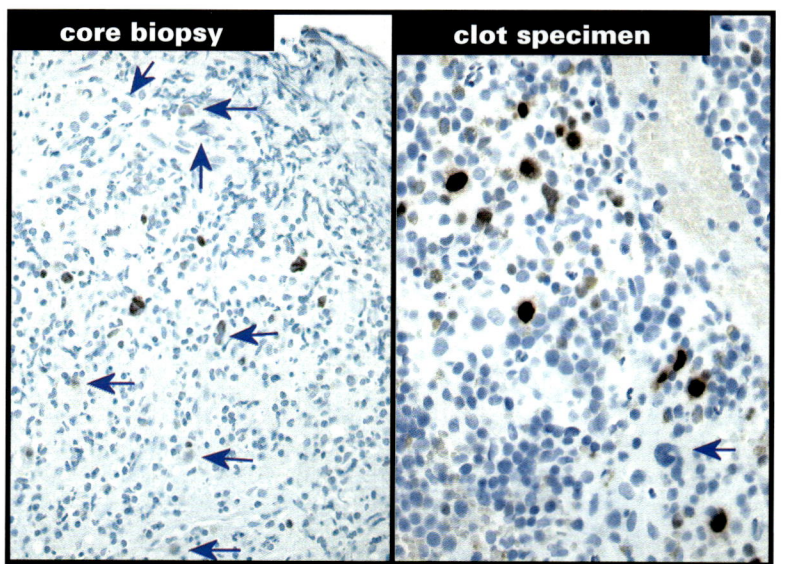

F4.16.3 MUM1 in classical Hodgkin lymphoma (cHL)

MUM1 is a good marker of cHL. The blue arrows indicate Hodgkin cells with weak or no detectable expression of MUM1. In the bone marrow, there may be stronger expression in the clot specimens than in the core biopsy. It is not clear if this is the result of the decalcification step in the processing of the core biopsy specimen, which is most probable, or lower expression of MUM1 in fibrotic areas because clot specimens usually show less fibrosis.

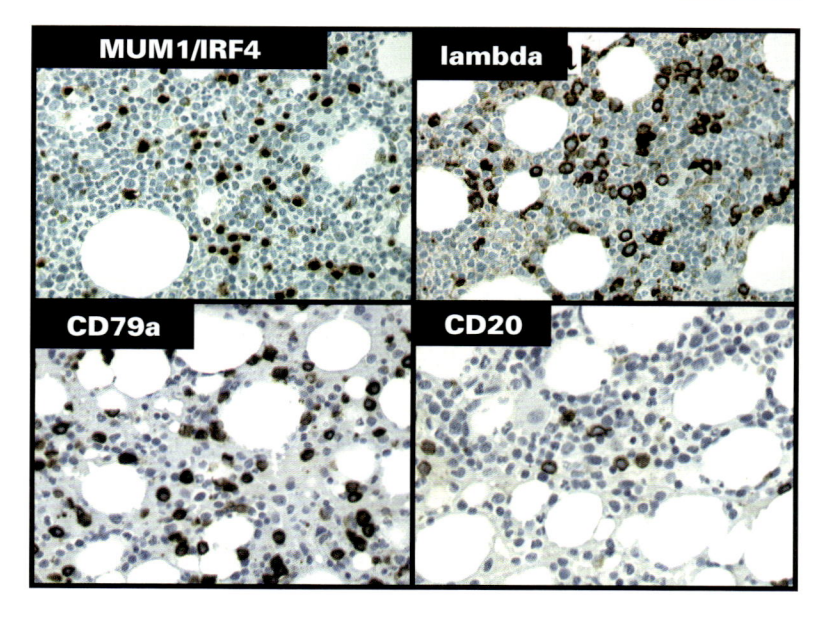

F4.16.4 MUM1 in lymphoplasmacytic lymphoma (LPL)

MUM1 expression is compared with cytoplasmic Ig, CD79a, and CD20 in LPL. MUM1 expression is common in at least a subpopulation of lymphoma cells in LPL because of its variable terminal B-cell differentiation. Its expression correlates well with cytoplasmic Ig expression. CD79a highlights lymphoma cells with all stages of differentiation and therefore CD79a always shows the largest number of lymphoma cells in LPL.

4.15 MUM1

F4.16.5 MUM1 in follicular lymphoma (FL)

This biopsy specimen is from a 66-year-old woman with stage IV FL. MUM1 is not expressed in FL except in some cases of grade 3 FL. In the bone marrow, just as in the lymph node involved by FL, it is common to detect a few larger positive cells.

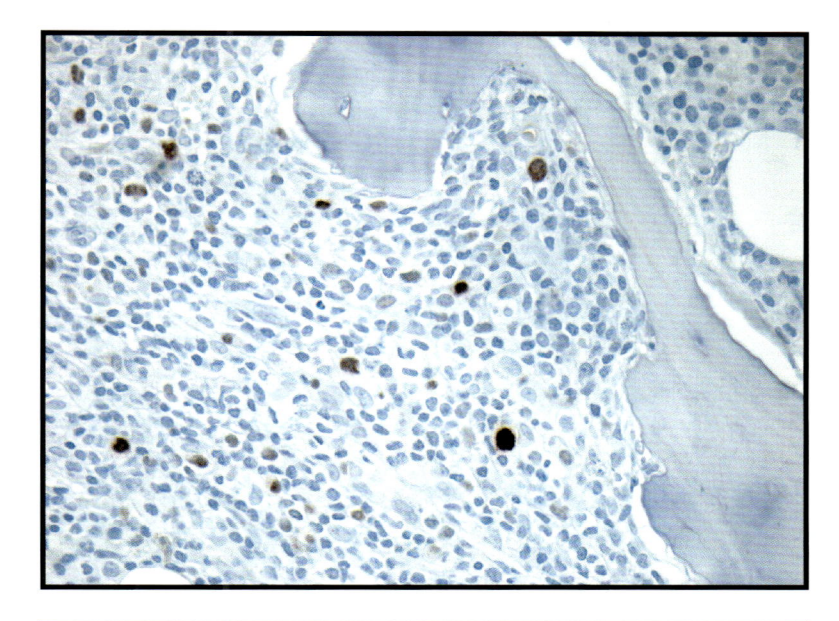

F4.16.6 MUM1 in diffuse large B-cell lymphoma (DLBCL) involving bone marrow

In DLBCL, MUM1 is often used for subtyping into germinal center type, which is CD10+ or Bcl6+/MUM1– and activated B-cell (ABC) type, which is CD10– and Bcl6– or Bcl6+/MUM1+. The same approach can be used in the BM biopsy. The cases are considered positive if 30% or more of the tumor cells are stained with an antibody.

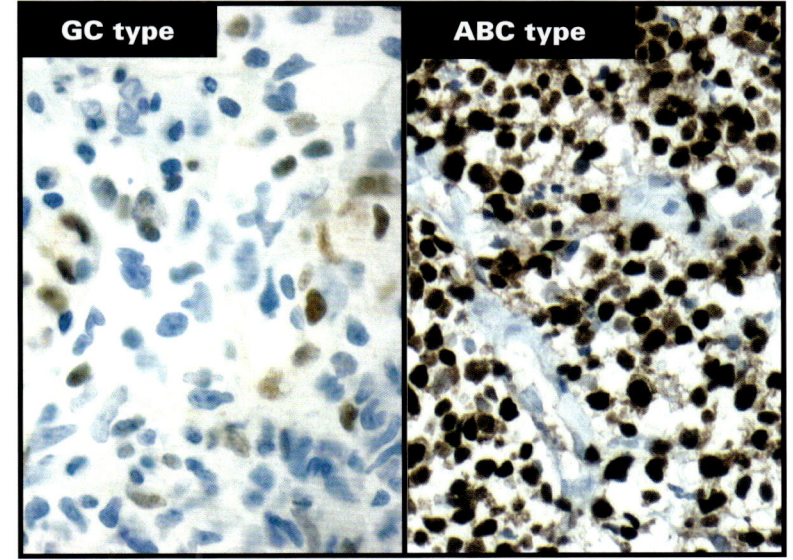

4.17 TRAP

Hairy cell leukemia (HCL) is usually diagnosed by correlating clinical presentation (splenomegaly, pancytopenia, dry BM tap) and flow cytometric findings as well morphologic findings in the peripheral blood and BM. However, some markers have been suggested to be useful for the identification of HCL in the BM biopsy specimen. These include TRAP, CD25, and CD72 (DBA.44) [Went 2005; Hoyer 1997; Akkaya 2005; Riccioni 2007; Burke 1984]. Even if flow cytometric results are not available, a correct diagnosis can be made based on characteristic clinical presentation, morphologic/cytologic appearance of the neoplastic cells in the blood or BM imprints, typical BM fibrosis with cells with relatively low nuclear-cytoplasmic ratio, and very high expression of CD20. Historically TRAP was demonstrated by cytochemistry for decades, and it has been used for the specific identification of HCL. TRAP has been used longer for identification of osteoclasts [Hayman 2001; Cole 1987; Marks 1987]. The enzyme, which is critical for normal bone development in mice, is also characteristic of monohistiocytes, including alveolar macrophages [Burke 1984]. TRAP shows widespread expression and is identified in skin, thymus, gut epithelia, and isolated dendritic cells, suggesting a possible role in immunity [Burke 1984]. Primary Abs that work in the BM core biopsy aspirate clot specimen from the BM have been developed and can be used to confirm the diagnosis of HCL. Hoyer et al [Hoyer 1997] showed that in the cases of HCL, TRAP immunostaining is highly sensitive, but somewhat less specific. Interestingly, TRAP detection with IHC is not highly sensitive, and generally detects less than 50% of the hairy cells in each individual case, while CD20 and DBA.44 detect 100% and about 95% respectively. Marginal zone lymphomas can show weak immunoreactivity to the TRAP antibody. TRAP may be detected in Gaucher cells and in mastocytosis in the macrophages and mast cells. Of note, only HCL is TRAP+ and DBA.44+. Therefore, in very few cases that are diagnostically equivocal, an antibody to TRAP is a useful addition to the diagnosis of HCL, but should be used in conjunction with CD20 and DBA.44 [Went 2005; Hoyer 1997; Akkaya 2005. It has been reported that HCL can be diagnosed by TRAP immunoreactivity in BM trephine biopsy materials and has a specificity of 98.27% and a sensitivity of 100% [Akkaya 2005].

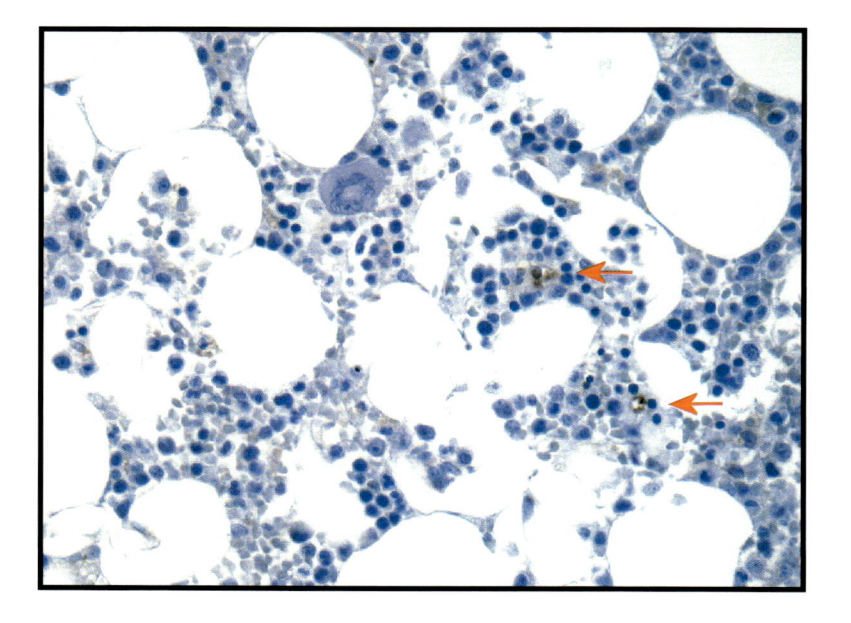

F4.17.1 TRAP in histologically normal bone marrow

Rare cells with a low nuclear-cytoplasmic ratio show weak cytoplasmic positivity (arrows). These cells are compatible with macrophages. Otherwise, osteoclasts (see **F4.17.3**) and rare dendritic cells also are normal structures that express TRAP.

F4.17.2 TRAP in hairy cell leukemia (HCL)

In most cases of HCL, about 50% or less of leukemic cells are positive; most leukemic cells show weak or borderline positivity, which is occasionally difficult to interpret. Immunohistochemistry does not have the reliability of the cytochemical detection of TRAP.

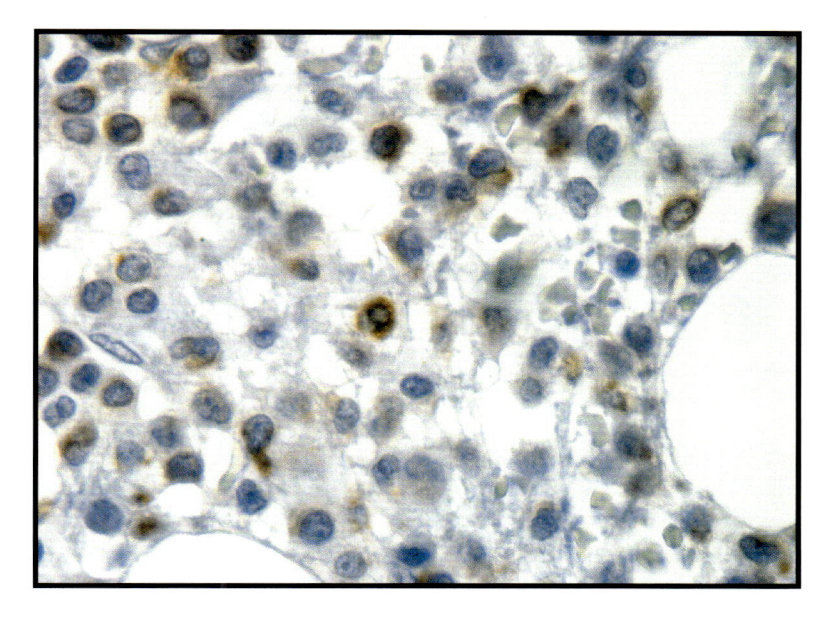

F4.17.3 TRAP in hairy cell leukemia (HCL)

No neoplastic cells are positive in this HCL. This is one of the 20% of cases that show no immunoreactivity with anti-TRAP primary antibody. The arrow points to a rare osteoclast in adult bone marrow. TRAP demonstration with immunohistochemistry is not required for the diagnosis of HCL.

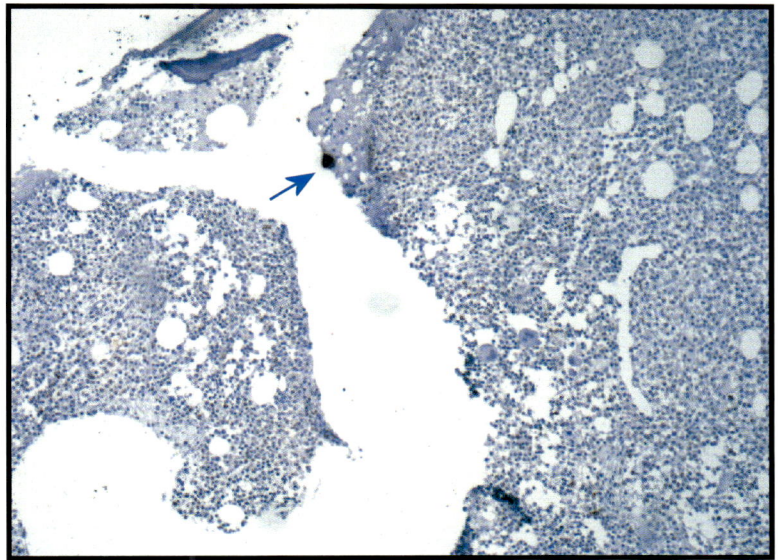

4.18 Bcl-2

B-cell leukemia/lymphoma 2 (Bcl-2) is an integral outer mitochondrial membrane protein that blocks the apoptotic death of some cells (Entrez Gene). It is considered to be a proto-oncogene because constitutive expression of BCL2 is highly associated with some malignancies. In up to 90% of FLs, the promoter of the *IGH* gene is translocated to the *BCL2* gene by t(14;18)(q32;q21), which leads to constitutive expression of Bcl-2. The same translocation is found in about 30% of DLBCLs [Tsujimoto 1985; Tsujimoto 1984]. Bcl-2 is not expressed by the great majority of cells in the BM. Occasional lymphoid cells express Bcl-2 in normal BM. Bcl-2 can be used to detect not only FL in the BM, but any small B-cell lymphoproliferative disorder. Importantly, Bcl-2 is typically negative in Burkitt lymphoma. It is controversial whether its expression could be compatible with a diagnosis of Burkitt-like lymphoma [McClure 2005; Hutchison 2000; Spina 1997]. In Burkitt (or "blastic") transformation of FL, Bcl-2 is expressed. In the presence of c-myc upregulation, this Bcl-2 expression results in a rapid accumulation of tumor volume because tumor cells that are in perpetual cycling due to *c-myc* die slower because of Bcl-2 [Brito-Babapulle 1991; Wong 2007]. Also, expression of Bcl-2 is significantly higher in precursor B-ALL than in hematogones [Hartung 2004]. The percentage of BM cells expressing Bcl-2 and Bcl-xL was reported higher in refractory anemia with excess blasts (RAEB), RAEB in transformation (RAEB-T), and CMML than in refractory anemia (RA) and RA with ringed sideroblasts (RAS) [Delia 1992; Boudard 2002]. Bcl-2 is expressed highly in normal myeloid blasts and in most AMLs, with the exception of t(8;21) AML [Shikami 1999; Porwit-MacDonald 1995]. For the most part, Bcl-2 expression in AML correlates with a differentiation stage similar to that of normal hematopoiesis [Porwit-MacDonald 1995]. The blasts in ALL also overexpress Bcl-2 [Gala 1994; Campana 1993]. The emergence of resistance to imatinib in CML is associated with a higher expression of Bcl-2 compared with parental sensitive cells [Baran 2007]. Bcl-2 is also increased in polycythemia vera [Fernández-Luna 1999]. Bcl-2 can be identified in cutaneous mastocytosis. However, BM mastocytosis typically does not show Bcl-2 expression, but marked expression of Bcl-xL [Hartmann 2003; Chaidos 2002]. Bcl-2 immunostaining occasionally may help detect morphologically undetectable abnormal cells in the bone marrow [Chetty 1995].

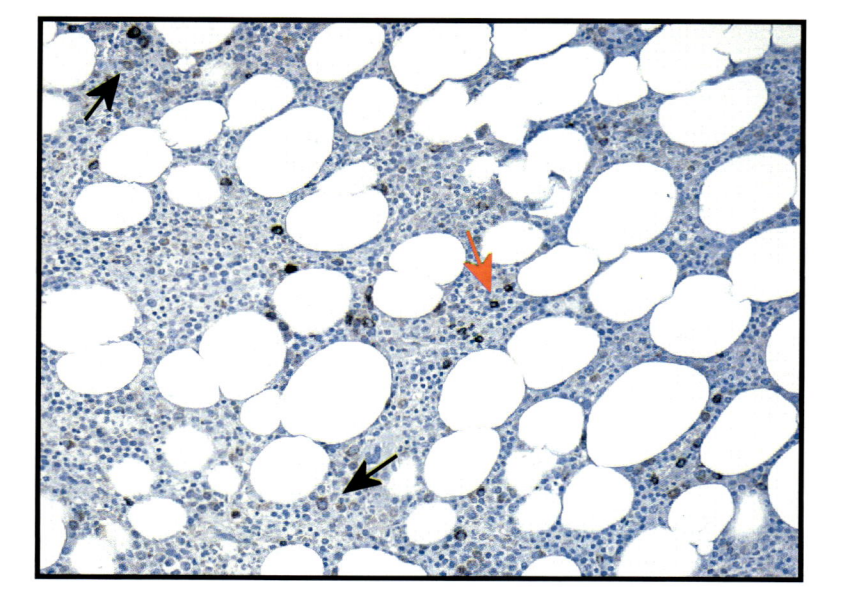

F4.18.1 Bcl-2 in histologically normal bone marrow
Occasional small lymphoid cells show strong expression (red arrow). Weak expression is detected in myeloid cells (black arrows). Bcl-2 expression in myeloid cells decreases with maturation.

4.18 Bcl-2

F4.18.2 Bcl-2 in histologically normal bone marrow

Perivascular benign plasma cells show weak Bcl-2 expression (red arrows). Immature appearing cells with high nuclear-cytoplasmic ratio also express Bcl-2 and are compatible with early hematopoietic precursors. Small lymphoid cells show strong expression (black arrows). The expression of Bcl-2 is cytoplasmic as illustrated here.

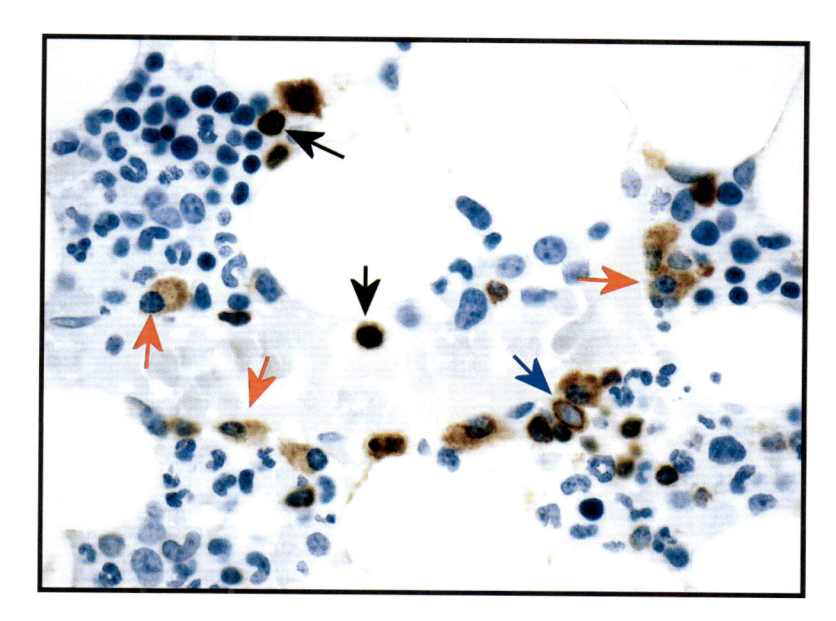

F4.18.3 Bcl-2 expression in myeloid precursors

Early myeloid precursors normally express Bcl-2. Blasts and promyelocytes are positive (blue arrows); appropriately 80% of the promyelocytes express Bcl-2. Red arrows point to possible plasma cells. Small lymphocytes are strongly positive as expected (green arrows). Occasional adipocyte may express Bcl-2 (black arrow).

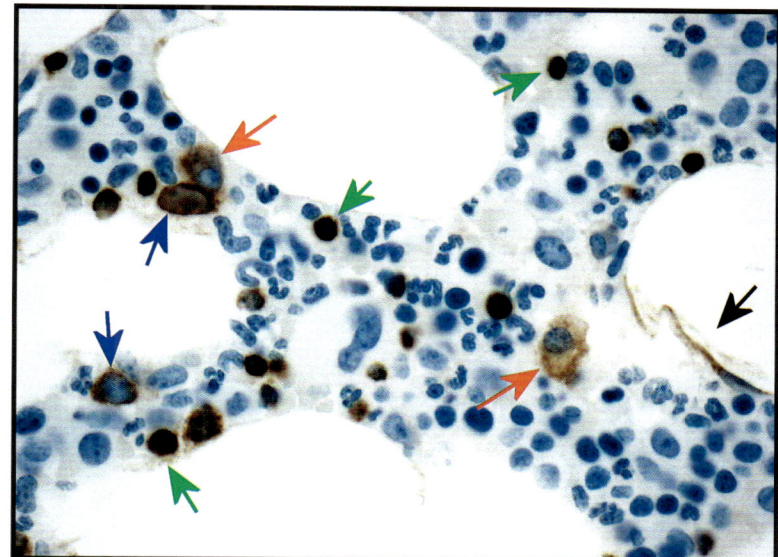

F4.18.4 Bcl-2 in small B-cell lymphoproliferative diseases

Bcl-2 expression in chronic lymphocytic leukemia is illustrated. Bcl-2 is sensitive, but a nonspecific marker of all small B-cell lymphoproliferative diseases.

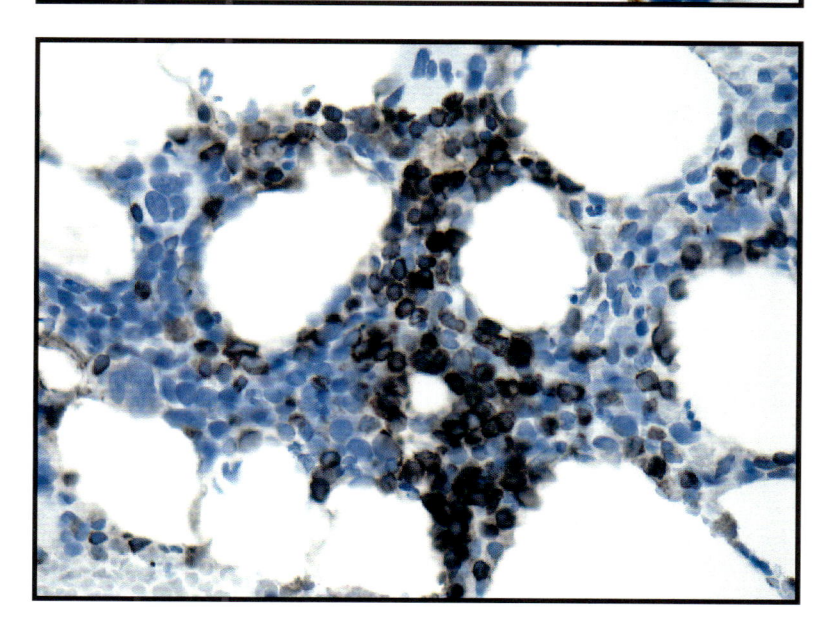

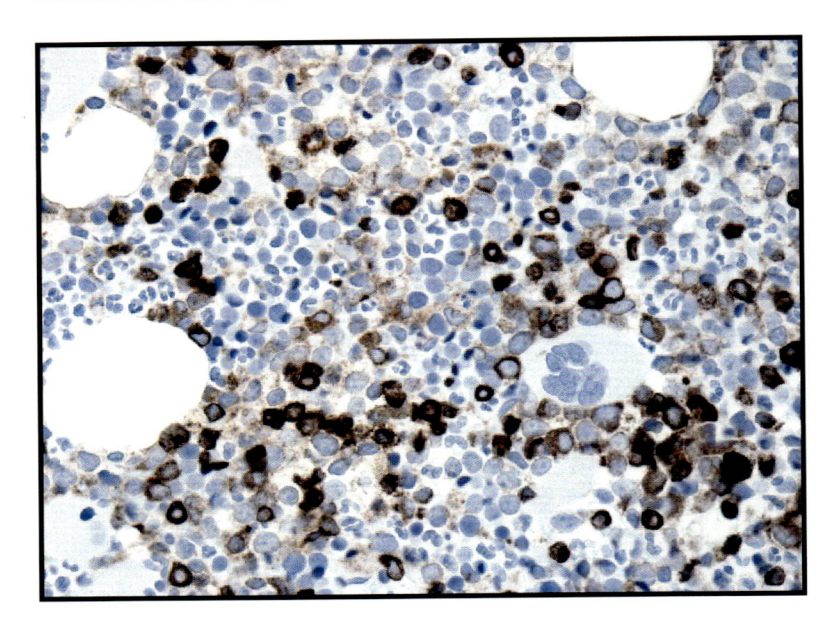

F4.18.5 Bcl-2 in chronic myelomonocytic leukemia (CMML)

This biopsy specimen is from a 66-year-old man with CMML type 2. Blasts are strongly positive and Bcl-2 expression is also upregulated in myeloid cells (compare with F4.18.1). Bcl-2 could be significantly increased in myeloproliferative, myelodysplastic/myeloproliferative, and myelodysplastic diseases.

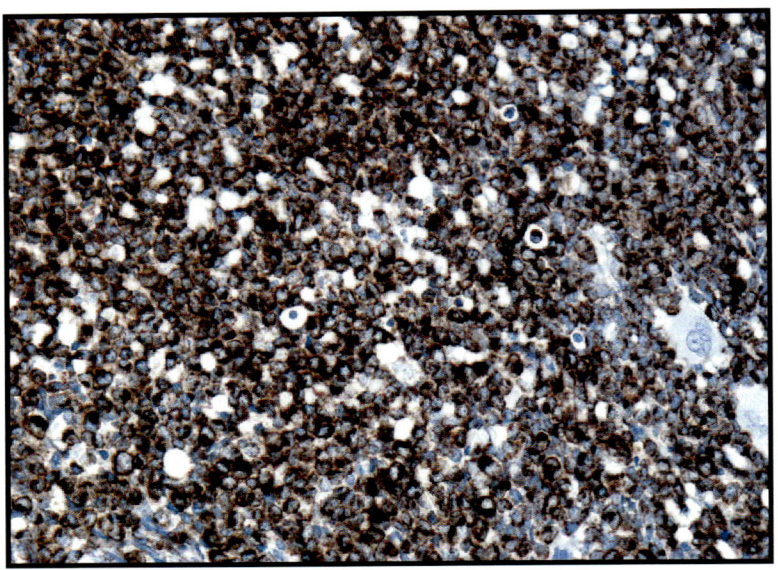

F4.18.6 Bcl-2 in precursor B-cell acute lymphoblastic leukemia (ALL)

This biopsy specimen is from a 10-year-old girl with CD10-negative precursor B-ALL. While Bcl-2 is generally known to be weakly expressed by normal CD34+/CD10+ lymphoid blasts, it is strongly expressed by blasts in precursor B and precursor T-ALL as illustrated here. In contrast, both benign and malignant myeloid blasts express high levels of Bcl-2. However, in both benign and malignant myeloid cells, its expression is downregulated with maturation.

References

Adams B, Dörfler P, Aguzzi A, et al. Pax-5 encodes the transcription factor BSAP and is expressed in B lymphocytes, the developing CNS, and adult testis. *Genes Dev* 1992;6(9):1589-607.

Adelstein DJ, Hines JD. Bone marrow morphologic changes after combination chemotherapy including VP-16. *Cancer* 1985;56(3):467-71.

Agis H, Sotlar K, Valent P, Horny HP. Ph-Chromosome-positive chronic myeloid leukemia with associated bone marrow mastocytosis. *Leuk Res* 2005 Oct;29(10):1227-32.

Akkaya H, Dogan O, Agan M, Dincol G. The value of tartrate resistant acid phosphatase (TRAP) immunoreactivity in diagnosis of hairy cell leukemia. *APMIS* 2005;113(3):162-6.

Anderson K, Rusterholz C, Månsson R, et al. Ectopic expression of PAX5 promotes maintenance of biphenotypic myeloid progenitors coexpressing myeloid and B-cell lineage-associated genes. *Blood* 2007;109(9):3697-705.

Anderson MK, Hernandez-Hoyos G, Diamond RA, Rothenberg EV. Precise developmental regulation of Ets family transcription factors during specification and commitment to the T-cell lineage. *Development* 1999;126(14):3131-48.

Anjos-Afonso F, Bonnet D. Flexible and dynamic organization of bone marrow stromal compartment [review]. *Br J Haematol* 2007;139(3):373-84.

Apaja-Sarkkinen M, Autio-Harmainen H, Alavaikko M, Risteli J, Risteli L. Immunohistochemical study of basement membrane proteins and type III procollagen in myelofibrosis. *Br J Haematol* 1986;63(3):571-80.

Apte SS. Expression of the cell proliferation-associated nuclear antigen reactive with the Ki-67 monoclonal antibody by cells of the skeletal system in humans and other species. *Bone Miner* 1990;10(1):37-50.

Athanasiou E, Kaloutsi V, Kotoula V, et al. Cyclin D1 overexpression in multiple myeloma: a morphologic, immunohistochemical, and in situ hybridization study of 71 paraffin-embedded BM biopsy specimens. *Am J Clin Pathol* 2001;116(4):535-42.

Aumeller C, Myer zum Bueschenfelde C, Koch I, et al. Changes of immunophenotype in B-NHL after rituximab treatment: impact for diagnostic evaluation and follow-up. Abstract 1124. *Mod Pathol* 2008;21(suppl 1):245A.

Bainton DF, Ullyot JL, Farquhar MG. The development of neutrophilic polymorphonuclear leukocytes in human bone marrow. *J Exp Med* 1971;134(4):907-34.

Balduino A, Hurtado SP, Frazão P, et al. Bone marrow subendosteal microenvironment harbours functionally distinct haemosupportive stromal cell populations. *Cell Tissue Res* 2005;319(2):255-66.

Ball LM, Pyesmany AF, Yhap M, et al. Apoptosis corrected proliferation fraction in childhood ALL is related to karyotype. *Adv Exp Med Biol* 1999;457:297-303.

Baran Y, Ural AU, Gunduz U. Mechanisms of cellular resistance to imatinib in human chronic myeloid leukemia cells [published online ahead of print 21, 2007]. *Hematology* 2007.

Bartl R, Frisch B, Burkhardt R. BM biopsies revisited: a new dimension for haematologic malignancies. Basel, Switzerland: S. Karger AG; 1982:15-32.

Benayahu D, Akavia UD, Shur I. Differentiation of bone marrow stroma-derived mesenchymal cells [review]. *Curr Med Chem* 2007;14(2):173-9.

Bendix-Hansen K, Nielsen HK. Myeloperoxidase-deficient polymorphonuclear leucocytes: II, longitudinal study in acute myeloid leukaemia, untreated, in remission and in relapse. *Scand J Haematol* 1983;31(1):5-8.

Bendix-Hansen K. Myeloperoxidase-deficient polymorphonuclear leucocytes: VII, incidence in untreated myeloproliferative disorders. *Scand J Haematol* 1986;36(1):8-10.

Berger F, Traverse-Glehen A, Felman P, et al. Clinicopathologic features of Waldenstrom's macroglobulinemia and marginal zone lymphoma: are they distinct or the same entity? *Clin Lymphoma* 2005;5(4):220-4.

Berti E, Tomasini D, Vermeer MH, Meijer CJ, Alessi E, Willemze R. Primary cutaneous CD8-positive epidermotropic cytotoxic T cell lymphomas: a distinct clinicopathological entity with an aggressive clinical behavior. *Am J Pathol* 1999;155(2):483-92.

Bianco P, Riminucci M, Gronthos S, Robey PG. Bone marrow stromal stem cells: nature, biology, and potential applications [review]. *Stem Cells* 2001;19(3):180-92.

Bock O, Hussein K, Neusch M, Schlué J, Wiese B, Kreipe H. Transcription factor Fli-1 expression by bone marrow cells in chronic myeloproliferative disorders is independent of an underlying JAK2 (V617F) mutation. *Eur J Haematol* 2006;77(6):463-70.

Bosch F, Campo E, Jares P, et al. Increased expression of the PRAD-1/CCND1 gene in hairy cell leukaemia. *Br J Haematol* 1995;91(4):1025-30.

Bosch F, Jares P, Campo E, et al. PRAD-1/cyclin D1 gene overexpression in chronic lymphoproliferative disorders: a highly specific marker of mantle cell lymphoma. *Blood* 1994;84(8):2726-32.

Boudard D, Vasselon C, Berthéas MF, et al. Expression and prognostic significance of Bcl-2 family proteins in myelodysplastic syndromes. *Am J Hematol* 2002;70(2):115-25.

Bousquet M, Broccardo C, Quelen C, et al. A novel PAX5-ELN fusion protein identified in B-cell acute lymphoblastic leukemia acts as a dominant negative on wild-type PAX5. *Blood* 2007;109(8):3417-23.

Brito-Babapulle V, Crawford A, Khokhar T, et al. Translocations t(14;18) and t(8;14) with rearranged bcl-2 and c-myc in a case presenting as B-ALL (L3) [review]. *Leukemia* 1991;5(1):83-7.

Burke JS, Rappaport H. The diagnosis and differential diagnosis of hairy cell leukemia in BM and spleen. *Semin Oncol* 1984;11(4):334-46.

Campana D, Coustan-Smith E, Manabe A, et al. Prolonged survival of B-lineage acute lymphoblastic leukemia cells is accompanied by overexpression of bcl-2 protein. *Blood* 1993;81(4):1025-31.

Capello D, Rossi D, Gaidano G. Post-transplant lymphoproliferative disorders: molecular basis of disease histogenesis and pathogenesis [review]. *Hematol Oncol* 2005;23(2):61-7.

Capello D, Vitolo U, Pasqualucci L, et al. Distribution and pattern of BCL-6 mutations throughout the spectrum of B-cell neoplasia. *Blood* 2000;95(2):651-9.

Carbone A, Gloghini A, Aldinucci D, Gattei V, Dalla-Favera R, Gaidano G. Expression pattern of MUM1/IRF4 in the spectrum of pathology of Hodgkin's disease. *Br J Haematol* 2002;117(2):366-72.

Cattoretti G, Chang CC, Cechova K, et al. BCL-6 protein is expressed in germinal-center B-cells. *Blood* 1995;86(1):45-53.

Cattoretti G, Orazi A, Gerdes J. Proliferating normal bone marrow cells do stain for Ki-67 antigen. *Br J Haematol* 1993;85(4):835-6.

Chaidos AI, Bai MC, Kamina SA, Kanavaros PE, Agnantis NJ, Bourantas KL. Incidence of apoptosis and cell proliferation in multiple myeloma: correlation with bcl-2 protein expression and serum levels of interleukin-6 (IL-6) and soluble IL-6 receptor. *Eur J Haematol* 2002;69(2):90-4.

Chang CC, Lorek J, Sabath DE, et al. Expression of MUM1/IRF4 correlates with clinical outcome in patients with B-cell chronic lymphocytic leukemia. *Blood* 2002;100(13):4671-5.

Chapiro E, Delabesse E, Asnafi V, et al. Expression of T-lineage-affiliated transcripts and TCR rearrangements in acute promyelocytic leukemia: implications for the cellular target of t(15;17) [published online ahead of print July 20, 2006]. *Blood* 2006;108(10):3484-93.

Chetty R, Echezarreta G, Comley M, Gatter K. Immunohistochemistry in apparently normal bone marrow trephine specimens from patients with nodal follicular lymphoma. *J Clin Pathol* 1995;48(11):1035-8.

Chetty R, Hlatswayo N, Muc R, Sabaratnam R, Gatter K. Plasmablastic lymphoma in HIV+ patients: an expanding spectrum. *Histopathology* 2003;42(6):605-9.

Choi JW, Fujino M, Ito M. F-blast is a useful marker for differentiating hypocellular refractory anemia from aplastic anemia. *Int J Hematol* 2002;75(3):257-60.

Chuang SS, Ye H, Du MQ, et al. Histopathology and immunohistochemistry in distinguishing Burkitt lymphoma from diffuse large B-cell lymphoma with very high proliferation index and with or without a starry-sky pattern: a comparative study with EBER and FISH. *Am J Clin Pathol* 2007;128(4):558-64.

Chuang SS, Jung YC, Li CY. von Willebrand factor is the most reliable immunohistochemical marker for megakaryocytes of myelodysplastic syndrome and chronic myeloproliferative disorders. *Am J Clin Pathol* 2000;113(4):506-11.

Claudio JO, Masih-Khan E, Tang H, et al. A molecular compendium of genes expressed in multiple myeloma. *Blood* 2002;100(6):2175-86.

Cobaleda C, Schebesta A, Delogu A, Busslinger M. Pax5: the guardian of B-cell identity and function [review]. *Nat Immunol* 2007;8(5):463-70.

Cole AA, Walters LM. Tartrate-resistant acid phosphatase in bone and cartilage following decalcification and cold-embedding in plastic. *J Histochem Cytochem* 1987;35(2):203-6.

Colomo L, Loong F, Rives S, et al. Diffuse large B-cell lymphomas with plasmablastic differentiation represent a heterogeneous group of disease entities. *Am J Surg Pathol* 2004;28(6):736-47.

Craig F, Soma L, Melan M, Kant J, Swerdlow S. MUM1/IRF4 expression in the circulating compartment of chronic lymphocytic leukemia. *Leuk Lymphoma* 2008;49(2):273-80.

Cramer EM, Berger G, Berndt MC. Platelet α-granule and plasma membrane share two new components: CD9 and PECAM-1. *Blood* 1994;84(6):1722-30.

d'Amore ES, Manivel JC, Gajl-Peczalska KJ, et al. B-cell lymphoproliferative disorders after bone marrow transplant: an analysis of ten cases with emphasis on Epstein-Barr virus detection by in situ hybridization. *Cancer* 1991;68(6):1285-95.

Dakic A, Wu L, Nutt SL. Is PU.1 a dosage-sensitive regulator of haemopoietic lineage commitment and leukaemogenesis? *Trends Immunol* 2007;28(3):108-14.

Dallegri F, Mela G, Patrone F. Myeloperoxidase-deficient neutrophils in chronic myelocytic leukemia. *Haematologica* 1978;63(2):163-7.

Datta NS, Pettway GJ, Chen C, Koh AJ, McCauley LK. Cyclin D1 as a target for the proliferative effects of PTH and PTHrP in early osteoblastic cells. *J Bone Miner Res* 2007;22(7):951-64.

Davis RE, Longacre TA, Cornbleet PJ. Hematogones in the bone marrow of adults. Immunophenotypic features, clinical settings, and differential diagnosis. *Am J Clin Pathol* 1994;102(2):202-11.

de Leval L, Savilo E, Longtine J, Ferry JA, Harris NL. Peripheral T-cell lymphoma with follicular involvement and a CD4+/bcl-6+ phenotype. *Am J Surg Pathol* 2001;25(3):395-400.

Delia D, Aiello A, Soligo D, et al. bcl-2 proto-oncogene expression in normal and neoplastic human myeloid cells. *Blood* 1992;79(5):1291-8.

Dellagi K, Vainchenker W, Vinci G, Paulin D, Brouet JC. Alteration of vimentin intermediate filament expression during differentiation of human hemopoietic cells. *EMBO J* 1983;2(9):1509-14.

Dennis JE, Merriam A, Awadallah A, Yoo JU, Johnstone B, Caplan AI. A quadripotential mesenchymal progenitor cell isolated from the marrow of an adult mouse. *J Bone Miner Res* 1999;14(5):700-9.

Diebold J, Anderson JR, Armitage JO, et al. Diffuse large B-cell lymphoma: a clinicopathologic analysis of 444 cases classified according to the updated Kiel classification. *Leuk Lymphoma* 2002;43(1):97-104.

Direkze NC, Alison MR. Bone marrow and tumour stroma: an intimate relationship [review]. *Hematol Oncol* 2006;24(4):189-95.

Dittel BN, LeBien TW. Reduced expression of vascular cell adhesion molecule-1 on bone marrow stromal cells isolated from marrow transplant recipients correlates with a reduced capacity to support human B lymphopoiesis in vitro. *Blood* 1995;86(7):2833-41.

References

Dogan A, Bagdi E, Munson P, Isaacson PG. CD10 and BCL-6 expression in paraffin sections of normal lymphoid tissue and B-cell lymphomas. *Am J Surg Pathol* 2000;24(6):846-52.

Dominici M, Le Blanc K, Mueller I, et al. Minimal criteria for defining multipotent mesenchymal stromal cells: the International Society for Cellular Therapy position statement. *Cytotherapy* 2006;8(4):315-7.

Dover GJ, Boyer SH. Quantitation of hemoglobins within individual red blood cells: asynchronous biosynthesis of fetal and adult hemoglobin during erythroid maturation in normal subjects. *Blood* 1980;56(6):1082-91.

Dunphy CH, Nies MK, Gabriel DA. Correlation of plasma cell percentages by CD138 immunohistochemistry, cyclin D1 status, and CD56 expression with clinical parameters and overall survival in plasma cell myeloma. *Appl Immunohistochem Mol Morphol* 2007a;15(3):248-54.

Dunphy CH, O'Malley DP, Perkins SL, Chang CC. Analysis of immunohistochemical markers in bone marrow sections to evaluate for myelodysplastic syndromes and acute myeloid leukemias. *Appl Immunohistochem Mol Morphol* 2007a;15(2):154-9.

Dunphy CH. Evaluation of mast cells in myeloproliferative disorders and myelodysplastic syndromes. *Arch Pathol Lab Med* 2005;129(2):219-22.

Eshoa C, Perkins S, Kampalath B, Shidham V, Juckett M, Chang CC. Decreased CD10 expression in grade III and in interfollicular infiltrates of follicular lymphomas. *Am J Clin Pathol* 2001;115(6):862-7.

Falini B, Fizzotti M, Pucciarini A, et al. A monoclonal antibody (MUM1p) detects expression of the MUM1/IRF4 protein in a subset of germinal center B cells, plasma cells, and activated T cells. *Blood* 2000;95(6):2084-92.

Falini B, Canino S, Sacchi S, et al. Immunocytochemical evaluation of the percentage of proliferating cells in pathological BM and peripheral blood samples with the Ki-67 and anti-bromo-deoxyuridine monoclonal antibodies. *Br J Haematol* 1988;69(3):311-20.

Fang W, An C, Jiang J, Czader MB, O'Malley DP, Orazi A. The stromal composition of myelofibrosis: differences between chronic myeloproliferative disorders and metastatic malignancies [abstract]. *Mod Pathol* 2003;16:232A.

Feiner HD, Rizk CC, Finfer MD, et al. IgM monoclonal gammopathy/Waldenström's macroglobulinemia: a morphological and immunophenotypic study of the bone marrow. *Mod Pathol* 1990;3(3):348-56.

Feldman AL, Arber DA, Pittaluga S, et al. Clonally related follicular lymphomas and histiocytic/dendritic cell sarcomas: evidence for transdifferentiation of the follicular lymphoma clone [published online ahead of print February 13, 2008]. *Blood*

Fernández-Luna JL. Apoptosis and polycythemia vera [review]. *Curr Opin Hematol* 1999;6(2):94-9.

Feyler S, O'Connor SJ, Rawstron AC, et al. IgM myeloma: a rare entity characterized by a CD20-CD56-CD117- immunophenotype and the t(11;14). *Br J Haematol* 2008;140(5):547-51.

Fitzsimmons D, Hodsdon W, Wheat W, Maira SM, Wasylyk B, Hagman J. Pax-5 (BSAP) recruits Ets proto-oncogene family proteins to form functional ternary complexes on a B-cell-specific promoter. *Genes Dev* 1996;10(17):2198-211.

Folpe AL, Chand EM, Goldblum JR, Weiss SW. Expression of Fli-1, a nuclear transcription factor, distinguishes vascular neoplasms from potential mimics. *Am J Surg Pathol* 2001;25(8):1061-6.

Folpe AL, Hill CE, Parham DM, O'Shea PA, Weiss SW. Immunohistochemical detection of FLI-1 protein expression: a study of 132 round cell tumors with emphasis on CD99-positive mimics of Ewing's sarcoma/primitive neuroectodermal tumor. *Am J Surg Pathol* 2000;24(12):1657-62.

Forni M, Meyer PR, Levy NB, Lukes RJ, Taylor CR. An immunohistochemical study of hemoglobin A, hemoglobin F, muramidase, and transferrin in erythroid hyperplasia and neoplasia. *Am J Clin Pathol* 1983;80(2):145-51.

Froelich CJ, Dixit VM, Yang X. Lymphocyte granule-mediated apoptosis: matters of viral mimicry and deadly proteases [review]. *Immunol Today* 1998 Jan;19(1):30-6.

Funk PE, Stephan RP, Witte PL. Vascular cell adhesion molecule 1-positive reticular cells express interleukin-7 and stem cell factor in the bone marrow. *Blood* 1995;86(7):2661-71.

Gala JL, Vermylen C, Cornu G, et al. High expression of bcl-2 is the rule in acute lymphoblastic leukemia, except in Burkitt subtype at presentation, and is not correlated with the prognosis. *Ann Hematol* 1994;69(1):17-24.

Gerdes J, Schwab U, Lemke H, Stein H. Production of a mouse monoclonal antibody reactive with a human nuclear antigen associated with cell proliferation. *Int J Cancer* 1983;31(1):13-20.

Gibson SE, Dong HY, Advani AS, Hsi ED. Expression of the B-cell-associated transcription factors PAX5, OCT-2, and BOB.1 in acute myeloid leukemia: associations with B-cell antigen expression and myelomonocytic maturation. *Am J Clin Pathol* 2006;126(6):916-24.

Hagman J, Wheat W, Fitzsimmons D, Hodsdon W, Negri J, Dizon F. Pax-5/BSAP: regulator of specific gene expression and differentiation in B lymphocytes [review]. *Curr Top Microbiol Immunol* 2000;245(1):169-94.

Hans CP, Weisenburger DD, Greiner TC, et al. Confirmation of the molecular classification of diffuse large B-cell lymphoma by immunohistochemistry using a tissue microarray. *Blood* 2004;103(1):275-82.

Harashima A, Matsuo Y, Drexler HG, et al. Transcription factor expression in B-cell precursor-leukemia cell lines: preferential expression of T-bet. *Leuk Res* 2005;29(7):841-8.

Hart A, Melet F, Grossfeld P, et al. Fli-1 is required for murine vascular and megakaryocytic development and is hemizygously deleted in patients with thrombocytopenia. *Immunity* 2000;13(2):167-77.

Hartmann K, Artuc M, Baldus SE, et al. Expression of Bcl-2 and Bcl-xL in cutaneous and BM lesions of mastocytosis. *Am J Pathol* 2003;163(3):819-26.

Hartung L, Bahler DW. Flow cytometric analysis of BCL-2 can distinguish small numbers of acute lymphoblastic leukaemia cells from B-cell precursors. *Br J Haematol* 2004;127(1):50-8.

Hayman AR, Macary P, Lehner PJ, Cox TM. Tartrate-resistant acid phosphatase (Acp 5): identification in diverse human tissues and dendritic cells. *J Histochem Cytochem* 2001;49(6):675-84.

Heintel D, Zojer N, Schreder M, et al. Expression of MUM1/IRF4 mRNA as a prognostic marker in patients with multiple myeloma [published online ahead of print August 9, 2007]. *Leukemia* 2008;22(2):441-5

Herling M, Jones D. CD4+/CD56+ hematodermic tumor: the features of an evolving entity and its relationship to dendritic cells [review]. *Am J Clin Pathol* 2007 May;127(5):687-700.

Hirt A, Werren EM, Luethy AR, Gerdes J, Wagner HP. Cell cycle analysis in lymphoid neoplasia of childhood: differences among immunologic subtypes and similarities in the proliferation of normal and leukaemic precursor B-cells. *Br J Haematol* 1992;80(2):189-93.

Horny HP, Sotlar K, Valent P. Mastocytosis: state of the art [review]. *Pathobiology* 2007;74(2):121-32.

Horny HP, Sotlar K, Stellmacher F, et al. The tryptase positive compact round cell infiltrate of the BM (TROCI-BM): a novel histopathological finding requiring the application of lineage specific markers. *J Clin Pathol* 2006;59(3):298-302.

Horny HP, Sillaber C, Menke D, et al. Diagnostic value of immunostaining for tryptase in patients with mastocytosis. *Am J Surg Pathol* 1998;22(9):1132-40.

Hoyer JD, Li CY, Yam LT, Hanson CA, Kurtin PJ. Immunohistochemical demonstration of acid phosphatase isoenzyme 5 (tartrate-resistant) in paraffin sections of hairy cell leukemia and other hematologic disorders. *Am J Clin Pathol* 1997;108(3):308-15.

Hsu SM, Jaffe ES. Phenotypic expression of T lymphocytes in thymus and peripheral lymphoid tissues. *Am J Pathol* 1985;121(1):69-78.

Hutchison RE, Finch C, Kepner J, et al. Burkitt lymphoma is immunophenotypically different from Burkitt-like lymphoma in young persons. *Ann Oncol* 2000;11(suppl 1):35-8.

Hyjek E, Chadburn A, Liu YF, Cesarman E, Knowles DM. BCL-6 protein is expressed in precursor T-cell lymphoblastic lymphoma and in prenatal and postnatal thymus. *Blood* 2001;97(1):270-6.

Iida S, Rao PH, Butler M, Corradini P, et al. Deregulation of MUM1/IRF4 by chromosomal translocation in multiple myeloma. *Nat Genet* 1997;17(2):226-30.

Irani AM, Goldstein SM, Wintroub BU, Bradford T, Schwartz LB. Human mast cell carboxypeptidase: selective localization to MCTC cells. *J Immunol* 1991;147(1):247-53.

Irani AM, Schwartz LB. Mast cell heterogeneity [review]. *Clin Exp Allergy* 1989;19(2):143-55.

Ito M, Tsurusawa M, Kawai S, Fujimoto T. Expression of a proliferation associated-nuclear antigen defined by Ki-67 monoclonal antibody in childhood acute leukemia [in Japanese]. *Rinsho Ketsueki* 1995;36(8):713-9.

Ito M, Tsurusawa M, Zha Z, Kawai S, Takasaki Y, Fujimoto T. Cell proliferation in childhood acute leukemia: comparison of Ki-67 and proliferating cell nuclear antigen immunocytochemical and DNA flow cytometric analysis. *Cancer* 1992;69(8):2176-82.

Iwama A, Osawa M, Hirasawa R, et al. Reciprocal roles for CCAAT/enhancer binding protein (C/EBP) and PU.1 transcription factors in Langerhans cell commitment. *J Exp Med* 2002;195(5):547-58.

Iwasaki T, Murakami M, Sugisaki C, et al. Characterization of myelodysplastic syndrome and aplastic anemia by immunostaining of p53 and hemoglobin F and karyotype analysis: differential diagnosis between refractory anemia and aplastic anemia. *Pathol Int* 2008;58(6):353-60.

Jaffe EA, Hoyer LW, Nachman RL. Synthesis of von Willebrand factor by cultured human endothelial cells. *Proc Natl Acad Sci U S A* 1974;71(5):1906-9.

Janeway CA, Travers P, Walport M, Shlomchik M. The development of mature lymphocyte receptor repertoires. In: *Immunobiology: The Immune System in Health and Disease* 5th ed. New York and London: Garland Science; 2001;pt III. Available at: http://www.ncbi.nlm.nih.gov/books/bv.fcgi?rid=imm.TOC&depth=2. Accessed April 20, 2008.

Jordan JH, Walchshofer S, Jurecka W, et al. Immunohistochemical properties of bone marrow mast cells in systemic mastocytosis: evidence for expression of CD2, CD117/Kit, and bcl-x(L). *Hum Pathol* 2001;32(5):545-52.

Khalil F, Cualing H, Cogburn J, Miles L. The criteria for bone marrow recovery post-myelosuppressive therapy for acute myelogenous leukemia: a quantitative study. *Arch Pathol Lab Med* 2007;131(8):1281-9.

Kim HS, Hausman GJ, Hausman DB, Martin RJ, Dean RG. The expression of cyclin D1 during adipogenesis in pig primary stromal-vascular cultures. *Obes Res* 2001;9(9):572-8.

Kinner B, Spector M. Expression of smooth muscle actin in osteoblasts in human bone. *J Orthop Res* 2002;20(3):622-32.

Kinney MC, Jones D. Cutaneous T-cell and NK-cell lymphomas: the WHO-EORTC classification and the increasing recognition of specialized tumor types [review]. *Am J Clin Pathol* 2007;127(5):670-86.

Knapp W, Strobl H, Majdic O. Flow cytometric analysis of cell-surface and intracellular antigens in leukemia diagnosis. *Cytometry* 1994;18(4):187-98.

Knowles DM. Immunodeficiency-associated lymphoproliferative disorders. *Mod Pathol* 1999;12(2):200-17.

Kozmik Z, Wang S, Dörfler P, Adams B, Busslinger M. The promoter of the CD19 gene is a target for the B-cell-specific transcription factor BSAP. *Mol Cell Biol* 1992;12(6):2662-72.

Kröber SM, Horny HP, Steinke B, Kaiserling E. Adult hypocellular acute leukaemia with lymphoid differentiation. *Leuk Lymphoma* 2003;44(10):1797-801.

References

Kumar S, Krenacs L, Medeiros J, et al. Subcutaneous panniculitic T-cell lymphoma is a tumor of cytotoxic T lymphocytes. *Hum Pathol* 1998;29(4):397-403.

Landau NR, St John TP, Weissman IL, Wolf SC, Silverstone AE, Baltimore D. Cloning of terminal transferase cDNA by antibody screening. *Proc Natl Acad Sci U S A* 1984;81(18):5836-40.

Lehtonen A, Veckman V, Nikula T, et al. Differential expression of IFN regulatory factor 4 gene in human monocyte-derived dendritic cells and macrophages. *J Immunol* 2005;175(10):6570-9.

Li WV, Kapadia SB, Sonmez-Alpan E, Swerdlow SH. Immunohistochemical characterization of mast cell disease in paraffin sections using tryptase, CD68, myeloperoxidase, lysozyme, and CD20 antibodies. *Mod Pathol* 1996;9(10):982-8.

Lisignoli G, Toneguzzi S, Monaco MC, Bertollini V, Facchini A. Immunohistochemical analysis of extracellular matrix components and cytoskeletal products of bone marrow stromal cells. *Boll Soc Ital Biol Sper* 1996;72(1-2):9-14.

Lisse I, Hasselbalch H, Junker P. Bone marrow stroma in idiopathic myelofibrosis and other haematological diseases: an immunohistochemical study. *APMIS* 1991;99(2):171-8.

Liu H, Wang J, Epner EM. Cyclin D1 activation in B-cell malignancy: association with changes in histone acetylation, DNA methylation, and RNA polymerase II binding to both promoter and distal sequences. *Blood* 2004;104(8):2505-13.

Liu CC, Walsh CM, Young JD. Perforin: structure and function [review]. *Immunol Today* 1995;16(4):194-201.

Llombart-Bosch A, Navarro S. Immunohistochemical detection of EWS and FLI-1 proteinss in Ewing sarcoma and primitive neuroectodermal tumors: comparative analysis with CD99 (MIC-2) expression. *Appl Immunohistochem Mol Morphol* 2001;9(3):255-60.

Loddenkemper C, Anagnostopoulos I, Hummel M, et al. Differential Emu enhancer activity and expression of BOB.1/OBF.1, Oct2, PU.1, and immunoglobulin in reactive B-cell populations, B-cell non-Hodgkin lymphomas, and Hodgkin lymphomas. *J Pathol* 2004;202(1):60-9.

Loyson SA, Rademakers LH, Joling P, Vroom TM, van den Tweel JG. Immunohistochemical analysis of decalcified paraffin-embedded human bone marrow biopsies with emphasis on MHC class I and CD34 expression. *Histopathology* 1997;31(5):412-9.

Mansoor A, Akbari M, Auer I, Lai R. Cyclin D1 and t(11;14)-positive B-cell neoplasms resembling marginal zone B-cell lymphoma: a morphological variant of mantle cell lymphoma [published online ahead of print February 20, 2007]. *Hum Pathol* 2007;38(5):797-802.

Marafioti T, Paterson JC, Ballabio E, et al. Novel markers of normal and neoplastic human plasmacytoid dendritic cells [published online ahead of print January 28, 2008]. *Blood* 2008;111(7):3778-92.

Marafioti T, Mancini C, Ascani S, et al. Leukocyte-specific phosphoprotein-1 and PU.1: two useful markers for distinguishing T-cell-rich B-cell lymphoma from lymphocyte-predominant Hodgkin's disease. *Haematologica* 2004;89(8):957-64.

Marks SC Jr, Grolman ML. Tartrate-resistant acid phosphatase in mononuclear and multinuclear cells during the bone resorption of tooth eruption. *J Histochem Cytochem* 1987;35(11):1227-30.

McClure RF, Remstein ED, Macon WR, et al. Adult B-cell lymphomas with Burkitt-like morphology are phenotypically and genotypically heterogeneous with aggressive clinical behavior. *Am J Surg Pathol* 2005;29(12):1652-60.

McKenna RW, Washington LT, Aquino DB, Picker LJ, Kroft SH. Immunophenotypic analysis of hematogones (B-lymphocyte precursors) in 662 consecutive bone marrow specimens by 4-color flow cytometry. *Blood* 2001;98(8):2498-507.

Mhawech-Fauceglia P, Herrmann FR, et al. Friend leukaemia integration-1 expression in malignant and benign tumours: a multiple tumour tissue microarray analysis using polyclonal antibody. *J Clin Pathol* 2007;60(6):694-700.

Miranda RN, Briggs RC, Kinney MC, Veno PA, Hammer RD, Cousar JB. Immunohistochemical detection of cyclin D1 using optimized conditions is highly specific for mantle cell lymphoma and hairy cell leukemia. *Mod Pathol* 2000;13(12):1308-14.

Morice WG, Kurtin PJ, Tefferi A, Hanson CA. Distinct BM findings in T-cell granular lymphocytic leukemia revealed by paraffin section immunoperoxidase stains for CD8, TIA-1, and granzyme B. *Blood* 2002;99(1):268-74.

Muehleck SD, McKenna RW, Gale PF, Brunning RD. Terminal deoxynucleotidyl transferase (TdT)-positive cells in bone marrow in the absence of hematologic malignancy. *Am J Clin Pathol* 1983;79(3):277-84.

Mueller BU, Pabst T, Fos J, et al. ATRA resolves the differentiation block in t(15;17) acute myeloid leukemia by restoring PU.1 expression. *Blood* 2006;107(8):3330-8.

Mullighan CG, Goorha S, Radtke I, et al. Genome-wide analysis of genetic alterations in acute lymphoblastic leukaemia. *Nature* 2007;446(7137):758-64.

Nachman R, Levine R, Jaffe EA. Synthesis of factor VIII antigen by cultured guinea pig megakaryocytes. *J Clin Invest* 1977;60(4):914-21.

Nagata D, Suzuki E, Nishimatsu H, et al. Transcriptional activation of the cyclin D1 gene is mediated by multiple cis-elements, including SP1 sites and a cAMP-responsive element in vascular endothelial cells. *J Biol Chem* 2001;276(1):662-9.

Naresh KN. MUM1 expression dichotomises follicular lymphoma into predominantly, MUM1-negative low-grade and MUM1-positive high-grade subtypes. *Haematologica* 2007;92(2):267-8.

Nilsson SK, Debatis ME, Dooner MS, Madri JA, Quesenberry PJ, Becker PS. Immunofluorescence characterization of key extracellular matrix proteins in murine bone marrow in situ. *J Histochem Cytochem* 1998;46(3):371-7.

Nomura Y, Karube K, Suzuki R, et al. High-grade mature B-cell lymphoma with Burkitt-like morphology: results of a clinicopathological study of 72 Japanese patients. *Cancer Sci* 2008;99(2):246-52.

Nowicki M, Miśkowiak B, Kaczmarek-Kanold M. Correlation between early treatment failure and Ki67 antigen expression in blast cells of children with acute lymphoblastic leukaemia before commencing treatment: a retrospective study. *Oncology* 2002;62(1):55-9.

O'Malley DP, Sen J, Juliar BE, Orazi A. Evaluation of stroma in human immunodeficiency virus/acquired immunodeficiency syndrome-affected bone marrows and correlation with CD4 counts. *Arch Pathol Lab Med* 2005;129(9):1137-40.

Orazi A, Chiu R, O'Malley DP, Czader M, Allen SL, An C, Vance GH. Chronic myelomonocytic leukemia: the role of bone marrow biopsy immunohistology [published online ahead of print October 13, 2006]. *Mod Pathol* 2006;19(12):1536-45.

Orazi A, Cattoretti G, John K, Neiman RS. Terminal deoxynucleotidyl transferase staining of malignant lymphomas in paraffin sections. *Mod Pathol* 1994;7(5):582-6.

Pangalis GA, Kyrtsonis MC, Kontopidou FN, et al. Differential diagnosis of Waldenstrom's macroglobulinemia and other B-cell disorders. *Clin Lymphoma* 2005;5(4):235-40.

Papadopoulos N, Simopoulos C, Kotini A, Lambropoulou M, Tolparidou I, Tamiolakis D. Differential expression of α-smooth muscle actin molecule in a subset of bone marrow stromal cells, in B-cell chronic lymphocytic leukemia, autoimmune disorders and normal fetuses. *Eur J Gynaecol Oncol* 2001;22(6):447-50.

Pellegrini W, Facchetti F, Marocolo D, et al. Assessment of cell proliferation in normal and pathological bone marrow biopsies: a study using double sequential immunophenotyping on paraffin sections. *Histopathology* 1995;27(5):397-405.

Pereira R, Quang CT, Lesault I, Dolznig H, Beug H, Ghysdael J. FLI-1 inhibits differentiation and induces proliferation of primary erythroblasts. *Oncogene* 1999;18(8):1597-608.

Peterson LC, Brown BA, Crosson JT, Mladenovic J. Application of the immunoperoxidase technique to bone marrow trephine biopsies in the classification of patients with monoclonal gammopathies. *Am J Clin Pathol* 1986;85(6):688-93.

Pileri SA, Zinzani PL, Gaidano G, et al; International Extranodal Lymphoma Study Group. Pathobiology of primary mediastinal B-cell lymphoma [review]. *Leuk Lymphoma* 2003a;44(suppl 3):S21-6.

Pileri SA, Gaidano G, Zinzani PL, et al. Primary mediastinal B-cell lymphoma: high frequency of BCL-6 mutations and consistent expression of the transcription factors OCT-2, BOB.1, and PU.1 in the absence of immunoglobulins. *Am J Pathol* 2003b;162(1):243-53.

Pinkus GS, Said JW. Intracellular hemoglobin-a specific marker for erythroid cells in paraffin sections: an immunoperoxidase study of normal, megaloblastic, and dysplastic erythropoiesis, including erythroleukemia and other myeloproliferative disorders. *Am J Pathol* 1981;102(3):308-13.

Polli M, Dakic A, Light A, Wu L, Tarlinton DM, Nutt SL. The development of functional B lymphocytes in conditional PU.1 knock-out mice. *Blood* 2005;106(6):2083-90.

Porwit-MacDonald A, Ivory K, Wilkinson S, Wheatley K, Wong L, Janossy G. Bcl-2 protein expression in normal human bone marrow precursors and in acute myelogenous leukemia. *Leukemia* 1995;9(7):1191-8.

Prasad DD, Rao VN, Reddy ES. Structure and expression of human Fli-1 gene. *Cancer Res* 1992;52(20):5833-7.

Preud'Homme JL, Hurez D, Danon F, Brouet JC, Seligmann M. Intracytoplasmic and surface-bound immunoglobulins in "nonsecretory" and Bence-Jones myeloma. *Clin Exp Immunol* 1976;25(3):428-36.

Pryzwansky KB, Martin LE, Spitznagel JK. Immunocytochemical localization of myeloperoxidase, lactoferrin, lysozyme and neutral proteases in human monocytes and neutrophilic granulocytes. *J Reticuloendothel Soc* 1978;24(3):295-310.

Pryzwansky KB, Martin LE, Spitznagel JK. Immunocytochemical localization of myeloperoxidase, lactoferrin, lysozyme and neutral proteases in human monocytes and neutrophilic granulocytes. *J Reticuloendothel Soc* 1978;24(3):295-310.

Pusztaszeri MP, Seelentag W, Bosman FT. Immunohistochemical expression of endothelial markers CD31, CD34, von Willebrand factor, and Fli-1 in normal human tissues. *J Histochem Cytochem* 2006;54(4):385-95.

Quick CM, Smoller BR, Hiatt KM. Fli-1 expression in mycosis fungoides. *J Cutan Pathol* 2006;33(9):642-5.

Reuss-Borst MA, Ning Y, Klein G, Müller CA. The vascular cell adhesion molecule (VCAM-1) is expressed on a subset of lymphoid and myeloid leukaemias. *Br J Haematol* 1995;89(2):299-305.

Riccioni R, Galimberti S, Petrini M. Hairy cell leukemia [review]. *Curr Treat Options Oncol* 2007;8(2):129-34.

Riggi N, Stamenkovic I. The biology of Ewing sarcoma [review]. *Cancer Lett* 2007;254(1):1-10.

Rimsza LM, Viswanatha DS, Winter SS, Leith CP, Frost JD, Foucar K. The presence of CD34+ cell clusters predicts impending relapse in children with acute lymphoblastic leukemia receiving maintenance chemotherapy. *Am J Clin Pathol* 1998;110(3):313-20.

Ruck P, Horny HP, Greschniok A, Wehrmann M, Kaiserling E. Nonspecific immunostaining of blast cells of acute leukemia by antibodies against nonhemopoietic antigens. *Hematol Pathol* 1995;9(1):49-56.

Rüdiger T, Ott G, Ott MM, Müller-Deubert SM, Müller-Hermelink HK. Differential diagnosis between classical Hodgkin's lymphoma, T-cell-rich B-cell lymphoma, and paragranuloma by paraffin immunohistochemistry [review]. *Am J Surg Pathol* 1998;22(10):1184-91.

Sadler JE. Biochemistry and genetics of von Willebrand factor [review]. *Annu Rev Biochem* 1998;67:395-424.

References

Samorapoompichit P, Kiener HP, Schernthaner GH, et al. Detection of tryptase in cytoplasmic granules of basophils in patients with chronic myeloid leukemia and other myeloid neoplasms. *Blood* 2001;98(8):2580-3.

Schlimok G, Funke I, Bock B, Schweiberer B, Witte J, Riethmüller G. Epithelial tumor cells in bone marrow of patients with colorectal cancer: immunocytochemical detection, phenotypic characterization, and prognostic significance. *J Clin Oncol* 1990;8(5):831-7.

Schlüter C, Duchrow M, Wohlenberg C, et al. The cell proliferation-associated antigen of antibody Ki-67: a very large, ubiquitous nuclear protein with numerous repeated elements, representing a new kind of cell cycle-maintaining proteins. *J Cell Biol* 1993;123(3):513-22.

Schotte R, Nagasawa M, Weijer K, Spits H, Blom B. The ETS transcription factor Spi-B is required for human plasmacytoid dendritic cell development. *J Exp Med* 2004;200(11):1503-9.

Scott EW, Simon MC, Anastasi J, Singh H. Requirement of transcription factor PU.1 in the development of multiple hematopoietic lineages. *Science* 1994;265(5178):1573-7.

Sen F, Lai R, Albitar M. Chronic lymphocytic leukemia with t(14;18) and trisomy 12. *Arch Pathol Lab Med* 2002;126(12):1543-6.

Sening W, Lisner R, Niedobitek G. Rare detection of phenotypically immature lymphocytes in Hashimoto thyroiditis and rheumatoid arthritis. *J Autoimmun* 2004;22(2):147-52.

Shikami M, Miwa H, Nishii K, et al. Low BCL-2 expression in acute leukemia with t(8;21) chromosomal abnormality. *Leukemia* 1999;13(3):358-68.

Simonitsch-Klupp I, Hauser I, Ott G, et al. Diffuse large B-cell lymphomas with plasmablastic/plasmacytoid features are associated with TP53 deletions and poor clinical outcome. *Leukemia* 2004;18(1):146-55.

Skinnider BF, Horsman DE, Dupuis B, Gascoyne RD. Bcl-6 and Bcl-2 protein expression in diffuse large B-cell lymphoma and follicular lymphoma: correlation with 3q27 and 18q21 chromosomal abnormalities. *Hum Pathol* 1999;30(7):803-8.

Smith RG, Kitchens RL. Phenotypic heterogeneity of TDT+ cells in the blood and BM: implications for surveillance of residual leukemia. *Blood* 1989;74(1):312-9.

Smyth MJ, Trapani JA. Granzymes: exogenous proteinases that induce targeT-cell apoptosis [review]. *Immunol Today* 1995;16(4):202-6.

Sperr WR, Jordan JH, Baghestanian M, et al. Expression of mast cell tryptase by myeloblasts in a group of patients with acute myeloid leukemia. *Blood* 2001;98(7):2200-9.

Spina D, Leoncini L, Megha T, et al. Cellular kinetic and phenotypic heterogeneity in and among Burkitt's and Burkitt-like lymphomas. *J Pathol* 1997;182(2):145-50.

Sporn LA, Marder VJ, Wagner DD. Inducible secretion of large, biologically potent von Willebrand factor multimers. *Cell* 1986;46(2):185-90.

Stavem P, Froland SS, Haugen HF, Lislerud A. Nonsecretory myelomatosis without intracellular immunoglobulin. Immunofluorescent and ultramicroscopic studies. *Scand J Haematol* 1976;17(2):89-95.

Strauchen JA, Miller LK. Lymphoid progenitor cells in human tonsils. *Int J Surg Pathol* 2003;11(1):21-4.

Strauchen JA, Miller LK. Terminal deoxynucleotidyl transferase-positive cells in human tonsils. *Am J Clin Pathol* 2001;116(1):12-6.

Sur M, AlArdati H, Ross C, Alowami S. TdT expression in Merkel cell carcinoma: potential diagnostic pitfall with blastic hematological malignancies and expanded immunohistochemical analysis. *Mod Pathol* 2007;20(11):1113-20.

Teruya-Feldstein J. Diffuse large B-cell lymphomas with plasmablastic differentiation. *Curr Oncol Rep* 2005;7(5):357-63.

Thaler J, Denz H, Gattringer C, et al. Diagnostic and prognostic value of immunohistological bone marrow examination: results in 212 patients with lymphoproliferative disorders. *Blut* 1987;54(4):213-22.

Thiele J, Kvasnicka HM. Myelofibrosis in chronic myeloproliferative disorders: dynamics and clinical impact [review]. *Histol Histopathol* 2006 Dec;21(12):1367-78.

Thiele J, Fischer R. Bone marrow tissue and proliferation markers: results and general problems. *Virchows Arch A Pathol Anat Histopathol* 1993;423(6):409-16.

Tiacci E, Pileri S, Orleth A, et al. PAX5 expression in acute leukemias: higher B-lineage specificity than CD79a and selective association with t(8;21)-acute myelogenous leukemia. *Cancer Res* 2004;64:7399-7404.

Toney LM, Cattoretti G, Graf JA, et al. BCL-6 regulates chemokine gene transcription in macrophages. *Nat Immunol* 2000;1(3):214-20.

Torlakovic E, Bilalovic N, Golouh R, Zidar A, Angel S. Prognostic significance of PU.1 in follicular lymphoma. *J Pathol* 2006a;209(3):352-9.

Torlakovic E, Slipicevic A, Florenes V, Chibbar R, Bilalovic N. Fli-1 expression in malignant melanoma. *Mod Pathol* 2006b;19(suppl 1):88A.

Torlakovic E, Tenstad E, Funderud S, Rian E. CD10+ stromal cells form B-lymphocyte maturation niches in the human bone marrow. *J Pathol* 2005a;205(3):311-7.

Torlakovic E, Nielsen S, Vyberg M. Antibody selection in immunohistochemical detection of cyclin D1 in mantle cell lymphoma. *Am J Clin Pathol* 2005b;124(5):782-9.

Torlakovic E, Torlakovic G, Nguyen PL, Brunning RD, Delabie J. The value of anti-Pax-5 immunostaining in routinely fixed and paraffin-embedded sections: a novel pan pre-B and B-cell marker. *Am J Surg Pathol* 2002;26(10):1343-50.

Torlakovic E, Tierens A, Dang HD, Delabie J. The transcription factor PU.1, necessary for B-cell development is expressed in lymphocyte predominance, but not classical Hodgkin's disease. *Am J Pathol* 2001;159(5):1807-14.

Troussard X, Avet-Loiseau H, Macro M, et al. Cyclin D1 expression in patients with multiple myeloma. *Hematol J* 2000;1(3):181-5.

Truong AH, Ben-David Y. The role of Fli-1 in normal cell function and malignant transformation [review]. *Oncogene* 2000;19(55):6482-9.

Tsuboi K, Iida S, Inagaki H, et al. MUM1/IRF4 expression as a frequent event in mature lymphoid malignancies. *Leukemia* 2000;14(3):449-56.

Tsujimoto Y, Cossman J, Jaffe E, Croce CM. Involvement of the bcl-2 gene in human follicular lymphoma. *Science* 1985;228(4706):1440-3.

Tsujimoto Y, Finger LR, Yunis J, Nowell PC, Croce CM. Cloning of the chromosome breakpoint of neoplastic B-cells with the t(14;18) chromosome translocation. *Science* 1984;226(4678):1097-9.

Ulyanova T, Priestley GV, Nakamoto B, Jiang Y, Papayannopoulou T. VCAM-1 ablation in nonhematopoietic cells in MxCre+ VCAM-1f/f mice is variable and dictates their phenotype. *Exp Hematol* 2007;35(4):565-71.

Vago JF, Hurtubise PE, Redden-Borowski MM, Martelo OJ, Swerdlow SH. Follicular center-cell lymphoma with plasmacytic differentiation, monoclonal paraprotein, and peripheral blood involvement. Recapitulation of normal B-cell development. *Am J Surg Pathol* 1985;9(10):764-70.

Valbuena JR, Medeiros LJ, Rassidakis GZ, et al. Expression of B-cell-specific activator protein/PAX5 in acute myeloid leukemia with t(8;21) (q22;q22). *Am J Clin Pathol* 2006;126(2):235-40.

Valent P, Horny H-P, Li CY, et al. Mastocytosis. In: Jaffe ES, Harris NL, Stein H, Vardiman JW, eds. *WHO Classification of Tumours: Tumours of Haematopoietic and lymphid tissues—Pathology and Genetics* Lyon, France: IARC Press; 2001:291-300.

Vasef MA, Medeiros LJ, Koo C, McCourty A, Brynes RK. Cyclin D1 immunohistochemical staining is useful in distinguishing mantle cell lymphoma from other low-grade B-cell neoplasms in BM. *Am J Clin Pathol* 1997;108(3):302-7.

Vega F, Chang CC, Medeiros LJ, et al. Plasmablastic lymphomas and plasmablastic plasma cell myelomas have nearly identical immunophenotypic profiles. *Mod Pathol* 2005;18(6):806-15.

Vermeer MH, Geelen FA, Kummer JA, Meijer CJ, Willemze R. Expression of cytotoxic proteins by neoplastic T cells in mycosis fungoides increases with progression from plaque stage to tumor stage disease. *Am J Pathol* 1999;154(4):1203-10.

Viswanatha DS, Foucar K, Berry BR, Gascoyne RD, Evans HL, Leith CP. Blastic mantle cell leukemia: an unusual presentation of blastic mantle cell lymphoma. *Mod Pathol* 2000;13(7):825-33.

Wagner DD, Olmsted JB, Marder VJ. Immunolocalization of von Willebrand protein in Weibel-Palade bodies of human endothelial cells. *J Cell Biol* 1982;95(1):355-60.

Walsh JC, DeKoter RP, Lee HJ, et al. Cooperative and antagonistic interplay between PU.1 and GATA-2 in the specification of myeloid cell fates. *Immunity* 2002;17(5):665-76.

Went PT, Zimpfer A, Pehrs AC, et al. High specificity of combined TRAP and DBA.44 expression for hairy cell leukemia. *Am J Surg Pathol* 2005;29(4):474-8.

West RB, Warnke RA, Natkunam Y. The usefulness of immunohistochemistry in the diagnosis of follicular lymphoma in BM biopsy specimens [published correction appears in *Am J Clin Pathol* 2002;118(1):145]. *Am J Clin Pathol* 2002;117(4):636-43.

White DM, Smith AG, Smith JL. Assessment of proliferative activity in leukaemic bone marrow using the monoclonal antibody Ki-67. *J Clin Pathol* 1994;47(3):209-13.

Wong KF. Transformed follicular lymphoma with concurrent t(2;3), t(8;14) and t(14;18). *Cancer Genet Cytogenet* 2007;173(1):68-70.

Wong KF, So CC, Chan JC, Kho BC, Chan JK. Gain of chromosome 3/3q in B-cell chronic lymphoproliferative disorder is associated with plasmacytoid differentiation with or without IgM overproduction. *Cancer Genet Cytogenet* 2002;136(1):82-5.

Xu W, Li JY, Wu YJ, Sheng RL, Lu FX. Expression of Ki-67 and Bcl-2 in adults and children with acute lymphoblastic leukemia and its clinical significance [in Chinese]. *Zhongguo Shi Yan Xue Ye Xue Za Zhi* 2006;14(5):887-90.

Yamada M, Asanuma K, Kobayashi D, et al. Quantitation of multiple myeloma oncogene 1/interferon-regulatory factor 4 gene expression in malignant B-cell proliferations and normal leukocytes. *Anticancer Res* 2001;21(1B):633-8.

Yamochi T, Kitabayashi A, Hirokawa M, et al. Regulation of BCL-6 gene expression in human myeloid/monocytoid leukemic cells. *Leukemia* 1997;11(5):694-700.

Yang F, Tran TA, Carlson JA, Hsi ED, Ross CW, Arber DA. Paraffin section immunophenotype of cutaneous and extracutaneous mast cell disease: comparison to other hematopoietic neoplasms. *Am J Surg Pathol* 2000;24(5):703-9.

Yatabe Y, Suzuki R, Matsuno Y, et al. Morphological spectrum of cyclin D1-positive mantle cell lymphoma: study of 168 cases. *Pathol Int* 2001;51(10):747-61.

Yu RY, Wang X, Pixley FJ, et al. BCL-6 negatively regulates macrophage proliferation by suppressing autocrine IL-6 production. *Blood* 2005;105(4):1777-84.

Chapter 5
SPECIAL DIAGNOSTIC CONSIDERATIONS

5.1 Acute Leukemia

The laboratory approach to acute leukemia should conform to the clinical need for prompt recognition and initiation of appropriate therapy. Therefore, this is a state of medical emergency which requires a separate discussion on the most appropriate use of immunohistochemistry (IHC) methods in evaluating a bone marrow (BM) biopsy to diagnose acute leukemia.

There are 4 different clinical settings in which the need for IHC analysis may be considered:

1. clinically overt acute leukemia with a well-sampled BM aspirate that is available for ancillary studies;
2. clinically overt acute leukemia and BM aspirate that is not available or is technically suboptimal and not suitable for all ancillary studies;
3. acute leukemia slowly evolving from a myelodysplastic syndrome; and
4. the need for nucleophosmin (NPM1) or CXC chemokine receptor 4 (CXCR4) immunostaining (or other emerging prognostic IHC markers [Falini 2007; Konoplev 2008]) in acute myelogenous leukemia (AML).

In the evaluation of an overt acute leukemia, the tissue samples are evaluated with morphologic studies, immunophenotyping by flow cytometry, and cytogenetics and/or molecular methods to integrate the laboratory results and clinical data and arrive at a specific diagnosis. Although a BM aspirate clot and/or core biopsy specimen are also available, there are no a priori clear indications for IHC testing in the BM biopsy. In some patients, particular morphologic observation may prompt for the IHC evaluation because of additional findings or discrepancy between morphologic findings and flow cytometric findings [Jaffe 2001]. Occasionally, characterization of bilineal and biphenotypic leukemias may benefit from additional IHC evaluation.

The BM core biopsy specimen is very useful and indispensable in the analysis of acute leukemia when a BM aspirate cannot be obtained because of BM fibrosis. It is also occasionally difficult to obtain a good aspirate from the BM in hypocellular acute leukemia. In some institutions, in particular in Europe, pathologists do not have access to the BM aspirate smears or flow cytometry specimens, and must make a specific diagnosis by evaluating only BM core biopsy specimens. Several markers may be needed for complete immunoprofiling and correct classification/subclassification of acute leukemia. Therefore, because of the clinical urgency to quickly diagnose and classify acute leukemia, a step-by-step approach is not recommended. Immunophenotyping of acute leukemia by IHC should be approached in a manner similar to that used in flow cytometry. However, the extent of the evaluation may vary from case to case. It will be determined by the hematopathologists in order to accumulate as much relevant information as possible. Myeloperoxidase (MPO) positivity that has been demonstrated with cytochemistry does not need to be evaluated with IHC. The clinical status of the patient may also determine the extent of the evaluation. It might be of little interest to find out whether acute myeloid leukemia, as morphologically diagnosed in the BM aspirate smears, also shows expression of Pax-5, TdT, or CD79a in an 89-year-old person who, for various reasons, was found not to be a candidate for aggressive chemotherapy or rejects any treatement. Several studies describe the work up of the paraffin-embedded BM biopsy specimen for acute leukemia [Pileri 1999; Toth 1999; Horny 1990; Horny 1994; Arber 1996; Kröber 2000; Islam 1985; Casasnovas 2003; Ngo 2008].

In contrast to overt acute leukemia, IHC analyses are very valuable in the evaluation of myelodysplastic syndrome, particularly in cases with increased blasts. IHC enables very accurate determination of the percentage of blasts cells when they are CD34+, which is very common, but not invariant. A 500-cell count using a cell counter and 1000X magnification (oil lens) establishes very accurate CD34+ blast percentage [Torlakovic 2002; Dunphy 2007]. Because of the large number of more mature cells, additional immunophenotyping of blasts may not be successful.

Nucleophosmin is a ubiquitously expressed nucleolar phosphoprotein. NPM1 mutations occur specifically in about 30% of adult de novo AML, and cause aberrant cytoplasmic expression of NPM (NPMc+ AML) [Falini 2006; Alcalay 2005]. The favorable impact of NPM1 mutations on overall survival and event-free survival has been reported in a large number of normal-karyotype AML cases. This positive effect was lost in the presence of a concomitant FLT3-LM. NPMc+ AML is associated with normal karyotype in about 50% of AML cases with normal karyotype, which usually have NPM gene exon 12 mutations [Boissel 2005; Falini 2006a]. The NPMc+ can be detected on IHC and unfixed specimens are not suitable for this type of analysis because of problems with antigen (Ag) localization, which is critical for the interpretation of the results [Falini 2006a]. NPMc+ AML with normal karyotype can be provisionally regarded as a separate AML with favorable prognosis [Falini 2006a; Falini 2007]. The cytoplasmic localization is the result of the NPM protein C-terminus modification secondary to mutations that create a new nuclear export signal motif [Falini 2006b; Bolli 2007]. IHC is the first choice of technique used in the diagnosis of NPMc+ AML in the case of dry-tap or biopsy specimens from extramedullary sites [Bolli 2006]. However, molecular analysis is the first choice of assay for monitoring minimal residual disease [Gorello 2006].

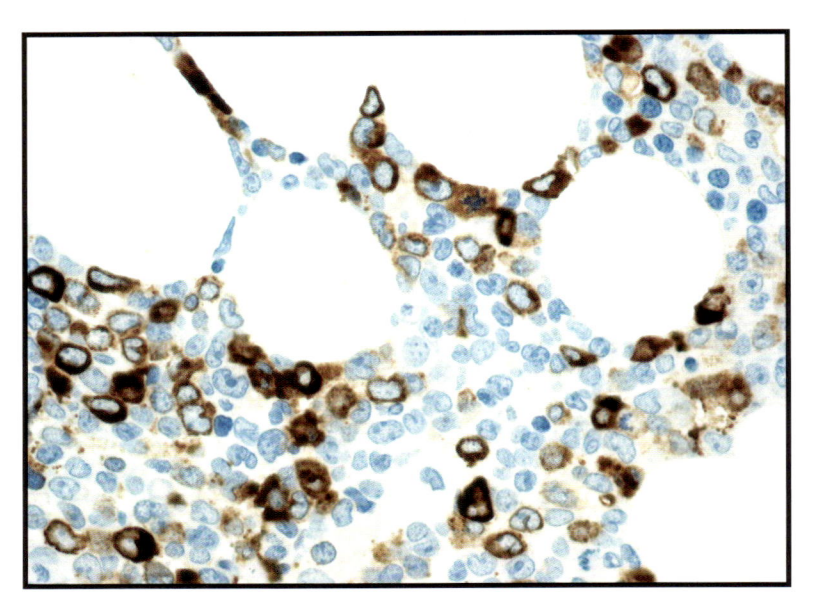

F5.1.1 Myeloperoxidase (MPO) in acute myelomonocytic leukemia

This BM biopsy specimen is from an 84-year old woman with acute myelomonocytic leukemia. Most of the cells in the BM are blasts. While MPO is widely expressed in acute myelogenous leukemia (AML), it varies from case to case in its distribution and intensity. In this type of acute leukemia, one typically finds only a subpopulation of cells strongly positive for MPO. Cells with monoblastic differentiation express less MPO and may be negative.

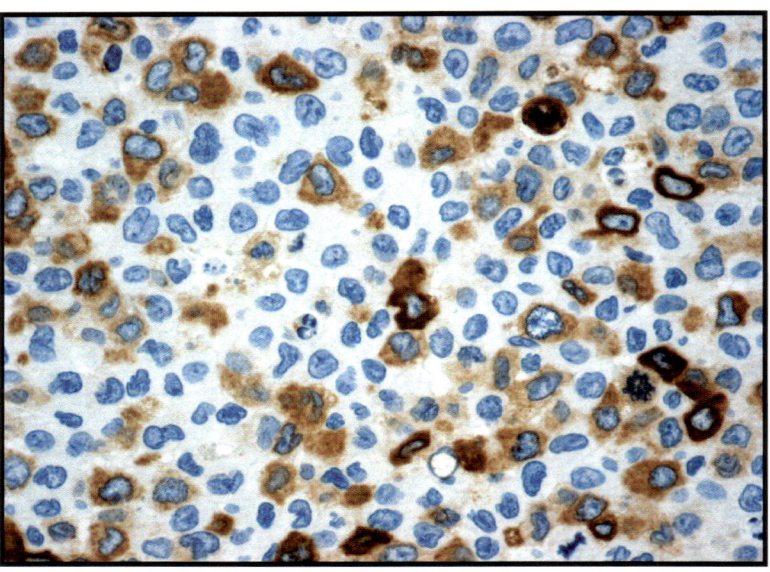

F5.1.2 Myeloperoxidase (MPO) in acute monocytic leukemia

Monocytic leukemias often show variable expression. In contrast, in acute monoblastic leukemia, the monoblasts are usually MPO-negative on immunohisochemistry and cytochemical stains. The opposite is true for the CD117 expression.

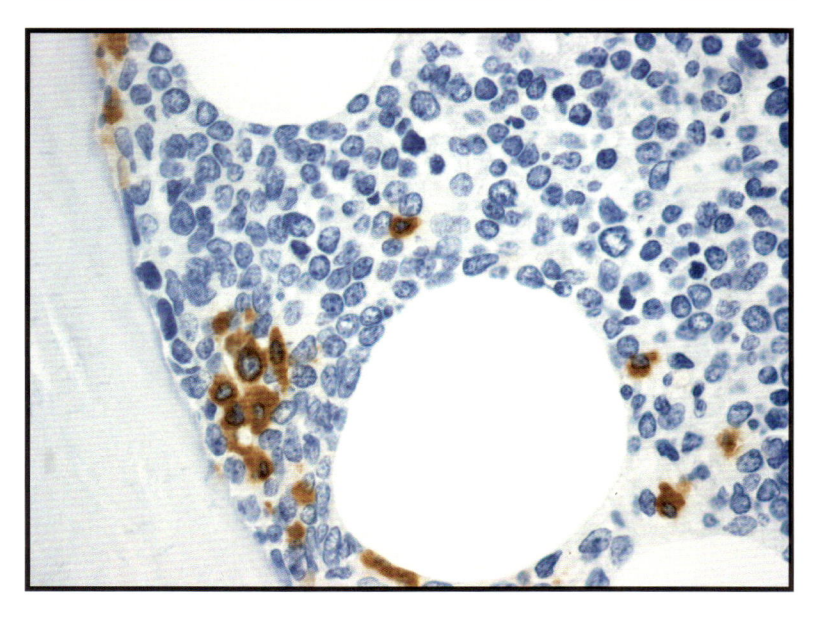

F5.1.3 Myeloperoxidase (MPO) in acute undifferentiated leukemia

In this acute leukemia, the leukemic blasts are negative for MPO on immunohistochemistry and flow cytometric analysis. Only rare MPO+ cells are found in the vicinity of the bone trabeculae. These cells represent small residual hematopoietic foci and should not be interpreted as evidence of myeloid differentiation of this leukemia. This is of particular importance in partial involvement of the bone marrow by leukemic cells, when large number of positive cells can be found.

F5.1.4 CD117 in acute myelogenous leukemia (AML)

Moderately strong expression of CD117 in AML blasts is shown, which is easily appreciated even on low power magnification. CD117 may be a useful marker even in bone marrow that is only partly involved by AML, because its expression is often higher in leukemic cells than in normal myeloid blasts. CD117 is often easily demonstrated in acute leukemia on immunohistochemistry, but the number of blasts may be underestimated because the expression can be quite variable from cell to cell.

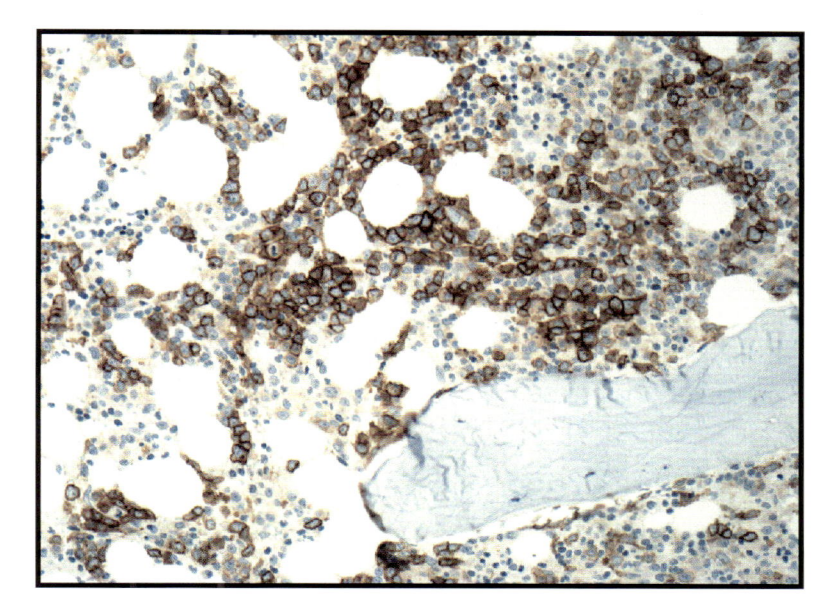

F5.1.5 CD117 in acute myelomonocytic leukemia

CD117 is an excellent marker of myeloid differentiation and its expression is not always proportional to myeloperoxidase (MPO) expression. In this case of acute myelomonocytic leukemia (same as F5.1.1), the expression of CD117 is higher that that of MPO and CD117 is expressed in all blasts. The level of expression is quite strong compared with its expression in normal myeloid blasts (see F3.32.1). Similar results would be expected for CD33 expression.

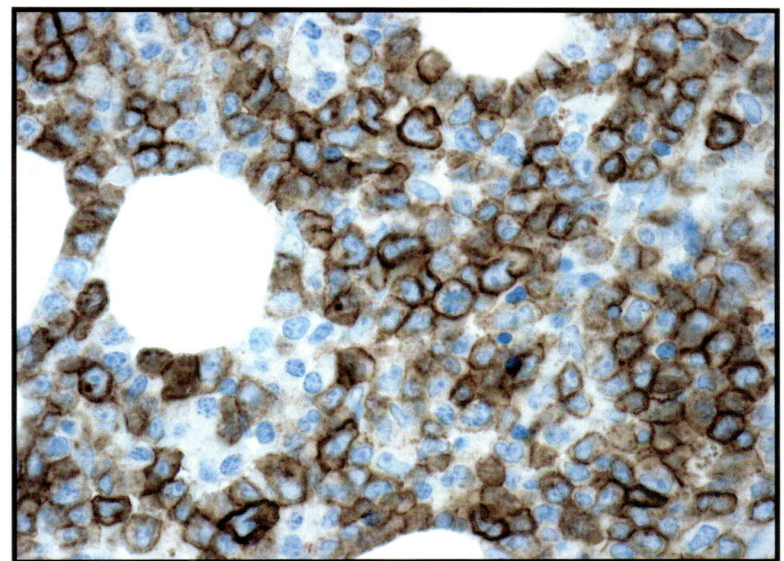

F5.1.6 Myeloid markers in acute myelomonocytic leukemia

In myelomonocytic leukemia, cells with monocytic differentiation may be closely intermixed with cells with neutrophil differentiation or they reside in their own areas as illustrated here. Both lysozyme (LZ) and KP-1 are expressed by the normal neutrophil population, but LZ+ and KP-1+ cells colocalize only with monocytic cells in this case and are not present in areas with MPO+ cells.

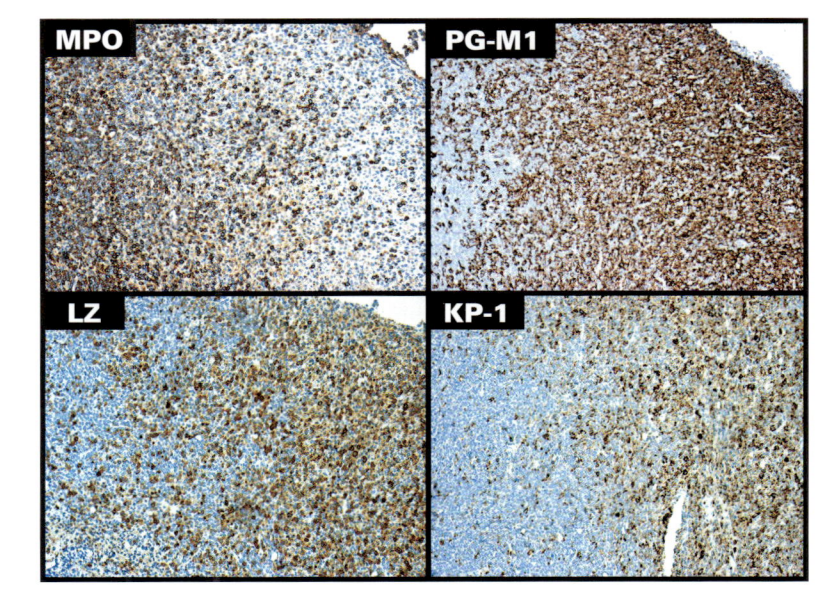

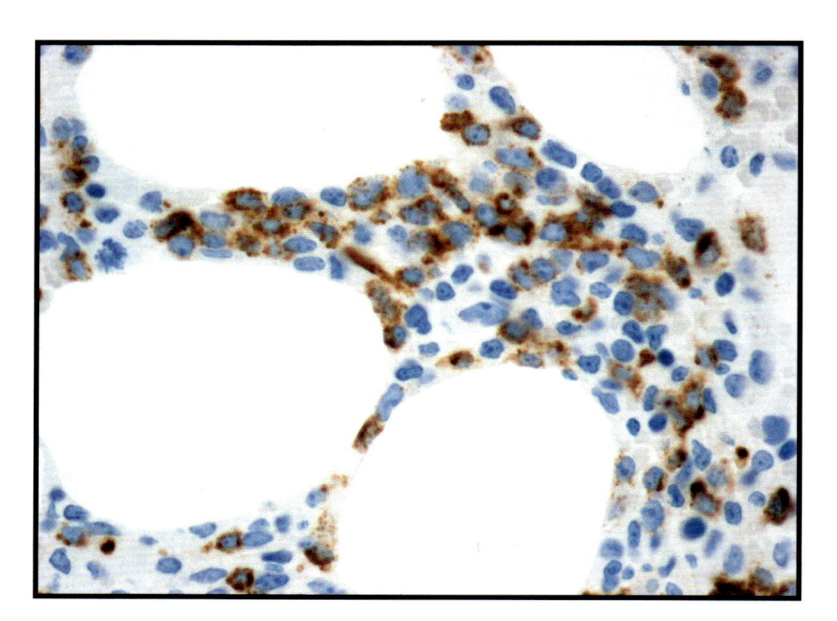

F5.1.7 CD34 in acute myeloid leukemia

This biopsy specimen shows about 70% blasts with CD34 expression, while flow cytometric analysis shows only 34% blasts to be positive. Because flow cytometric methods evaluate only surface expression of CD34, some discrepancy may be expected if the leukemic cells express predominantly cytoplasmic CD34 which is regularly detected on immunohistochemistry as illustrated in this case.

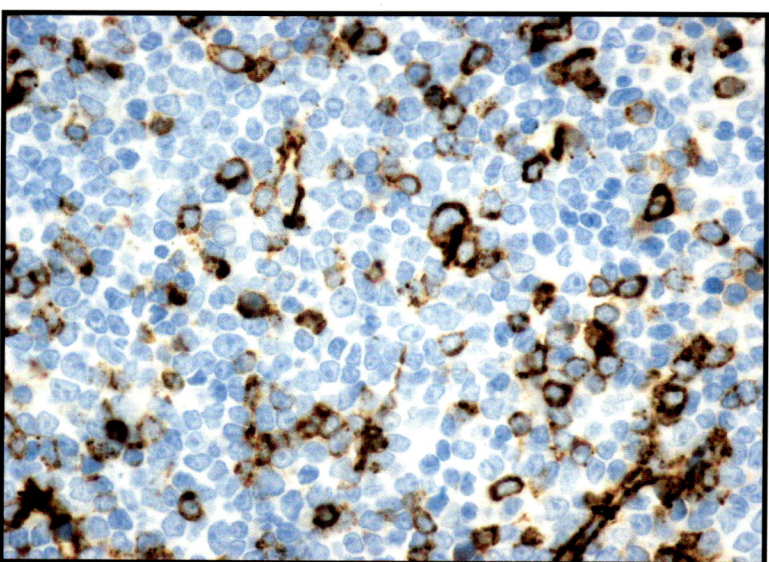

F5.1.8 CD34 in acute megakaryoblastic leukemia

Most of the illustrated cells in this area are leukemic blasts that expressed von Willebrand factor and CD61. Myeloperoxidase (MPO) was detected in very few cells and CD34, as shown here, was present in a small subpopulation of cells. Strong cytoplasmic positivity is seen in many cells. Again, immunohistochemistry appeared to show more CD34+ blasts than flow cytometric analysis.

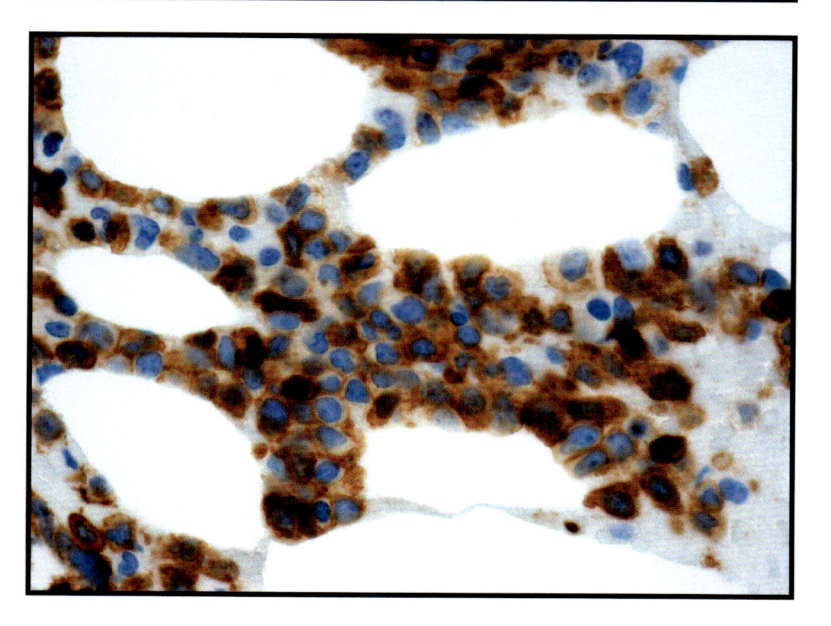

F5.1.9 CD45 in acute myeloid leukemia

CD45RA (CD45) is a membranous marker. In some acute leukemias, CD45RA may be expressed in the cytoplasm, which is seen in about 30% blasts in this case. While such cells appear intensely positive on immunohistochemistry, flow cytometric analysis revealed dim expression of CD45 in all CD34+ cells because only surface CD45 expression is analyzed with flow cytometry.

5.1 Acute Leukemia

F5.1.10 CD235a in erythroleukemia

A subpopulation of blasts shows strong expression of CD235a (glycophorin A). Some blasts are negative and occasional blasts show weak expression (red arrow). Non-nucleated red blood cells are also detected (blue arrows showing few circulating red blood cells).

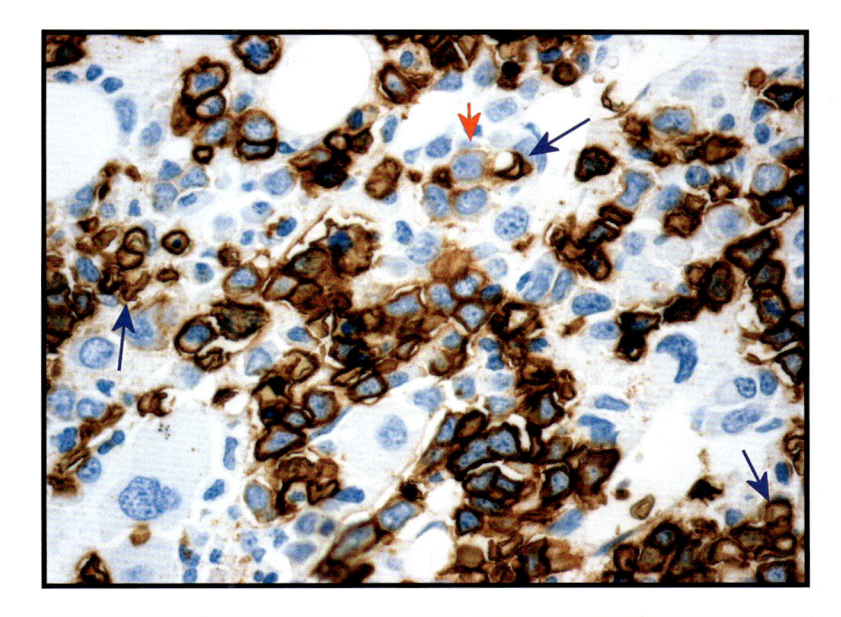

F5.1.11 Hemoglobin in acute myeloid leukemia with maturation

Residual normal hematopoiesis is compressed by leukemic cells in this bone marrow specimen. Arrows point to residual erythroid maturation. This finding should not be interpreted as partial erythroid differentiation of leukemic cells.

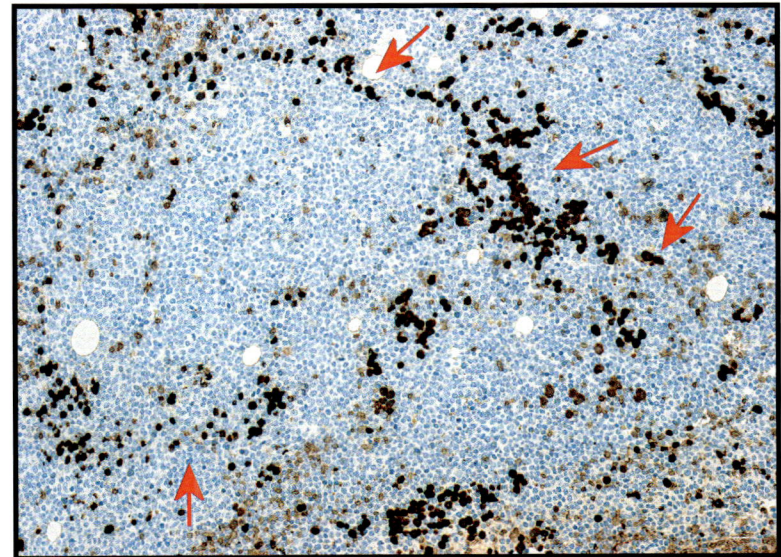

F5.1.12 TdT in acute myelomonocytic leukemia

TdT is expressed in some cases of AML, most of the time in the minimally differentiated subtype. However, any AML can express some TdT, particularly t(8;21) associated AML. In this case of myelomonocytic subtype, the expression is present in most blasts, but there is great variation in the intensity of TdT expression. This is in contrast to lymphoblastic leukemia in which there is more uniform and diffuse expression.

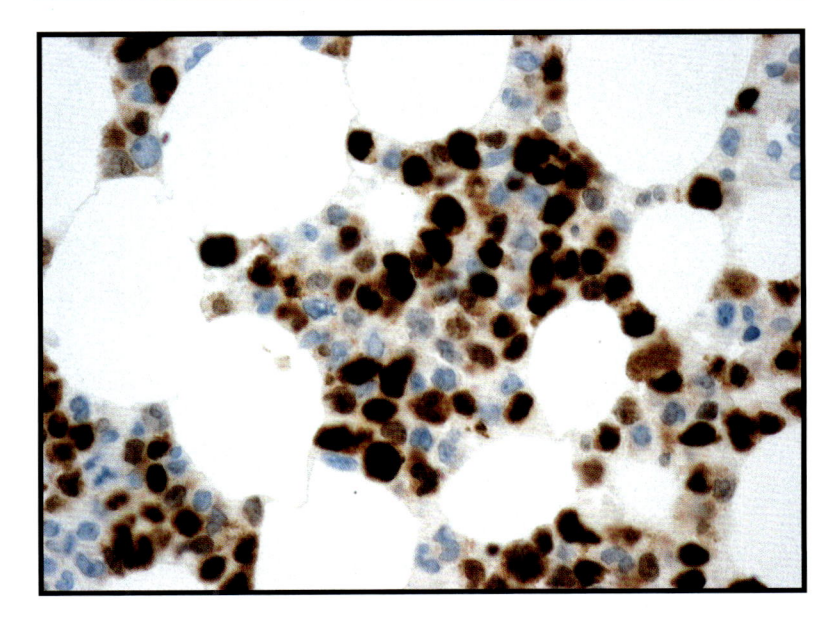

5: Special Diagnostic Considerations

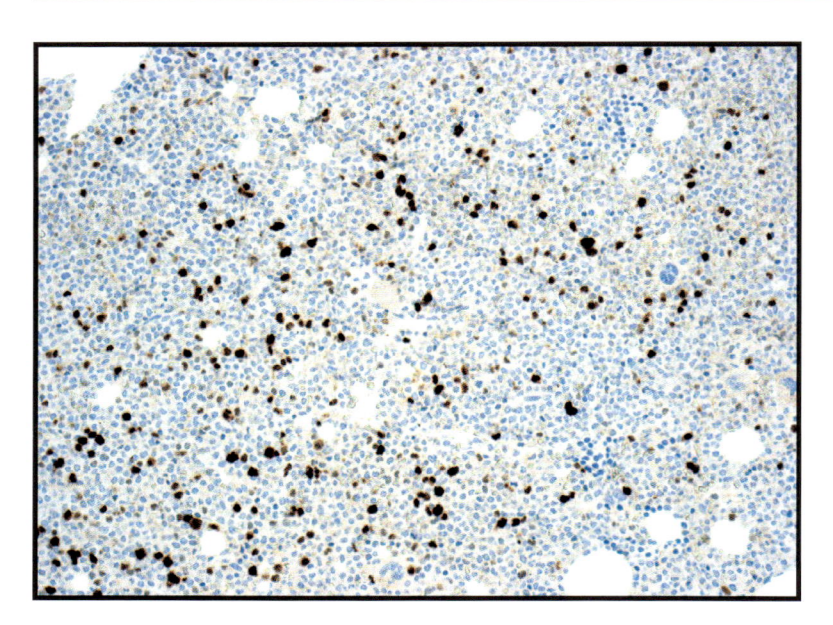

F5.1.13 TdT in acute myeloid leukemia with maturation

TdT+ cells are increased in this myeloid leukemia. However, the number of cells is less than 10%. Such a finding should not be interpreted as "positive" and it should not be used for classification of acute leukemia (it does not suffice for 0.5 score in the European Group for the Immunological Characterization of Leukemias [EGIL]).

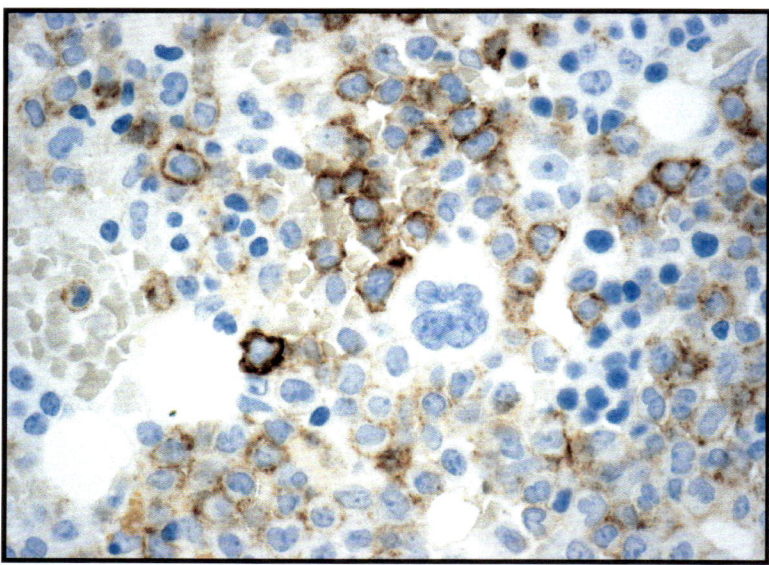

F5.1.14 CD123 in acute myeloid leukemia

While expression of CD123 is considered as evidence of plasmacytoid dendritic cells, it also is relatively common in acute myeloid leukemia and has been linked with more aggressive disease. Variable and relatively weak expression is common.

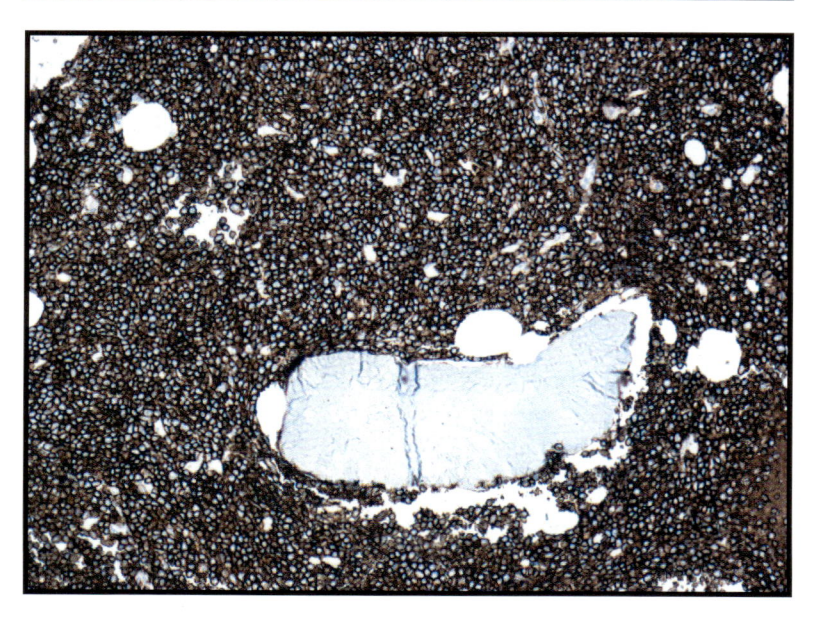

F5.1.15 CD43 (MT-1)

CD43, a leukocyte sialoglycoprotein, is an antiadhesive molecule mediating repulsion between leukocytes and other cells. It is expressed typically at high levels on all leukocytes except most resting B lymphocytes. Expression on platelets is weak. It should not be used as a T-cell marker. It is commonly expressed in acute leukemias and often at higher levels than CD45RA.

F5.1.16 Pancytokeratin (AE1/AE3) in chronic myelogenous leukemia (CML) blast crisis with megakaryoblastic differentiation

This biopsy specimen is from a 55-year old man with CML in blast crisis. In addition to CD34 and von Willebrand factor, the blasts expressed cytokeratin. The distribution of positivity mimics a dotlike pattern in neuroendocrine carcinomas (ie, Merkel cell carcinoma). Anaplastic large cell lymphoma and diffuse large B-cell lymphoma can also express cytokeratin(s). In addition, positive E-cadherin IHC in the bone marrow should not be regarded as evidence of metastatic carcinoma since it is also expressed in normal early erythroid precursors and is largely preserved in erythroid precursors in MDS and pure erythroid leukemia [Morosan 2008].

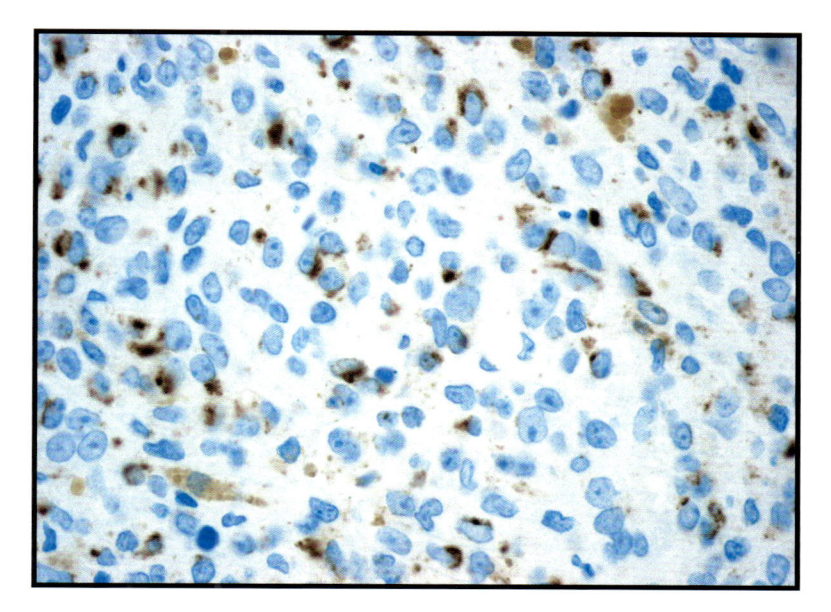

F5.1.17 Epithelial membrane antigen (EMA) in acute erythroid leukemia

EMA was considered a marker of erythroid differentiation as well as plasmacytic differentiation when only less specific markers were available for use in paraffin-embedded tissues. Even with improved immunohistochemistry methods and optimized protocols, EMA is a suboptimal marker of erythroid leukemia and it generally should not be used for acute leukemia classification. Instead, glycophorin C and hemoglobin A are recommended as erythroid markers.

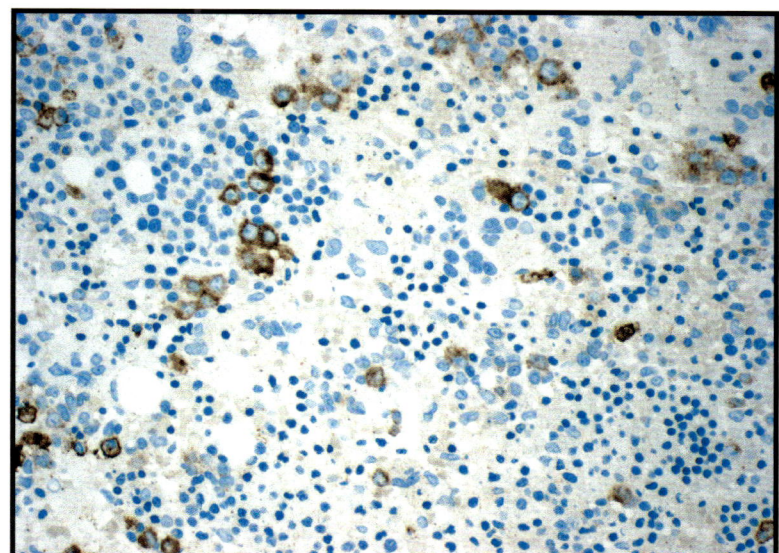

F5.1.18 Vimentin expression in blasts of acute leukemia

Vimentin is strongly expressed in many myeloid leukemias because it is normally found in early hematopoietic precursors. The only exception is megakaryoblastic leukemia, because megakaryocytes downregulate vimentin earlier than other cells in the bone marrow. Because vimentin is an intermediate filament, it is localized in the cytoplasm and its filamentous nature can be observed.

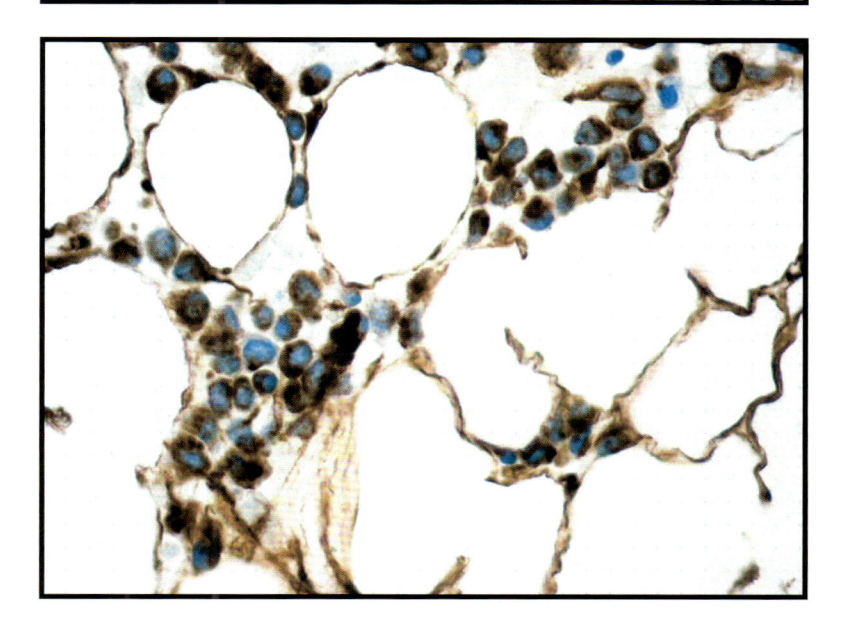

5: Special Diagnostic Considerations

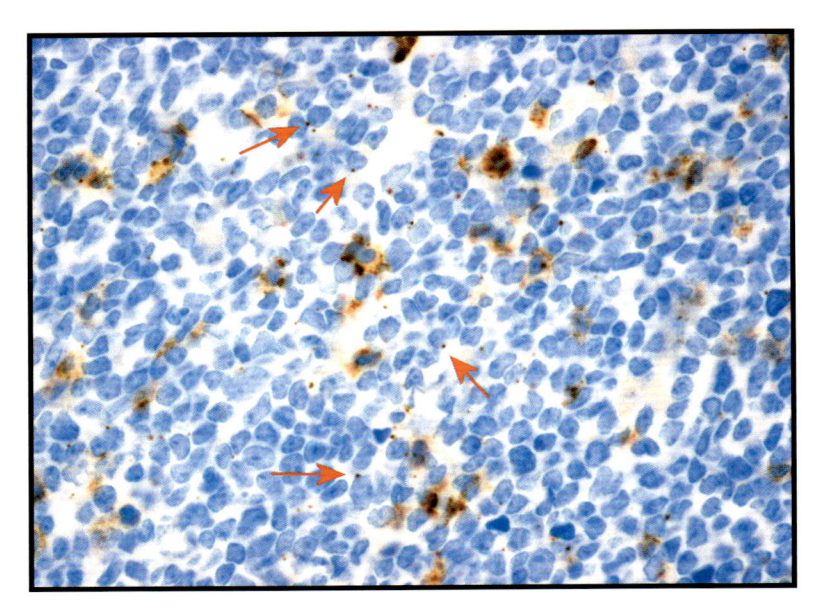

F5.1.19 CD2 in an undifferentiated acute leukemia

This biopsy specimen is from a 57-year old woman with pancytopenia. Extensive evaluation of the leukemic cells revealed expression of CD34, CD38, and HLA-DR, while CD45, CD99, and vimentin were strongly positive. All lineage-specific markers were negative on flow cytometry. Immunohistochemistry demonstrated very weak dotlike CD2 positivity in some leukemic cells (arrows). The significance of this finding is not clear and should be ignored.

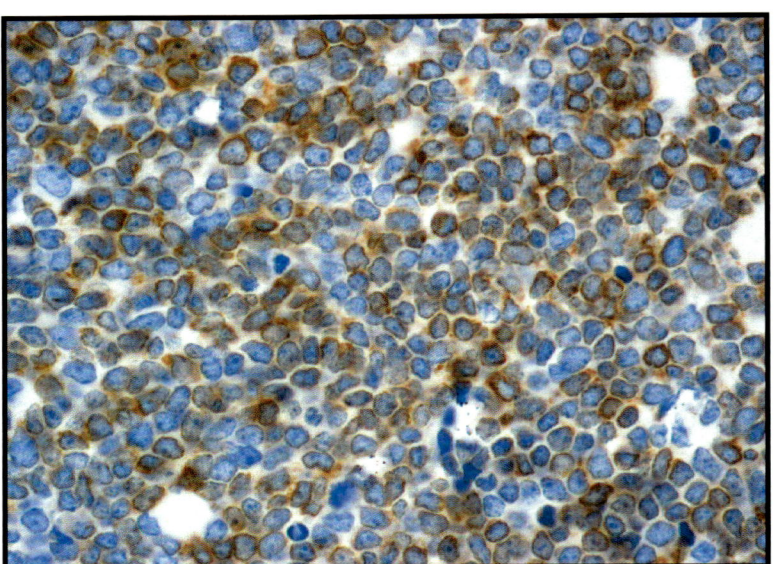

F5.1.20 CD79a in acute myelogenous leukemia (AML)

CD79a is expressed in B cells from an early stage of B-cell development and is a rare B-cell marker expressed in plasma cells. It is typically downregulated at germinal center stage of B-cell development. In acute leukemia, cytoplasmic expression is typical, but it can be expressed in some cases of both precursor T-ALL and AML. Despite its lineage infidelity, its expression accounts for a score of 2 in the European Group for the Classification of Acute Leukemia (EGIL) scoring system.

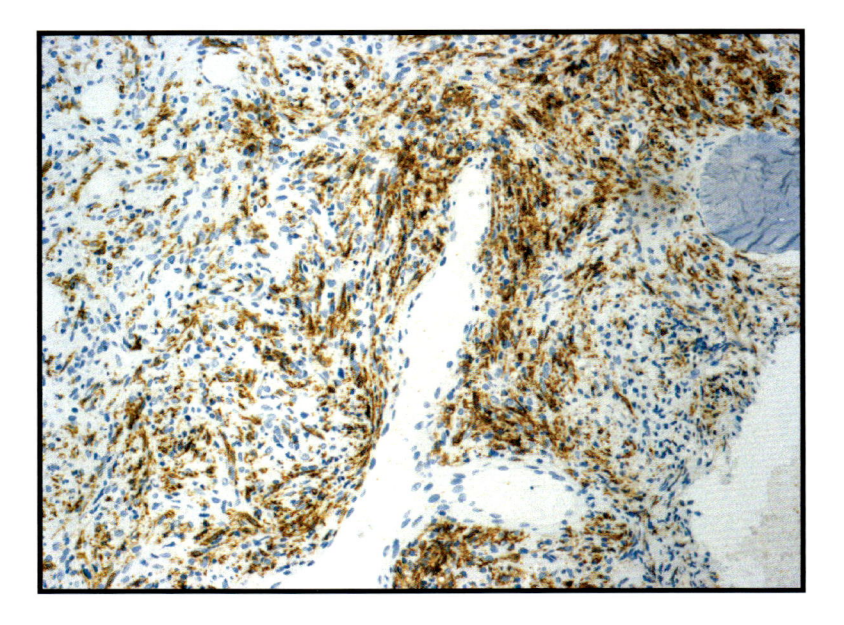

F5.1.21 CD20 in acute megakaryoblastic leukemia

CD20 is a pan-B cell marker, but it may be aberrantly expressed by various myeloid leukemias. It can be found in acute myelogenous leukemia with maturation and such cases also often express Pax-5, CD19, and CD79a. However, in this acute megakaryoblastic leukemia, this was the only detected B-cell Ag. In the European Group for the Classification of Acute Leukemia (EGIL) scoring system, CD20 expression accounts for a score of 1.

F5.1.22 Ki-67 in acute myelogenous leukemia (AML) with minimal differentiation

Ki-67 expression correlates with proliferation fraction. Despite the "acute" nature of AML, the proliferation fraction is often similar to that seen in normal bone marrow or lower. Fewer than 50% cells are positive in this case, which is a common finding in AML.

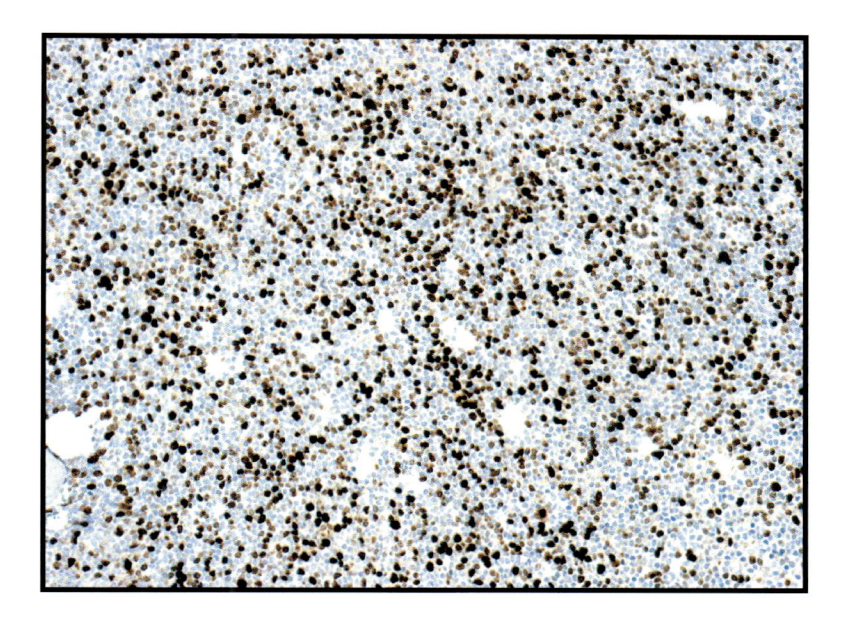

F5.1.23 Ki-67 in undifferentiatiated acute leukemia

Ki-67 in myeloid leukemia is higher than in lymphoblastic leukemia and also is higher in adults than in children. This acute leukemia shows very high Ki-67 expression, which is uncommon.

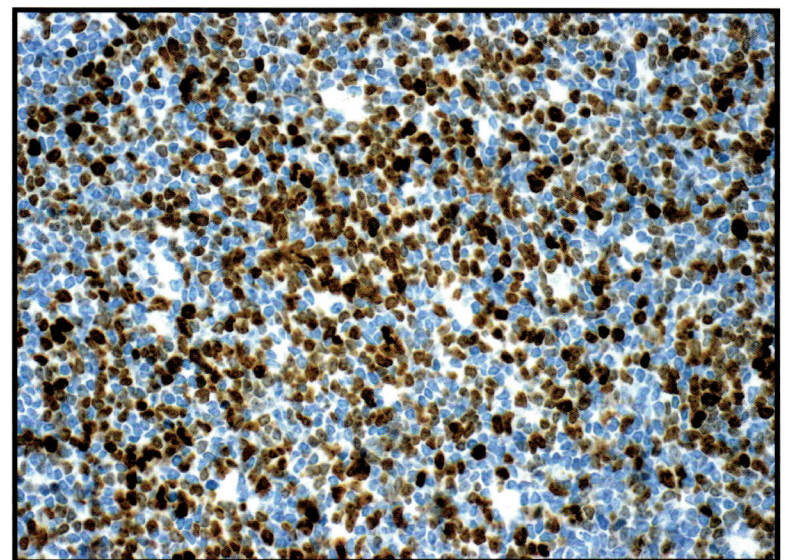

F5.1.24 CD23 in acute myelogenous leukemia (AML) without maturation

This image illustrates predominant cytoplasmic expression of CD23 in AML. CD23 expression has been described in eosinophilic and monocytic cell lines as well as in some cases of AML. It can also be upregulated in tissue macrophages in atopic subjects. Biological significance or potential diagnostic usefulness of CD23 detection in subtyping of AML has not been systematically evaluated.

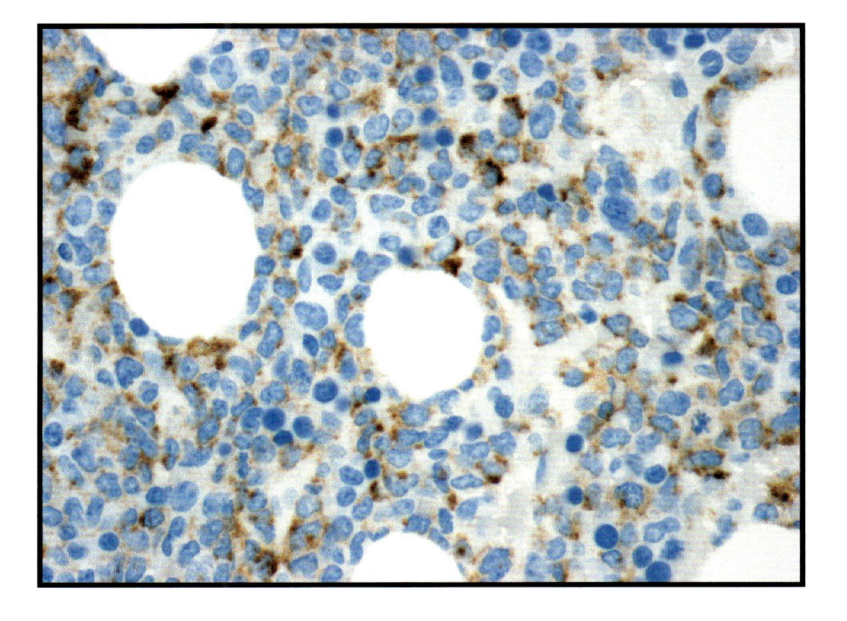

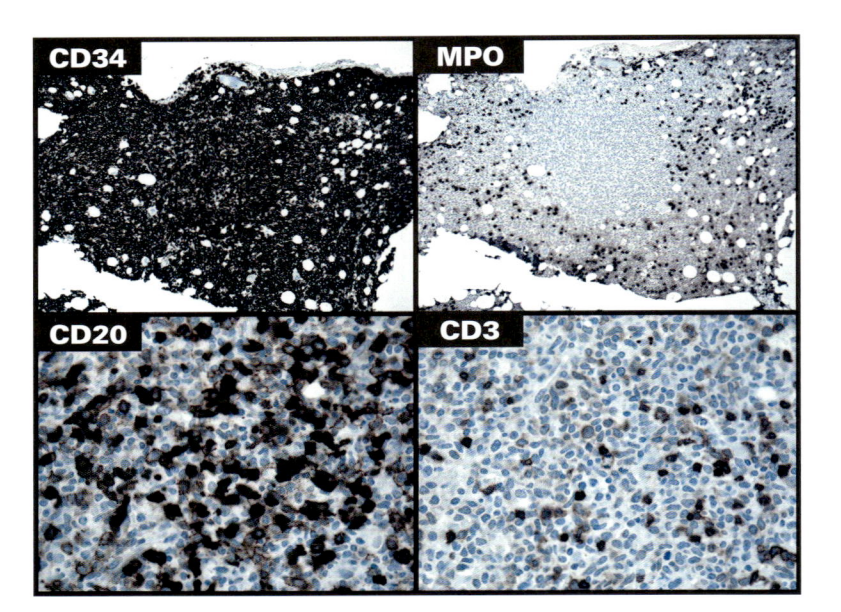

F5.1.25 Acute bilineal leukemia

Flow cytometric analysis suggested an acute biphenotypic leukemia (CD34+, cCD3+, cMPO+, CD2+, CD7+, CD79a+, CD33+, CD11b+, HLA-DR+, CD10−). The bone marrow core biopsy specimen was hypercellular with focal evidence of even more cellular clusters of MPO− blasts. CD34+/MPO+ areas did not express any lymphoid antigens. Most MPO− hypercellular areas with CD34+/CD20+ cells also contained cells with cCD3 expression. Unexpectedly, these MPO− areas did not express TdT.

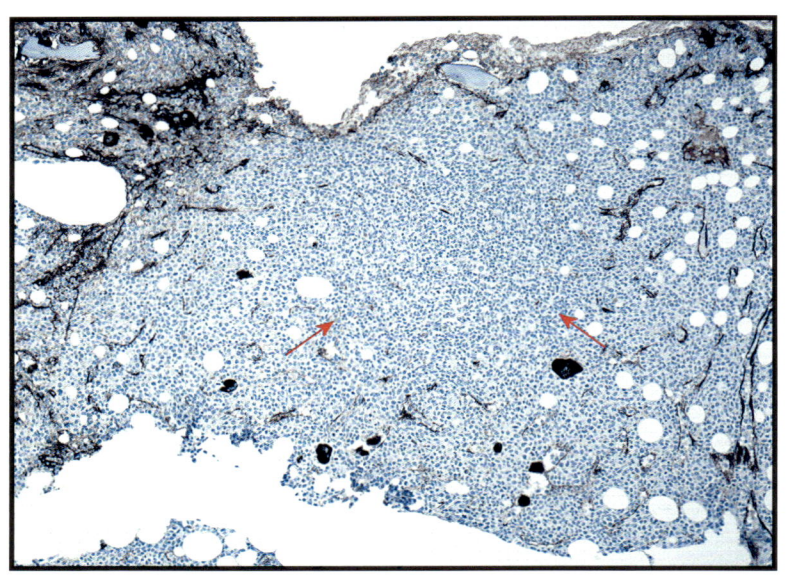

F5.1.26 Von Willebrand factor in acute bilineal leukemia

In the foci, the sinusoids are not present, suggesting an expansion of a new, possibly more aggressive subclone. The red arrows indicate the border between the new subclone and the rest of the bone marrow. Note that residual strongly positive megakaryocytes are present only in areas in which sinusoids are preserved. Blasts in all areas are negative for von Willebrand factor.

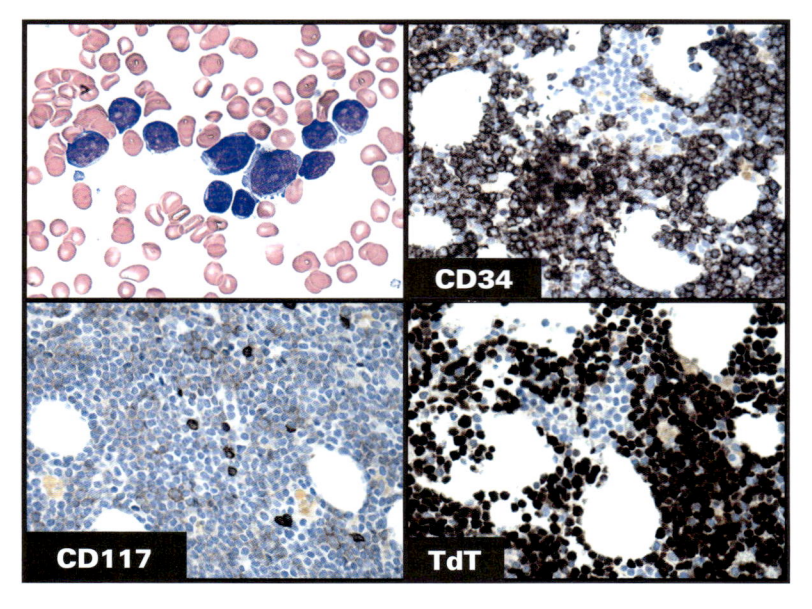

F5.1.27 Acute biphenotypic leukemia

In contrast to bilineal leukemias, biphenotypic leukemia is characterized by a single neoplastic clone that shows significant evidence of differentiation into more than one one lineage. In this case, the immunophenotype with immunohistochemistry (IHC) was as follows: myeloid markers included myeloperoxidase and CD117 (EGIL score of 3), and B-lymphoid markers included CD79a and TdT (European Group for the Classification of Acute Leukemia [EGIL] score of 2.5). In some cases, biphenotypic leukemia can be diagnosed only with IHC without the help of flow cytometry. There was no evidence of t(8;21) in this case.

5.2 Metastatic Tumors

Specimens of BM core biopsy are occasionally evaluated for metastatic tumors. However, bone biopsy specimens, which undergo all the same steps of tissue processing, are more commonly evaluated by surgical pathologists than by hematopathologists. Immunohistochemical analyses of such specimens present unique problems. While many of these specimens are processed similar to a BM core biopsy specimen, the size of the tissue is variable and the tissue processing method is generally less standardized. The decalcification step is usually longer than that in BM core biopsy because of the large size of the bone biopsy specimen. Because of predictably longer decalcification, some specimens are placed in decalcification solution too early before they are well fixed. This combination of suboptimal fixation with prolonged aggressive decalcification may be detrimental to antigen preservation. As a result, IHC staining can be suboptimal or unsatisfactory. In optimally processed BM core biopsies, IHC can produce excellent results with almost any test that would be used in the analysis of metastatic tumors and undifferentiated malignancies [Krishnan 2007].

The most common primary tumor types giving rise to bone metastases are, in order of frequency: breast, lung, and prostate carcinomas in adults and neuroblastoma, rhabdomyosarcoma, and Ewing sarcoma in children [Krishnan 2007]. Immunohistochemical panels are useful in identifying the primary tumor site [Krishnan 2007]. The same guidelines should be used as for any other presentation site.

Cytokeratin (CK) typing is important. CK7 and CK20 are widely used. So-called "double negative" tumors include hepatoma, renal cell carcinoma, prostate carcinoma, and some squamous carcinomas, all of which can be confirmed with HepPar, RCC antigen, prostate specific antigen (PSA)/prostatic acid phosphatase (PSAP), and p63 or CK10 or CK14 respectively. "Double positive" tumors include transitional cell carcinoma, pancreatic carcinoma, ovarian mucinous carcinoma, and some mucinous breast carcinomas. Classic CK7-positive tumors include breast, lung, pancreas, and biliary duct carcinomas. CK7 is also present in trophoblast in germ cell tumors. Classic CK20-positive tumors include colon, Merkel cell carcinoma, and transitional cell carcinoma of the urinary bladder. In contrast to transitional carcinoma of the urinary bladder, the transitional cell carcinoma of the ovary is CK20-negative as well as thrombomodulin-negative [Tot 2002; Wick 2008; Park 2007; Tot 2003; Rubin 2001; Tot 1999; Lagendijk 1998; Perry 1997].

Vimentin is a nonspecific marker, but is very useful in addition to CK7 and CK20. Vimentin-positive tumors include renal cell carcinoma, thyroid, lung, stomach, salivary gland, ovary, endometrial/endometrioid carcinoma, and choroid plexus carcinoma. Vimentin is also consistently strongly positive in metastatic melanoma. Classic vimentin-negative tumors are adenocarcinomas of the colon, small intestine, prostate, gallbladder, pancreas, and endocervix. Seminoma and embryonal carcinoma, hepatoma, and transitional cell carcinoma are also typically negative for vimentin.

Monoclonal carcinoembryonic antigen CEA (mCEA) is often positive in many tumors. However, some tumors are typically mCEA negative. They include hepatoma, renal cell carcinoma, and adrenal carcinoma. In contrast to a monoclonal (mCEA) that is not expressed in hepatoma, a polyclonal CEA (pCEA) is characteristically expressed in biliary capillaries in hepatoma.

Metastic breast carcinoma can be studied for estrogen receptor (ER), progesterone receptor (PR), and HER2/*neu*. However, no guidelines are provided for HER2/neu testing in the decalcified bone specimens. In many centers the results of breast carcinoma markers are reported. If the tests were not specifically validated for use in the bone marrow biopsy, the negative results for ER and PR should be reported with comments on possible false-negative results because of the decalcification step in tissue processing and possibly use of different fixative. Similarly, the HER2/*neu* test also must be validated before it is reported as either positive or negative. While Solomayer et al [Solomayer 2006] report significant discrepancies in Her2/*neu* expression between the primary tumor and disseminated tumor cells in the BM, analyzing BM aspirates, Gancberg et al [Gancberg 2002] found good concordance between the primary tumor and distant metastases by using routine IHC. These authors recommended assessment of HER-2/*neu* status in one of the distant metastatic sites only in some patients with easily accessible metastases and for whom HER-2/*neu* evaluation with IHC, performed in a primary tumor sample collected many years before, shows a negative score [Gancberg 2002]. Therefore, it is often not necessary to perform the HER2/*neu* test in the bone marrow biopsy specimen involved by metastatic breast carcinoma. It appears that antigen deterioration in this case is more a function of the length of storage than the type of tissue processing because most discrepancies were between positive bone metastases and negative primary tumors [Gancberg 2002]. This contention is consistent with a previous study which showed no systematic differences between HER-2/*neu* assessments in fresh and paraffin-embedded material [Press 1994]. However, significant loss at an average of 50% antigenicity was noted for stored, unstained cut sections for several Ags including p53, ER, Bcl-2, and F8-ra [van Diest 1991; Jacobs 1996].

Metastatic lung carcinomas express CK7, TTF-1, and low-molecular-weight CK (CK8) and/or high-molecular-weight CK (34βE12 or CK5/6). Small cell carcinomas express neuroendocrine markers in addition to cytokeratin expression. Most have at least focal cytoplasmic dotlike positivity for chromogranin, similar to cytokeratin and may also have the same pattern of expression for CD57. CD57 and CD56 are both good markers for neuroendocrine differentiation. However, if chromogranin is negative, at least 2 other less specific markers of neuroendocrine differentiation should be detected to classify the tumor as neuroendocrine with high certainty.

Prostate carcinomas are usually morphologically obvious and there is usually an appropriate history of prostate carcinoma. PSA and PSAP are usually positive, but in metastatic tumors their expression may be weak and focal or even totally absent. Prostate carcinomas are so-called "double negative" tumors (CK7−/CK20−), but up to 30% of cells may be weakly positive for 1 or both cytokeratins to be still considered as negative for the purpose of CK typing.

In children, as in adults, if the primary tumor is known, very little or no IHC testing is necessary for the diagnosis. Markers of neural differentiation for neuroblastoma, Fli-1 for Ewing sarcoma, and myoglobin may be used to confirm the respective diagnoses, but occasionally, and in particular when the tumor presents in the BM, a large number of markers will be necessary to classify pediatric tumors [Crary 1992; Brahmi 2001; Jambhekar 2006; Hicks 2005; López-Terrada 2006]. However, if the primary tumor is unknown, one should first consider the possibility of primary hematopoietic tumors that morphologically may mimic metastatic tumor. Acute megakaryoblastic leukemia, particularly the t(1;22)(p13;q13)–associated type in very young children, needs to be considered in the differential diagnosis.

5: Special Diagnostic Considerations

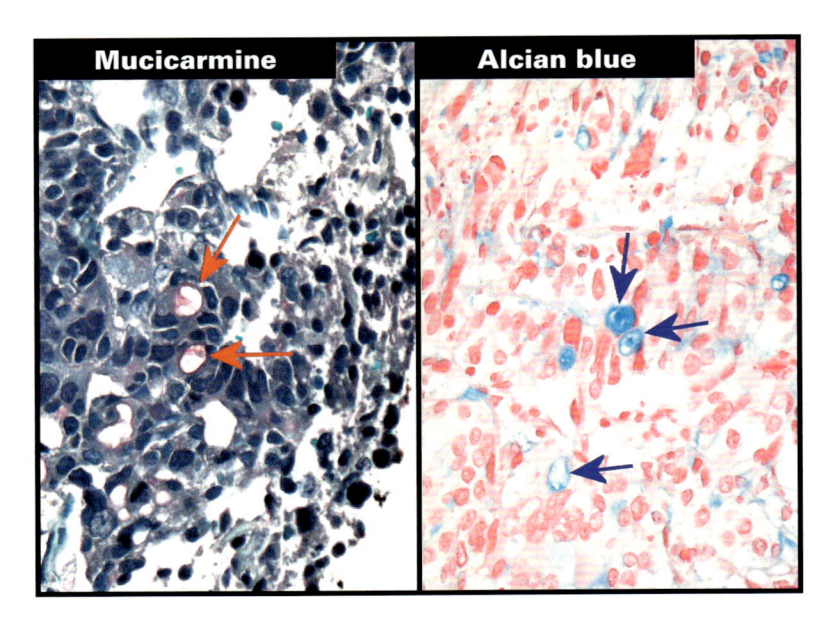

F5.2.1 Mucin staining in metastatic adenocarcinoma

In a patient with known primary tumor, morphologic evaluation is usually sufficient to confirm the diagnosis. Histochemical stains for mucin work well in decalcified tissues including bone and bone marrow biopsies and may be used to confirm the diagnosis of metastatic adenocarcinoma.

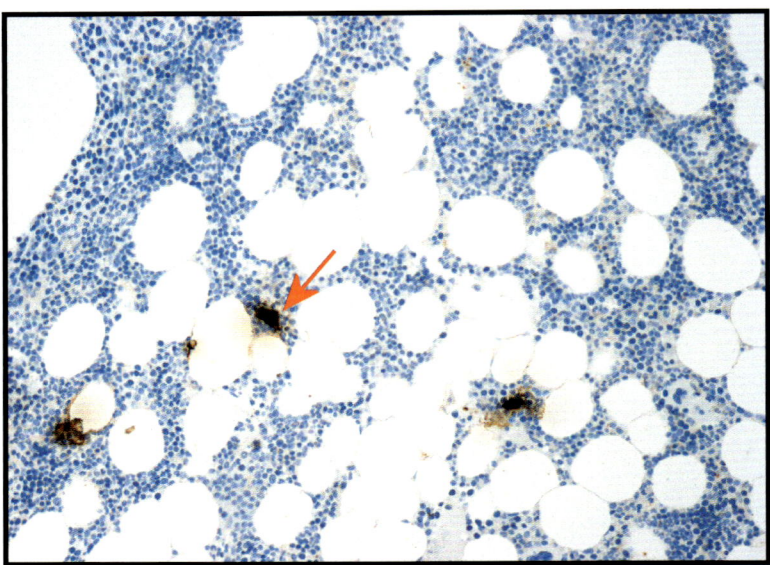

F5.2.2 AE1/AE3 (pankeratin) in histologically normal bone marrow

Similar to other tissue, AE1/AE3 and other pankeratin antibody cocktails may produce focal positivity secondary to contamination by desquamated cells from skin by histotechnologists who are processing the tissue. It is almost impossible to avoid this artefact, but it is easily recognizable.

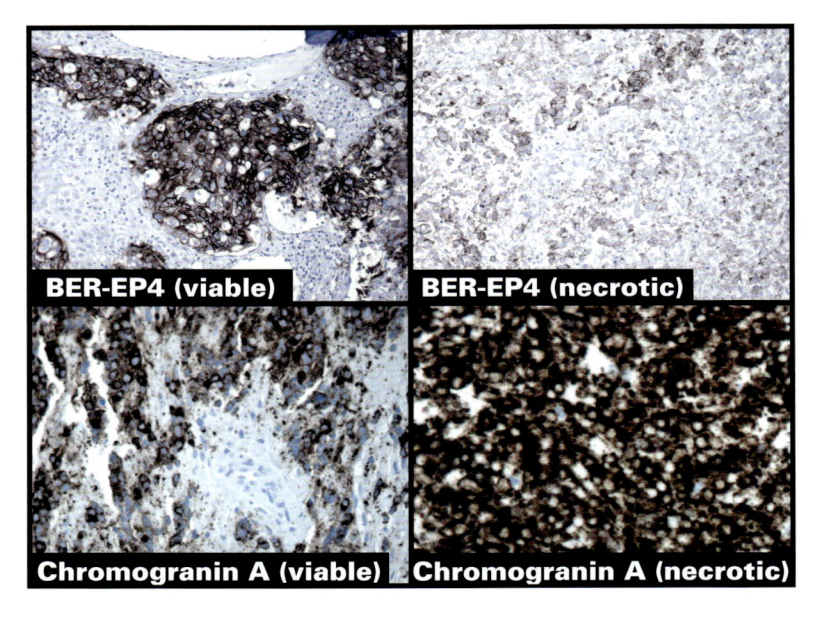

F5.2.3 Immunohistochemical (IHC) staining of necrotic tissues

Many antigens can be demonstrated with IHC even in necrotic tissues. These may include chromogranin, melan-A, HMB-45, vimentin, myeloperoxidase, mast cell tryptase, CD20, CD3, and many others. However, some antigens can be more rapidly degraded. Ber-EP4, an excellent epithelial marker, is poorly preserved in necrotic tissue. Many nuclear antigens are degraded and therefore negative results with Ki-67, TdT, Pax-5, and other markers should be considered uninformative, rather than truly negative.

5.2   Metastatic Tumors

F5.2.4 CD15 in metastatic lung carcinoma

CD15 is a myeloid marker and a good marker of classical Hodgkin lymphoma. It is also commonly expressed in many adenocarcinomas. CD15 has been used in the past in a mesothelioma vs. adenocarcinoma panel to favor adenocarcinoma. Because of its low sensitivity, it has been replaced by other more sensitive and more specific markers in the later panel, but it continues to be widely used for Hodgkin lymphoma immunophenotyping.

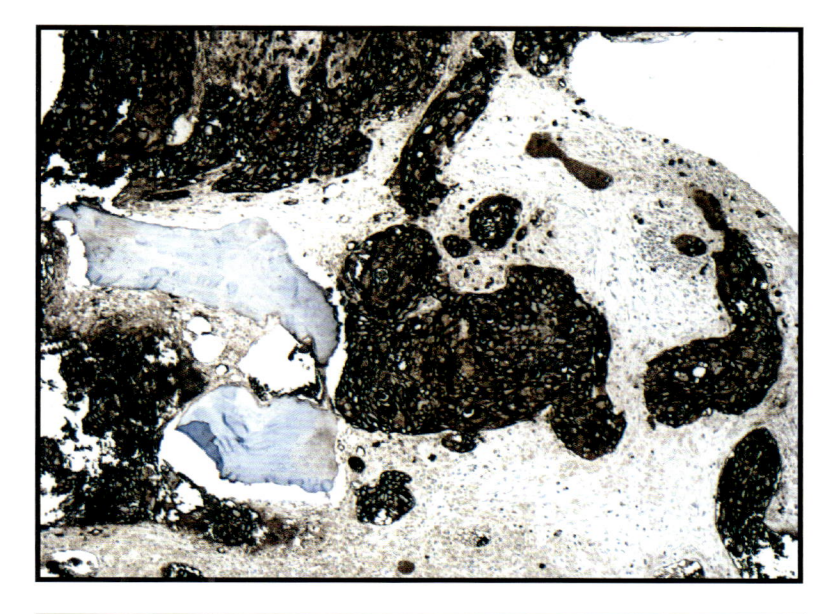

F5.2.5 CD56 in neuroblastoma

This natural killer (NK) cell marker, which is commonly expressed in multiple myeloma, is also a marker of neural/neuroendocrine differentiation (CD56 is a neural cell adhesion molecule [NCAM]). It is a very sensitive marker of neuroendocrine differentiation, possibly the most sensitive one, in small cell carcinoma. It is highly expressed in neuroblastoma because it is implicated in neural development.

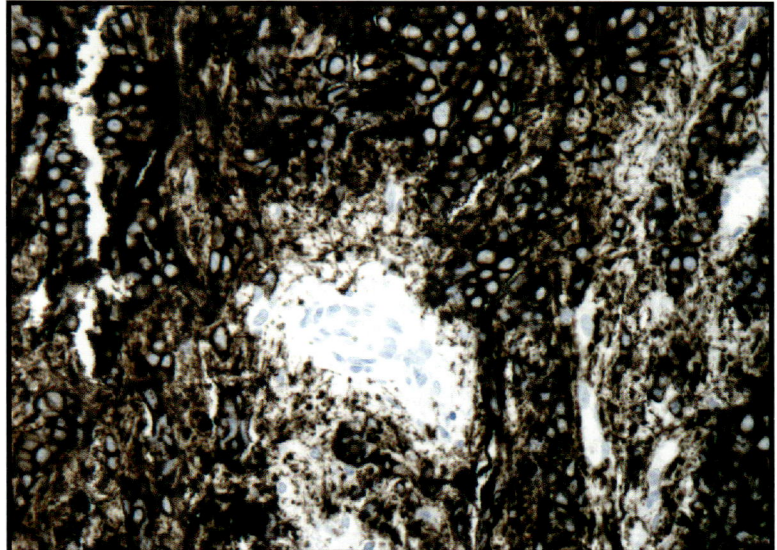

F5.2.6 CK7 in metastatic colon carcinoma

CK is demonstrated in fewer than 30% of cells and it is only weakly expressed in positive cells. This result should be interpreted as "negative" for the purpose of cytokeratin typing. The same rule needs to be applied to CK20 expression. The cutoff point depends on the sensitivity of the test. If less sensitive detection methods are used, a cutoff point may be set at 10% rather than 30% positivity. Such diagnostic cutoff points may be validated by participation in extralaboratory testing.

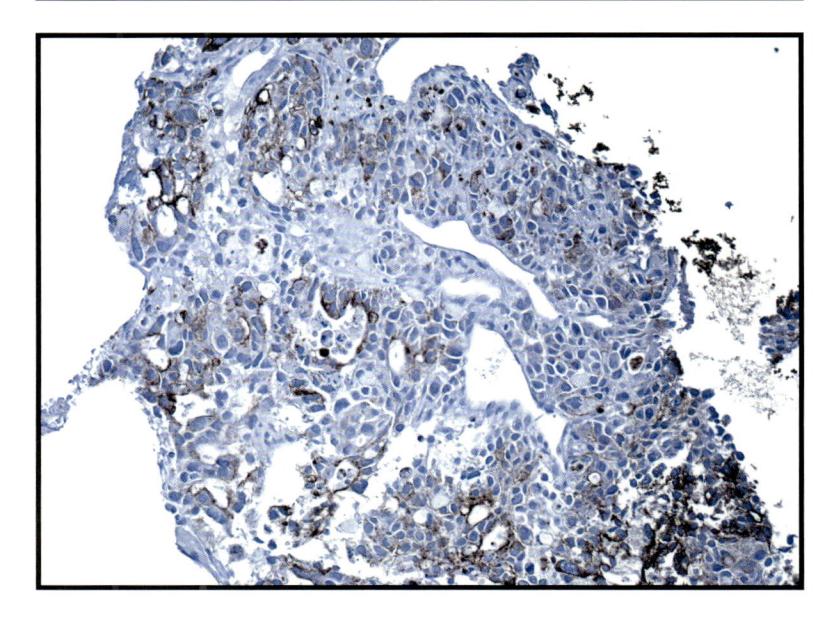

5: Special Diagnostic Considerations

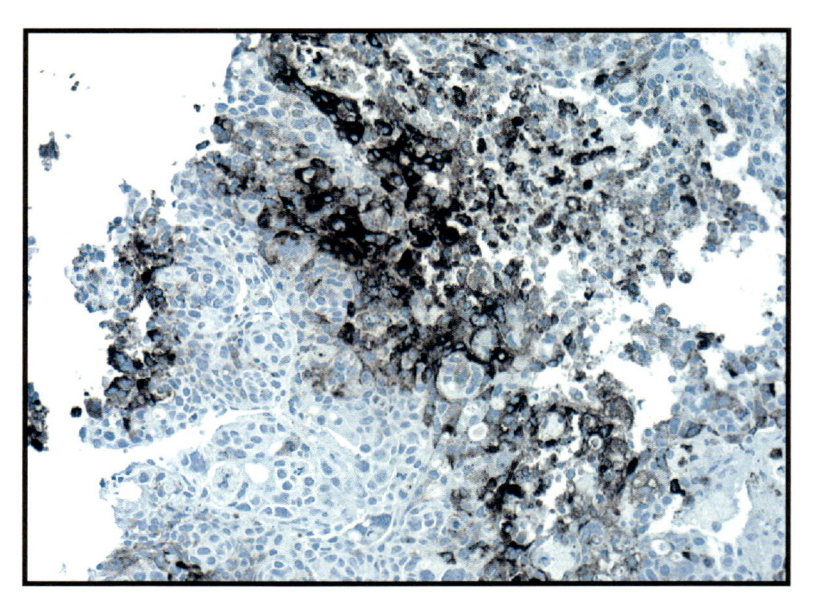

F5.2.7 TAG72 (B72.3) in metastatic breast carcinoma

Only about 20% of tumor cells were positive. Focal, rather than diffuse, expression of B72.3 in adenocarcinomas is common. B72.3 antibody was developed by using breast carcinoma cell line with TAG72 tumor antigen. The vast majority of breast carcinomas are positive, but most other adenocarcinomas express TAG72 as well. Tumors negative for B72.3 are unlikely to be a primary tumor in the breast. B72.3 antibody is used in a mesothelioma vs. adenocarcinoma panel.

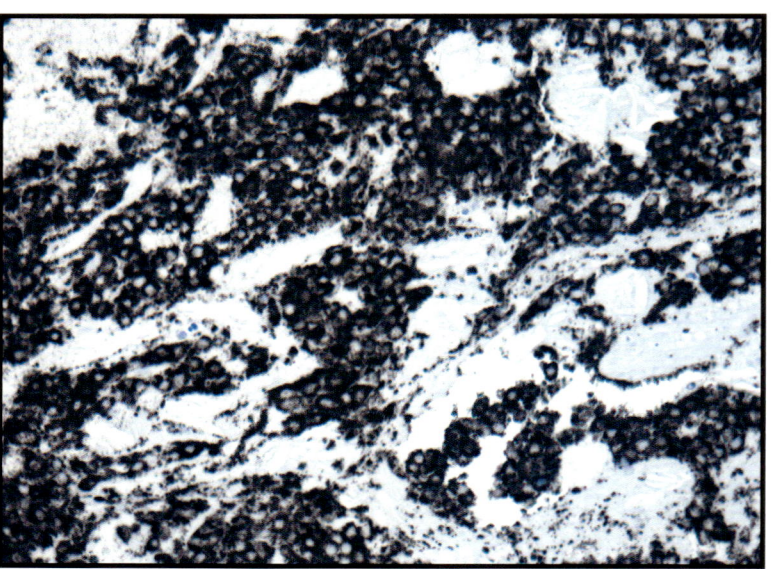

F5.2.8 Chromogranin A in neuroblastoma

This biopsy specimen is from a 13-year old girl with neuroblastoma. The tumor shows strong expression of chromogranin A. PgP 9.5, neuron-specific enolase (NSE), NPY, substance P, and other neural markers can be expressed in the bone marrow with neuroblastoma. Chromogranin A expression in metastatic neuroblastoma was linked with early relapse in one study. Chromogranin A is a pan-neuroendocrine marker, in which detection in various lesions critically depends on selection of the primary antibody and the method of antigen retrieval.

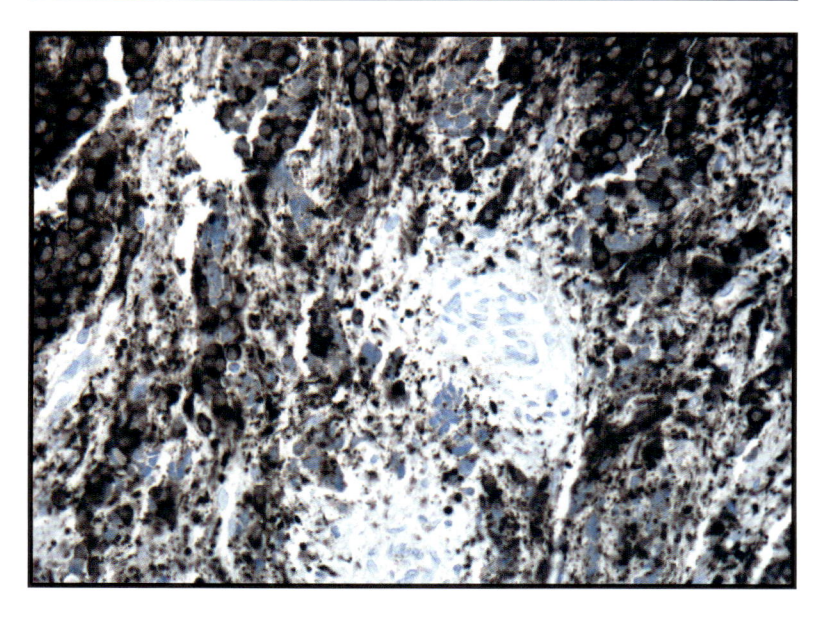

F5.2.9 Neuron-specific enolase (NSE) in neuroblastoma

Detection of NSE in paraffin-embedded tissues has been in use for decades as a marker of neural/neuroendocrine differentiation despite its low specificity. However, in neuroblastoma, this is a very sensitive marker that is detected in all cases in contrast to many other neuroendocrine tumors, in which specificity and sensitivity of the NSE are less than optimal.

5.2 Metastatic Tumors

F5.2.10 Neuron-specific enolase (NSE) in osteoblasts and osteocytes

In the bone marrow, NSE staining can be detected in osteoblasts and osteocytes as illustrated herein. Also, several stromal cells may show some NSE expression. Results of NSE staining should always be interpreted with caution.

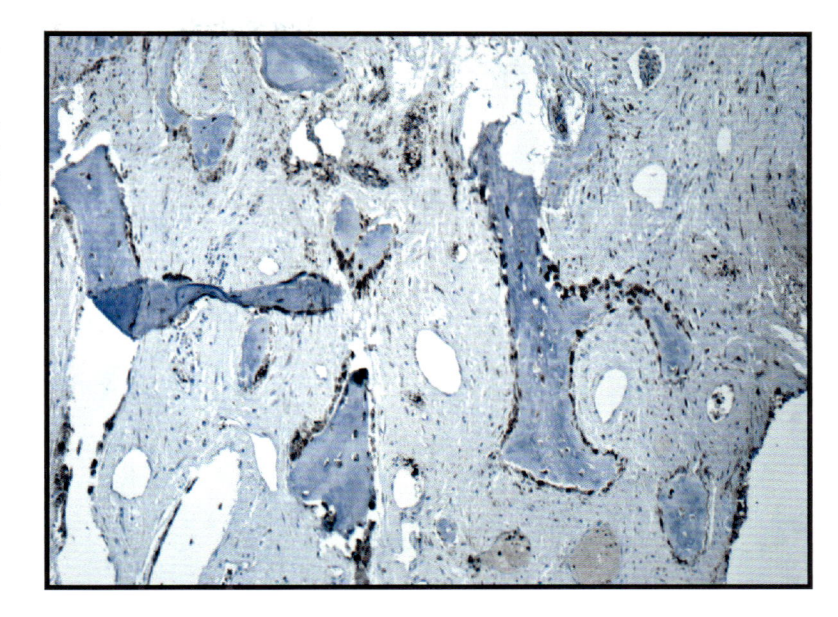

F5.2.11 Vimentin and neurofilaments in large cells in neuroblastoma

More differentiated areas with larger cells show strong expression of vimentin (left) and neurofilaments (right). The immunophenotype of neuroblastoma changes with differentiation.

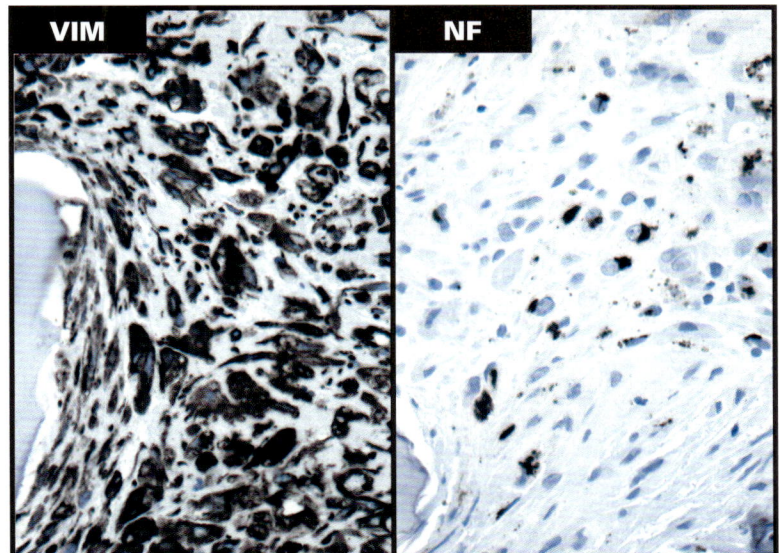

F5.2.12 Vimentin and neurofilaments in small cells in neuroblastoma

Undifferentiated areas show no expression of vimentin (left) or neurofilaments (right). The arrow points to a single NF+ cytoplasmic extension in this area. Same biopsy specimen as in F5.2.11.

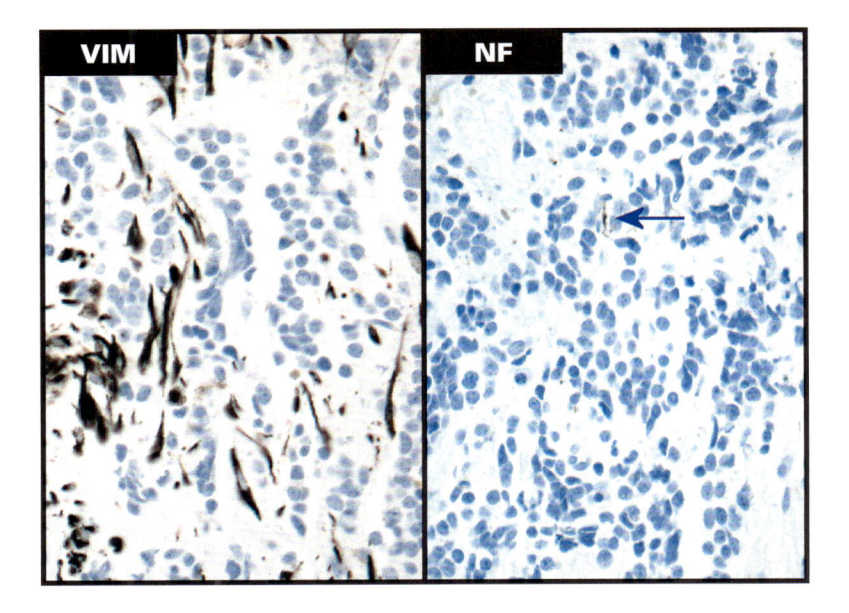

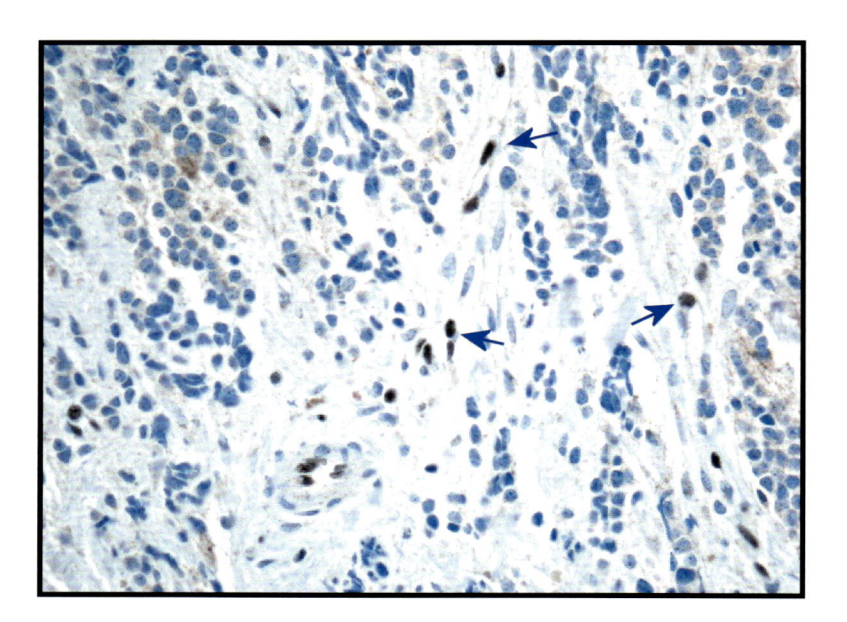

F5.2.13 Fli-1 in neuroblastoma

Neuroblastomas are typically Fli-1 negative. However, when there is no staining, a false-negative result needs to be excluded. This is important in decalcified specimens including bone biopsies for either primary or metastatic tumors. Fli-1 weak to moderate positivity needs to be identified in most endothelial cells to be certain that this is not an artefact. When bone marrow cells are present in the biopsy specimen, all hematopoietic cells except erythroid precursors should be strongly positive.

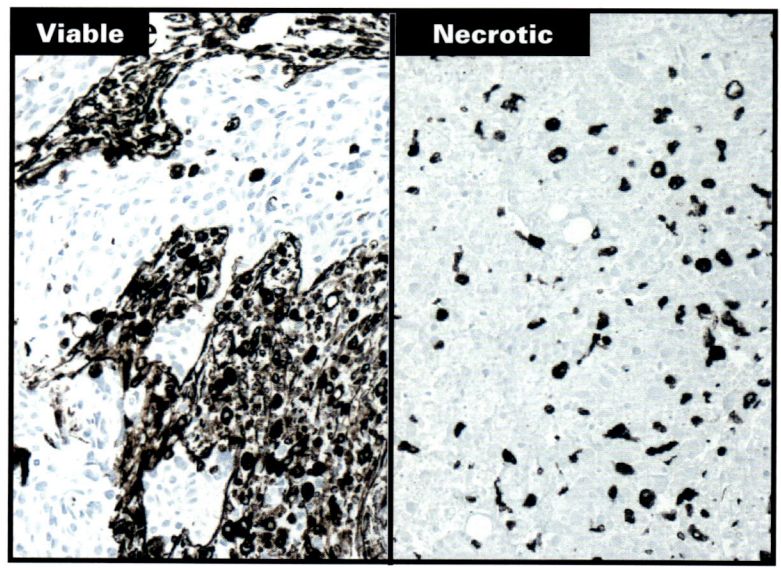

F5.2.14 Vimentin in vimentin-negative tumors

Stromal reactions in the BM are highlighted by vimentin staining. This metastatic prostate carcinoma shows no evidence of vimentin expression (left). Vimentin can usually be demonstrated even in necrotic tissues (right). Stromal elements are staining and can be used as an internal positive control. In this area, only necrotic tumor tissue was present. Colon, small intestinal, prostate, gallbladder, pancreas, and endocervical adenocarcinomas, and also seminoma, hepatoma, and transitional cell carcinomas are all typically vimentin-negative tumors.

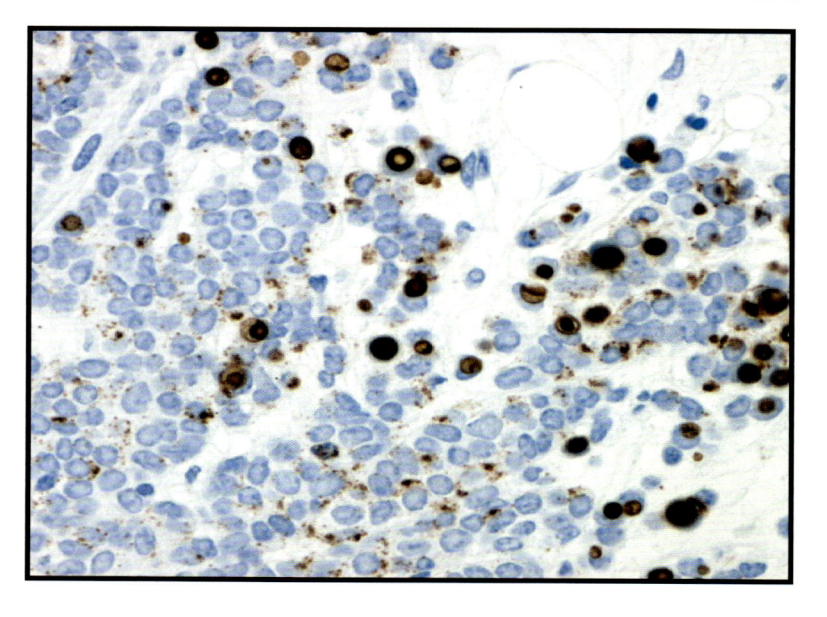

F5.2.15 CA-125 in metastatic lobular breast carcinoma

Metastatic breast carcinoma, in particular lobular carcinoma, may show strong focal expression of CA-125. This peculiar pattern results from the formation of intracytoplasmic glandular lumens in this histological subtype of breast carcinoma. Similar patterns may be seen with GCDFP-15, mucin stains, and TAG72 (B72.3). This pattern is highly specific and has important diagnostic value even when fewer than 10% show positivity.

Special Diagnostic Considerations

5.3 Recommended Panels

Every patient's BM sample represents a unique biological material in a setting of specific clinical and laboratory findings. Therefore, the panels recommended herein for immunohistochemical testing should not be considered either obligatory or inflexible **T5.1**. They need to be adapted to suit the clinicopathological setting and provide useful information. The extent of the panels may also reflect the need for evidence-based medicine; IHC tests may be used to confirm or further characterize an already known diagnosis.

Experts agree that the appropriate number of markers for complete characterization of acute leukemia would average 20 to 25 in flow cytometry, but not every marker would be useful in all cases [Bain 2002; Béné 2005]. Experts also agree that a significant reduction in the number of antibodies in the diagnostic specimens could significantly compromise the diagnostic accuracy, appropriate monitoring, or treatment of these disorders.

A similar number of markers is probably needed in IHC, but often a smaller number of markers is used [Pileri 1999]. Smaller number of markers is clearly justified in evaluation of patients with available flow cytometric results, but one should not hesitate to use larger panels in evaluation of the specimens where tissue biopsy is the only material available. In any disease, fewer reagents are needed in the monitoring or staging of patients with previously characterized disease. The selection and the number of markers required for the work up of other disease, in the bone marrow is less defined than for acute leukemia.

The IHC panels also depend on the extent of the previous training in hematopathology or IHC, individual experience, budgetary considerations, and technical success of the procedures. All of the aforementioned factors may work either way to produce bias in ordering either large or small panels in any particular BM biopsy.

T5.1. Recommended Panels for Bone Marrow Immunohistochemistry

Panel	Antibodies
Acute leukemia	CD34, TdT, MPO, CD33, CD117, F8-ra, CD61 (or CD42b), Hgb-A, Gly-C (or Gly-A), Pax-5, CD10, CD79a, CD20, CD45, CD3 *To consider:* NPM1, CD68, CD63, lysozyme, CD15, CD123, CD99, CD31
Myelodysplatic syndromes and myelodysplastic/myeloproliferative diseases	CD34, CD117, CD61 (or CD42b), MCT *To consider:* MPO, CD33, MCT, Hgb-A, Parvovirus B19
Chronic myeloproliferative diseases	CD34, MPO, CD61 (or CD42b or F8-ra), PG-M1, Hgb-A *To consider:* CD33, TdT, CD3, CD20, Pax-5
Mature B-cell neoplasms	CD3, CD20, CD10, CD5, cyclin D1, CD23, Bcl-6 *To consider:* CD79a, IgM, CD25, Bcl-2, κ, λ, CD138, CD72. TRAP, Bcl-3, ZAP70
Mature T-cell neoplasms	CD2, CD3, CD4, CD5, CD7, CD8, CD56, CD57, TIA-1, granzyme B, EBV *To consider:* MUM1, CD45RO, Bcl-6, CD30, ALK-1, perforin
Hodgkin lymphoma	A. For presentation in the BM: CD30, CD15, CD3, CD20, Pax-5, and to consider MUM1, EBV, PU.1, OCT2, BOB1 B. For staging when abnormal cells morphologically present: CD30, CD15 C. For staging when abnormal cells not morphlogically obvious: CD3, Pax-5, CD30
Plasma cell disorders	CD138, κ, λ, CD45, CD56, CD20 *To consider:* Ki-67, EBV, IgM, IgD, IgA, IgG, IgE, Pax-5, CD117
Histiocytic and dendritic cell neoplasms	CD68, CD163, PU.1, CD45, CD21, CD23, CD35, CD123, S-100, CD1a
Mastocytosis	MCT, CD25, CD117 *To consider:* CD34, CD3, CD20

References

Alcalay M, Tiacci E, Bergomas R, et al. Acute myeloid leukemia bearing cytoplasmic nucleophosmin (NPMc+ AML) shows a distinct gene expression profile charwacterized by up-regulation of genes involved in stem-cell wmaintenance [published online ahead of print April 14, 2005]. *Blood* 2005;106(3):899-902.

Arber DA, Jenkins KA. Paraffin section immunophenotyping of acute leukemias in bone marrow specimens. *Am J Clin Pathol* 1996;106(4):462-8.

Bain BJ, Barnett D, Linch D, Matutes E, Reilly JT; General Haematology Task Force of the British Committee for Standards in Haematology (BCSH), British Society of Haematology. Revised guideline on immunophenotyping in acute leukaemias and chronic lymphoproliferative disorders. *Clin Lab Haematol* 2002;24(1):1-13.

Béné MC. Immunophenotyping of acute leukaemias [review]. *Immunol Lett* 2005;98(1):9-21.

Boissel N, Renneville A, Biggio V, et al. Prevalence, clinical profile, and prognosis of NPM mutations in AML with normal karyotype. *Blood* 2005;106(10):3618-20.

Bolli N, Nicoletti I, De Marco MF, et al. Born to be exported: COOH-terminal nuclear export signals of different strength ensure cytoplasmic accumulation of nucleophosmin leukemic mutants. *Cancer Res* 2007;67(13):6230-7.

Bolli N, Galimberti S, Martelli MP, et al. Cytoplasmic nucleophosmin in myeloid sarcoma occurring 20 years after diagnosis of acute myeloid leukaemia. *Lancet Oncol* 2006;7(4):350-2.

Brahmi U, Rajwanshi A, Joshi K, et al. Flow cytometric immunophenotyping and comparison with immunocytochemistry in small round cell tumors. *Anal Quant Cytol Histol* 2001;23(6):405-12.

Casasnovas RO, Slimane FK, Garand R, et al. Immunological classification of acute myeloblastic leukemias: relevance to patient outcome. *Leukemia* 2003;17(3):515-27.

Crary GS, Singleton TP, Neglia JP, Swanson PE, Strickler JG. Detection of metastatic neuroblastoma in bone marrow biopsy specimens with an antibody to neuron-specific enolase. *Mod Pathol* 1992;5(3):308-11.

Dunphy CH, O'Malley DP, Perkins SL, Chang CC. Analysis of immunohistochemical markers in bone marrow sections to evaluate for myelodysplastic syndromes and acute myeloid leukemias. *Appl Immunohistochem Mol Morphol* 2007;15(2):154-9.

Falini B, Martelli MP, Bolli N, et al. Immunohistochemistry predicts nucleophosmin (NPM) mutations in acute myeloid leukemia [published online ahead of print May 23, 2006]. *Blood* 2006a;108(6):1999-2005.

Falini B, Bolli N, Shan J, Martelli MP, et al. Both carboxy-terminus NES motif and mutated tryptophan(s) are crucial for aberrant nuclear export of nucleophosmin leukemic mutants in NPMc+ AML [published online ahead of print February 2, 2006]. *Blood* 2006b;107(11):4514-23.

Falini B, Nicoletti I, Martelli MF, Mecucci C. Acute myeloid leukemia carrying cytoplasmic/mutated nucleophosmin (NPMc+ AML): biologic and clinical features [review] [published online ahead of print September 28, 2007]. *Blood* 2007;109(3):874-85.

Gancberg D, Di Leo A, Cardoso F, et al. Comparison of HER-2 status between primary breast cancer and corresponding distant metastatic sites. *Ann Oncol* 2002;13(7):1036-43.

Gorello P, Cazzaniga G, Alberti F, et al. Quantitative assessment of minimal residual disease in acute myeloid leukemia carrying nucleophosmin (NPM1) gene mutations. *Leukemia* 2006;20(6):1103-8.

Hicks J, Mierau GW. The spectrum of pediatric tumors in infancy, childhood, and adolescence: a comprehensive review with emphasis on special techniques in diagnosis [review]. *Ultrastruct Pathol* 2005;29(3-4):175-202.

Horny HP, Wehrmann M, Steinke B, Kaiserling E. Assessment of the value of immunohistochemistry in the subtyping of acute leukemia on routinely processed bone marrow biopsy specimens with particular reference to macrophage-associated antibodies. *Hum Pathol* 1994;25(8):810-4.

Horny HP, Campbell M, Steinke B, Kaiserling E. Acute myeloid leukemia: immunohistologic findings in paraffin-embedded bone marrow biopsy specimens. *Hum Pathol* 1990;21(6):648-55.

Islam A, Catovsky D, Goldman JM, Galton DA. Bone marrow biopsy changes in acute myeloid leukaemia: I, observations before chemotherapy. *Histopathology* 1985;9(9):939-57.

Jacobs TW, Prioleau JE, Stillman IE, Schnitt SJ. Loss of tumor marker-immunostaining intensity on stored paraffin slides of breast cancer. *J Natl Cancer Inst* 1996;88(15):1054-9.

Jaffe E, Harris N, Stain H, Vardiman J, ed. *World Health Organization Classification of Tumours Pathology and Genetics of Tumours of Haematopoietic and Lymphoid Tissues* Lyon, France: IARC Press; 2001.

Jambhekar NA, Bagwan IN, Ghule P, et al. Comparative analysis of routine histology, immunohistochemistry, reverse transcriptase polymerase chain reaction, and fluorescence in situ hybridization in diagnosis of Ewing family of tumors. *Arch Pathol Lab Med* 2006;130(12):1813-8.

Konoplev S, Lu H, Rubin JB, et al. CXCR4 overexpression is associated with poor prognosis in AML patients independently of NPM1 mutations. Abstract 1193. *Mod Pathol* 2008;21(suppl 1):261A.

References

Krishnan C, George TI, Arber DA. BM metastases: a survey of nonhematologic metastases with immunohistochemical study of metastatic carcinomas. *Appl Immunohistochem Mol Morphol* 2007;15(1):1-7.

Kröber SM, Greschniok A, Kaiserling E, Horny HP. Acute lymphoblastic leukaemia: correlation between morphological/immunohistochemical and molecular biological findings in bone marrow biopsy specimens. *Mol Pathol* 2000;53(2):83-7.

Lagendijk JH, Mullink H, Van Diest PJ, Meijer GA, Meijer CJ. Tracing the origin of adenocarcinomas with unknown primary using immunohistochemistry: differential diagnosis between colonic and ovarian carcinomas as primary sites. *Hum Pathol* 1998;29(5):491-7.

López-Terrada D. Integrating the diagnosis of childhood malignancies [review]. *Adv Exp Med Biol* 2006;587:121-37.

Morosan CG, Allan RW. E-cadherin immunohistochemical stain is a useful specific marker of early erythroid elements in bone marrow core biopsies and has utility in MDS and erythroleukemia. Abstract 1220. *Mod Pathol* 2008;21(suppl 1):267A.

Ngo N, Lampert IA, Naresh KN. Bone marrow trephine findings in acute myeloid leukaemia with multilineage dysplasia [published online ahead of print October 31, 2007]. *Br J Haematol* 2008;140(3):279-86.

Park SY, Kim BH, Kim JH, Lee S, Kang GH. Panels of immunohistochemical markers help determine primary sites of metastatic adenocarcinoma. *Arch Pathol Lab Med* 2007;131(10):1561-7.

Perry A, Parisi JE, Kurtin PJ. Metastatic adenocarcinoma to the brain: an immunohistochemical approach. *Hum Pathol* 1997;28(8):938-43.

Pileri SA, Ascani S, Milani M, et al. Acute leukaemia immunophenotyping in bone-marrow routine sections. *Br J Haematol* 1999;105(2):394-401.

Press MF, Hung G, Godolphin W, Slamon DJ. Sensitivity of HER-2/neu antibodies in archival tissue samples: potential source of error in immunohistochemical studies of oncogene expression. *Cancer Res* 1994;54(10):2771-7.

Rubin BP, Skarin AT, Pisick E, Rizk M, Salgia R. Use of cytokeratins 7 and 20 in determining the origin of metastatic carcinoma of unknown primary, with special emphasis on lung cancer. *Eur J Cancer Prev* 2001;10(1):77-82.

Solomayer EF, Becker S, Pergola-Becker G, et al. Comparison of HER2 status between primary tumor and disseminated tumor cells in primary breast cancer patients [published online ahead of print March 22, 2006]. *Breast Cancer Res Treat* 2006;98(2):179-84.

Torlakovic G, Langholm R, Torlakovic E. CD34/QBEND10 immunostaining in the bone marrow trephine biopsy: a study of CD34-positive mononuclear cells and megakaryocytes. *Arch Pathol Lab Med* 2002;126(7):823-8.

Tot T, Samii S. The clinical relevance of cytokeratin phenotyping in needle biopsy of liver metastasis. *APMIS* 2003;111(12):1075-82.

Tot T. Cytokeratins 20 and 7 as biomarkers: usefulness in discriminating primary from metastatic adenocarcinoma [review]. *Eur J Cancer* 2002;38(6):758-63.

Tot T. Adenocarcinomas metastatic to the liver: the value of cytokeratins 20 and 7 in the search for unknown primary tumors. *Cancer* 1999;85(1):171-7.

Toth B, Wehrmann M, Kaiserling E, Horny HP. Immunophenotyping of acute lymphoblastic leukaemia in routinely processed bone marrow biopsy specimens. *J Clin Pathol* 1999;52(9):688-92.

van Diest PJ, Baak JP, Chin D, Theeuwes JW, Bacus SS. Quantitation of HER-2/neu oncoprotein overexpression in invasive breast cancer by image analysis: a study comparing fresh and paraffin-embedded material. *Anal Cell Pathol* 1991;3(4):195-202.

Wick MR. Immunohistochemical approaches to the diagnosis of undifferentiated malignant tumors [review]. *Ann Diagn Pathol* 2008;12(1):72-84.

INDEX

Numbers in *italics* refer to pages on which tables appear. Numbers in **boldface** refer to pages on which images appear.

A

acetic acid-zinc-formalin
  fixation time and implications, *4*
  sample results, **7–10**
  turnaround time and diagnostic implications, *6*
acids, decalcification applications, *5*
actin
  association with adipocytes, **217**
  association with dendritic cells, **217**
  association with stromal cells, **217** in non-Hodgkin lymphoma staging, in endosteal lining cells, and in classical Hodgkin lymphoma sample, **218**
actin smooth muscle, in pericytes; contrasted with desmin **217, 218**
activated lymphocytes, CD25 in, **77**
activated T cells
  CD3 in, **18**
  CD5 in, **28**
acute bilineal leukemia
  acute leukemia diagnostic considerations with CD34, myeloperoxidase, CD20, CD3, TdT, von Willebrand factor, and CD117, **246**
  terminal deoxynucleotidyltransferase (TdT) in, **172**
acute biphenotypic leukemia
  acute leukemia diagnostic considerations with CD34, myeloperoxidase, CD20, CD3, TdT, von Willebrand factor, and CD118, **246**
  CD3 in, **19**
  CD117 in, **129**
  terminal deoxynucleotidyltransferase (TdT) in, **171**
acute erythroid leukemia
  acute leukemia diagnostic considerations with epithelial membrane antigen, **243**
  CD15 in, **53**
  CD117 in, **131**
  CD138 in, **138**
  CD235a in, **141**
  Fli-1 in, **193**
  glycophorin A expression, **141**
  hemoglobin A in, **160**
  lysozyme vs myeloperoxidase in, **200**
  myeloperoxidase vs lysozyme in, **200**
  Pax-5 in, **181**
  vimentin in, **215**
acute hypocellular leukemia, myeloperoxidase in, **155**
acute leukemia, undifferentiated
  acute leukemia diagnostic considerations with CD2 negativity, **244**
  acute leukemia diagnostic considerations with Ki-67, **245**
  CD4 in, **56**
  CD16 in, **56**
  CD16 in, **57**
  CD68 vs CD16 in, **57**
  PU.1 in, **187**
  terminal deoxynucleotidyltransferase (TdT) in, **173**
acute leukemias
  diagnostic considerations, 237–246
  flow cytometry diagnostic role, *3*
  recommended panels, *253*
acute lymphoblastic leukemia
  CD10 in, **41**
  CD15 in, **53**
  CD34 14 days after chemotherapy, **93**
  myeloperoxidase in, **157**
  terminal deoxynucleotidyltransferase (TdT) in, **168**
acute megakaryoblastic leukemia
  acute leukemia diagnostic considerations with CD20, **244**
  acute leukemia diagnostic considerations with CD34, **240**
  acute leukemia diagnostic considerations with vimentin **243**
  CD31 in, **83**
  CD61 in, **110, 112**
  von Willebrand factor in, **177, 178**
acute monoblastic leukemia
  CD33 in, **87**
  CD45RA in, **101**
  CD99 in, **124**
  myeloperoxidase expression in, **87**
acute monocytic leukemia, acute leukemia diagnostic considerations with myeloperoxidase, **238**
acute myeloid leukemia
  acute leukemia diagnostic considerations with CD34 and CD45, **240**
  acute leukemia diagnostic considerations with CD79a, **244**
  acute leukemia diagnostic considerations with CD117, **239**
  acute leukemia diagnostic considerations with hemoglobin **241**
  acute leukemia diagnostic considerations with Ki-67, CD23, **245**
  acute leukemia diagnostic considerations with TdT, CD123, **242**
  acute leukemia diagnostic considerations with vimentin **243**
  biopsy sample with AZF fixative, **8**
  CD15 in, **53**
  CD31 in, **83**
  CD34 in, **89, 90, 92**
  CD34 in, 14 days after chemotherapy, **93**
  CD45RO in, **103**
  CD56 in, **107**
  CD61 in, **112**
  CD117 in, **129, 130, 131**
  CD117 in after chemotherapy, **94, 132**
  CD138 in, **135, 138**
  CD235a in, **141**
  false negatives with myeloperoxidase, **155**
  Fli-1 in, **193**
  glycophorin A expression, **141**
  hemoglobin A in, **160**
  immunoglobulins in, **208**
  lysozyme vs myeloperoxidase in, **200**
  myeloperoxidase in, **156**
  myeloperoxidase vs CD15 in, **155**
  myeloperoxidase vs lysozyme in, **200**
  Pax-5 in, **182**
  PU.1 in, **187, 188**
  terminal deoxynucleotidyltransferase (TdT) in, **171, 172**
  vimentin in, **215**

Index

acute myeloid leukemia, undifferentiated, CD10 stromal induction in, **42**
acute myelomonoblastic leukemia
    CD31 in, **82, 83**
    CD99 in, **125**
    CD117 in, **130**
acute myelomonocytic leukemia
    acute leukemia diagnostic considerations with CD117, myeloperoxidase, PG-M1, lysozyme, and KP-1, **239**
    acute leukemia diagnostic considerations with myeloperoxidase, **238**
    acute leukemia diagnostic considerations with TdT, **241**
    CD34 in, **92**
    terminal deoxynucleotidyltransferase (TdT) in, **173**
acute panmyelosis with myelofibrosis, CD61 in, **111**
acute promyelocytic leukemia
    biopsy sample with AZF fixative, **7**
    CD3 in, **21**
    CD14 in, **48, 50**
    CD68 vs CD14 in, **50**
    CD117 in, **130**
    terminal deoxynucleotidyltransferase (TdT) in, **172**
    von Willebrand factor in, **176**
acute undifferentiated leukemia, acute leukemia diagnostic considerations with myeloperoxidase, **238**
adenocarcinoma
    CD3 in metastatic, **19**
    metastatic tumor diagnostic considerations, **248**
adenocarcinoma of the stomach, CD20 in, **61**
adipocytes
    actin association with, **217**
    CD10 in, **38**
    CD25 in, **76**
    Cyclin D1 in, **195**
    EnVision CD10 sensitivity, **39**
    S-100 protein in, **219**
    TdT+ cell associational with, **168**
AE1
    acute leukemia diagnostic considerations with acute myeloid leukemia, **243**
    metastatic tumor diagnostic considerations, **248**
AE3
    acute leukemia diagnostic considerations with acute myeloid leukemia, **243**
    metastatic tumor diagnostic considerations, **248**
alcohol, tissue processing considerations, 4
ALK-1, recommended panel applications, 253
AML. See acute myeloid leukemia.
anemia, von Willebrand factor in, **175**
anemia, aplastic, CD14 in, **47**
angioimmunoblastic T-cell lymphoma, Bcl-6 in, **202**
antigen diffusion, with CD15, **52**
antigen retrieval, methods and recommendations, 5–6
APL. See acute promyelocytic leukemia.
aplastic anemia
    CD14 in, **47**
    hemoglobin A in, **160**
APMF (acute panmyelosis with myelofibrosis), CD61 in, **111**
artifacts, analytical, diagnostic implications, 1
atypical lymphoid aggregates, Cyclin D1 in, **196**
AZF (acetic acid-zinc-formalin)
    fixation time and implications, 4
    sample results, **7–10**
    turnaround time and diagnostic implications, 6

B

B cells, vimentin in, **215**
B1, 57–63
B1 thymoma and myasthenia gravis, CD1a in, **14**
B5 fixative, fixation time and implications, 4
B6, 69–74
B72.3
    localization in diagnosis, 2
    metastatic tumor diagnostic considerations, **250**
B220, 97–103
bands, CD16 in, **55**
B-cell leukemia/lymphoma 2 (Bcl-2), 226–228
B-cell lymphoma
    CD5 expression interpretation, **28–29**
    interpretation with CD5 and CD3, **28–29**
    mature, Pax-5 highlighting of intrasinusoidal distribution, **184**
    mature, Pax-5 vs CD20 in, **183**
B-cell lymphoma-6, 201–203
B-cell neoplasms, recommended panels, 253
B-cell precursor, CD22 and CD10 in, **69**
B-cell-specific activator protein, 178–185
Bcl-1, 194–199
Bcl-2, 226–228
    in blasts, **227**
    in chronic myelomonocytic leukemia, **228**
    localization in diagnosis, 2
    in myeloid precursors, **227**
    in normal bone marrow, **226, 227**
    in precursor B-cell lymphoblastic leukemia, **228**
    in promyelocytes, **227**
    recommended panel applications, 253
    in small B-cell lymphoproliferative diseases, **227**
Bcl-3, recommended panel applications, 253
Bcl-6, 201–203
    in angioimmunoblastic T-cell lymphoma, **202**
    biopsy sample with AZF fixative, **10**
    in diffuse large B-cell lymphoma, **202–203**
    in endothelial cells, **201**
    in follicular lymphoma, **202**
    localization in diagnosis, 2
    in marginal zone lymphoma, **201**
    in monocytic cells, **201**
    in normal bone marrow, **201**
    in peripheral T-cell lymphoma, **202**
    in perivascular monocytic cells, **202**
    recommended panel applications, 253
benign lymphoid aggregate, CD4 in, **25**
benign mast cells, CD33 in, **86**
benign plasma cells, CD99 in, **126**
benign T cells
    CD5 in with hairy cell leukemia, **30**
    infiltrating lymphoplasmacytic lymphoma, CD3 in, **23**
    infiltrating mantle cell lymphoma, CD3 in, **24**
BER-EP4, metastatic tumor diagnostic considerations, **248**
Ber-H2 antigen, 78–81

Index

biphenotypic leukemia, acute,
    CD3 in, **19**
    CD15 in, **53**
BLAST-2, 69–74
blasts, Bcl-2 in, **227**
B-lymphoid cells, interstitial infiltration example, **9**
BOB1
    biopsy sample with AZF fixative, **10**
    localization in diagnosis, *2*
    recommended panel applications, *253*
bone marrow, hypoplastic, hemoglobin A in, **160**
bone marrow, reactive, mast cell tryptase in, **162**
bone marrow sinusoids, megakaryocyte-endothelial cell association, **177**
Bouin fixative, fixation time and implications, *4*
Bp35, 57–63
breast carcinoma, metastatic tumor diagnostic considerations, **250, 252**
BSAP (B-cell-specific activator protein), 178–185
buffered formal-saline, fixation time and implications, *4*

C

C3bR, 95–97
C4bR, 95–97
CA-125
    localization in diagnosis, *2*
    metastatic tumor diagnostic considerations, **252**
calcium chelator EDTA
    decalcification applications, *5*
    decalcification time and processing implications, *5*
    turnaround time and diagnostic implications, *6*
CD nomenclature, 13
CD1a, 13–15
    in B1 thymoma and myasthenia gravis, **14**
    in Langerhans cell histocytosis, **14, 15**
    in precursor T-cell acute lymphoblastic leukemia, **14**
    recommended panel applications, *253*
    in thrombocytopenia with no definite bone pathology, **13**
CD2, 16–17
    acute leukemia diagnostic considerations with undifferentiated acute leukemia, **244**
    recommended panel applications, *253*
CD2R, 16–17
CD3, 17–24
    in activated T cells, **18**
    acute leukemia diagnostic considerations with acute bilineal leukemia, **246**
    in acute promyelocytic leukemia, **21**
    in adenocarcinoma, metastatic, **19**
    in atypical lymphoid aggregate, **22**
    in atypical T cells, nonmalignant, **20**
    in benign T cells infiltrating lymphoplasmacytic lymphoma, **23**
    in benign T cells infiltrating mantle cell lymphoma, **24**
    biopsy sample with AZF fixative, **10**
    in biphenotypic leukemia, acute, **19**
    in CD5 expression interpretation, **28**
    in chronic myeloid leukemia, **23**
    in classical Hodgkin lymphoma, **20**
    in CML (chronic myeloid leukemia), **23**
    vs cytotoxic maerks in T-cell large granular lymphocytic leukemia, **213**
    in follicular lymphoma, **18, 19**
    in HIV+ patient with atypical lymphoid aggregate, **22**
    in hypocellular bone marrow with increased hematogones, **22**
    in interstitial lymphoid aggregates, **22**
    in lymphoplasmacytic lymphoma infiltrated by benign T cells, **23**
    in multiple myeloma, **18**
    in myelogenous leukemia, after induction chemotherapy, **18**
    in nodal diffuse large B-cell lymphoma, **22**
    in normal bone marrow, **17**
    in peripheral T-cell lymphoma, **21**
    in perivascular T cells, **20**
    in precursor T-lymphoblastic leukemia, **23**
    in peripheral T-cell lymphoma, **21**
    in reactive T cells, **18, 19**
    recommended panel applications, *253*
CD4, 24–26
    in benign lymphoid aggregate, **25**
    in epithelioid histiocytes, **26**
    in hemophagocytic histiocytes, **26**
    recommended panel applications, *253*
    in sinusoidal endothelial cells, **25**
    in T lymphocytes in normal bone marrow, **25**
CD5, 27–30
    in activated T cells, **28**
    in B-cell lymphoma, interpretation of, **28–29**
    in benign T cells, **30**
    biopsy sample with AZF fixative, **9**
    cytoplastic and membranous expression of, **28**
    in diffuse large B-cell lymphoma, **30**
    in follicular lymphoma, **30**
    in hairy cell leukemia, **30**
    in hemophagocytic syndrome, **30**
    in histologically normal bone marrow, **27**
    in mantle cell lymphoma, **29**
    mebranous and cytoplastic expression of, **28**
    in peripheral T-cell lymphoma, **29–30**
    recommended panel applications, *253*
CD7, 31–32
    in peripheral T-cell lymphoma, **32**
    in reactive T cells, **31**
    recommended panel applications, *253*
    in refractory anemia with excess blasts, **31**
CD8, 32–35
    in classical Hodgkin lymphoma staging, **34**
    in endosteal lining cells, **34**
    in endothelial cells, **33**
    Golgi-type expression, **35**
    in histologically normal bone marrow, **33**
    in interstitial T cells, **33**
    lymphocytosis, **35**
    membranous expression, **35**
    in normal bone marrow, **33**
    peripheral T-cell lymphoma, **35**
    recommended panel applications, *253*
    refractory anemia with excess blasts, **35**
    in T cells, interstitial, **33**
    T-cell large granular lymphocytic leukemia, **35**

Index

CD9, 36–38
    in endothelial cells, **37**
    in lymphoid cells, small, **37**
    in mast cells, **37**
    in pericytes, **36, 37**
    in perivascular plasma cells, **37**
    in plasma cells, **37**
    in platelets, **36**
    in stromal bone marrow cells, **38**
    in vascular smooth muscle, **36**

CD10, 38–44
    in acute lymphoblastic leukemia, **41**
    in adipocytes, **38**
    vs CD68 (via PG-M1) in precursor B-cell lymphoblastic leukemia, **117**
    in dendritic stromal cells, **43**
    in double-stained specimen with CD22, **69**
    in endosteal lining cells, **44**
    EnVision sensitivity, **39**
    in follicular lymphoma, **43, 44**
    in hematogones, **41**
    in lymphoid cells, immature, **38**
    in maturing lymphocytes, **39**
    in neoplastic lymphoid aggregates, **41**
    in neutrophils, **38, 39, 40**
    in plasma cells, **41**
    in precursor B-cell lymphoblastic leukemia, **40**
    recommended panel applications, *253*
    in stromal cell dendritic extensions, **38**
    stromal induction in various neoplasms, **42**

CD14, 44–50
    in acute promyelocytic leukemia, **48**
    in chronic myeloid leukemia, **50**
    in chronic myelomonocytic leukemia, **48**
    in circulating monocytes, **46**
    in classical Hodgkin lymphoma, **45**
    cytoplasmic ruffles with, **45**
    in dendritic cells, **48**
    in endothelial cells, **46**
    in hemophagocytic syndrome, **48, 49**
    in histologically normal bone marrow, **45, 46**
    in interstitium, **45**
    in macrophages, **48**
    in macrophages, **45, 46**
    in monocytes, **45**
    in normal bone marrow, **45, 46**
    in peripheral T-cell lymphoma, **48, 49**
    in promyelocytic leukemia, acute, **48**
    in stromal dendritic cells, **45, 46**

CD15, 51–53
    in acute erythroid leukemia, **53**
    in acute lymphoblastic leukemia, **53**
    in acute myeloid leukemia, **53**
    in antigen diffusion, **52**
    in biphenotypic leukemia, acute, **53**
    in classical Hodgkin lymphoma, **52**
    in dendritic cells, **52**
    in erythroid hyperplasia, **51**
    in histiocytic cells, **52**
    in histologically normal bone marrow, **51**
    metastatic tumor diagnostic considerations, **249**
    CD15, vs myeloperoxidase in acute myeloid leukemia, **155**
    in normal bone marrow, **51**
    recommended panel applications, *253*

CD16, 54–56
    in bands, **55**
    in dendritic cells, **56**
    in histologically normal bone marrow, **54–55**
    in macrophages, **56**
    in macrophages, **57**
    in metamyelocytes, **55**
    in segmented neutrophils, **55**
    in stromal cells, **56**
    in undifferentiated acute leukemia, **56**
    in undifferentiated acute leukemia, **57**

CD19, acute leukemia diagnostic considerations with acute megakaryoblastic leukemia, **244**

CD20, 57–63
    acute leukemia diagnostic considerations with acute bilineal leukemia, **246**
    acute leukemia diagnostic considerations with acute megakaryoblastic leukemia, **244**
    in adenocarcinoma of the stomach, **61**
    biopsy sample with AZF fixative, **9**
    biopsy sample with AZF fixative, **10**
    in bone marrow with Pax-5+ cells in linear arrangements, **180**
    vs CD79a in hairy cell leukemia, **122**
    vs CD79a in lymphoplasmacytic lymphoma, **122**
    in chronic myeloid leukemia, **23**
    in CML (chronic myeloid leukemia), **23**
    in crushed bone marrow specimen, **63**
    cytoplasmic ruffles with, **59**
    in diffuse large B-cell lymphoma, **63**
    in fibrotic bone marrow specimen, **63**
    in follicular lymphoma, **60, 61**
    in interstitial lymphoid aggregates, **22**
    in large lymphoid aggregates, **60**
    in lymphoid aggregates, large, **63**
    in lymphoid aggregates, very small, **61**
    in lymphoplasmacytic lymphoma, **62**
    in mantle cell lymphoma, **60, 61**
    in marginal zone lymphoma, **62**
    in myeloproliferative disease, **63**
    in nodal classical Hodgkin lymphoma, **58**
    in nodal diffuse large B-cell lymphoma, **22**
    in nodular lymphocyte predominance Hodgkin lymphoma, **58**
    in normal bone marrow, **58, 59**
    vs Pax-5 in follicular lymphoma, **183**
    in precursor B-cell lymphoblastic leukemia, **63**
    in reactive bone marrow, **59**
    recommended panel applications, *253*
    in systemic lupus erythematosus, **59**

CD21, 64–67
    vs CD35 demonstration of follicular dendritic cells, **96**
    in follicular lymphoma, **66, 67**
    in marginal zone lymphoma, **66, 67**
    in mononuclear bone marrow cell, **65**
    in normal bone marrow, **64, 65**
    in reactive lymphoid aggregate, **65**
    recommended panel applications, *253*

CD22, 68–69
    in B-cell precursor, **69**
    in bone marrow with mild reactive changes, **68**
    in cytoplastic and membranous expression, **69**
    in hematogones, **68**

Index

CD23, 69–74
    acute leukemia diagnostic considerations with acute myeloid leukemia, **245**
    vs CD35 demonstration of follicular dendritic cells, **96**
    in chronic lymphocytic leukemia, **72–74**
    in follicular dendritic cells, **70**
    in follicular lymphoma, **71**
    in hairy cell leukemia, **72**
    in interstitial chronic lymphocytic leukemia, **73, 74**
    in interstitium, **70**
    in lymphoid aggregates, reactive, **70**
    in lymphoid clusters, **74**
    in marginal zone lymphoma, **71**
    in normal bone marrow, **70**
    in normochromic normocytic anemia, **71**
    recommended panel applications, *253*

CD25, 75–77
    in activated lymphocytes, **77**
    in adipocytes, **76**
    histologically normal bone marrow, **75**
    in mastocytosis, **76**
    normal bone marrow, **75**
    recommended panel applications, *253*
    in systemic mastocytosis, **77**

CD30, 78–81
    biopsy sample with AZF fixative, **10**
    in classical Hodgkin lymphoma, **80**
    Golgi-type expression in cHL, **80**
    in marginal zone lymphoma, **81**
    in myeloproliferative disease, **79**
    in normal bone marrow, **78–79**
    recommended panel applications, *253*

CD31, 81–84
    in acute megakaryoblastic leukemia, **84**
    in acute myeloid leukemia, **84**
    in acute myelomonoblastic leukemia, **82, 83**
    CD61 expression contrasted, **110**
    in normal bone marrow, **81–82**
    in precursor B-cell lymphoblastic leukemia, **84**
    recommended panel applications, *253*
    vs von Willebrand factor in myelodysplastic syndrome, **82**

CD33, 84–87
    in acute monoblastic leukemia, **87**
    in benign mast cells, **86**
    in intestinal myeloid sarcoma, **87**
    in mast cell disease, **87**
    in normal bone marrow, **85–86**
    recommended panel applications, *253*

CD34, 88–95
    acute leukemia diagnostic considerations with acute bilineal and biphenotypic leukemias, **246**
    acute leukemia diagnostic considerations with acute myeloid and megakaryoblastic leukemias, **240**
    acute leukemia diagnostic considerations with undifferentiated acute leukemia, **244**
    in acute lymphoblastic leukemia 14 days after chemotherapy, **93**
    in acute myeloid leukemia, **89**
    in acute myeloid leukemia 14 days after chemotherapy, **93**
    in acute myelomonocytic leukemia, **92**
    biopsy sample with AZF fixative, **7**
    in chronic lymphocytic leukemia, **94**
    in chronic myeloid leukemia, **89**
    in chronic myelomonocytic leukemia, **94**
    in clotted blood, **90, 91**
    in endothelial cells in direct contact with CD22+ cells, **69**
    in endothelial cells, with mantle cell lymphoma, **94**
    in hyperblastic bone marrow, **90**
    in hypocellular acute myeloid leukemia, **91**
    in hypocellular bone marrow with increased hematogones, **22**
    in lymphoid aggregates, with mantle cell lymphoma, **94**
    vs lysozyme, myeloperoxidase, and CD117 in acute myeloid leukemia, **200**
    in mantle cell lymphoma, **94**
    in megakaryocytes, **89**
    in megakaryocytes, **95**
    in normal bone marrow, **88**
    in precursor B-cell acute lymphoblastic leukemia 14 days after induction chemotherapy, **92**
    in precursor B-cell acuute lymphoblastic leukemia, **91**
    recommended panel applications, *253*
    recommended panel applications, *253*
    in refractory anemia with excess blasts, **88**
    in serous atrophy, **93**
    vs VCAM-1 expression in endothelial cells, **220**

CD35, 95–97
    in erythroid precursors, **97**
    in follicular colonization of benign interstitial aggregates, **96**
    in follicular dendritic cells, vs CD21 and CD23, **96**
    in follicular dendritic cells, with lymphoplasmacytic lymphoma, **97**
    in follicular lymphoma, **96**
    in interstitial aggregates colonized by follicular lymphoma, **96**
    in lymphoplasmacytic lymphoma, **97**
    in normal bone marrow, **95**
    recommended panel applications, *253*

CD38
    acute leukemia diagnostic considerations with undifferentiated acute leukemia, **244**
    biopsy sample with AZF fixative, **8**

CD42b, 109, 113
    in normal bone marrow, **113**
    in platelets, **113**
    recommended panel applications, *253*

CD43, acute leukemia diagnostic considerations, **242**

CD45
    acute leukemia diagnostic considerations with acute myeloid leukemia, **240**
    acute leukemia diagnostic considerations with undifferentiated acute leukemia, **244**
    biopsy sample with AZF fixative, **10**
    recommended panel applications, *253*

CD45RA, 97–103
    in acute monoblastic leukemia, **101**
    in classical Hodgkin lymphoma, **99**
    in IgA multiple myeloma, **100**
    in IgM+ myeloma, **100**
    in lymphoplasmacytic lymphoma, **101**
    in myelomonocytic leukemia, **100**
    in normal bone marrow, **98–99**
    in precursor B-cell acute lymphoblastic leukemia, **101**
    in transformed essential thrombocythemia, **99**

Index

CD45RO, 102–103
    in acute myeloid leukemia, **103**
    mebranous expression in peripheral T-cell lymphoma, **103**
    in myeloid cells, **103**
    in peripheral T-cell lymphoma, **102**
    in plasma cells, **103**
    recommended panel applications, 253

CD56, 104–107
    in acute myeloid leukemia, **107**
    in benign plasma cells, **105**
    contrasted with CD57 on endosteal lining cells, **108**
    in endosteal localization, **106**
    in hematodermic neoplasm, **106**
    in lymphoid cells, **105**
    metastatic tumor diagnostic considerations, 249
    in monoclonal gammopathy, **105**
    in natural killer cells, **105**
    in neoplastic plasma cells, **106**
    in normal bone marrow, **104**
    in paratrabecular localization, **106, 107**
    in plasmacytoid dendritic cells, **106**
    recommended panel applications, 253
    in stromal dendritic cells, **106, 107**

CD57, 107–109
    in chronic normochromic normocytic anemia, **108**
    in classical Hodgkin lymphoma, **107–108**
    contrasted with CD56 on endosteal lining cells, **108**
    in hypocellular bone marrow, **108**
    in normal bone marrow, **107–108**
    in peripheral T-cell lymphoma, **108–109**
    recommended panel applications, 253
    in T-cell large granular lymphocytic leukemia, **109**

CD61, 109–113
    in acute megakaryoblastic leukemia, **110, 112**
    in acute myeloid leukemia, **112**
    in acute panmyelosis with myelofibrosis, **111**
    CD31 expression contrasted, **110**
    in chronic idiopathic myelofibrosis, **113**
    cytoplasmic expression of, **110**
    dysplastic megakaryocytes expressing, **112**
    in endothelial cells, **110**
    in histologically normal bone marrow, **110**
    in megakaryoblasts, **110, 111, 112**
    membranous expression of, **110, 111**
    in myelodysplastic syndrome, **110, 111**
    in normal bone marrow, **110**
    in platelets, **110**
    recommended panel applications, 253
    in refractory anemia with excess blasts, **111**
    in systemic mastocytosis, **111**
    in trilinear dyshematopoiesis associated with myelodysplastic syndrome and acute panmyelosis, **111**
    von Willebrand factor expression contrasted, **110**

CD68, 114–118
    biopsy sample with AZF fixative, **8**
    vs CD14 in acute promyelocytic leukemia, **50**
    in chronic myeloid leukemia, **116**
    in chronic myelomonocytic leukemia, **116**
    in hemophagocytic syndrome, **117, 118**
    localization in diagnosis, 2
    in marginal zone lymphoma, **115**
    in normal bone marrow, **114, 115**
    in peripheral T-cell lymphoma, **117**
    in precursor B-cell lymphoblastic leukemia, **116, 117**
    recommended panel applications, 253

CD72, recommended panel applications, 253

CD79a, 119–123
    acute leukemia diagnostic considerations with acute megakaryoblastic leukemia, **244**
    acute leukemia diagnostic considerations with acute myeloid leukemia, **244**
    biopsy sample with AZF fixative, **10**
    in classical Hodgkin lymphoma, **119**
    in focally hypocellular bone marrow, **120**
    in follicular lymphoma, **120, 121**
    in hairy cell leukemia, **122**
    in hematogones, **120, 121**
    in hypocellular bone marrow, **120**
    intrasinusoidal localization of, **121**
    in lymphoplasmacytic lymphoma, **122**
    paratrabecular localization of, **120**
    in plasma cell myeloma, **121**
    in plasma cells, **120**
    in precursor B-cell lymphoblastic leukemia, **122, 123**
    in pure erythroid acute leukemia, **123**
    in reactive bone marrow, **119**
    recommended panel applications, 253
    reliability after rituximab therapy, **180**
    vs terminal deoxynucleotidyltransferase (TdT) in showing maturational rows of hematogones, **168**

CD99, 123–127
    acute leukemia diagnostic considerations with undifferentiated acute leukemia, **244**
    in acute monoblastic leukemia, **124**
    in acute myelomonoblastic leukemia, **125**
    in endothelial cells, **125**
    in hematopoietic precursor cells, **125**
    in megakaryocytes, **126**
    in multiple myeloma, **126**
    in myeloid leukemias, **125**
    negativity in erythroid precursors, **127**
    negativity in mature granulocytes, **127**
    in nodular sclerosis Hodgkin lymphoma, **126**
    in normal bone marrow, **124**
    in osteoblasts, **125**
    in osteosarcoma, **125**
    in pancytopenia, **125**
    in plasma cells, **126**
    in precursor B-cell lymphoblastic leukemia, **127**
    recommended panel applications, 253
    in sinusoidal endothelial cells, **125**
    in stromal cells, **127**

Index

CD99R, 123–127
CD117, 128–133
    in acute biphenotypic leukemia, **129**
    in acute erythroid leukemia, **131**
    acute leukemia diagnostic considerations with acute bilineal and biphenotypic leukemias, **246**
    acute leukemia diagnostic considerations with acute myelogenous and myelomonocytic leukemias, **239**
    in acute myeloid leukemia, **129, 130, 131**
    in acute myeloid leukemia, after chemotherapy, 94, **132**
    in acute myelomonoblastic leukemia, **130**
    in acute promyelocytic leukemia, **130**
    biopsy sample with AZF fixative, **7**
    in chronic myeloid leukemia, **131**
    in hypocellular acute myeloid leukemia, **132**
    in indolent systemic mastocytosis, **132**
    vs lysozyme, myeloperoxidase, and CD34 in acute myeloid leukemia, **200**
    in myeloproliferative disease, **133**
    in normal bone marrow, **128**
    in pancytopenia, **131**
    paratrabecular localization after chemotherapy, **132**
    in polycythemia vera, **133**
    in precursor B-cell lymphoblastic leukemia, **129**
    in reactive bone marrow, **129**
    recommended panel applications, 253
CD123, 133–134
    acute leukemia diagnostic considerations with acute myeloid leukemia, **242**
    in classical Hodgkin lymphoma, **133**
    in hairy cell leukemia, **134**
    in normal bone marrow, **133–134**
    recommended panel applications, 253
CD138, 134–139
    in acute erythroid leukemia, **138**
    in acute myeloid leukemia, 135, **138**
    vs CD79a in follicular lymphoma, **120**
    in chronic myelomonocytic leukemia, **139**
    in diffuse large B-cell lymphoma, **139**
    in IgA myeloma, **135**
    in lymphoplasmacytic lymphoma, **139**
    in marginal zone lymphoma, **139**
    in multiple myeloma, **136, 137**
    in normal bone marrow, **135**
    in paratrabecular localization, **138**
    perivascular distribution of, **135**
    in plasma cells, **135**
    in reactive plasma cells, **135**
    recommended panel applications, 253
    in stromal cells, **138**
CD163
    biopsy sample with AZF fixative, **8**
    localization in diagnosis, 2
    recommended panel applications, 253

CD235a, 140–141
    in acute erythroid leukemia, **141**
    acute leukemia diagnostic considerations with erythroleukemia, **241**
    in acute myeloid leukemia, **141**
    in erythroid precursors, **140**
    in myelodysplastic syndrome, **140, 141**
chain restriction, demonstrating monoclonality after plasma cell transplantation, **138**
chemical reaction, in biopsy fixation, 4
cHL: See classical Hodgkin lymphoma.
chromogranin
    localization in diagnosis, 2
    metastatic tumor diagnostic considerations, **248, 250**
chronic idiopathic myelofibrosis, CD61 in, **113**
chronic lymphocytic leukemia
    biopsy sample with AZF fixative, **8, 9**
    CD23 in, **72–74**
    CD34 in, **94**
    Cyclin D1 in, **197**
chronic myelogenous leukemia: See chronic myeloid leukemia.
chronic myeloid leukemia
    acute leukemia diagnostic considerations with pancytokeratin 243
    CD3 in, **23**
    CD14 in, **50**
    CD20 in, **23**
    CD34 in, **89, 90**
    CD68 (via KP-1) in, **116**
    CD68 (via PG-M1) in, **116**
    CD117 in, **131**
    mast cell tryptase in, **165–166**
    myeloperoxidase in, **153**
    myeloperoxidase in, **154**
    PU.1 in, **190**
chronic myelomonocytic leukemia
    Bcl-2 in, **228**
    biopsy sample with AZF fixative, **8**
    CD14 in, **48**
    CD34 in, **94**
    CD68 (via KP-1) in, **116**
    CD68 (via PG-M1) in, **116**
    CD138 in, **139**
    immunoglobulins in, **208**
    lysozyme vs myeloperoxidase in, **200**
    mast cell tryptase in, **166**
    myeloperoxidase in, **154**
    myeloperoxidase vs lysozyme in, **200**
    Pax-5 in, **179**
    PU.1 in, **189**
chronic normochromic normocytic anemia, CD57 in, **108**
CIMF (chronic idiopathic myelofibrosis), CD61 in, **113**
circulating monocytes, CD14 in, **46**
CK7, metastatic tumor diagnostic considerations, **249**
c-KIT, 128–133

Index

CLA (common leukocyte antigen), 97–103
classical Hodgkin lymphoma
    actin presence in sample, **218**
    biopsy sample with AZF fixative, **10**
    CD3 in, **20**
    CD10 stromal induction in, **42**
    CD14 in, **45**
    CD15 in, **52**
    CD30 in, **80**
    CD45RA in, **99**
    CD57 in, **107–108**
    CD79a in, **119**
    CD123 in, **133**
    desmin in, **217**
    Fli-1 in, **191**
    MUM1 in, **222**
    Pax-5 in, **182**
    staging with CD8, **34**
    terminal deoxynucleotidyltransferase (TdT) in, **167**
CLL (chronic lymphocytic leukemia)
    CD23 in, **72–74**
    CD34 in, **94**
clotted blood
    CD34 in, **90, 91**
    proper fixation for hemoglobin A staining, **159**
cluster of differentiation, of markers, 13–141
CML: See chronic myeloid leukemia.
CMML: See chronic myelomonocytic leukemia.
colon carcinoma, metastatic tumor diagnostic considerations, **249**
common leukocyte antigen, 97–103
CR1, 95–97
crush artifacts, tissue processing considerations, 3
crushed bone marrow specimen, CD20 in, **63**
Cyclin D1, 194–199
    in adipocytes, **195**
    in atypical lymphoid aggregates, **196**
    biopsy sample with AZF fixative, **9**
    in chronic lymphocytic leukemia, **197**
    in dendritic cells, **196**
    as Dutcher body marker, **199**
    in follicular lymphoma, **196**
    in hairy cell leukemia, **197**
    in IgA myeloma, **199**
    localization in diagnosis, *2*
    in lymphoid aggregates, **196**
    in mantle cell lymphoma, **197–198**
    in normal bone marrow, **194–195**
    in osteoblasts, **195**
    in peripheral T-cell lymphoma, **196**
    in pleomorphic mantle cell lymphoma, **198**
    recommended panel applications, 253
cymase, in mast cells, **164**
cytokeratin
    acute leukemia diagnostic considerations with acute myeloid leukemia, **243**
    localization in diagnosis, *2*
cytologic details, tissue processing implications for, 3
cytoplasmic antigens, flow cytometry diagnostic role, 3

cytoplasmic antigens, in reactive T cells, **18**
cytoplasmic expression
    of CD5, **28**
    of CD22, **69**
    of CD30 in normal bone marrow, **79**
    of CD61, **110**
cytoplasmic granules, biopsy sample with AZF fixative, **8**
cytoplasmic localization, of immunohistochemical markers, *2*
cytoplasmic ruffles
    with CD14, **45**
    with CD20, **59**
cytoplasmic staining, biopsy sample with AZF fixative, **8**
cytotoxic molecules, 211–213

D

D11S287E, 194–199
DBA.44, biopsy sample with AZF fixative, **9**
DeCal Retrieval Solution, for, decalcification, 6
decalcification, diagnostic significance, *3, 5*
dendritic cell neoplasms, recommended panels, 253
dendritic cells
    actin association with, **217**
    CD14 in, **48**
    CD15 in, **52**
    CD16 in, **56**
    Cyclin D1 in, **196**
    follicular, CD23 in, **70**
    identified in precursor B-cell lymphoblastic leukemia with CD68 marker (PG-M1) and lysozyme, **117**
    vascular cell adhesion molecule in, **220**
dendritic extensions of stromal cells, CD10 in, **38, 39**
dendritic histiocytes, biopsy sample with AZF fixative, **8**
dendritic pattern, of CD14 in normal bone marrow, **47**
dendritic stromal cells
    CD10 positivity in some neoplasms, **42**
    CD10 vs reticulin staining, **43**
desmin
    in bone marrow, classical Hodgkin lymphoma present, **217**
    in classical Hodgkin lymphoma, **217**
    localization in diagnosis, *2*
differentiation, cluster of, 13
diffuse large B-cell lymphoma
    Bcl-6 in, **202–203**
    CD5 in, **30**
    CD20 in, **63**
    CD138 in, **139**
    immunoglobulins in, **206**
    MUM1 in, **223**
DNA deoxynucleotidylexotransferase, 167–173
DNA nucleotidylexotransferase, 167–173
DRAP-27, 36–38
Dutcher bodies, Cyclin D1 as marker for, **199**
dysplastic megakaryocytes
    concentration of von Willebrand factor in, **176**
    expressing CD61, **112**

Index

E

E2, 123–127
EBER1 probe, Epstein-Barr virus demonstration in AZF-fixated biopsy, 10
EBV, recommended panel applications, 253
EC 3.1.3.4, 97–103
ELFT, 51–53
EMA (epithelial membrane antigen)
    acute leukemia diagnostic considerations with acute erythroid leukemia, 243
    localization in diagnosis, 2
embedding, diagnostic implications, 5
endocam, 81–84
endosteal lining cells
    actin expression in, 218
    CD8 in, 34
    CD10 in, 44
    CD56 and CD57 contrasted, 108
    Fli-1 in, 192
    Ki-67 negativity in adult bone marrow, 209
endosteal localization, CD56 in, 106
endothelial cells
    Bcl-6 in, 201
    CD8 in, 33
    CD9 in, 37
    CD14 in, 46
    CD34 in with mantle cell lymphoma, 94
    CD61 in, 110
    CD99 in, 125
    Fli-1 in, 192
    megakaryocyte association with, 177
    von Willebrand factor in, 175
EnVision, CD10 sensitivity, 39
eosinophils, in biopsy sample with AZF fixative, 10
epithelial membrane antigen
    acute leukemia diagnostic considerations with acute erythroid leukemia, 243
    localization in diagnosis, 2
epithelioid histiocytes, CD4 in, 26
epitope antigenicity, tissue processing implications for, 3
Epstein-Barr virus, in biopsy sample with AZF fixative, 10
E-rosette receptor, 16–17
erythroid acute leukemia, CD79a in, 123
erythroid hyperplasia
    CD15 in, 51
    hemoglobin A in, 160
erythroid hypoplasia, biopsy sample with AZF fixative, 7
erythroid leukemia, PU.1 in, 190
erythroid maturation, differential expression of hemoglobin A, 159
erythroid precursors, biopsy sample with AZF fixative, 7
erythroid precursors
    CD35 in, 97
    CD99 negativity in, 127
    CD235a in, 140
    glycophorin A expression, 140
erythroleukemia, acute leukemia diagnostic considerations with CD235a, 241
essential thrombocythemia, Fli-1 in, 193

F

F8-related antigen: See von Willebrand factor.
FcεRII, 69–74
FCT3A, 51–53
fibrotic bone marrow specimen, CD20 in, 63
fixation
    biopsy preparation for diagnosis, 1
    diagnostic significance, 3–4
    recent progress, 10
FL: See follicular lymphoma.
Fli-1, 191–193
    in acute erythroid leukemia, 193
    in acute myeloid leukemia, 193
    in classical Hodgkin lymphoma, 191
    in endosteal lining cells, 192
    in endothelial cells, 192
    in essential thrombocythemia, 193
    localization in diagnosis, 2
    metastatic tumor diagnostic considerations, 252
    in normal bone marrow, 191–192
    overexpression in abnormal megakaryocytes, 193
flow cytometry, diagnostic role, 1, 3
focal bone marrow involvement in CLL, CD23 in, 73
focally hypocellular bone marrow, CD79a in, 120
follicular colonization of benign interstitial aggregates, CD35 in, 96
follicular dendritic cells
    CD21 and CD23 vs CD35 demonstration, 96
    CD23 in, 70
    CD35 in with lymphoplasmacytic lymphoma, 97
follicular lymphoma
    Bcl-2 positivity in, 44
    Bcl-6 in, 202
    BcL-6 positivity in, 44
    CD3 in, 18
    CD5 in, 30
    CD10 in, 43, 44
    CD20 in, 60, 61
    CD21 in, 66, 67
    CD23 in, 71
    CD35 in, 96
    CD79a in, 120, 121
    CD138 vs CD79a in, 120
    Cyclin D1 in, 196
    mast cell tryptase in, 161
    MUM1 in, 223
    Pax-5 highlighting of intrasinusoidal B-cell distribution, 184
    Pax-5 in, 179
    Pax-5 vs CD20 in, 183
formaldehyde, tissue processing considerations, 4
formalin
    in biopsy fixation, 4
    implications for decalcification in tissue processing, 6
FUC-TIV, 51–53
FUT4, 51–53

Index

G

glycocalicin, 109, 113
glycophorin A, 140–141
    in acute erythroid leukemia, **141**
    in acute myeloid leukemia, **141**
    in erythroid precursors, **140**
    vs hemoglobin A staining, **158**
    in myelodysplastic syndrome, **140, 141**
    recommended panel applications, 253
glycophorin B, 140–141
glycophorin-C
    biopsy sample with AZF fixative, **7**
    recommended panel applications, 253
glycophorins, localization in diagnosis, 2
glycoprotein IIIa, 109–113
Golgi area, vascular cell adhesion molecule in, **220**
Golgi-type
    CD8 expression, **35**
    CD30 expression, **80**
    concentration of von Willebrand factor in dysplastic megakaryocytes, **176**
Golgi-type localization, of immunohistochemical markers, 2
Gooding and Stewart decalcification fluid, decalcification time and processing implications, 5, 6s
GP3A (platelet glycoprotein IIIA), 109–113
gp67, 84–87
gp105-120, 88–95
gp110, 114–118
GPIb[alpha], 109, 113
GPIba, 109, 113
Gpiia, 81–84
granzyme B
    localization in diagnosis, 2
    in normal bone marrow, **212**
    in peripheral T-cell lymphoma, **212**
    recommended panel applications, 253
    in T-cell large granular lymphocytic leukemia, **213**
GYPA (glycophorin A), 140–141
GYPB (glycophorin B), 140–141

H

hairy cell leukemia
    biopsy sample with AZF fixative, **9**
    CD5 in, **30**
    CD20 vs CD79a in, **122**
    CD23 in, **72**
    CD79a in, **122**
    CD123 in, **134**
    Cyclin D1 in, **197**
    κ–λ immunoglobulin comparison to detect, **204**
    Ki-67 in, **210**
    Pax-5 in, **184**
    TRAP in, **225**
Hammersmith protocol, turnaround time implications, 6
HCDM, vs HLDA nomenclature, 13

HCL: See hairy cell leukemia.
hematodermic neoplasm
    CD56 in, **106**
    PU.1 in, **188**
hematogones
    CD10 in, **41**
    CD22 in, **68**
    CD79a in, **120**
    CD79a in, **121**
    CD79a vs TdT in demonstrating maturational rows, **168**
    maturational rows demonstrated with TdT, **168**
hematopoietic precursor cells, CD99 in, **125**
hemoglobin
    acute leukemia diagnostic considerations with acute myeloid leukemia, **241**
    localization in diagnosis, 2
    recommended panel applications, 253
hemoglobin A staining, 157–160
    in acute erythroid leukemia, **160**
    in acute myeloid leukemia, **160**
    in aplastic anemia, **160**
    in bone marrow, hypoplastic, **160**
    to determine myeloid-erythroid ratio, **154**
    in erythroid hyperplasia, **160**
    in erythroid maturation, **159**
    vs glycophorin A, **158**
    in hypercellular bone marrow, **158**
    in hypoplastic bone marrow, **160**
    in myelodysplastic syndrome, **160**
    in myeloid hyperplasia, **158**
    in neutrophil hyperplasia, **158**
    proper fixation for, in clotted blood sections, **159**
    in thin tissue sections, **159**
hemophagocytic histiocytes, CD4 in, **26**
hemophagocytic syndrome
    CD5 in, **30**
    CD14 in, **48, 49**
    CD68 (via PG-M1) in, 117, **118**
    vimentin in, **216**
hemorrhage artifacts, tissue processing considerations, 3
histiocytic cells, CD15 in, **52**
histiocytic neoplasms, recommended panels, 253
histologically unremarkable bone marrow, CD2 in, **16**
HIV+ patient with atypical lymphoid aggregate, CD3 in, **22**
HLA-DR
    acute leukemia diagnostic considerations with undifferentiated acute leukemia, **244**
    biopsy sample with AZF fixative, **7**
    localization in diagnosis, 2
HLDA, vs HCDM nomenclature, 13
HNK-1 (human natural killer-1), 107–109
Hodgkin cells, Pax-5 to distinguish from megakaryocytes, **182**
Hodgkin lymphoma, recommended panels, 253
human natural killer-1, 107–109
hydrochloric-formic acid, decalcification time and processing implications, 5
hyperblastic bone marrow, CD34 in, **90**
hypercellular bone marrow, hemoglobin A staining in, **158**

Index

hypocellular bone marrow
    in biopsy sample with AZF fixative, **9**
    CD34 in, **91**
    CD57 in, **108**
    CD79a in, **120**
    CD117 in, **132**
    κ–λ immunoglobulin comparison to detect, **204**
    MUM1 in, **221**
    with increased hematogones, CD3 in, 22, CD34 in, **22**
hypoplastic bone marrow, hemoglobin A in, **160**

I

Ig-α, 119–123
IgA, recommended panel applications, 253
IgA multiple myeloma, CD45RA in, **100**
IgA myeloma
    CD138 in, **135**
    Cyclin D1 in, **199**
IgD, recommended panel applications, 253
IgE, recommended panel applications, 253
IgG, recommended panel applications, 253
IgG-κ multiple myeloma, MUM1 in, **222**
IgM, recommended panel applications, 253
IgM+ myeloma, CD45RA in, **100**
IL3RA, 133–134
immunoglobulins, 203–208
    in acute myeloid leukemia, **208**
    in chronic myelomonocytic leukemia, **208**
    in diffuse large B-cell lymphoma, **206**
    in hairy cell leukemia, **204**
    in hypocellular bone marrow, **204**
    immunoglobulins, localization in diagnosis, *2*
    in lymphoplasmacytic lymphoma, **206, 207**
    in mantle cell lymphoma, 207, **208**
    in marginal zone lymphoma, **207**
    in monotypic plasma cells, **204**
    in multiple myeloma, **205**
    in non-Hodgkin lymphoma, **204**
    in plasmacytosis, **205**
    in reactive plasmacytosis, **205**
immunohistochemistry, diagnostic role, 1, 3
in situ hybridization, in biopsy sample with AZF fixative, **10**
indented nuclei, residual disease demonstration, **9**
indolent systemic mastocytosis, CD117 in, **132**
integrin [beta]4, 109–113
interferon regulatory factor 4, 221–223
interpretation, diagnostic implications, 1
interstitial B-lymphoid cell infiltrate example, **9**
interstitial aggregates, CD35 and follicular lymphoma colonization of, **96**
interstitial chronic lymphocytic leukemia, CD23 in, **73, 74**
interstitial lymphoid aggregates, CD3 in, 22, CD20 in, **22**
interstitial T cells, CD8 in, **33**
interstitium, CD14 in, 45, CD23 in, **70**
intestinal myeloid sarcoma
    CD33 in, **87**
    myeloperoxidase expression in, **87**

intrasinusoidal localization
    of CD79a, **121**
    Pax-5 highlighting in B-cell lymphoma, **184**
IRF4, 221–223
ISM (indolent systemic mastocytosis), CD117 in, **132**
ITGB3, 109–113

K

κ, recommended panel applications, 253
κ Ig light chain mRNA, biopsy sample with AZF fixative, **9**
Ki-1 antigen, 78–81
Ki-67, 209–210
    acute leukemia diagnostic considerations with acute myeloid leukemia, **245**
    biopsy sample with AZF fixative, **10**
    in hairy cell leukemia, **210**
    localization in diagnosis, *2*
    in multiple myeloma, **210**
    in normal bone marrow, **209**
    in precursor B-cell lymphoblastic leukemia, **210**
    recommended panel applications, 253
KP-1
    acute leukemia diagnostic considerations with acute myelomonocytic leukemia, **239**
    to demonstrate CD68 in chronic myeloid leukemia, **116**
    to demonstrate CD68 in chronic myelomonocytic leukemia, **116**
    to demonstrate CD68 in normal bone marrow, **115**

L

λ, recommended panel applications, 253
λ mRNA, biopsy sample with AZF fixative, **9**
L3T4, 24–26
laboratory, procedure variability, 1
laboratory, processing volume turnaround time implications, 6
lactoferrin, 153
laminin in normal bone marrow, **221**
Langerhans cell histocytosis, CD1a in, 14, **15**
LAZ3 (lymphoma-associated zinc finger gene on chromosome 3), 201–203
LCH (Langerhans cell histocytosis), CD1a in, **14, 15**
Leu-1, 27–30
Leu-7, CD57 in, **107**
Leu-16, 57–63
Leu-19, 104–107
Leu-20, 69–74
Lewis x, 51–53
LFA-2, 16–17
light chain demonstration, in biopsy sample with AZF fixative, **9**
lobular breast carcinoma, metastatic tumor diagnostic considerations, **252**
localization, of immunohistochemical markers, 2
low-affinity IgE receptor, 69–74
Lowy formalin mercuric chloride
    decalcification applications, 5
    fixation time and implications, *4*

LPL: See lyphoplasmacytic lymphoma.
lung carcinoma, metastatic tumor diagnostic considerations, **249**
lupus erythematosus, systemic, CD20 in, **59**
Ly-1, 27–30
Ly5, 97–103
lymphoblastic leukemia, acute, CD34 14 in days after chemotherapy, **93**
lymphocyte-function antigen-2, 16–17
lymphocytes, activated, CD25 in, **77**
lymphocytes, maturing, CD10 in, **39**
lymphocytosis, CD8 in, **35**
lymphoid aggregates
    atypical, CD3 in, **22**
    benign, CD4 in, **25**
    CD34 in with mantle cell lymphoma, **94**
    Cyclin D1 in, **196**
    large, CD20 in, 60, **63**
    mast cell tryptase around, **164**
    reactive, CD23 in, **70**
    S-100 protein in, **219**
    terminal deoxynucleotidyltransferase (TdT) induction around, **169**
    very small, CD20 in, **61**
lymphoid cells
    CD56 in, **105**
    immature, CD10 in, **38**
    small, CD9 in, **37**
lymphoid clusters, CD23 in, **74**
lymphoma-associated zinc finger gene on chromosome 3, 201–203
lymphoplasmacytic lymphoma
    CD20 in, **62**
    CD20 vs CD79a in, **122**
    CD35 in follicular dendritic cells with, **97**
    CD45RA in, **101**
    CD79a in, **122**
    CD138 in, **139**
    immunoglobulins in, **206, 207**
    infiltrated by benign T cells, CD3 in, **23**
    MUM1 in, **222**
lysozyme, 153, 199–200
    in acute erythroid leukemia, **200**
    acute leukemia diagnostic considerations with acute myelomonocytic leukemia, **239**
    in acute myeloid leukemia, **200**
    in chronic myelomonocytic leukemia, **200**
    to identify precursor B-cell lymphoblastic leukemia, **117**
    localization in diagnosis, 2
    recommended panel applications, 253

M

mAbs (monoclonal antibodies), CD nomenclature of, 13
macronucleoli, to identify tumor cells, **138**
macrophages
    CD14 in, 45, 46, **48**
    CD16 in, 56, **57**
    CD68 vs CD16 in, **57**

mantle cell lymphoma
    CD5 in, **29**
    CD20 in, **60, 61**
    CD23 in, **72**
    CD34 in, **94**
    Cyclin D1 in, **197–198**
    immunoglobulins in, **207, 208**
    infiltrated by benign T cells, CD3 in, **24**
    Pax-5 in, **184–185**
marginal zone lymphoma
    Bcl-6 in, **201**
    CD138 in, **139**
    CD20 in, **62**
    CD21 in, **66, 67**
    CD23 in, **71**
    CD30 in, **81**
    CD68 (via PG-M1) in, **115**
    immunoglobulins in, **207**
    Pax-5 in, **178, 185**
markers, cluster of differentiation, 13–141
mast cell disease
    CD33 in, **87**
    myeloperoxidase expression in, **87**
mast cell tryptase, 161–166
    in chronic myeloid leukemia, **165–166**
    in chronic myelomonocytic leukemia, **166**
    in follicular lymphoma, **161**
    localization in diagnosis, 2
    around lymphoid aggregates, **164**
    in normal bone marrow, **161**
    in postmortem specimens, **162**
    in reactive bone marrow, **162**
    in rheumatoid arthritis, **162**
    in systemic mastocytosis, **162–164**
mast cells
    benign, CD33 in, **86**
    CD9 in, **37**
    CD117 positivity in acute erythroid leukemia, **131**
    chymase in, **164**
mastocytosis
    CD25 in, **76, 77**
    recommended panels, 253
mature B-cell lymphoma, Pax-5 vs CD20 in, **183**
mature granulocytes, CD99 negativity in, **127**
maturing lymphocytes, CD10 in, **39**
MB1, 119–123
MCL: See mantle cell lymphoma.
MCT, recommended panel applications, 253
megakaryoblastic leukemia, acute
    acute leukemia diagnostic considerations with vimentin **243**
    CD31 in, **83**
megakaryoblasts, CD61 in, **111**
megakaryocytes
    acute leukemia diagnostic considerations with vimentin **243**
    association with endothelial cells of marrow sinusoids, **177**
    CD9 in, **36**
    CD34 in, 89, 90, **95**
    CD61 in, 110, 111, **112**
    CD99 in, **126**
    concentration of von Willebrand factor in dysplastic, **176**
    dendritic pattern of CD14 positivity, **47**
    Fli-1 overexpression in abnormal, **193**
    Pax-5 to distinguish from Hodgkin cells, **182**
    staining for von Willebrand factor, **174, 175**

Index

megaloblastoid dyserythropoiesis, biopsy sample with AZF fixative, **7**
membranous expression
    of CD5, **28**
    of CD8, **35**
    of CD9, **36**
    of CD22, **69**
    of CD45RO in peripheral T-cell lymphoma, **103**
    membranous expression, of CD61, **110, 111**
membranous localization, of immunohistochemical markers, *2*
mercurial fixatives, in biopsy fixation, 4
Merkel cell carcinoma, acute leukemia diagnostic considerations with pancytokeratin **243**
metamyelocytes, CD16 in, **55**
metastatic tumors, diagnostic considerations, 247–252
MGC3969, 57–63
MGUS (monoclonal gammopathy of unknown significance), CD56 in, **105**
MIC2, 123–127
MIC2X, 123–127
MIC2Y, 123–127
monoblastic leukemia, acute
    CD33 in, **87**
    myeloperoxidase expression in, **87**
monoclonal antibodies (mAbs), CD nomenclature of, 13
monoclonal gammopathy, CD56 in, **105**
monoclonality, chain restriction as support for, **138**
monocytes
    biopsy sample with AZF fixative, **8**
    CD14 in, **45**
    dendritic pattern of CD14 positivity, **47**
    circulating, CD14 in, **46**
monocytic cells, Bcl-6 in, **201**
monocytoid nuclei, residual disease demonstration, **9**
mononuclear bone marrow cell, CD21 in, **65**
monotypic plasma cells, κ–λ immunoglobulin comparison to detect, **204**
MPO: See myeloperoxidase.
MRP-1, 36–38
MS4A1, 57–63
mucin metastatic tumor diagnostic considerations, **248**
multiple myeloma
    CD10 stromal induction in, **42**
    CD3 in, **18**
    CD99 in, **126**
    CD138 in, **136, 137**
    immunoglobulin G in, **205**
    Ki-67 in, **210**
    metastatic tumor diagnostic considerations, **249**
    MUM1 in, **222**
multiple myeloma oncogene 1, 221–223
MUM1, 221–223
    biopsy sample with AZF fixative, 8, **10**
    in classical Hodgkin lymphoma, **222**
    in diffuse large B-cell lymphoma, **223**
    in follicular lymphoma, **223**
    in hypocellular bone marrow, **221**
    in IgG-κ multiple myeloma, **222**
    localization in diagnosis, *2*
    in lymphoplasmacytic lymphoma, **222**
    in multiple myeloma, 137, **222**
    in reactive plasmacytosis, **221**
    recommended panel applications, *253*

myelodysplastic syndrome
    biopsy sample with AZF fixative, **7**
    CD31 vs von Willebrand factor in, **82**
    CD61 in, **110**
    CD61 in, **111**
    CD235a in, **140, 141**
    glycophorin A expression, 140, **141**
    hemoglobin A in, **160**
    recommended panels, *253*
    von Willebrand factor in, **177**
myelogenous leukemia, after induction chemotherapy, CD3 in, **18**
myeloid cells, CD45RO in, **103**
myeloid hyperplasia, hemoglobin A staining in, **158**
myeloid hypoplasia, vimentin in, **215**
myeloid leukemia, PU.1 in, **190**
myeloid leukemia, acute. See acute myeloid leukemia.
myeloid leukemia, undifferentiated acute. See undifferentiated acute myeloid leukemia.
myeloid leukemias, CD99 in, **125**
myeloid precursors
    Bcl-2 in, **227**
    CD138 and MUM-1 negativity, **137**
    myeloperoxidase in, **154**
myeloid sarcoma, intestinal
    CD33 in, **87**
    myeloperoxidase expression in, **87**
myeloid-erythroid ratio, determined with myeloperoxidase and hemoglobin A staining, **154**
myeloma, multiple, CD99 in, **126**
myelomonoblastic leukemia, acute, CD31 in, 82, **83**
myelomonocytic cells, biopsy sample with AZF fixative, **8**
myelomonocytic leukemia, CD45RA in, **100**
myeloperoxidase, 153–157
    in acute hypocellular leukemia, **155**
    acute leukemia diagnostic considerations with acute bilineal leukemia, **246**
    acute leukemia diagnostic considerations in acute myelomonocytic, monocytic, and undifferentiated leukemias, **238**
    in acute lymphoblastic leukemia, **157**
    in acute monoblastic leukemia, **87**
    in acute myeloid leukemia, **155, 156**
    biopsy sample with AZF fixative, **7**
    vs CD15 in acute myeloid leukemia, **53**
    vs CD117 in acute myeloid leukemia, **130**
    in chronic myeloid leukemia, 153, **154**
    in chronic myelomonocytic leukemia, **154**
    to determine myeloid-erythroid ratio, **154**
    false negatives with, **155**
    in intestinal myeloid sarcoma, **87**
    localization in diagnosis, *2*
    vs lysozyme in CMML, AML, and acute erythroid leukemia, **200**
    in mast cell disease, **87**
    in myeloid precursors, **154**
    in neutropenia, **154**
    in neutrophil precursors, **154**
    in normal bone marrow, **153**
    in paratrabecular localization, **154**
    in precursor B-cell lymphoblastic leukemia, **157**
    recommended panel applications, *253*

myeloproliferative disease
    CD20 in, **63**
    CD30 in, **79**
    CD117 in, **133**
    recommended panels, 253
MZL. See marginal zone lymphoma.
natural killer cells, CD56 in, **105**

N

NCAM (neural cell adhesion molecule), 104–107
necrotic tissue, metastatic tumor diagnostic considerations, **248**
neoplastic lymphoid aggregates, CD10 in, **41**
neoplastic plasma cells, CD56 in, **106**
neural cell adhesion molecule, 104–107
neuroblastoma
    metastatic tumor diagnostic considerations, 249, 250, 251, **252**
neurofilaments
    localization in diagnosis, 2
    metastatic tumor diagnostic considerations, **251**
neuron-specific enolase
    localization in diagnosis, 2
    metastatic tumor diagnostic considerations, 250, **251**
neutropenia, myeloperoxidase in, **154**
neutrophil hyperplasia, hemoglobin A staining in, **158**
neutrophil precursors, myeloperoxidase in, **154**
neutrophils
    CD10 in, 38, 39, **40**
    CD16 in, **55**
nitric acid, decalcification time and processing implications, 5
NK (natural killer) cells, CD56 in, **105**
NKH1, 104–107
NLPHL (nodular lymphocyte predominance Hodgkin lymphoma), CD20 in, **58**
nodal classical Hodgkin lymphoma, CD20 in, **58**
nodal diffuse large B-cell lymphoma
    CD3 in, **22**
    CD20 in, **22**
nodal peripheral T-cell lymphoma, CD5 in, **29**
nodular lymphocyte predominance Hodgkin lymphoma, CD20 in, **58**
nodular sclerosis Hodgkin lymphoma, CD99 in, **126**
non-Hodgkin lymphoma
    κ–λ immunoglobulin comparison in diagnosis, **204**
    staging with actin, **218**
nonmalignant atypical T cells, CD3 in, **20**
non-neoplastic hematopoiesis, Pax-5 in, **179**
normal bone marrow
    Bcl-2 in, 226, **227**
    Bcl-6 in, **201**
    CD3 in, **17**
    CD4 in T lymphocytes in, **24–25**
    CD5 in, **27**
    CD8 in, **33**
    CD14 in, 45, **46**
    CD15 in, **51**
    CD16 in, **54–55**
    CD20 in, 58, **59**
    CD21 in, 64, **65**
    CD23 in, **70**
    CD25 in, **75**
    CD30 in, **78–79**
    CD31 in, **81–82**
    CD33 in, **85–86**
    CD34 in, **88**
    CD35 in, **95**
    CD42b in, **113**
    CD45RA in, **98–99**
    CD56 in, **104**
    CD57 in, **107–108**
    CD61 in, **110**
    CD68 in, 114, **115**
    CD99 in, **124**
    CD117 in, **128**
    CD123 in, **133–134**
    CD138 in, **135**
    Cyclin D1 in, **194–195**
    dendritic pattern of CD14 positivity, **47**
    Fli-1 in, **191–192**
    granzyme B in, **212**
    Ki-67 in adult, **209**
    laminin in, **221**
    mast cell tryptase in, **161**
    myeloperoxidase in, **153**
    Pax-5 in, **178**
    PU.1 in, **186**
    S-100 protein in, **219**
    terminal deoxynucleotidyltransferase (TdT) in, **167–169**
    TRAP in, **224**
    vascular cell adhesion molecule in, **220**
    vimentin in, **214**
    von Willebrand factor in, **174**
normochromic normocytic anemia, CD23 in, **71**
NPM1, localization in diagnosis, 2
NPM1, recommended panel applications, 253
NSE (neuron-specific enolase)
    localization in diagnosis, 2
    metastatic tumor diagnostic considerations, 250, **251**
nuclear antigens, flow cytometry diagnostic role, 3
nuclear localization, of, immunohistochemical markers, 2
nuclear staining pattern, in biopsy sample with AZF fixative, **9**
nucleic acid, tissue processing considerations, 4
nucleophosmin biopsy sample with AZF fixative, **8**
nucleosidetriphosphate, 167–173

O

OCT2
    biopsy sample with AZF fixative, **10**
    localization in diagnosis, 2
    recommended panel applications, 253
osteoblasts
    CD99 in, **125**
    Cyclin D1 in, **195**
    metastatic tumor diagnostic considerations, **251**
osteocytes, metastatic tumor diagnostic considerations, **251**
osteosarcoma, CD99 in, **125**

Index

P

p24, 36–38
p53, biopsy sample with AZF fixative, 8
p53, localization in diagnosis, 2
p67, 84–87
pancytokeratin
    acute leukemia diagnostic considerations with acute myeloid leukemia, 243
    metastatic tumor diagnostic considerations, 248
pancytopenia
    CD99 in, 125
    CD117 in, 131
panels, recommended, 253
paraffin embedding
    biopsy preparation for diagnosis, 1
    diagnostic implications, 5
    turnaround time and diagnostic implications, 6
paratrabecular lining cells, actin presence in classical Hodgkin lymphoma sample, 218
paratrabecular localization
    CD56 in, 106, 107
    of CD79a, 120
    of CD117 after chemotherapy, 132
    CD138 in, 138
    myeloperoxidase in, 154
parvovirus B19
    biopsy sample with AZF fixative, 7
    localization in diagnosis, 2
    recommended panel applications, 253
Pax-5, 178–185
    in acute erythroid leukemia, 181
    acute leukemia diagnostic considerations with acute megakaryoblastic leukemia, 244
    in acute myeloid leukemia, 182
    biopsy sample with AZF fixative, 10
    vs CD20 in follicular lymphoma, 183
    in chronic myelomonocytic leukemia, 179
    in classical Hodgkin lymphoma, 182
    in follicular lymphoma, 183, 184
    in hairy cell leukemia, 184
    intrasinusoidal localization, 184
    in linear arrangement of, 179, 180
    localization in diagnosis, 2
    in mantle cell lymphoma, 184–185
    in marginal zone lymphoma, 178, 185
    in mature B-cell lymphoma, 183, 184
    in non-neoplastic hematopoiesis, 179
    in normal bone marrow, 178
    in precursor B-cell lymphoblastic leukemia, 180–181
    recommended panel applications, 253
    reliability after rituximab therapy, 180
    vs terminal deoxynucleotidyltransferase (TdT) in non-neoplastic hematopoiesis, 179
PECAM-1, 81–84
perforin
    localization in diagnosis, 2
    recommended panel applications, 253
pericytes, CD9 in, 36, 37
peripheral blood lymphocytosis, biopsy sample with AZF fixative, 9
peripheral T-cell lymphoma
    Bcl-6 in, 202
    CD2 in, 16–17
    CD3 in, 21
    CD5 in, 29
    CD7 in, 32
    CD8 in, 35
    CD14 in, 48, 49
    CD45RO in, 102–103
    CD57 in, 108–109
    CD68 (via PG-M1) in, 117
    Cyclin D1 in, 196
    granzyme B in, 212
    TIA-1 (T-cell intracellular antigen-1) in, 212
perivascular distribution, CD138 in, 135
perivascular monocytic cells
    Bcl-6 in, 202
    CD14 in, 47
perivascular plasma cells, CD9 in, 36
perivascular T cells, CD3 in, 20
PG-M1
    acute leukemia diagnostic considerations with acute myelomonocytic leukemia, 239
    to demonstrate CD68 in chronic myeloid leukemia, 116
    to demonstrate CD68 in chronic myelomonocytic leukemia, 116
    to demonstrate CD68 in hemophagocytic syndrome, 117, 118
    to demonstrate CD68 in marginal zone lymphoma, 115
    to demonstrate CD68 in peripheral T-cell lymphoma, 117
    to demonstrate CD68 in precursor B-cell lymphoblastic leukemia, 116–117
    recommended panel applications, 253
phagocytic histiocytes, biopsy sample with AZF fixative, 8
phosphate buffer, in biopsy fixation, 4
plasma cell disorders, recommended panels, 253
plasma cell myeloma, CD79a in, 121
plasma cells
    CD9 in, 37
    CD10 in, 41
    CD45RO in, 103
    CD56 in benign, 105
    CD79a in, 120
    CD99 in, 126
    CD138 in, 135
    plasma cells, CD138 marking after transplantation, 138
plasmacytoid dendritic cells, CD56 in, 106
plasmacytosis, immunoglobulin A vs G in, 205
platelet glycoprotein IIIA, 109–113
platelets
    CD9 in, 36
    CD42b in, 113
    CD61 in, 110
pleomorphic mantle cell lymphoma, Cyclin D1 in, 198
polycythemia vera, CD117 in, 133
postmortem specimens, mast cell tryptase in, 162
PRAD1, 194–199

Index

precursor B-cell acute lymphoblastic leukemia
    Bcl-2 in, **228**
    CD10 contrasted with CD68 (via PG-M1) in, **117**
    CD10 in, **40**
    CD20 in, **63**
    CD31 in, **84**
    CD34 in, 91, 14 days after induction chemotherapy, **92**
    CD45RA in, **101**
    CD68 (via PG-M1) in, **116–117**
    CD79a in, **122, 123**
    CD99 in, **127**
    CD117 in, **129**
    Ki-67 in, **210**
    myeloperoxidase in, **157**
    Pax-5 in, **180–181**
    PU.1 in, **189**
    terminal deoxynucleotidyltransferase (TdT) in, **169–171**
    von Willebrand factor in, **176**
precursor T-cell acute lymphoblastic leukemia, CD1a in, **14**
precursor T-lymphoblastic leukemia, CD3 in, **23**
preparation of tissue for diagnosis, 3
processing of tissue for diagnosis, 3
proerythroblasts, giant, biopsy sample with AZF fixative, **7**
promonocytes
    biopsy sample with AZF fixative, **8**
    Bcl-2 in, **227**
promyelocytic leukemia, acute
    CD3 in, **21**
    CD14 in, **48**
    von Willebrand factor in, **176**
PTCL. See peripheral T-cell lymphoma.
PU.1, 185–190
    in acute myeloid leukemia, **187**
    in chronic myeloid leukemia, **190**
    in chronic myelomonocytic leukemia, **189**
    in erythroid leukemia, **190**
    in hematodermic neoplasm, **188**
    localization in diagnosis, 2
    in myeloid leukemia, **190**
    in normal bone marrow, **186**
    in precursor B-cell lymphoblastic leukemia, **189**
    in pure erythroid acute leukemia, **190**
    recommended panel applications, 253
    in undifferentiated acute leukemia, **187**
pure erythroid acute leukemia
    CD79a in, **123**
    PU.1 in, **190**

R

RDO, decalcification time and processing implications, 5
reactive bone marrow
    CD20 in, **59**
    CD20 in, **59**
    CD22 in mild, **68**
    CD79a in, **119**
    CD117 in, **129**
    mast cell tryptase in, **162**
reactive lymphoid aggregate, CD21 in, **65**

reactive plasma cells, CD138 in, **135**
reactive plasmacytosis
    immunoglobulin A vs G in, **205**
    MUM1 in, **221**
reactive T cells
    CD3 in, **18, 19**
    CD7 in, **31**
recommended panels, 253
Reed-Sternberg cells, in biopsy sample with AZF fixative, **10**
refractory anemia with excess blasts
    CD7 in, **31**
    CD8 in, **35**
    CD34 in, **88**
    CD61 in, **111**
    TIA-1 (T-cell intracellular antigen-1) in, **211**
refractory anemia with myeloid hyperplasia, vimentin in, **216**
residual disease, in biopsy sample with AZF fixative, **9**
resin embedding
    diagnostic implications, 5
    turnaround time and diagnostic implications, 6
reticulin staining, vs CD10 marker in dendritic stromal cells, **43**
retrieval, of antigens, methods and recommendations, 5–6
rheumatoid arthritis, mast cell tryptase positivity in, **162**
rituximab therapy, CD20, CD79a, and Pax-5 followup, **180**
rosebud, 272
ruffles, cytoplasmic
    with CD14, **45**
    with CD20, **59**

S

S-100 protein
    localization in diagnosis, 2
    in normal bone marrow, adipocytes, and small stromal cells, **219**
    recommended panel applications, 253
S7, 57–63
sampling, diagnostic implications, 1
SCFR (stem cell factor receptor), 128–133
Schäfer's fixative, fixation time and implications, 4
sectioning, diagnostic implications, 5
segmented neutrophils, CD16 in, **55**
serous atrophy, CD34 in, **93**
sinusoidal endothelial cells
    CD4 in, **25**
    CD99 in, **125**
small B-cell lymphoproliferative diseases
    Bcl-2 in, **227**
    flow cytometry diagnostic role, 3
smooth muscle actin
    localization in diagnosis, 2
    in pericytes; contrasted with desmin **217, 218**
SPI1, 185–190
staining
    of megakaryocytes for von Willebrand factor, **174, 175**
    of PU.1 in extracellular spaces, **187**

Index

stem cell factor receptor, 128–133
stromal bone marrow cells, CD9 in, **38**
stromal cell dendritic extensions, CD10 in, **38, 39**
stromal cells
    actin association with, **217**
    CD16 in, **56**
    CD99 in, **127**
    CD138 in, **138**
    S-100 protein in, **219**
    vascular cell adhesion molecule in, **220**
stromal dendritic cells
    CD10 positivity, **42**
    CD14 in, **45, 46**
    CD56 in, 106, **107**
stromal induction, of CD10 positivity, **42**
stromal markers, 213–221
Surgipath decalcifier, decalcification time and processing implications, 5
syndecan-1, 134–139
systemic lupus erythematosus, CD20 in, **59**
systemic mastocytosis
    CD25 in, **77**
    CD61 in, **111**
    mast cell tryptase in, **162–164**
    von Willebrand factor in, **177**

T

T cells
    activated, CD3 in, **18**
    benign, CD5 in with hairy cell leukemia, **30**
    interstitial, CD8 in, **33**
    reactive, CD3 in, **18**
T lymphocytes in normal bone marrow, CD4 in, **24–25**
T lymphocytosis, TIA-1 (T-cell intracellular antigen-1) in, **211**
T1, 27–30
T11, 16–17
T200, 97–103
T3, 17–24
TAG72, metastatic tumor diagnostic considerations, **250**
T-cell intracellular antigen-1 (TIA-1)
    localization in diagnosis, 2
    in peripheral T-cell lymphoma, **212**
    recommended panel applications, **253**
    in refractory anemia with excess blasts, **211**
    in T-cell large granular lymphocytic leukemia, **213**
T-cell large granular lymphocytic leukemia
    CD8 in, **35**
    CD57 in, **109**
    TIA-1 vs granzyme B diagnosis, **213**
T-cell neoplasms, recommended panels, **253**
TdT: See terminal deoxynucleotidyltransferase.
temperature, tissue processing considerations, 3
terminal deoxynucleotidyltransferase (TdT), 167–173
    in acute bilineal leukemia, **172**
    in acute biphenotypic leukemia, **171**

acute leukemia diagnostic considerations with acute bilineal and biphenotypic leukemias, **246**
acute leukemia diagnostic considerations with acute myeloid leukemia, **242**
acute leukemia diagnostic considerations with acute myelomonocytic leukemia, **241**
    in acute leukemia, undifferentiated, **173**
    in acute lymphoblastic leukemia, **168**
    in acute myeloid leukemia, 171, **172**
    in acute myelomonocytic leukemia, **173**
    in acute promyelocytic leukemia, **172**
    in classical Hodgkin lymphoma, **167**
    localization in diagnosis, 2
    terminal deoxynucleotidyltransferase (TdT), around lymphoid aggregates, **169**
    in normal bone marrow, **167–169**
    vs Pax-5 in non-neoplastic hematopoiesis, **179**
    positive cell association with adipocytes, **168**
    in precursor B-cell lymphoblastic leukemia, **169–171**
    recommended panel applications, **253**
thin tissue sections, hemoglobin A in, **159**
thrombocytopenia with no definite bone pathology, CD1a in, **13**
thrombocytosis, von Willebrand factor in, **177**
TIA-1. See T-cell intracellular antigen-1.
time of day, tissue processing considerations, 3
timing, of decalcification in tissue processing, 5
tissue processing, for diagnosis, 3
Tp41, 31–32
Tp67, 27–30
transformed essential thrombocythemia, CD45RA in, **99**
TRAP, 224–225
    biopsy sample with AZF fixative, **9**
    in hairy cell leukemia, **225**
    localization in diagnosis, 2
    in normal bone marrow, **224**
    recommended panel applications, **253**
trilinear dyshematopoiesis, CD61 in myelodysplastic syndrome and acute panmyelosis, **111**
tungsten carbide knives, for sectioning, diagnostic implications, 5
turnaround time
    diagnostic implications, 6
    implications for decalcification in tissue processing, 5

U

U21B31, 194–199
undifferentiated acute leukemia
    acute leukemia diagnostic considerations with CD2 negativity, **244**
    acute leukemia diagnostic considerations with Ki-67, **245**
    CD4 in, **56**
    CD10 stromal induction in, **42**
    CD16 in, 56 (illus.,) **57**
    CD68 vs CD16 in, **57**
    PU.1 in, **187**
    terminal deoxynucleotidyltransferase (TdT) in, **173**

V

vascular cell adhesion molecule, in normal marrow, endothelial cells, and dendritic cells, **220**

vascular smooth muscle, CD9 in, **36**

VCAM-1 (vascular cell adhesion molecule), in normal marrow, endothelial cells, and dendritic cells, **220**

vimentin
- in acute erythroid leukemia, **215**
- acute leukemia diagnostic considerations with megakaryoblastic leukemia, **243**
- acute leukemia diagnostic considerations with undifferentiated acute leukemia, **244**
- in acute myeloid leukemia, **215–216**
- in B cells (lymph node), **215**
- in hemophagocytic syndrome, **216**
- localization in diagnosis, *2*
- metastatic tumor diagnostic considerations, **251**
- metastatic tumor diagnostic considerations, **252**
- in myeloid hypoplasia, **215–216**
- in normal bone marrow, **214**
- in refractory anemia with myeloid hyperplasia, **216**

von Willebrand factor, 174–178
- acute leukemia diagnostic considerations with acute biphenotypic leukemia, **246**
- in acute megakaryoblastic leukemia, 177, **178**
- in acute promyelocytic leukemia, **176**
- in anemia, **175**
- vs CD31 in myelodysplastic syndrome, **82**
- CD61 expression contrasted, **110**
- in dysplastic megakaryocytes, **176**
- in endothelial cells, **175**
- Golgi-type concentration in dysplastic megakaryocytes, **176**
- localization in diagnosis, *2*
- megakaryocyte staining for, 174, **175**
- in myelodysplastic syndrome, **177**
- in normal bone marrow, **174**
- in precursor B-cell lymphoblastic leukemia, **176**
- recommended panel applications, *253*
- staining for, 174, **175**
- in systemic mastocytosis, **177**
- in thrombocytosis, **177**

W

W3/25, 24–26

Z

ZAP70, recommended panel applications, *253*

Zenker fixative, fixation time and implications, *4*

zinc finger protein 51, 201–203